Berquist's Musculoskeletal Imaging
COMPANION

Berquist's Musculoskeletal Imaging
COMPANION

THIRD EDITION

Jeffrey J. Peterson, MD

Professor of Radiology
Vice Chairman for Education
Diagnostic Radiology Residency Program Director
Mayo Clinic
Jacksonville, Florida

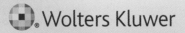
. Wolters Kluwer

Philadelphia • Baltimore • New York • London
Buenos Aires • Hong Kong • Sydney • Tokyo

Senior Acquisitions Editor: Sharon Zinner
Editorial Coordinator: Lauren Pecarich
Production Project Manager: David Saltzberg
Design Coordinator: Holly McLaughlin
Manufacturing Coordinator: Beth Welsh
Marketing Manager: Dan Dressler
Prepress Vendor: S4Carlisle Publishing Services

Third Edition

9 8 7 6 5 4 3 2 1

Printed in China

Library of Congress Cataloging-in-Publication Data

Names: Peterson, Jeffrey J., author. | Preceded by (work): Berquist, Thomas
  H. (Thomas Henry), 1945– . Musculoskeletal imaging companion.
Title: Berquist's musculoskeletal imaging companion / Jeffrey J. Peterson.
Other titles: Musculoskeletal imaging companion
Description: Third edition. | Philadelphia: Wolters Kluwer Health, [2018] |
  Preceded by Musculoskeletal imaging companion / Thomas H. Berquist. 2nd
  ed. c2007. | Includes bibliographical references and index.
Identifiers: LCCN 2017043484 | ISBN 9781496314994
Subjects: | MESH: Musculoskeletal Diseases—diagnostic imaging |
  Musculoskeletal System—diagnostic imaging
Classification: LCC RC925.7 | NLM WE 141 | DDC 616.7/0757—dc23 LC record available at
  https://lccn.loc.gov/2017043484

RRS1709

*Thank you to my musculoskeletal colleagues Laura Bancroft,
Tom Berquist, Joe Bestic, Hillary Garner, Mark Kransdorf,
and Daniel Wessell. I have learned so much from each of you.
Thank you for your encouragement and contributions.*

*Thank you to my parents Mary Kay and Jim
for their inspiration and reassurance.*

*Thank you to Brianne, Addison, and Charlotte
for your love and support.*

Contributors

Laura W. Bancroft, MD, FACR
Chief of Musculoskeletal Imaging
Florida Hospital Orlando
Department Chair of Radiology and
    Professor
University of Central Florida College of
    Medicine
Orlando, Florida
Professor of Radiology
Florida State University College of Medicine
Orlando, Florida

Francesca D. Beaman, MD
Associate Professor
Departments of Radiology and Orthopedics &
    Sports Medicine
Chief Division of Musculoskeletal Imaging and
    Intervention
Musculoskeletal Fellowship
    Program Director
University of Kentucky
Lexington, Kentucky

Stephanie A. Bernard, MD
Associate Professor Radiology
Penn State Hershey Medical Center
Hershey, Pennsylvania

Thomas H. Berquist, MD
Professor of Radiology
Mayo Clinic
Jacksonville, Florida

Joseph M. Bestic, MD
Assistant Professor of Radiology
Mayo Clinic
Jacksonville, Florida

William E. Clifton, MD
Neurosurgery Resident
Mayo Clinic Florida
Jacksonville, Florida

Madhura A. Desai, MD
Radiology Consultant
Mayo Clinic
Jacksonville, Florida

Hillary W. Garner, MD
Assistant Professor of Radiology
Mayo Clinic
Jacksonville, Florida

Vivek Gupta, MD
Consultant
Division of Neuroradiology
Mayo Clinic
Jacksonville, Florida

Mark J. Kransdorf, MD
Professor of Radiology
Mayo Clinic Arizona
Phoenix, Arizona

Thomas Magee, MD, FACR
NSI Radiology
Melbourne, Florida

Jeffrey J. Peterson, MD
Professor of Radiology
Vice Chairman for Education
Diagnostic Radiology Residency Program Director
Mayo Clinic
Jacksonville, Florida

Prasanna G. Vibhute, MD
Assistant Professor of Radiology
Mayo Clinic
Jacksonville, Florida

Daniel E. Wessell, MD
Assistant Professor of Radiology
Musculoskeletal Fellowship Program Director
Mayo Clinic
Jacksonville, Florida

Preface

Tom Berquist is one of the founders of modern musculoskeletal radiology. Over his remarkable career, his contributions to the field of radiology have been immeasurable. His work in early musculoskeletal MR helped lay the foundation for the field's success today. Tom has authored numerous texts and has composed an amazing array of books and enduring learning materials that will continue to educate future generations of radiologists. It has been a highlight of my career to train under and subsequently work alongside one of the giants of radiology education.

This is the third edition of Tom's iconic Musculoskeletal Imaging Companion. Previous editions have provided a foundation of musculoskeletal knowledge for radiology trainees, as well as a quick reference for more experienced musculoskeletal radiologists. In this edition, we have expanded the text, updated the material and references, and refreshed a majority of the images and figures. Each chapter is again designed to provide the key points on each disorder followed by high-quality imaging examples depicting key features of each disease process. As with previous editions, we seek to provide a quick, easy-to-utilize learning resource covering most of the common entities affecting the musculoskeletal system. We have renamed this book, Berquist's Musculoskeletal Imaging Companion to honor Tom and his invaluable contributions to our field.

Contents

1 Temporomandibular Joint 1

Anatomy   1
Internal Derangement   2
Anterior Disc Displacement   4
Lateral and Medial Disc Displacement   8
Trauma   9
Osteoarthritis   10
Miscellaneous Arthropathies   11
Tumors   13

2 Spine 14

Trauma: Cervical Spine—Basic Concepts   14
Trauma: Cervical Spine—Atlanto-Occipital Fracture Dislocations   21
Trauma: Cervical Spine—C1 Fractures   22
Trauma: Cervical Spine—Atlantoaxial Dislocations   25
Trauma: Cervical Spine—Axis (C2)   28
Trauma: Cervical Spine—Lower Cervical Spine: Vertebral Arch Fractures   32
Trauma: Cervical Spine—Lower Cervical Spine: Vertebral Body Fractures   35
Trauma: Cervical Spine—Lower Cervical Spine: Subluxation,
    Fracture/Dislocation   38
Trauma: Thoracolumbar Spine—Basic Concepts   42
Trauma: Thoracolumbar Spine—Hyperflexion Injuries   45
Trauma: Thoracolumbar Spine—Flexion–Rotation Injuries   47
Trauma: Thoracolumbar Spine—Vertical Compression Injuries   48
Trauma: Thoracolumbar Spine—Hyperextension Injuries   50
Trauma: Thoracolumbar Spine—Shearing Injuries   51
Trauma: Thoracolumbar Spine—Minor Fractures   53
Spondylolysis/Spondylolisthesis   54
Scoliosis: Basic Concepts   59
Scoliosis: Imaging   60
Degenerative Disc Disease   63
Disc Herniation   66
Synovial Cysts   71
Infection (Infectious Discospondylitis or Spondylodiscitis)   72
Arthropathies   76
Tumors and Tumorlike Conditions: Bone Lesions   80
Tumors and Tumorlike Conditions: Soft Tissue Masses   88
Inflammatory Conditions of Spinal Cord and Nerve Roots   92
Miscellaneous Conditions   97
Congenital Anomalies   99
Congenital Anomalies: Spinal Dysraphism   99
Congenital Anomalies: Caudal Regression Syndrome   102

Congenital Anomalies: Chiari Malformation   103
Congenital Anomalies: Segmentation Anomalies   105

3   Pelvis, Hips, and Thighs **107**

Trauma: Pelvic Fractures—Minor   107
Trauma: Pelvic Fractures—Single Break in Pelvic Ring   109
Trauma: Pelvic Fractures—Complex   110
Trauma: Acetabular Fractures—Simple   115
Trauma: Acetabular Fractures—Complex   116
Trauma: Fracture/Dislocation—Dislocation of the Hip   121
Trauma: Femoral Neck Fractures   123
Trauma: Trochanteric Fractures   126
Trauma: Insufficiency Fractures   128
Trauma: Soft Tissue Trauma   130
Trauma: Soft Tissue Trauma—Muscle/Tendon Tears   131
Trauma: Soft Tissue Trauma—Bursitis   133
Trauma: Soft Tissue Trauma—Greater Trochanteric Pain Syndrome   135
Trauma: Soft Tissue Trauma—Acetabular Labral Tears   137
Trauma: Soft Tissue Trauma—Femoroacetabular Impingement   139
Osteonecrosis   141
Osteonecrosis: Avascular Necrosis   143
Osteonecrosis: Bone Infarcts   147
Bone Marrow Edema   148
Transient Osteoporosis of the Hip   149
Neoplasms   151
Arthropathies   155
Arthropathies: The Hip   156
Arthropathies: Sacroiliac Joints   160
Infection   162
Pediatric Hip Disorders: Legg–Calvé–Perthes Disease   164
Pediatric Hip Disorders: Developmental Dysplasia of the Hip   167
Pediatric Hip Disorders: Slipped Capital Femoral Epiphysis   171
Pediatric Hip Disorders: Rotational/Orientation Abnormalities—Coxa Vara
    And Coxa Valga   174
Pediatric Hip Disorders: Rotational/Orientation Abnormalities—Femoral
    Anteversion   176

4   Knee **178**

Skeletal Trauma: Osteochondral Fractures   178
Skeletal Trauma: Patellar Fractures   179
Skeletal Trauma: Supracondylar Fractures   182
Skeletal Trauma: Proximal Tibial Fractures   186
Skeletal Trauma: Miscellaneous Fractures   189
Meniscal Lesions: Meniscal Tears   197
Meniscal Lesions: Postoperative Meniscus   203
Meniscal Lesions: Meniscal Cysts   205
Meniscal Lesions: Discoid Menisci   206
Ligament and Tendon Injuries: Basic Concepts   208
Ligament and Tendon Injuries: Anterior Cruciate Ligament—Acute
    (Primary Features)   210

Ligament and Tendon Injuries: Anterior Cruciate Ligament—Acute
(Secondary Features)   212
Ligament and Tendon Injuries: Anterior Cruciate
Ligament—Chronic Tears   214
Ligament and Tendon Injuries: Posterior Cruciate Ligament   215
Ligament and Tendon Injuries: Medial and Lateral Collateral Ligaments   216
Ligament and Tendon Injuries: Quadriceps Tendon   218
Ligament and Tendon Injuries: Patellar Tendon   220
Ligament and Tendon Reconstruction   222
Plicae   226
Patellar Disorders: Patellofemoral Relationships   228
Patellar Disorders: Patellar Tracking and Instability   230
Patellar Disorders: Chondromalacia Patella   232
Loose Bodies   234
Osteochondritis Dissecans   236
Osteonecrosis   239
Osteochondroses   242
Arthropathies   244
Neoplasms: Bone Tumors and Tumorlike Conditions   249
Neoplasms: Soft Tissue Tumors and Masses   252
Chronic Overuse/Miscellaneous Conditions: Bursitis   255
Chronic Overuse/Miscellaneous Conditions: Iliotibial Band Syndrome   257
Chronic Overuse/Miscellaneous Conditions: Muscle Tears   258

5   Foot, Ankle, and Calf 260

Fractures/Dislocations: Ankle Fractures—Pediatric   260
Fractures/Dislocations: Ankle Fractures—Pediatric: Triplane Fracture   262
Fractures/Dislocations: Ankle Fractures—Pediatric: Juvenile Tillaux   264
Fractures/Dislocations: Ankle Fractures—Pediatric Complications   266
Fractures/Dislocations: Ankle Fractures—Adult   268
Fractures/Dislocations: Ankle Adult—Supination–Adduction Injuries   269
Fractures/Dislocations: Ankle Adult—Supination Lateral
Rotation Injuries   271
Fractures/Dislocations: Ankle Adult—Pronation–Abduction Injuries   273
Fractures/Dislocations: Ankle Adult—Pronation Lateral Rotation Injuries   275
Fractures/Dislocations: Ankle Adult—Plafond Fractures (Pilon)   277
Fractures/Dislocations: Ankle Adult—Complications   278
Fractures/Dislocations: Talar Fractures—Talar Neck   279
Fractures/Dislocations: Talar Fractures—Body, Head, Process Fractures   281
Fractures/Dislocations: Talar Fractures—Talar Dome Fractures   283
Fractures/Dislocations: Talar and Subtalar Dislocations   285
Fractures/Dislocations: Calcaneal Fractures—Intra-Articular   287
Fractures/Dislocations: Calcaneal Fractures—Extra-Articular   289
Fractures/Dislocations: Midfoot Injuries   291
Fractures/Dislocations: Forefoot Injuries—Fifth Metatarsal Fractures   294
Fractures/Dislocations: Forefoot Injuries—Metatarsophalangeal
Fracture/Dislocations   296
Fractures/Dislocations: Stress Fractures   298
Soft Tissue Trauma/Overuse Syndromes: Ligament Injuries   301
Soft Tissue Trauma/Overuse Syndromes: Peroneal Tendon Injuries   304

Soft Tissue Trauma/Overuse Syndromes: Achilles Tendon 307
Soft Tissue Trauma/Overuse Syndromes: Medial Tendon Injuries 309
Soft Tissue Trauma/Overuse Syndromes: Anterior Tendon Injuries 312
Soft Tissue Trauma/Overuse Syndromes: Plantar Fasciitis 314
Soft Tissue Trauma/Overuse Syndromes: Bursitis 317
Soft Tissue Trauma/Overuse Syndromes: Os Trigonum Syndrome 319
Soft Tissue Trauma/Overuse Syndromes: Tarsal Tunnel Syndrome 321
Soft Tissue Trauma/Overuse Syndromes: Sinus Tarsi Syndrome 323
Soft Tissue Trauma/Overuse Syndromes: Impingement Syndromes 325
Soft Tissue Trauma/Overuse Syndromes: Midfoot and
    Forefoot Syndromes 327
Neoplasms/Tumorlike Conditions: Skeletal Lesions—Benign 329
Neoplasms/Tumorlike Conditions: Soft Tissue Lesions—Benign 332
Arthritis: Osteoarthritis (Degenerative Joint Disease) 334
Arthritis: Rheumatoid Arthritis 335
Arthritis: Psoriatic Arthritis 337
Arthritis: Reactive Arthritis 338
Arthritis: Ankylosing Spondylitis 339
Arthritis: Neurotrophic Arthropathy 340
Arthritis: Gout 341
Arthritis: Calcium Pyrophosphate Deposition Disease 342
Infection: Osteomyelitis 343
Infection: Soft Tissue Infection 345
Infection: Joint Space Infection 346
Infection: Diabetic Foot 348
Pediatric Disorders: Terminology 350
Pediatric Disorders: Normal Angles of the Foot and Ankle 351
Pediatric Disorders: Hindfoot Abnormalities 354
Pediatric Disorders: Plantar Arch Abnormalities 358
Pediatric Disorders: Forefoot Abnormalities 360
Pediatric Disorders: Talipes Equinovarus 362
Pediatric Disorders: Congenital Vertical Talus 363
Pediatric Disorders: Pes Planovalgus 364
Pediatric Disorders: Tarsal Coalitions 365
Pediatric Disorders: Overgrowth/Hypoplasia/Aplasia 367
Pediatric Disorders: Freiberg Infraction 369
Pediatric Disorders: Köhler Disease 370

6   Shoulder/Arm **372**

Fractures/Dislocations: Proximal Humeral Fractures 372
Fractures/Dislocations: Glenohumeral Dislocations 374
Fractures/Dislocations: Acromioclavicular Dislocation 378
Fractures/Dislocations: Sternoclavicular Dislocations 381
Fractures/Dislocations: Clavicle Fractures 383
Fractures/Dislocations: Posttraumatic Osteolysis 385
Fractures/Dislocations: Scapular Fractures 388
Fracture/Dislocations: Humeral Shaft Fractures 389
Rotator Cuff Disease: Basic Concepts 391
Rotator Cuff Disease: Impingement 393
Rotator Cuff Disease: Rotator Cuff Tears—Full Thickness Tears 395

Rotator Cuff Disease: Partial Thickness Tears   399
Rotator Cuff Disease: Tendinosis   401
Rotator Cuff Disease: Postoperative Changes   403
Instability: Basic Concepts   405
Instability: Recurrent Subluxation/Dislocations—Capsular Abnormalities   406
Instability: Labral Tears   408
Instability: Humeral Osteochondral or Ligament Avulsions   411
Instability: Posterior Instability   413
Instability: Multidirectional Instability   414
Instability: Labral Variants   415
Biceps Tendon   416
Adhesive Capsulitis   419
Nerve Entrapment Syndromes   422
Inflammatory Arthropathies   424
Osteonecrosis   428
Neoplasms   430
Brachial Plexus   434

7   Elbow/Forearm **436**

Fractures/Dislocations: Distal Humeral Fractures   436
Fractures/Dislocations: Epicondylar Fractures   438
Fractures/Dislocations: Adult Distal Humeral Fractures   439
Fractures/Dislocations: Capitellar Fractures   444
Fractures/Dislocations: Fractures of the Proximal Radius   445
Fractures/Dislocations: Ulnar Fractures   447
Fractures/Dislocations: Coronoid Fractures   448
Fracture/Dislocations: Elbow Dislocations   449
Fractures/Dislocations: Monteggia Fractures   450
Fractures/Dislocations: Forearm Fractures   451
Osteochondritis Dissecans   454
Soft Tissue Trauma: Biceps Tendon   455
Soft Tissue Trauma: Triceps Tendon Injuries   457
Soft Tissue Trauma: Flexor/Extensor Tendon Injuries   458
Soft Tissue Trauma: Muscle Injuries   460
Soft Tissue Trauma: Ligament Injuries   461
Neoplasms: Bone Tumors   463
Neoplasms: Soft Tissue Tumors   464
Infection   465
Arthropathies   467
Nerve Entrapment Syndromes   470

8   Hand and Wrist **476**

Fractures/Dislocations: Distal Radius/Ulnar Fractures—Colles Fracture   476
Fractures/Dislocations: Distal Radius/Ulnar Fractures—Smith Fracture   480
Fractures/Dislocations: Distal Radius/Ulnar Fractures—Barton Fracture   481
Fractures/Dislocations: Distal Radius/Ulnar Fractures—Chauffeur's
    Fracture   483
Fractures/Dislocations: Galeazzi Fractures   484
Fractures/Dislocations: Distal Radioulnar Joint Subluxation/Dislocations   486
Fractures/Dislocations: Scaphoid Fractures   487

Fractures/Dislocations: Other Carpal Fractures   492
Fractures/Dislocations: Carpal and Carpometacarpal Dislocations   494
Fractures/Dislocations: Metacarpal Fractures   497
Fractures/Dislocations: Phalangeal Fractures/Dislocations   501
Carpal Instability   503
Soft Tissue Trauma/Miscellaneous Conditions: Ligament Injuries   506
Soft Tissue Trauma/Miscellaneous Conditions: Tendon Injuries   509
Soft Tissue/Miscellaneous Conditions: De Quervain Tenosynovitis and
   Intersection Syndrome   512
Neoplasms: Bone Tumors   514
Neoplasms: Soft Tissue Masses   516
Arthropathies   518
Avascular Necrosis   522
Nerve Compression Syndromes: Carpal Tunnel Syndrome   524
Nerve Compression Syndromes: Ulnar Nerve Compression   526
Ulnar Lunate Abutment Syndrome   528

9   Musculoskeletal Neoplasms **530**

Bone Tumors/Tumorlike Conditions: Imaging Approaches   530
Bone Tumors/Tumorlike Conditions: Radiographic Features   531
Bone Tumors/Tumorlike Conditions: Magnetic Resonance
   Imaging Protocols   535
Bone Tumors/Tumorlike Conditions: Osteoid Osteoma   536
Bone Tumors/Tumorlike Conditions: Osteoblastoma   538
Bone Tumors/Tumorlike Conditions: Osteochondroma   540
Bone Tumors/Tumorlike Conditions: Enchondroma   542
Bone Tumors/Tumorlike Conditions: Chondroblastoma   545
Bone Tumors/Tumorlike Conditions: Chondromyxoid Fibroma   547
Bone Tumors/Tumorlike Conditions: Nonossifying Fibroma   549
Bone Tumors/Tumorlike Conditions: Solitary Bone Cyst   551
Bone Tumors/Tumorlike Conditions: Aneurysmal Bone Cyst   553
Bone Tumors/Tumorlike Conditions: Fibrous Dysplasia   555
Bone Tumors/Tumorlike Conditions: Giant Cell Tumor   557
Bone Tumors/Tumorlike Conditions: Eosinophilic Granuloma/Langerhans Cell
   Histiocytosis   559
Bone Tumors/Tumorlike Conditions: Osteosarcoma   561
Bone Tumors/Tumorlike Conditions: Parosteal Osteosarcoma   563
Bone Tumors/Tumorlike Conditions: Periosteal Osteosarcoma   565
Bone Tumors/Tumorlike Conditions: Telangiectatic Osteosarcoma   568
Bone Tumors/Tumorlike Conditions: Ewing Sarcoma   570
Bone Tumors/Tumorlike Conditions: Chondrosarcoma (Primary, Central)   571
Bone Tumors/Tumorlike Conditions: Chondrosarcoma (Secondary)   573
Bone Tumors/Tumorlike Conditions: Fibrosarcoma and Malignant Fibrous
   Histiocytoma of Bone   575
Bone Tumors/Tumorlike Conditions: Adamantinoma   576
Bone Tumors/Tumorlike Conditions: Paget Sarcoma   577
Bone Tumors/Tumorlike Conditions: Metastasis   578
Bone Tumors/Tumorlike Conditions: Myeloma   579
Bone Tumors/Tumorlike Conditions: Lymphoma   581
Soft Tissue Masses: Lipoma   583

Soft Tissue Masses: Liposarcoma   585
Soft Tissue Masses: Myxoma (Intramuscular)   588
Soft Tissue Masses: Simple Venous Malformation (Previously
  Called Hemangioma)   590
Soft Tissue Masses: Simple Common Cystic Lymphatic
  Malformation/Lymphangioma   592
Soft Tissue Masses: Benign Peripheral Nerve Sheath Tumor   594
Soft Tissue Masses: Malignant Peripheral Nerve Sheath Tumor   597
Soft Tissue Masses: Deep Fibromatosis (Desmoid Tumor)   599
Soft Tissue Masses: Elastofibroma   601
Soft Tissue Masses: Ganglion   603
Soft Tissue Masses: Giant Cell Tumor of Tendon Sheath   605
Soft Tissue Masses: Hematoma   607
Soft Tissue Masses: Myositis Ossificans   611
Soft Tissue Masses: Undifferentiated-Unclassified Tumor
  (Previously Known as Undifferentiated Pleomorphic Sarcoma)   613
Soft Tissue Masses: Synovial Sarcoma   615
Soft Tissue Masses: Rhabdomyosarcoma   618

10   Musculoskeletal Infection **620**

Basic Concepts   620
Osteomyelitis   622
Chronic Recurrent Multifocal Osteomyelitis   626
SAPHO (Synovitis, Acne, Pustulosis, Hyperostosis, Osteitis)   628
Osteomyelitis—Violated Tissue   630
Joint Space Infection   632
Soft Tissue Infection   635
Brodie Abscess   638
Tuberculosis/Atypical Mycobacterial Infections   641
Fungal Infections   643

11   Marrow Disorders **645**

Normal Marrow: Basic Concepts   645
Marrow Reconversion   647
Myeloid Depletion   648
Marrow Ischemia   650
Marrow Infiltration: Basic Concepts   652
Marrow Infiltration: Lipidosis   653
Langerhans Cell Histiocytosis   654
Erdheim–Chester Disease   655
Hyperlipoproteinemias   657
Myelofibrosis   659
Compression Fractures: Benign versus Malignant   661

12   Arthropathies/Connective Tissue Diseases **662**

Rheumatoid Arthritis   662
Psoriatic Arthritis   666
Reactive Arthritis   668
Ankylosing Spondylitis   670
Osteoarthritis   673

Enteric Arthropathies 677
Systemic Lupus Erythematosus 679
Scleroderma 680
Dermatomyositis/Polymyositis 681
Mixed Connective Tissue Disease/Overlap Syndromes 683
Juvenile Chronic Arthropathy 685
Hemophilia 688
Gout 690
Hemochromatosis 693
Calcium Pyrophosphate Deposition Disease 695
Wilson Disease 697
Ochronosis 698
Neurotrophic Arthropathy 699
Synovial Chondromatosis/Osteochondromatosis 702
Pigmented Villonodular Synovitis 704
Amyloid Arthropathy 705

13 Metabolic Diseases **707**

Osteoporosis: Basic Concepts 707
Osteoporosis: Generalized 708
Osteoporosis: Regional Osteoporosis 713
Rickets and Osteomalacia: Basic Concepts 716
Rickets and Osteomalacia: Rickets 718
Rickets and Osteomalacia: Osteomalacia 720
Renal Osteodystrophy 722
Parathyroid Disorders: Hyperparathyroidism 725
Parathyroid Disorders: Hypoparathyroidism, Pseudohypoparathyroidism,
    and Pseudo-Pseudohypoparathyroidism 728
Thyroid Disorders 730
Pituitary Disorders 732
Paget Disease 733

14 Miscellaneous Conditions **736**

Bone Islands (Enostosis) 736
Osteopoikilosis 738
Osteopathia Striata 739
Melorheostosis 740
Progressive Diaphyseal Dysplasia (Engelmann Disease) 742
Cleidocranial Dysplasia (Cleidocranial Dysostosis) 743
Osteopetrosis 744
Mastocytosis 746
Tuberous Sclerosis 747
Neurofibromatosis 749
Ollier Disease (Enchondromatosis) 753
Maffucci Syndrome 754
Hereditary Multiple Exostosis 755
Epiphyseal Dysplasias 757
Metaphyseal Dysplasias 760
Marfan Syndrome 761
Ehlers–Danlos Syndrome 762

Osteogenesis Imperfecta   763
Achondroplasia   765
Mucopolysaccharidoses   767
Dyschondrosteosis (Leri–Weill Syndrome)   771
Pachydermoperiostosis   773
Secondary Hypertrophic Osteoarthropathy   775
Vitaminosis: Vitamin A   777
Vitaminosis: Vitamin C   778
Vitaminosis: Vitamin D   780
Tumoral Calcinosis   782
Heavy Metal Disorders   783
Hemoglobinopathies/Anemias: Basic Concepts   785
Hemoglobinopathies/Anemias: Sickle Cell Anemia   786
Emoglobinopathies/Anemias: Thalassemia   788
Sarcoidosis   790
Diffuse Idiopathic Skeletal Hyperostosis   793
Gorham Disease (Massive Osteolysis)   795
Nonaccidental Trauma (Battered Child Syndrome)   796

Index   799

CHAPTER

1

Temporomandibular Joint

Jeffrey J. Peterson and Thomas H. Berquist

■ ANATOMY

KEY FACTS

- The temporomandibular joint (TMJ) is a synovial joint divided by a disc into superior and inferior compartments.
- The normal disc is biconcave.
- The posterior band is thicker and separated from the anterior band by the thin intermediate zone, giving the disc a "bow-tie" configuration.
- The posterior attachment (bilaminar zone) contains the neurovascular supply for the disc.
- When the mouth is closed, the disc is at the apex of the mandibular condyle.
- With opening of the mouth, the mandibular condyle translates forward.
- The normal disc remains centered over the condyle as the mouth opens.

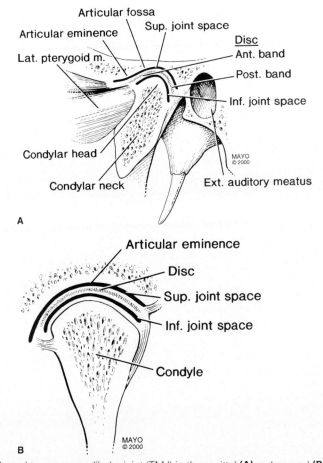

FIGURE 1-1. Normal temporomandibular joint (TMJ) in the sagittal **(A)** and coronal **(B)** planes.

■ INTERNAL DERANGEMENT

KEY FACTS

The disc is normally at the 12-o'clock position, with the mouth in the closed position. There is some degree of displacement in up to 34% of asymptomatic patients.

- Internal derangement is defined as an abnormal relationship or position of the disc to the condyle and articular eminence.
- The cause is unknown, but trauma, malocclusion, bruxism, hypermotility, ligament laxity, condylar abnormalities, and stress are implicated.
- Females outnumber males by a ratio of 5:1.
- Internal derangement is a progressive process.
  - Initially anterior, medial, or lateral displacement occurs when the mouth is closed, which reduces with opening.
  - The disc no longer reduces as elasticity decreases.
  - The disc becomes deformed with secondary bony changes.
  - Anterior displacement is most common, and 80% to 90% are bilateral. Medial or lateral displacement occurs in 5%, and posterior displacement occurs in 1%.
- Clinical symptoms include pain, clicking, and reduced motion.

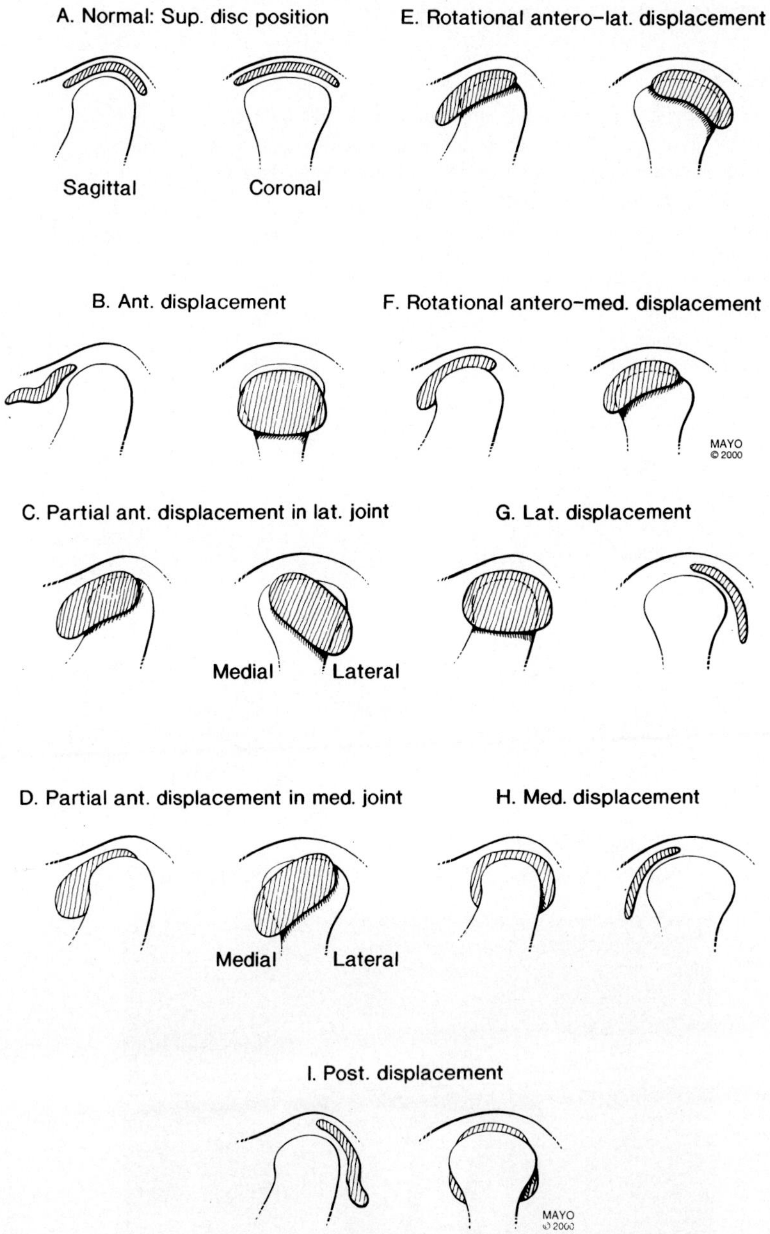

A. Normal: Sup. disc position   E. Rotational antero–lat. displacement

Sagittal   Coronal

B. Ant. displacement   F. Rotational antero–med. displacement

MAYO
© 2000

C. Partial ant. displacement in lat. joint   G. Lat. displacement

Medial   Lateral

D. Partial ant. displacement in med. joint   H. Med. displacement

Medial   Lateral

I. Post. displacement

MAYO
© 2000

FIGURE 1-2. Disc displacement categories: normal **(A)**, anterior displacement **(B)**, partial anterior displacement in lateral joint **(C)**, partial anterior displacement in medial joint **(D)**, rotational antero-lateral displacement **(E)**, rotational anteromedial displacement **(F)**, lateral displacement **(G)**, medial displacement **(H)**, and posterior displacement **(I)**.

SUGGESTED READING

Aiken A, Bouloux G, Hudgins P. MR imaging of the temporomandibular joint. *Mag Reson Imaging Clin N Am.* 2012;20(3):397–412.

Milano V, Desiate A, Bellin R, et al. Magnetic resonance imaging of temporomandibular disorders: classification, prevalence, interpretation of disc displacement and deformation. *Dentomaxillofac Radiol.* 2000;29:353–361.

Sale H, Bryndahl F, Isberg A. Temporomandibular joints in asymptomatic and symptomatic volunteers: a prospective 15-year follow-up clinical and MR imaging study. *Radiology.* 2013;267(1):183–194.

■ ANTERIOR DISC DISPLACEMENT

KEY FACTS

■ Anterior disc displacement occurs most commonly; 80% to 90% are bilateral.
■ Ninety percent of nondeformed anteriorly displaced discs reduce with opening.
■ Seventy-six percent of distorted discs do not reduce with opening.
■ Symptoms increase as disc deformity progresses.
■ Secondary signs of internal derangement.
  ● Joint effusion
  ● Joint space asymmetry
  ● Marrow edema
  ● Condylar erosion
  ● Lateral pterygoid abnormalities

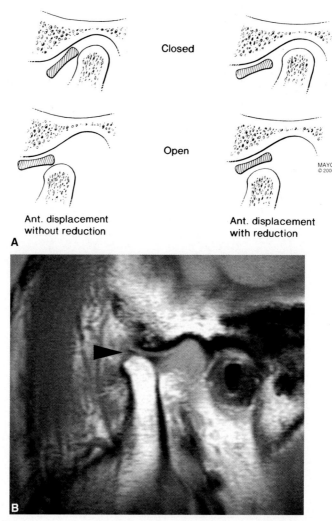

FIGURE 1-3. (A) Schematic diagrams depicting anterior disc displacement without (*left*) and with (*right*) reduction. Sagittal T1-weighted magnetic resonance (MR) images show the normal imaging appearance of the disc (*arrowhead*) with open-mouth position **(B)** and closed-mouth positioning **(C)**. Anterior disc dislocation without reduction (*arrowhead*) seen with open-mouth **(D)** and closed-mouth positioning **(E)**. Anterior disc dislocation with reduction (*arrowhead*) seen with open-mouth **(F)** and closed-mouth positioning **(G)**.

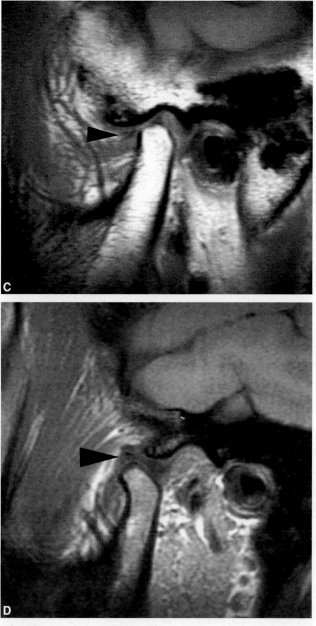

FIGURE 1-3. *(continued)*

(continued)

■ ANTERIOR DISC DISPLACEMENT   *(Continued)*

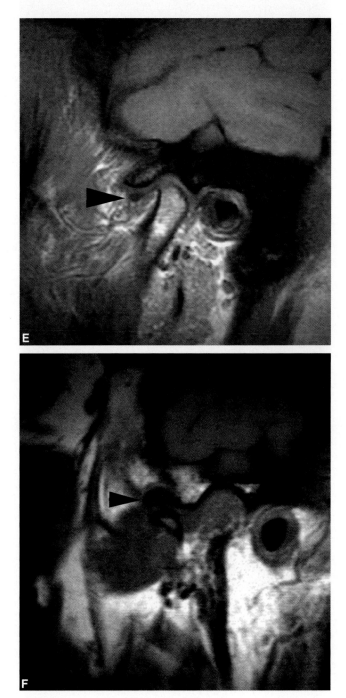

FIGURE 1-3. *(continued)*

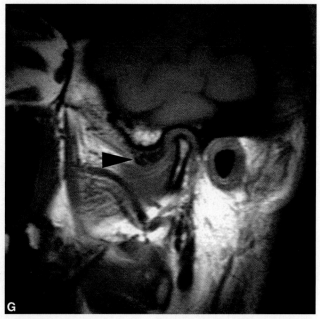

FIGURE 1-3. *(continued)*

SUGGESTED READING

Aiken A, Bouloux G, Hudgins P. MR imaging of the temporomandibular joint. *Mag Reson Imaging Clin N Am.* 2012;20(3):397–412.

Amaral Rde O, Damasceno NN, de Souza LA, et al. Magnetic resonance images of patients with temporomandibular disorders: prevalence and correlation between disk morphology and displacement. *Eur J Radiol.* 2013;82(6):990–994.

Kurita H, Ohtsuka A, Kobayashi H, et al. Resorption of the lateral pole of the mandibular condyle in temporomandibular disc displacement. *Dentomaxillofac Radiol.* 2001;39:88–91.

Yang X, Pernu H, Pyhtinen J, et al. MRI findings concerning the lateral pterygoid muscle in patients with symptomatic TMJ hypermotility. *Cranio.* 2001;19:260–268.

■ LATERAL AND MEDIAL DISC DISPLACEMENT

KEY FACTS

■ Anterior and anterolateral displacements account for 46% to 52% of disc displacements.
■ Rotational displacement was associated with 34% of displacements that did not reduce with open-ing and 53% of reducing discs.
■ Additional categories of internal derangement include 11% with partial displacement, 4% with stuck discs (disc does not move with condylar motion), and 1% with posterior displacements.
■ Magnetic resonance imaging (MRI) is 95% accurate for disc position and classification, and 93% accurate for osseous abnormalities.

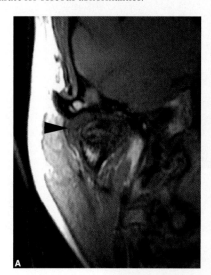 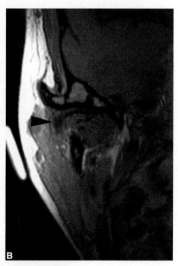

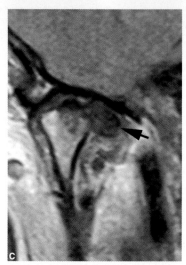

FIGURE 1-4. Coronal **(A)** and sagittal **(B)** magnetic resonance (MR) images depict an anterior and lateral disc dislocation with lateral displacement of the degenerative disc (*arrowheads*). Coronal MR image **(C)** demonstrates a medial disc dislocation (*arrow*).

SUGGESTED READING

Aoyama S, Kino K, Amagasa T, et al. Clinical and magnetic resonance imaging study of unilateral sideways disc displacements of the temporomandibular joint. *J Med Dent Sci.* 2002;49:89–94.
Foucart JM, Carpenter P, Pajoni D, et al. MR of 732 TMJs: anterior, rotational, partial, and sideways disc displace-ments. *Eur J Radiol.* 1998;28:86–94.

■ TRAUMA

KEY FACTS

- ■ Injury to the mandible and TMJ is usually secondary to a blow to the chin.
- ■ Injuries are most common in 15- to 30-year-old persons.
- ■ Multiple injuries to the mandible and TMJs are common.
- ■ TMJ injuries may involve soft tissues (subluxation and dislocation) or osseous and articular structures.

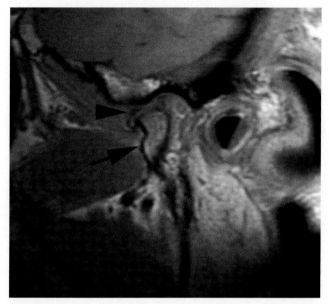

FIGURE 1-5. Sagittal magnetic resonance (MR) image in a patient with a prior fracture of the neck of the mandibular condyle (*arrow*) shows degeneration of the articular disc (*arrowhead*).

SUGGESTED READING

Cascone P, Leonardi R, Marino S, et al. Intracapsular fractures of the mandibular condyle: diagnosis, treatment, and anatomic and pathologic evaluations. *J Craniofacial Surg.* 2003;14(2):184–191.

Yu YH, Wang MH, Zhang SY, et al. Magnetic resonance imaging assessment of temporomandibular joint soft tissue injuries of intracapsular condylar fracture. *Br J Maxillofac Surg.* 2013;51(2):133–137.

■ OSTEOARTHRITIS

KEY FACTS

- Osteoarthritis is commonly associated with internal derangement.
- The condition may be posttraumatic.
- Sclerosis and osteophyte formation are commonly seen.
- Computed tomography and MRI are most useful for evaluation.

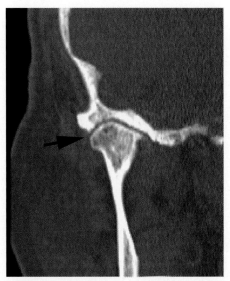

FIGURE 1-6. Coronal reformatted computed tomography (CT) of the temporomandibular joint (TMJ) depicting osteoarthritis of the right TMJ with narrowing, sclerosis, and remodeling of the mandibular condyle and mandibular fossa (*arrow*).

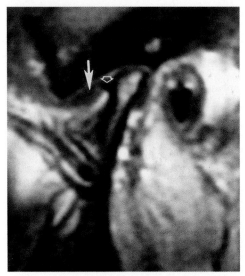

FIGURE 1-7. Sagittal T1-weighted magnetic resonance (MR) image with anterior disc displacement (*arrow*) and a condylar osteophyte (*open arrow*).

SUGGESTED READING

Westesson PL. Structural hard-tissue changes in temporomandibular joints with internal derangement. *Oral Surg Med Oral Pathol.* 1985;59:220–224.

■ MISCELLANEOUS ARTHROPATHIES

KEY FACTS

■ Multiple arthropathies can affect the TMJ: rheumatoid arthritis (RA), juvenile chronic arthritis, psoriatic arthritis, ankylosing spondylitis, systemic lupus erythematosus, gout, and other crystal arthropathies.

■ Some 28% to 63% of patients with juvenile chronic arthritis have TMJ involvement.

■ RA involving the TMJ is three times more common in females.

■ Up to 50% of patients with severe RA have TMJ involvement.

■ Patients may have joint erosions, laxity, and malocclusion.

■ MRI with contrast enhancement is most useful for complete evaluation of TMJ arthropathies.

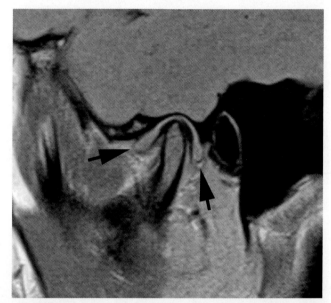

FIGURE 1-8. Sagittal magnetic resonance imaging (MRI) in a patient with rheumatoid arthritis (RA) with extensive pannus formation about the temporomandibular joint (TMJ; *arrows*).

(continued)

▪ MISCELLANEOUS ARTHROPATHIES   *(Continued)*

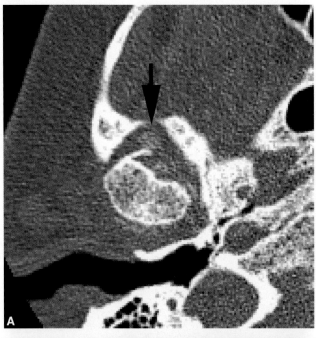

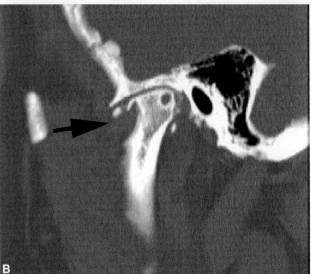

FIGURE 1-9. Axial **(A)** and sagittal **(B)** reformatted computed tomography (CT) images in a patient with synovial osteochondromatosis of the temporomandibular joint (TMB). High-density cartilaginous loose bodies (*arrow*) are seen within the joint, with erosion and remodeling of the mandibular condyle.

SUGGESTED READING

Kretapirom K, Okochi K, Nakamura S, et al. MRI characteristics of rheumatoid arthritis in the temporomandibular joint. *Dentomaxillofac Radiol.* 2013;42(4):31627230.

Kuseler A, Pedersen TK, Herlin T, et al. Contrast-enhanced magnetic resonance imaging as a method to diagnose early inflammatory changes in the temporomandibular joint in children with juvenile rheumatoid arthritis. *J Rheumatol.* 1998;25:1406–1412.

■ TUMORS

KEY FACTS

■ Primary tumors in the TMJ region are rare.
■ Metastasis can occur, especially from breast carcinoma.
■ Fifteen of 1,907 (0.7%) benign tumors and 119 of 6,035 (1.9%) malignant tumors involve the mandible.

BENIGN AND MALIGNANT OSSEOUS TUMORS OF THE MANDIBLE

Tumor	No. in mandible
Benign	
Giant cell tumor	7
Hemangioma	4
Neurolemmoma	4
Total	15
Malignant	
Lymphoma	12
Chondrosarcoma	24
Osteosarcoma	39
Fibrosarcoma	17
Total	119

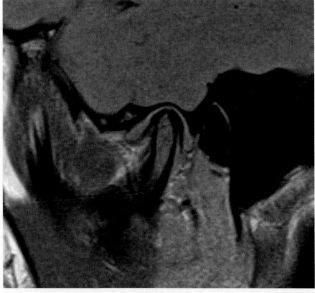

FIGURE 1-10. A 65-year-old patient with jaw swelling. Anteroposterior radiograph demonstrates a large benign osteoma.

SUGGESTED READING

Unni KK. *Dahlin's Bone Tumors: General Aspects and Data on 11,087 Cases.* 5th ed. Philadelphia: Lippincott-Raven; 1996.

CHAPTER
2

Spine
Thomas H. Berquist, William E. Clifton, Prasanna G. Vibhute,
Vivek Gupta, and Jeffrey J. Peterson

■ TRAUMA: CERVICAL SPINE—BASIC CONCEPTS

KEY FACTS

- Traumatic injuries to the cervical spine comprise approximately 65% of all spinal injuries.
- The incidence of cervical spine injury (CSI) after blunt trauma is 2% to 6%.
- Cervical spine immobilization is an important initial step in preventing neurologic injury after trauma. The immobilization may be "cleared" by a combination of physical examination findings and radiographic studies.
- Computed tomography (CT) has approximately 100% sensitivity for detection of fractures compared with 65% for radiographs, and therefore should be the first imaging modality in patients with suspected injury (Level I evidence).
- NEXUS (National Emergency X-Radiography Utilization Study) criteria and CCR (Canadian C-Spine Rule) are validated clinical decision tools to safely rule out CSI without the need to obtain radiographs in alert and stable trauma patients. Both have sensitivity of 90% to 100% for ruling out CSI (Table 2-1).
- ACR Appropriateness Criteria rating if imaging indicated by NEXUS criteria:
  - CT cervical spine without intravenous (IV) contrast—9
  - Radiographs—6
  - Magnetic resonance imaging (MRI) without IV contrast for myelopathy—9, and treatment planning for unstable spine—8
  - Computed tomography angiography head and neck if clinical or imaging findings suggest arterial injury—9
- Understanding the mechanism of injury is helpful for evaluating images and determining prognosis (Table 2-2).
- Stability of injuries is important to assess. This can be usually accomplished on the lateral view or reformatted CT images, although all images should be assessed.
- Indicators of instability include
  - More than one column involved (Fig. 2-7)
  - Subluxation greater than 3 mm
  - Increased interspinous distance
  - Facet joint widening
  - Narrowed disc or widened space
  - Vertebral compression greater than 25%
- Not all radiographically documented cervical spine injuries are clinically significant (Table 2-3)

Table 2-1

NEXUS (*N*ational *E*mergency *X*-Radiography *U*tilization *S*tudy)

Patient's neck can be clinically cleared safely without imaging if all five low-risk conditions are met:

No posterior midline neck pain or tenderness

No focal neurologic deficit

Normal level of alertness

No evidence of intoxication

No clinically apparent, painful other bodily injury distracting patient's attention away from neck injury

CCR (*C*anadian *C*-Spine *R*ules)

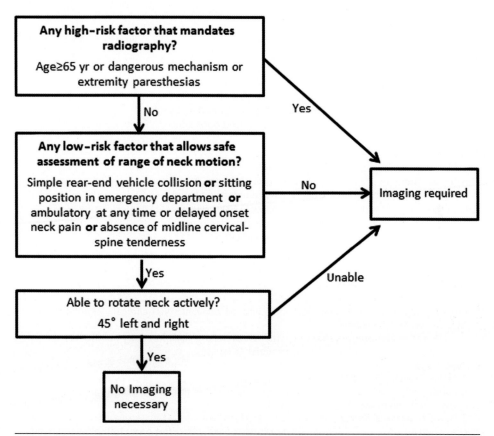

Adapted from Stiell IG, Clement CM, McKnight RD, et al. The Canadian C-Spine Rule versus the NEXUS low-risk criteria in patients with trauma. *N Engl J Med.* 2003; 349:2510–2518.

(continued)

■ TRAUMA: CERVICAL SPINE—BASIC CONCEPTS *(Continued)*

Table 2-2 CERVICAL SPINE TRAUMA: MECHANISMS OF INJURY

Type of Injury	Radiographic Features	Comments
Hyperflexion		Most common
Disruptive hyperflexion	Sprain, transient dislocation Locked facets Spinous process fractures	
Compressive hyperflexion	Vertebral wedge fractures Teardrop fractures Fracture/dislocations	
Shearing injuries	Anteriorly displaced odontoid fractures	
Hyperextension		Findings may be subtle
Disruptive hyperextension	Hangman's fractures Hyperextension sprain Anterior inferior body fractures	
Compressive hyperextension	Posterior arch fractures Hyperextension fracture/dislocation	
Shearing	Posteriorly displaced odontoid fractures	
Axial compression	Jefferson fractures Burst fractures	
Flexion–rotation	Rotary fixation of C1 on C2 Unilateral locked/perched facets	
Lateral flexion	Uncinate process fractures Transverse process fractures Lateral wedge fractures	

Table 2-3

Radiographically documented cervical spine injuries which are NOT clinically significant:
1. Spinous process fracture
2. Simple wedge compression fracture with less than 25% vertebral body height loss
3. Isolated avulsion without ligamentous injury
4. Type 1 odontoid fracture
5. Endplate fracture
6. Osteophyte fracture (should not include vertebral corner fracture or teardrop fracture)
7. Trabecular bone injury
8. Transverse process fracture

These, when occurring in isolation, are extremely unlikely to cause harm to the patient even if missed on the radiographs, and require no specific treatment.

Adapted from Hoffman JR et al. Validity of a set of clinical criteria to rule out injury to the cervical spine in patients with blunt trauma. *N Engl J Med.* 2000;343:94–99.

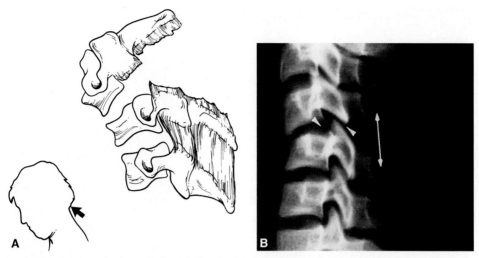

FIGURE 2-1. Disruptive hyperflexion injuries. **(A)** Mechanism (blow to the occipital region) that causes more posterior soft tissue injury compared with anterior compression. **(B)** Lateral radiograph shows widened interspinous distance (*double arrow*), subluxation of the facets (*posterior arrowhead*) and slight subluxation, and disc space widening (*anterior arrowhead*).

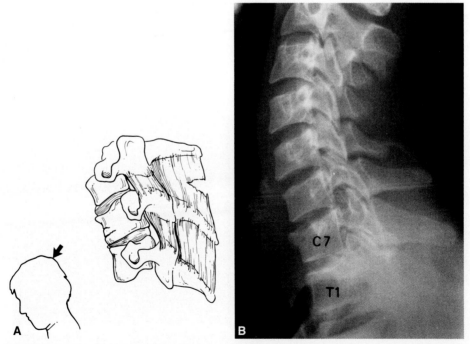

FIGURE 2-2. Compressive hyperflexion injuries. **(A)** Mechanism of injury with force transmitted to the anterior vertebral body. **(B)** Lateral radiograph demonstrates compression of C7 and T1 (*arrow*).

(continued)

■ TRAUMA: CERVICAL SPINE—BASIC CONCEPTS *(Continued)*

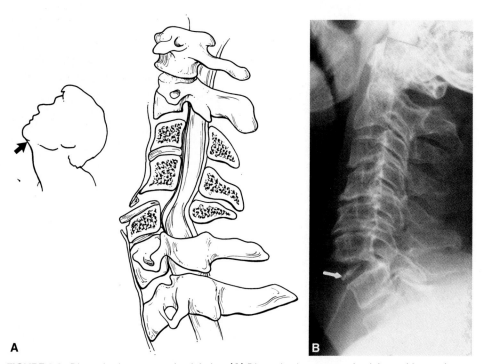

FIGURE 2-3. Disruptive hyperextension injuries. **(A)** Disruptive hyperextension injury with anterior distraction. The cord may be compressed. **(B)** Lateral radiograph shows anterior disc space widening and vertebral chip fracture *(arrow)*.

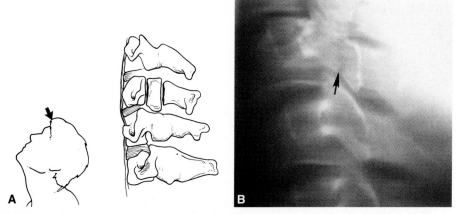

FIGURE 2-4. Compressive hyperextension injuries. **(A)** Mechanism resulting in posterior compression and less anterior distraction. **(B)** Lateral radiograph demonstrates a vertical posterior arch fracture *(arrow)*.

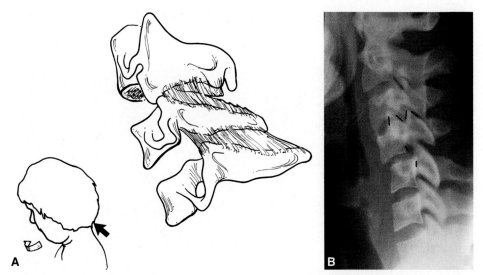

FIGURE 2-5. Flexion–rotation injuries. **(A)** Mechanism of injury. **(B)** Lateral radiograph shows a unilateral locked facet with subluxation and "bow-tie" configuration (*lines*) of the facets.

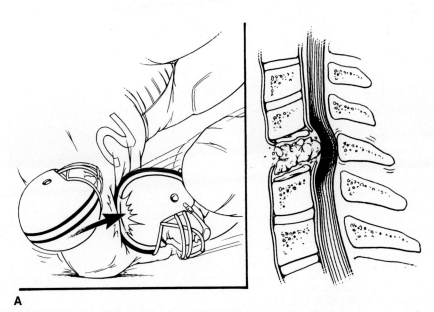

FIGURE 2-6. Vertical compression injuries. **(A)** Mechanism of injury. **(B, C)** Axial computed tomography (CT) images of a burst fracture.

(continued)

■ TRAUMA: CERVICAL SPINE—BASIC CONCEPTS *(Continued)*

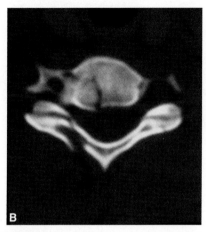
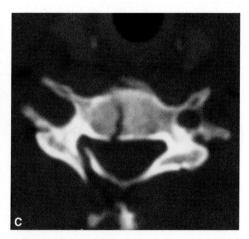

FIGURE 2-6. *(continued)*

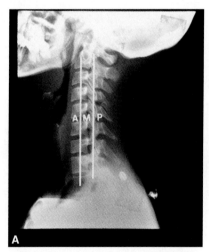
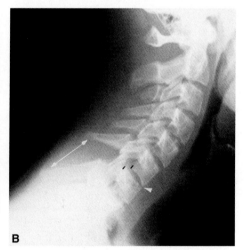

FIGURE 2-7. Instability. **(A)** Lateral radiograph demonstrates the anterior (anterior longitudinal ligament, body, and disc), middle (posterior body and disc and posterior longitudinal ligament), and posterior (facet joints and posterior ligaments) columns. When two columns are involved, the injury should be considered unstable. **(B)** Lateral view shows multiple column involvement with widened interspinous distance (*double arrow*), subluxation (*black lines*), and anterior disc space narrowing (*arrowhead*) caused by a disruptive hyperflexion injury.

SUGGESTED READING

Antevil JL, Sise MJ, Sack DI, et al. Spiral computed tomography for the initial evaluation of spine trauma: a new standard of care? *J Trauma.* 2006;61:382–387.

Barba CA, Taggert J, Morgan AS, et al. A new cervical spine clearance protocol using computed tomography. *J Trauma.* 2001;51:652–656, discussion 656–657.

Denis F. Spinal instability as defined by the three-column spine concept in acute spinal trauma. *Clin Orthop.* 1984;189:65–76.

Gehweiler JA, Osborne RL, Becker RF. *The Radiology of the Vertebral Trauma.* Philadelphia: WB Saunders; 1980.

Griffen MM, Frykberg ER, Kerwin AJ, et al. Radiographic clearance of blunt cervical spine injury: plain radiograph or computed tomography scans. *J Trauma.* 2003;55:222–227.

Sliker CW, Mirvis SE, Shanmuganathan K. Assessing cervical spine stability in obtunded blunt trauma patients: review of the medical literature. *Radiology.* 2005;234:733–739.

■ TRAUMA: CERVICAL SPINE
—ATLANTO-OCCIPITAL FRACTURE DISLOCATIONS

KEY FACTS

- Atlanto-occipital dislocations are usually fatal; therefore, imaging is rarely performed.
- The injury results from high-velocity shearing forces dislocating the head from C1.
- In children, the condyles are less well developed, making patients more susceptible to injury.
- Occur due to widespread ligamentous disruption between the occiput and upper cervical spine. Often without bony fractures and hence more ready missed by an inexperienced observer.
- If the patient survives the injury, treatment is occipital-C2 fusion.

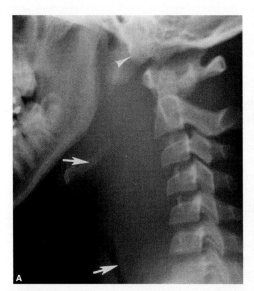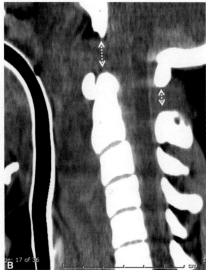

FIGURE 2-8. Atlanto-occipital dislocation. **(A)** Lateral radiograph shows a huge prevertebral hematoma (*arrows*) with anterior dislocation of the occipital condyles (*arrowhead*). **(B)** Sagittal computed tomography (CT) reconstruction in another patient following high-speed motor vehicle accident shows clear separation of the occipital condyles from the C1 with huge prevertebral and epidural hematomas and stretching to the cervicomedullary junction. Both patients did not survive.

SUGGESTED READING

Deliganis AV, Baxter AB, Hanson JA, et al. Radiologic spectrum of craniocervical distraction injuries. *Radiographics.* 2000;20:S237–S250.

Hall GC, Kinsman MJ, Nazar RG, et al. Atlanto-occipital dislocation. *World J Orthop.* 2015;6(2):236–243. doi:10.5312/wjo.v6.i2.236.

Hosalkar HS, Cain EL, Chin KR, et al. Traumatic atlanto-occipital dislocation in children. *J Bone Joint Surg.* 2005; 87A:2480–2488.

■ TRAUMA: CERVICAL SPINE— C1 FRACTURES

KEY FACTS

- Fractures of the atlas (C1) account for 25% of craniocervical injuries, 3% to 13% of cervical spine injuries, and 1% to 3% of all spinal injuries.
- Biomechanism: Distraction of C1 lateral masses and failure of the C1 ring at its weakest points adjacent to the lateral masses due to axial loading of occiput.
- Isolated posterior arch followed by anterior arch fractures are most common and are managed conservatively with excellent union rates.
- Isolated burst fractures (including classic Jefferson fracture) are second most common and seldom cause neurologic injury because the anatomy and mechanism of injury force the fragments away from the spinal canal.
- Injuries to transverse ligament are common and can occur without bony injury. Unless the occipital condyles are fractured, other ligaments are spared.
- Modified Jefferson Classification:
  - Type I: Posterior arch alone, most common (67%), bilateral, nondisplaced, and stable
  - Type II: Anterior arch
  - Type III: Bilateral posterior arch with unilateral or bilateral anterior arch; includes classic Jefferson burst fracture defined by bilateral fractures of both anterior and posterior arches; usually high-velocity loading mechanism
  - Type IV: Lateral mass; usually medial portion of lateral mass and unilateral; low-velocity loading mechanism
  - Type V: Transverse fractures of anterior arch, usually horizontal and in elderly
- Forty percent to forty-four percent atlas fractures can occur in combination with axis (C2) or subaxial cervical spine fractures. C2 fractures are usually Type II odontoid or isthmus (hangman's fractures).
- Treatment depends upon integrity of the transverse ligament and the presence or absence of other cervical spine injuries.
  - Isolated atlas fractures with intact transverse ligament or associated with avulsion of bony medial tubercle have a good union rate with external immobilization (hard collar vs. halo).
  - Isolated atlas fractures with disruption of mid-portion or nonbony avulsion from medial tubercle cannot heal and are treated with surgical fixation.
- Imaging:
  - Radiographs include open-mouth odontoid, lateral, and flexion-extension views. CT preferred for complete evaluation. MRI highly sensitive for evaluation of transverse ligament rupture.
  - Displacement of C1 lateral mass over C2 facets suggests burst fracture of atlas.
  - C1 lateral mass overhang upon C2 facets combined on both sides >7 mm (rule of Spence) is suggestive of ruptured transverse ligament. However, rule of Spence can miss transverse ligament disruption from avulsion of medial tubercle.
  - The amount of C1 lateral mass overhang is important for surgical planning and fixation approach (transarticular vs. lateral mass).
  - Atlantodental interspace >3 mm in adults and >5 mm in children highly suggestive of ruptured transverse ligament.
  - Retropharyngeal soft tissue swelling at C1–C3 suggestive of anterior arch fracture.

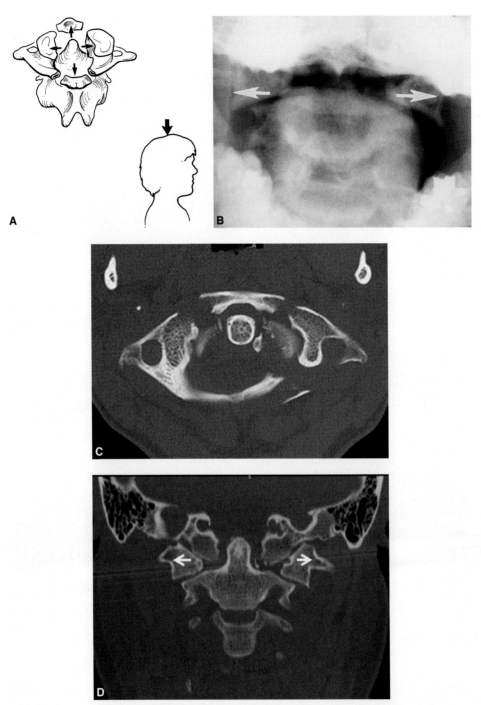

FIGURE 2-9. Jefferson fracture. **(A)** Mechanism of injury for Jefferson fractures. **(B)** Anteroposterior (AP) open-mouth odontoid view shows displacement of the lateral masses outward (*arrows*). The extent of injury is best appreciated on the axial **(C)** and coronal **(D)** computed tomography (CT) images.

(continued)

■ TRAUMA: CERVICAL SPINE—C1 FRACTURES *(Continued)*

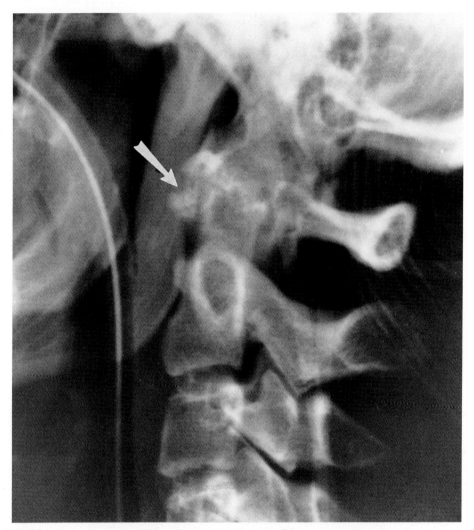

FIGURE 2-10. Hyperextension injury C1. Lateral radiograph of the upper cervical spine demonstrates an avulsion fracture of the anterior arch of C1 (*arrow*).

SUGGESTED READING

Dickman CA, Douglas RA, Sonntag VKH. Occipitocervical fusion: posterior stabilization of the craniovertebral junction and upper cervical spine. *BNI Q.* 1990;6(2):2–14.

Hadley MN, Dickman CA, Browner CM, et al. Acute traumatic atlas fractures: management and long term outcome. *Neurosurgery.* 1988;23(1):31–35.

Harris JH, Mirvis SE. *The Radiology of Acute Cervical Spine Trauma.* 3rd ed. Baltimore: Williams and Wilkins; 1996:340–366.

Jackson RS, Banit DM, Rhyne AL, et al. Upper cervical spine injuries. *J Am Acad Orthop Surg.* 2002;10:271–280.

Kakarla UK, Chang SW, Theodore N, et al. Atlas fractures. *Neurosurgery.* 2010; 66(suppl 3):A60–A67. doi:10.1227/01.NEU.0000366108.02499.8F.

Mead LB, Millhouse PW, Krystal J, et al. C1 fractures: a review of diagnoses, management options, and outcomes. *Curr Rev Musculoskelet Med.* 2016;9(3):255–262. doi:10.1007/s12178-016-9356-5.

■ TRAUMA: CERVICAL SPINE—ATLANTOAXIAL DISLOCATIONS

KEY FACTS

- ■ Traumatic dislocations of the atlantoaxial axis are rare.
- ■ The transverse ligament assists in maintaining the normal C1–C2 relationship. Subluxations may occur with conditions that affect the normal osseous or ligamentous integrity (rheumatoid arthritis, retropharyngeal infection, congenital abnormalities, and trauma).
- ■ Traumatic subluxation/dislocation may be anterior, posterior, or rotary in nature.
- ■ Normally, the space between the odontoid and lower anterior arch of C1 is 2 mm in adults and 4 mm in children.
- ■ Imaging can be accomplished with lateral and open-mouth odontoid views. However, thin-section CT with reformatting or three-dimensional reconstruction is most accurate for detection and classification.

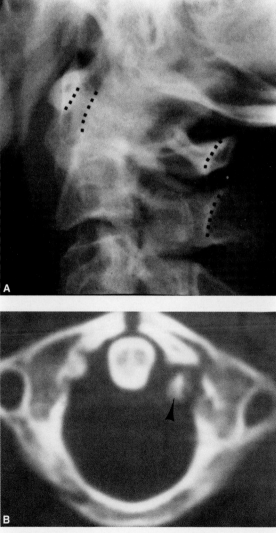

FIGURE 2-11. (A) Lateral radiograph of the upper cervical spine demonstrates anterior subluxation of C1 on C2. Odontoid-C1 and posterior arch relationships (*dotted lines*). **(B)** Axial computed tomography (CT) image demonstrates an anterior arch fracture (*arrow*) and avulsion (*arrowhead*) of the transverse ligament.

(continued)

▪ TRAUMA: CERVICAL SPINE—ATLANTOAXIAL DISLOCATIONS *(Continued)*

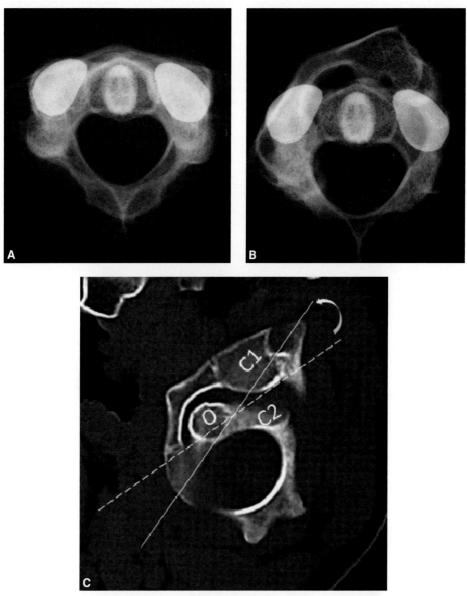

FIGURE 2-12. Rotary subluxation/fixation. Skeletal specimens with metal markers on the C2 facet demonstrate normal **(A)** and rotary fixation **(B)** of C1 on C2. Axial computed tomography (CT) **(C)** and three-dimensional surface rendered reconstructions, caudocranial **(D)** and craniocaudal **(E)** views show rotary fixation. The rotation of C1 (*solid line*) in relation to C2 (*broken line*) and (*O*) odontoid process in **(C)**.

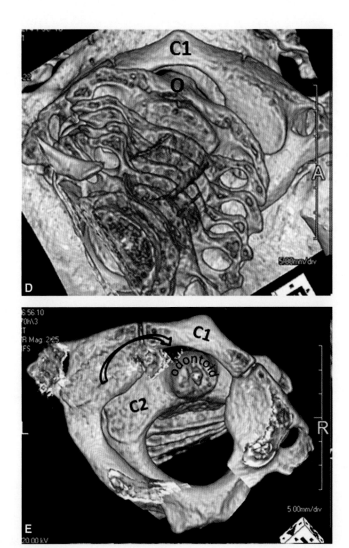

FIGURE 2-12. (*continued*)

SUGGESTED READING

Fielding JW, Hawkins RJ. Atlantoaxial rotary fixation. *J Bone Joint Surg.* 1977;57A:37–44.
Neumann U, Urbanski H, Riedel K. Posterior atlantoaxial dislocation without fracture of the odontoid. *J Bone Joint Surg.* 2003;85A:1343–1346.

▪ TRAUMA: CERVICAL SPINE—AXIS (C2)

KEY FACTS

- ▪ Fractures of C2 are common, accounting for 15% to 27% of cervical spine injuries (Table 2-4). Up to 25% have associated lower cervical fractures. Odontoid fractures account for 75% of cervical spine injuries in children.
- ▪ Ossification of the dens completes by 12 years of age; this must be considered in pediatric trauma cases.
- ▪ Fractures of the odontoid and neural arch (hangman's fracture) account for 80% of C2 fractures.
- ▪ Odontoid fractures are classified by location (Table 2-5). Fractures of the base of the odontoid (Type II) have a high incidence of nonunion (54% to 67%) and instability.
- ▪ Hangman's fractures (neural arch) are hyperextension injuries.
- ▪ Posterior C1–C2 fixation methods have a high fusion rate.
- ▪ Anterior odontoid screw placement is contraindicated in cases of chronic fracture, disruption of transverse ligament, or angulated displacement of dens.

Table 2-4 AXIS (C2) FRACTURES

Location	Incidence (%)
Odontoid	41
Hangman's	38
Anterior inferior body	13
Lamina, spinous process	8

Table 2-5 ODONTOID FRACTURE CLASSIFICATION

Type	Incidence (%)	Complications
I, odontoid tip	8	None
II, odontoid base	59	Nonunion 54%–67%
		Neurologic 20%
III, below odontoid	33	Nonunion in 40% if displaced >5 mm

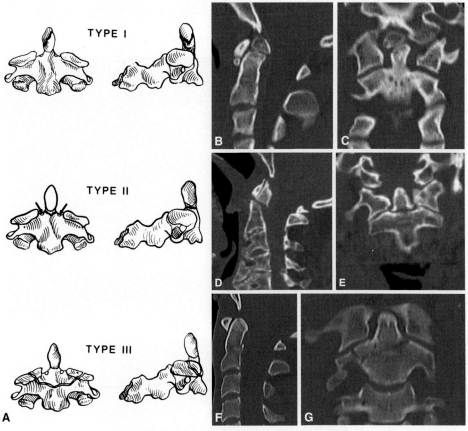

FIGURE 2-13. (A) Odontoid fracture classification: Type I—odontoid tip; Type II—odontoid base, above accessory ligament and vascular supply (*arrows*); and Type III—extend into body below vascular supply. Sagittal and coronal computed tomography (CT) images; **(B, C)** Type I (chronic) fracture; **(D, E)** Type II fracture with posterior subluxation of C1 and displacement of the odontoid process; and **(F, G)** Type III fracture.

(continued)

■ TRAUMA: CERVICAL SPINE—AXIS (C2) *(Continued)*

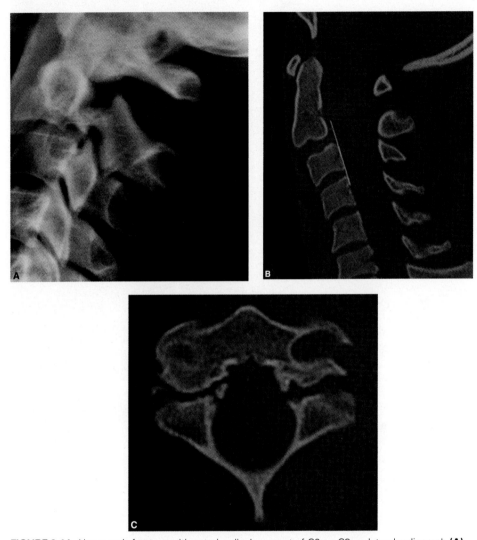

FIGURE 2-14. Hangman's fracture with anterior displacement of C2 on C3 on lateral radiograph **(A)** and sagittal computed tomography (CT) image **(B)**. Fracture of bilateral C2 pars on axial CT **(C)**.

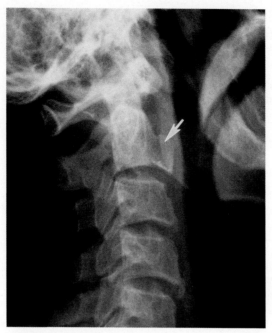

FIGURE 2-15. Anterior inferior body fracture of C2 (*arrow*).

SUGGESTED READING

Berquist TH. *Imaging of Orthopedic Trauma*. 2nd ed. New York: Raven Press; 1992:93–206.
Jackson RS, Banit DM, Rhyne AL, et al. Upper cervical spine injuries. *J Acad Orthop Surg*. 2002;10:271–280.
Sim HB, Lee JW, Park JT, et al. Biomechanical evaluations of various C1–C2 posterior fixation techniques. *Spine*. 2011;36:E401–E407.

■ TRAUMA: CERVICAL SPINE—LOWER CERVICAL SPINE: VERTEBRAL ARCH FRACTURES

KEY FACTS

■ Vertebral arch fractures are most frequently the result of hyperextension or lateral flexion injuries. Common sites and incidences in our experience are as follows:

Lamina	28%
Pedicle	25%
Spinous process	22%
Pillar	16%
Facets	9%
Transverse process	2%

■ Laminar fractures are commonly associated with spinous process fractures. The majority occur from C5–C7.
■ Pedicle fractures may occur at C2 (hangman's) or in the lower cervical spine. If nondisplaced, they may be easily overlooked on routine radiographs.
■ Spinous process fractures are most common from C5–T1. Injury may be the result of direct trauma, hyperextension, or hyperflexion.
■ Pillar fractures without displacement may be overlooked on radiographs. They are most common at C6.
■ Facet fractures are the result of flexion–rotation or hyperflexion injuries.
■ Transverse process fractures occur with direct trauma or lateral flexion, and are managed conservatively.
■ In general, isolated nondisplaced posterior element fractures have a high spontaneous union rate and are managed conservatively with bracing unless there is neurologic compromise.
■ Displaced fractures of the facet or pedicle are treated with surgical fixation; however, conservative treatment may be attempted.
■ Transverse process fractures are stable; however, it is important to assess for potential vertebral artery injury secondary to transverse foramen compromise (40% incidence).

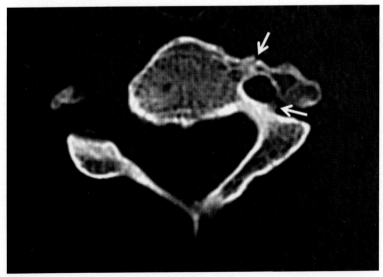

FIGURE 2-16. Computed tomography (CT) image of a remote fracture of the left transverse process through the foramen transversarium (*arrows*).

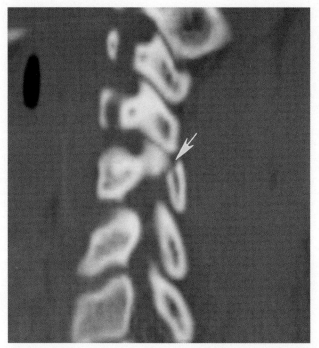

FIGURE 2-17. Sagittal computed tomography (CT) image of a C5 facet fracture (*arrow*).

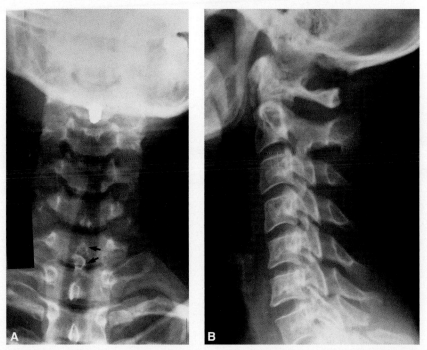

FIGURE 2-18. Spinous process fracture at C7 (Clay shoveler's fracture). **(A)** Anteroposterior (AP) view shows a double spinous process (*arrows*). This is a helpful sign because the lower cervical spine is often difficult to visualize on the lateral view. **(B)** Lateral view shows the C7 spinous process fracture clearly in this case.

(continued)

■ **TRAUMA: CERVICAL SPINE—LOWER CERVICAL SPINE: VERTEBRAL ARCH FRACTURES** *(Continued)*

SUGGESTED READING

Berquist TH. Imaging of adult cervical spine trauma. *Radiographics.* 1988;8:667–694.

Harris JH, Mirvis SE. *The Radiology of Acute Cervical Spine Trauma.* 3rd ed. Baltimore: Williams and Wilkins; 1996:408–419.

Inamasu J, Guiot BH. Vertebral artery injury after blunt cervical trauma: an update. *Surg Neurol.* 2006;65:238–245, discussion 245–246.

Kotani Y, Abumi K, Ito M, et al. Cervical spine injuries associated with lateral mass and facet joint fractures: new classification and surgical treatment with pedicle screw fixation. *Eur Spine J.* 2005;14:69–77.

Lee SH, Sung JK. Unilateral lateral mass-facet fractures with rotational instability: new classification and a review of 39 cases treated conservatively and with single segment anterior fusion. *J Trauma.* 2009;66:758–767.

Torg JS, Sennett B, Vegso JJ, et al. Axial loading injuries to the middle cervical spine segment. An analysis and classification of twenty-five cases. *Am J Sports Med.* 1991;19:6–20.

■ TRAUMA: CERVICAL SPINE—LOWER CERVICAL SPINE: VERTEBRAL BODY FRACTURES

KEY FACTS

- More than 31% of cervical spine injuries involve the vertebral body. Seventy-five percent of fractures occur from C5–C7.
- Flexion teardop fractures (avulsion injuries of inferior vertebral body) may have a benign appearance on plain radiographs; however, they have a high rate of spinal cord injury and are unstable injuries.
- Burst fractures usually occur in the lower cervical spine and have a high incidence of neurologic injury; however, they may be managed conservatively with bracing if there is no ligamentous disruption.
- Ligamentous disruption can be hidden by spontaneous reduction in plain radiographs taken in the supine position.
- Table 2-6 summarizes vertebral body fractures.

Table 2-6   VERTEBRAL BODY FRACTURES

Type	Mechanism of Injury	Comments
Chip fractures	Hyperextension (anterior inferior body) Hyperflexion (anterior superior body)	Usually stable
Teardrop fractures	Hyperflexion neurologic injury	Quadriplegia in 87%
	Hyperextension	C2 most common
Compression fracture	Flexion–compression	Look for posterior soft tissue injuries
Lateral wedge, uncinate process	Asymmetric vertical compression	
Burst fractures	Vertical compression	CT to assess spinal canal

CT, computed tomography.

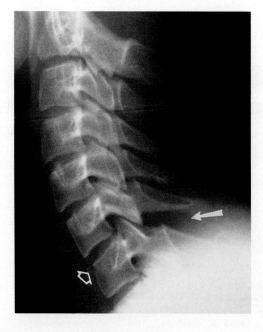

FIGURE 2-19. Flexion–compression injury with compression of C7 and an anterior chip fracture (*open arrow*). There is widening of the interspinous distance (*arrow*) indicating posterior ligament injury and instability.

(continued)

■ TRAUMA: CERVICAL SPINE—LOWER CERVICAL SPINE: VERTEBRAL BODY FRACTURES *(Continued)*

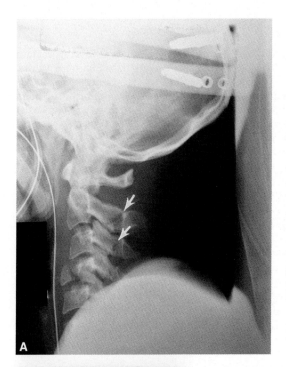
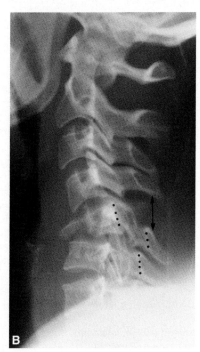
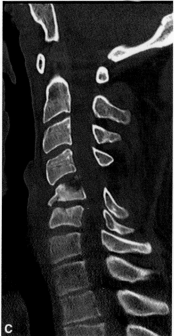
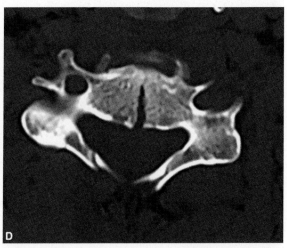

FIGURE 2-20. Teardrop fractures. **(A)** Hyperextension teardrop of C4. Note the posterior arch fractures of C2 and C3 (*arrows*) indicating the mechanism of injury. **(B)** Hyperflexion teardrop fracture of C5 with compromise of the spinal canal (*dotted lines*) and posterior ligament tears (*double arrow*)—finding best seen on sagittal computed tomography (CT) image **(C)**. Axial CT **(D)** shows the sagittal fracture commonly seen with flexion teardrop fracture.

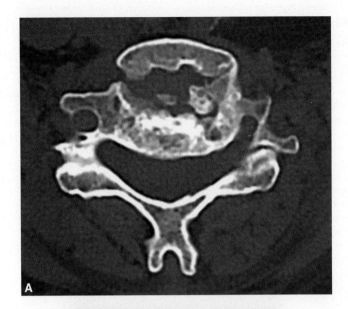

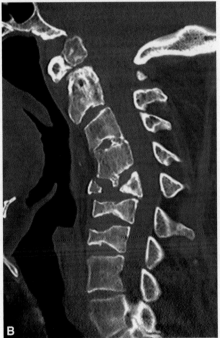

FIGURE 2-21. Axial **(A)** and sagittal **(B)** computed tomography (CT) images show chronic C5 vertebral body burst fracture with retropulsion which mildly narrows the spinal canal. Also noted are chronic compression deformities of C6 and C7 vertebral bodies and a nonunited Type II odontoid fracture.

SUGGESTED READING

Berquist TH. *Imaging of Orthopedic Trauma*. 2nd ed. New York: Raven Press; 1992:93–206.

Dvorak MF, Fisher CG, Fehlings MG, et al. The surgical approach to subaxial cervical spine injuries: an evidence-based algorithm based on the SLIC classification system. *Spine*. 2007;32:2620–2629.

Kwon BK, Vaccaro AR, Grauer JN, et al. Subaxial cervical spine trauma. *J Am Acad Orthop Surg*. 2006;14:78–89.

Lauweryns P. Role of conservative treatment of cervical spine injuries. *Eur Spine J*. 2010;19(suppl 1):S23–S26.

Sanchez B, Waxmann K, Jones T, et al. Cervical spine clearance in blunt trauma: evaluation of a computed tomography-based protocol. *J Trauma*. 2005;59:179–183.

■ TRAUMA: CERVICAL SPINE—LOWER CERVICAL SPINE: SUBLUXATION, FRACTURE/DISLOCATION

KEY FACTS

- Most significant ligament injuries involve the posterior column. Seventy-three percent occur at the C5–C7 levels. Anterior ligament injuries are most common at C2–C4 and C6–C7. Ligament injuries may occur alone or with fractures.
- The spectrum of injuries may be subtle, without obvious abnormality and normal bony alignment, or injuries may be grossly obvious, such as bilateral locked facets.
- Unilateral facet locking or perching may present with subtle radiographic findings. This flexion-rotation injury accounts for 12% of cervical injuries. Reformatted CT imaging is often required for detection and complete evaluation of these injuries.
- Flexion–distraction injuries may present with acute spinal cord injury, radiculopathy, or both.
- Magnetic resonance (MR) should be performed in stable patients who have suspected ligamentous injury and inconclusive findings on CT.
- Ligamentous injury (anterior longitudinal ligament [ALL] and posterior longitudinal ligament [PLL]) is an unstable injury, and open reduction/internal fixation is indicated.

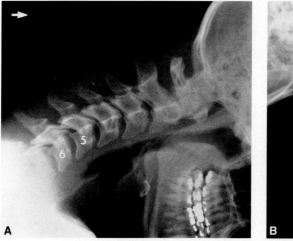 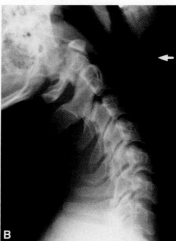

FIGURE 2-22. Flexion–distraction injury with posterior ligament tear at C5–C6. Flexion **(A)** and extension **(B)** views show subluxation and widening of the interspinous distance and facet joints with flexion that reduces with extension. Treatment—posterior fusion.

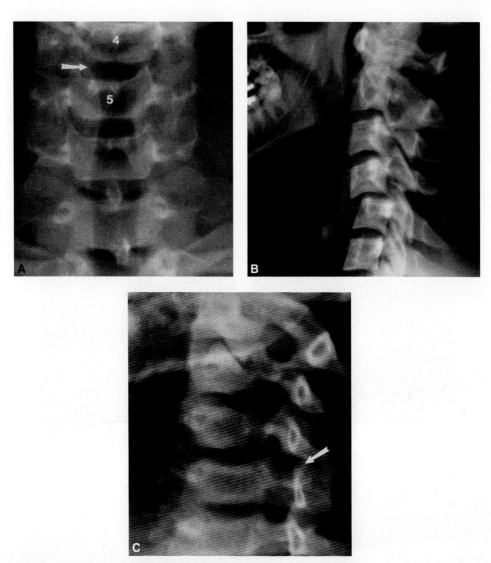

FIGURE 2-23. Unilateral locked facet. **(A)** Anteroposterior (AP) radiograph shows disc space asymmetry (*arrow*) at C4–C5 and rotation of the spinous process. **(B)** Lateral view shows subluxation, and the C4 facets form the "bow-tie" sign. **(C)** Oblique view shows the facet overlap (*arrow*).

(continued)

■ TRAUMA: CERVICAL SPINE—LOWER CERVICAL SPINE: SUBLUXATION, FRACTURE/DISLOCATION *(Continued)*

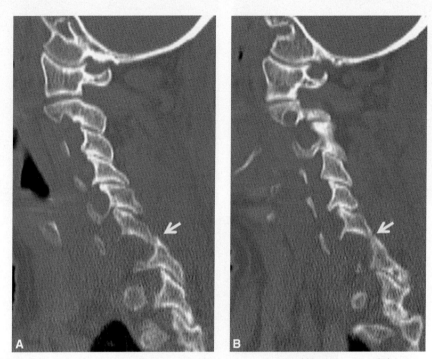

FIGURE 2-24. Sagittal computed tomography (CT) images of locked **(A)** and perched **(B)** facets *(arrow)*.

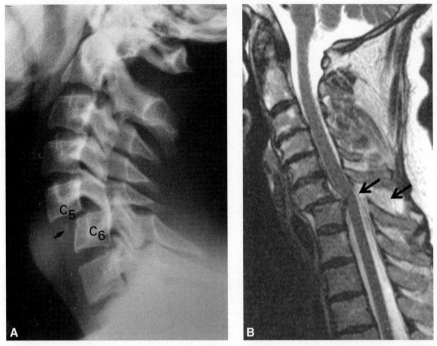

FIGURE 2-25. Lateral radiograph **(A)** demonstrates bilateral locked facets at C5–C6 with a chip fracture (*arrow*) of C6. Subluxation with bilateral locked facets must be equal or greater than 50%. Sagittal T2 magnetic resonance imaging (MRI) **(B)** in another patient with bilateral facet dislocation demonstrates spinal cord impingement, ligamentum flavum, and interspinous ligament injury (*black arrows*) with resultant fanning of the C6 and C7 spinous processes. Quadriplegia occurs in 72% of patients with this injury.

SUGGESTED READING

Brodke DS, Anderson PA, Newell DW, et al. Comparison of anterior and posterior approaches in cervical spinal cord injuries. *J Spinal Disord Tech.* 2003;16:229–235.

Harris JH, Mirvis SE. *The Radiology of Acute Cervical Spine Trauma.* 3rd ed. Baltimore: Williams and Wilkins; 1996:270–276, 291–304.

Scher AT. Anterior cervical subluxation: an unstable position. *Am J Roentgenol.* 1979;133:275–280.

Vaccaro AR, Hulbert RJ, Patel AA, et al. The subaxial cervical spine injury classification system: a novel approach to recognize the importance of morphology, neurology, and integrity of the disco-ligamentous complex. *Spine.* 2007;32:2365–2374.

Vaccaro AR, Nachwalter RS. Is magnetic resonance imaging indicated before reduction of a unilateral cervical facet dislocation? *Spine.* 2002;27:117–118.

▪ TRAUMA: THORACOLUMBAR SPINE—BASIC CONCEPTS

KEY FACTS

▪ Because of differences in range of motion, transition in the facet joints, and other anatomic factors, the thoracolumbar junction is most susceptible to injury (66% of injuries occur between T12 and L2).
▪ Mechanism of injury
  ● Hyperflexion (most common)
  ● Flexion–compression
  ● Flexion–distraction
  ● Flexion–rotation
  ● Lateral flexion
  ● Vertical compression
  ● Hyperextension
  ● Shearing/rotation forces
▪ Complete evaluation of bone and soft tissue structures is essential to assess stability.
▪ Thoracolumbar spine injuries are classified on the basis of radiographic and CT features.
▪ Instability: Three-column approach of Denis is most useful. If two columns (Fig. 2-26) are involved, the injury is unstable.
▪ Image evaluation: Routine radiographs remain the primary screening tool for thoracolumbar fractures. However, CT is almost 100% sensitive for fracture detection compared with 32% for radiographs. CT is also useful to fully evaluate fragment position and spinal canal compromise. MRI is useful in selected cases to evaluate the cord, nerve roots, and soft tissue injuries. Unsuspected posterior ligament injuries are evident on MRI, when not seen on radiographs or CT.
▪ Burst fractures (2-column injuries) are treated conservatively unless there is neural element compromise.
▪ Injury to the posterior ligamentous complex (PLC) is an unstable injury and requires surgical fixation in the majority of cases.
▪ The TLICS Score (Thoracolumbar Injury Classification and Severity Score) is an evidence-based method of determining which patients with TL injuries will benefit from surgery.

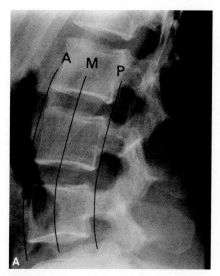 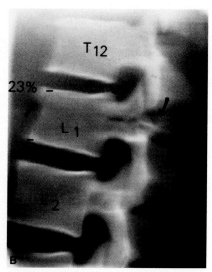

FIGURE 2-26. (A) Lateral radiographs demonstrate the three columns proposed by Denis. Anterior—anterior longitudinal ligament, anterior disc, and vertebral body. Middle—posterior disc, body, and posterior longitudinal ligament. Posterior—facet joints, ligamentum flavum, interspinous, and supraspinous ligaments. **(B)** Lateral radiograph shows mild compression of L1 (*arrow*) with splitting of the neural arch (*curved arrow*) caused by hyperflexion distraction injury. Unstable with three-column involvement.

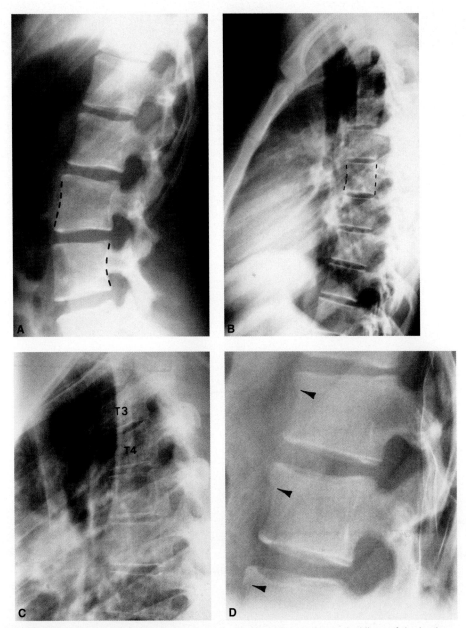

FIGURE 2-27. Anterior wedge fractures. Normal anterior and posterior cortical lines of the lumbar
(A) and thoracic **(B)** vertebral bodies. The lumbar vertebral body is concave anteriorly and posteriorly,
and the thoracic vertebral body is concave anteriorly and straight posteriorly. Lateral radiographs
of mild anterior wedge fractures of T3 and T4 **(C)** and T12–L2 **(D)**. Note the anterior buckling of the
cortex in **(D)** (*arrowheads*).

(continued)

■ TRAUMA: THORACOLUMBAR SPINE—BASIC CONCEPTS *(Continued)*

SUGGESTED READING

Denis F. The three-column spine and its significance in classification of thoraco-lumbar spinal injuries. *Spine.* 1983;8:817–831.

Lee HM, Kim HS, Suk KS, et al. Reliability of magnetic resonance imaging in detecting posterior ligament complex injuries in thoracolumbar spinal fractures. *Spine.* 2000;25:2079–2084.

Lee JY, Vaccaro AR, Lim MR, et al. Thoracolumbar Injury Classification and Severity Score: a new paradigm for the treatment of thoracolumbar spine trauma. *J Orthop Sci.* 2005;10:671–675.

Singh K, Vaccaro AR, Eichenbaum MD, et al. The surgical management of thoracolumbar injuries. *J Spinal Cord Med.* 2004;27:95–101.

Wintermark M, Moushine E, Theumann N, et al. Thoracolumbar spine fractures in patients who have sustained severe trauma: depiction with multi-detector row CT. *Radiology.* 2003;227:681–689.

■ TRAUMA: THORACOLUMBAR SPINE—HYPERFLEXION INJURIES

KEY FACTS

- Hyperflexion injuries are most common in the thoracolumbar spine.
- The axis of force centers in the middle of the intervertebral disc. Therefore, the appearance of injury may vary at different levels of the spine. The discs are larger in the lower thoracic and lumbar spine, so endplate fractures are more common.
- Types of fracture:
    - Anterior wedge fracture: Almost always visible on anteroposterior (AP) and lateral radiographs. Evaluate degree of compression and disc space narrowing (poorer prognosis) on the lateral view and paraspinal soft tissue swelling on the AP view.
    - Lateral wedge fracture: Caused by lateral compression. Best seen on AP radiograph. Typically a stable lesion.
    - Flexion–distraction injury: The majority are located at the thoracolumbar junction. Neurologic complications occur in 70%. When the posterior arch and ligaments are disrupted, the lesion is unstable. Radiographs may show minimal compression on the lateral view. The posterior arch injury may be seen more easily in the AP view. Multiplanar CT is important for complete assessment. Seat-belt injuries occur less frequently today, but present with the pattern described earlier. Neurologic injury occurs in 4%. Abdominal injuries are common, occurring in 80% of patients.
- It is important to rule out vascular injury in the initial trauma assessment in flexion–distraction injury.

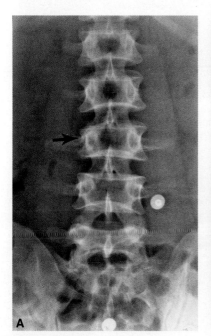 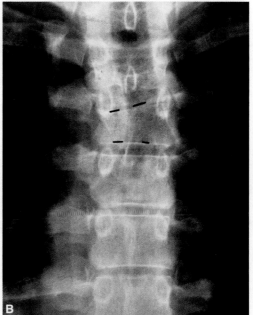

FIGURE 2-28. Lateral wedge fractures. Asymmetric compression of L3 **(A)** (*arrow*) and T5 **(B)** (*broken lines*).

(continued)

■ TRAUMA: THORACOLUMBAR SPINE—HYPERFLEXION INJURIES *(Continued)*

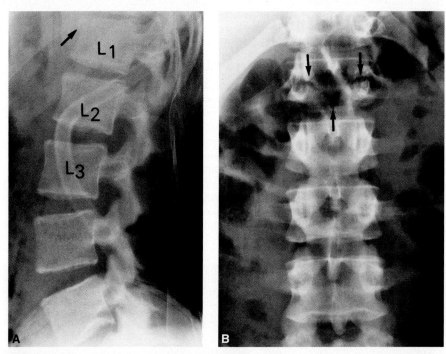

FIGURE 2-29. (A) Lateral radiograph demonstrates a Chance fracture (flexion–distraction injury). There is only mild compression (*arrow*) of L1. **(B)** Anteroposterior (AP) radiograph clearly demonstrates the fracture through the posterior elements (*arrows*).

SUGGESTED READING

Holdsworth F. Fractures, dislocations, and fracture-dislocations of the spine. *J Bone Joint Surg Am.* 1970; 52:1534–1551.

Rogers LF. The roentgenographic appearance of transverse or Chance fractures of the spine: the seat belt fracture. *Am J Roentgenol.* 1971;111:844–849.

Vialle LR, Vialle E. Thoracic spine fractures. *Injury.* 2005;36(suppl 2):B65–B72.

Wood KB, Khanne G, Vaccaro AR, et al. Assessment of two thoracolumbar fracture classification systems used by multiple surgeons. *J Bone Joint Surg.* 2005;87A:1423–1429.

■ TRAUMA: THORACOLUMBAR SPINE—FLEXION–ROTATION INJURIES

KEY FACTS

■ Flexion–rotation injuries are relatively uncommon (10% of thoracolumbar injuries), but among the most unstable.

■ The injury typically occurs at the thoracolumbar junction. Neurologic injury occurs in 70%.

■ Radiographic features may be subtle or similar to those described with this injury in the cervical spine. CT is essential to confirm the extent of injury and to plan reduction.

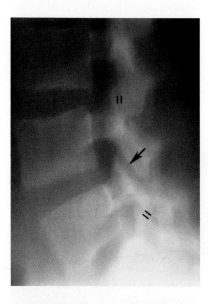

FIGURE 2-30. Lateral radiograph demonstrates separation of the L4–L5 facet joint (*arrow*) secondary to a flexion–rotation injury.

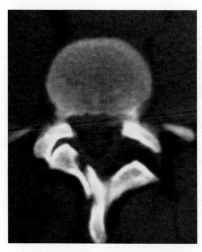

FIGURE 2-31. Computed tomography (CT) image demonstrates facet separation and neural arch fractures.

SUGGESTED READING

Manaster BJ, Osborne AG. CT patterns of facet dislocation at the thoracolumbar junction. *Am J Roentgenol.* 1987;148:335–340.

Pizones J, Izquierdo E, Alvarez P, et al. Impact of magnetic resonance imaging on decision making for thoracolumbar traumatic fracture diagnosis and treatment. *Eur Spine J.* 2011;20(suppl 3):390–396.

Saboe LA, Reid DC, Davis LA, et al. Spine trauma and associated injuries. *J Trauma.* 1991;31:43–48.

■ TRAUMA: THORACOLUMBAR SPINE—VERTICAL COMPRESSION INJURIES

KEY FACTS

- ■ The injury accounts for 1.5% of spinal injuries and is most common from T12–L2.
- ■ Vertical compression injuries result in axial compression with burst fractures.
- ■ Disc herniation into vertebral endplates and displaced fragments into the spinal canal occur to varying degrees.
- ■ Burst fractures can be identified on AP and lateral radiographs. There is increased interpedicular distance and paraspinal swelling on AP radiographs. In the lateral view, the vertebral body is compressed to a variable degree, and the posterior cortical line is convex instead of concave. CT is essential to assess the spinal canal and fragment position. The entire spine should be studied because separate injuries occur in 40%.
- ■ MRI may demonstrate posterior ligament injury not evident on CT or radiographs.
- ■ Anterior column injuries are stable and are usually managed conservatively.
- ■ Anterior and middle column injuries (burst fractures) are stable unless there is disruption of the PLC or neural element compromise.

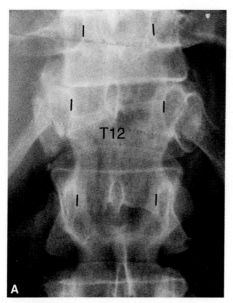 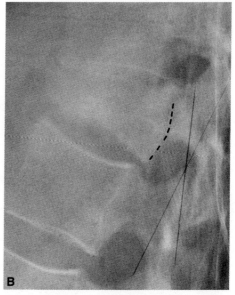

FIGURE 2-32. T12 burst fracture. **(A)** Anteroposterior (AP) radiograph demonstrates widening of the interpedicular distance (*lines* mark pedicles T11 to L1). **(B)** Lateral radiograph shows vertebral compression and posterior cortical convexity (*broken lines*).

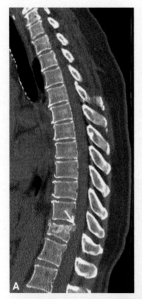
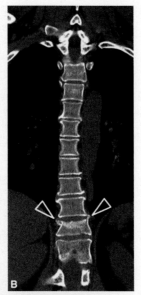

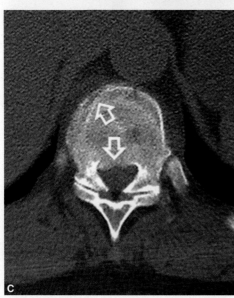

FIGURE 2-33. Lower thoracic burst fracture. Sagittal **(A)** and coronal **(B)** computed tomography (CT) images demonstrate vertebral compression with outward displacement of fragments on the coronal image (*arrowheads*) and posterior displaced fragments on the sagittal image (*arrow*). **(C)** Axial image demonstrates displaced anterior fragments and posterior extension into the spinal canal (*open arrow*).

SUGGESTED READING

Atlas SW, Regenbogen V, Rogers LF, et al. The radiographic characterization of burst fractures of the spine. *Am J Roentgenol.* 1986;147:575–582.

Ballock RT, Mackersie R, Abitbol JJ, et al. Can burst fractures be predicted from plain radiographs? *J Bone Joint Surg.* 1992:147–150.

Petersilge CA, Pathria MN, Emery SE, et al. Thoracolumbar burst fractures: evaluation with MR imaging. *Radiology.* 1995;194:49–54.

Qaiyum M, Tyrrell PN, McCall IW, et al. MRI detection of unsuspected vertebral injury in acute spinal trauma: incidence and significance. *Skeletal Radiol.* 2001;30:299–304.

Saboe LA, Reid DC, Davis LA, et al. Spine trauma and associated injuries. *J Trauma.* 1991;31:43–48.

■ TRAUMA: THORACOLUMBAR SPINE—HYPEREXTENSION INJURIES

KEY FACTS

■ Hyperextension injuries in the thoracolumbar spine are rare.

■ Posterior arch fractures are a hallmark of this injury, but the strong, broad anterior longitudinal ligament is difficult to disrupt in the lumbar spine compared with the cervical spine.

■ Features of hyperextension injuries are similar to those in the cervical spine and best demonstrated on lateral radiographs. CT should be performed with coronal and sagittal reformatting for complete evaluation.

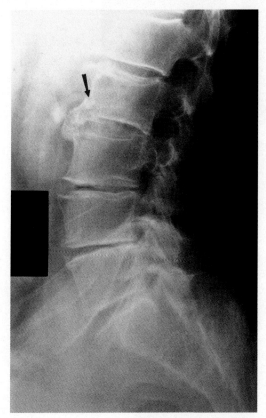

FIGURE 2-34. Lateral radiograph demonstrates an anterior inferior fracture of L2 (*arrow*) caused by hyperextension injury.

SUGGESTED READING

Berquist TH. *Imaging of Orthopedic Trauma.* 2nd ed. New York: Raven Press; 1992:93–206.
Roaf A. A study of the mechanism of spinal injuries. *J Bone Joint Surg.* 1960;42B:810–823.

■ TRAUMA: THORACOLUMBAR SPINE—SHEARING INJURIES

KEY FACTS

- ■ Shearing forces may cause dislocation (usually anterior displacement of the vertebra onto the vertebra below) in an AP or transverse direction.
- ■ This injury is most common in the thoracic spine.
- ■ Lesions usually are unstable, with significant cord injury.
- ■ Although routine radiographs (AP and lateral) are adequate for detection, CT scan, and in selected patients MRI, is essential for planning spinal instrumentation.

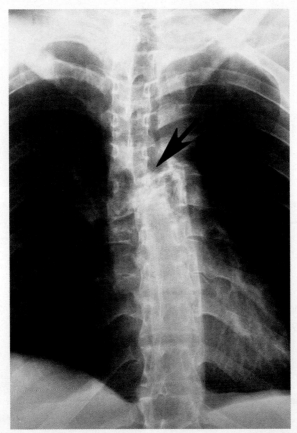

FIGURE 2-35. Anteroposterior (AP) radiograph of a transverse shearing fracture dislocation (*arrow*) of the thoracic spine.

(continued)

■ TRAUMA: THORACOLUMBAR SPINE—SHEARING INJURIES *(Continued)*

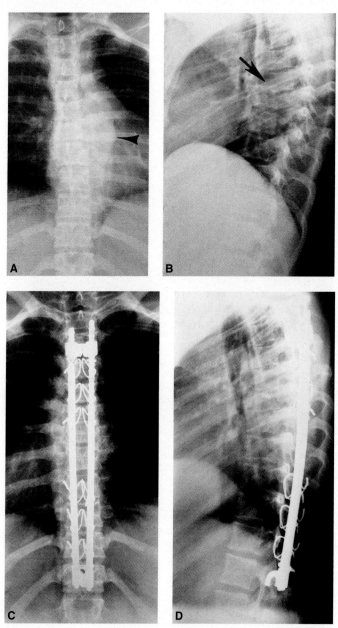

FIGURE 2-36. Posterior dislocation. **(A)** Anteroposterior (AP) radiograph demonstrates prominent paraspinal soft tissue swelling *(arrowhead)*. **(B)** Lateral radiograph shows posterior dislocation *(arrow)* in the mid-thoracic spine. AP **(C)** and lateral **(D)** radiographs after Harrington rod instrumentation with sublaminar wire augmentation.

SUGGESTED READING

Berquist TH. *Imaging Atlas of Orthopedic Appliances and Prostheses.* New York: Raven Press; 1995:109–215.
Holdsworth F. Fracture and fracture-dislocations of the spine. *J Bone Joint Surg.* 1970;52A:1534–1551.

■ TRAUMA: THORACOLUMBAR SPINE—MINOR FRACTURES

KEY FACTS

- Minor fractures include isolated neural arch fractures, spinous process fractures, facet fractures, and transverse process fractures.
- Spinous process fractures occur most frequently in the upper thoracic spine and are rare in the lumbar spine.
- Transverse process fractures are usually the result of direct trauma. They are not significant in and of themselves, but may be associated with retroperitoneal hematoma or renal injury.

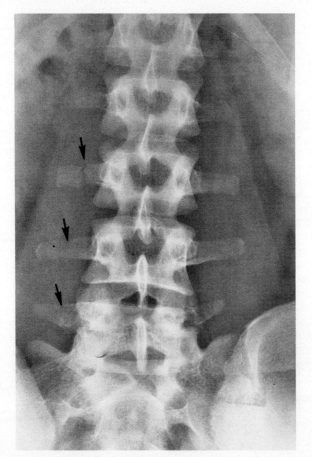

FIGURE 2-37. Anteroposterior (AP) radiograph of the lumbar spine demonstrates multiple transverse process fractures (*arrows*).

SUGGESTED READING

Berquist TH. *Imaging of Orthopedic Trauma.* 2nd ed. New York: Raven Press; 1992:93–206.

■ SPONDYLOLYSIS/SPONDYLOLISTHESIS

KEY FACTS

■ Spondylolisthesis is anterior subluxation of a vertebral body on the vertebral body below it. Wiltse classified this disorder into five categories:
  ● Congenital
  ● Fractures (stress, elongation of the pars, and acute fracture)
  ● Degenerative
  ● Trauma to neural arch other than the pars
  ● Pathologic bone disease
Repetitive trauma and degenerative disease are the most common. Patients present with chronic or intermittent low back pain.

■ Spondylolysis is a pars interarticularis defect that occurs in 2.3% to 7.2% of patients; 67% occur at L5 and 10% at L4. The condition is bilateral in 74%. The cause is unclear, but both inheritance and acquired risk factors are implicated. The condition increases with age and is more common in whites than African Americans.

■ Spondylolisthesis caused by bilateral pars defects is most common at L5–S1. Degenerative spondylolisthesis is most common at L4–L5.

■ There is frequent association of L5 hypoplasia with bilateral spondylolysis. The hypoplastic L5 vertebral body has smaller AP diameter than the L4 vertebral body with more pronounced posterior wedging. L5 hypoplasia and posterior wedging with bilateral spondylolysis lead to false sense of anterior vertebral slipping—pseudospondylolisthesis. True spondylolisthesis should be diagnosed only if both the anterior and posterior margins of the vertebral body are displaced forward.

■ Treatment depends on symptoms and the degree of subluxation and instability. Surgical intervention is most commonly required for higher grades of subluxation.

■ Spondylolisthesis without central stenosis usually presents with radiculopathy secondary to neural foramen compromise, especially in cases with concomitant disc degeneration.

■ Image features
  ● Radiographic features: Subluxation is easily appreciated on lateral radiographs. Flexion and extension studies are useful to evaluate stability. Oblique views may be necessary to define pars defects.
  ● CT: Axial and coronal and sagittal reformatted CT images are useful for defining pars defects and the extent of fragmentation and neuroforaminal evaluation.
  ● Radionuclide scans: Single-photon emission CT is useful for identification of stress injuries.
  ● MRI: Sagittal and axial MR images are useful for neural involvement. Bone changes are more easily assessed with CT, although reactive marrow changes, edema, and synovitis are best appreciated with fat-saturated T2-weighted MR images.

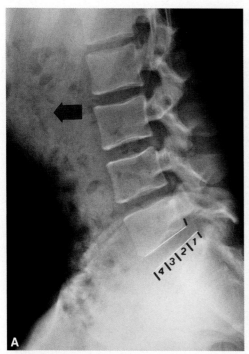
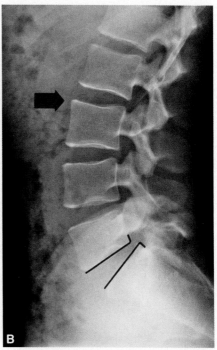

FIGURE 2-38. Flexion **(A)** and extension **(B)** radiographs demonstrate anterior subluxation of L5 on S1. The degree of subluxation is determined by dividing the lower vertebral endplate into four equal segments. Subluxation is graded 1 to 4. In this case, it is Grade 1 and reduces slightly with extension.

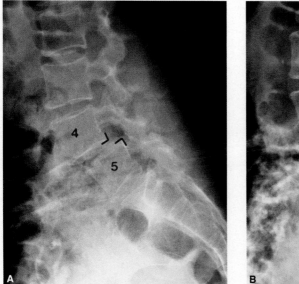
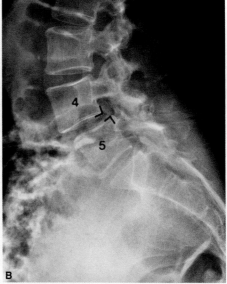

FIGURE 2-39. Flexion **(A)** and extension **(B)** radiographs of Grades 1 to 2 spondylolisthesis that increases with flexion. At this level, the subluxation is most commonly the result of facet degenerative disease.

(continued)

■ SPONDYLOLYSIS/SPONDYLOLISTHESIS *(Continued)*

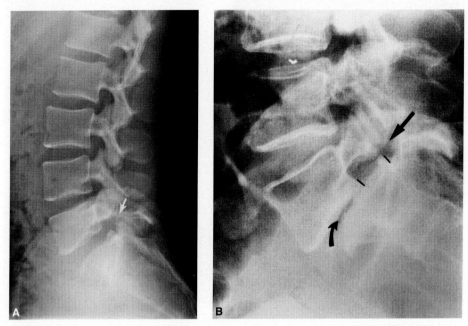

FIGURE 2-40. (A) Lateral radiograph demonstrates a pars defect at L5 *(arrow)* with slight subluxation of L5 on S1. **(B)** Lateral radiograph shows Grades 2 to 3 subluxation caused by a pars defect *(arrow)*. There is associated degenerative disc disease *(curved arrow)*.

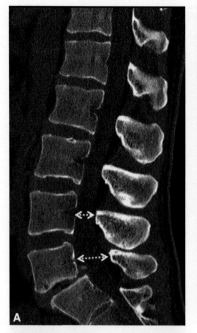

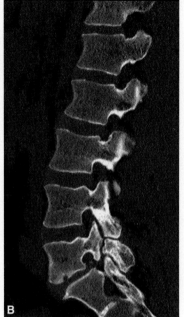

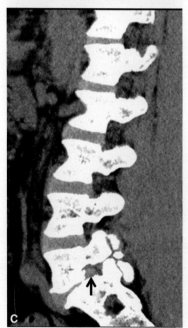

FIGURE 2-41. Spondylolysis with spondylolisthesis. Sagittal computed tomography (CT) images, **(A)** Grade 1 anterolisthesis of L5 vertebral body with anteroposterior (AP) widening of the spinal canal (*dotted arrows*) at L5 due to separation of the anterior and posterior elements by spondolysis. On the contrary, spondylolisthesis associated with facet osteoarthritis will cause spinal canal narrowing. **(B, C)** L5 pars defects. Note severe narrowing of L5 neural foramina is best appreciated on soft tissue windows (*black arrow* in **C**) and caused by combination of anterolisthesis, disc bulge, and height loss.

(continued)

■ SPONDYLOLYSIS/SPONDYLOLISTHESIS *(Continued)*

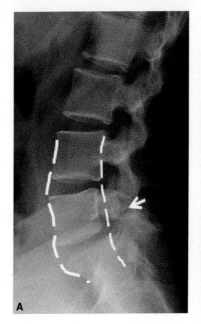

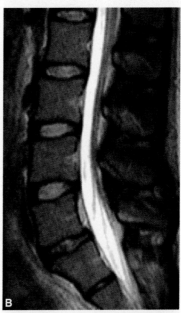

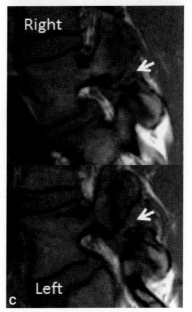

FIGURE 2-42. Pseudospondylolisthesis with spondylosis. Lateral radiograph **(A)** and midline sagittal T2 **(B)** magnetic resonance (MR) demonstrate L5 vertebral body hypoplasia (small anteroposterior [AP] diameter of L5 compared with L4 body) and posterior wedging creating a false sense of anterior slippage of L5 vertebral body (*broken lines* show step-off of the posterior spinal line with normally aligned anterior spinal line). **(C)** The parasagittal T1 MR shows bilateral pars defects (*arrow*). Again note the AP widening of spinal canal at L5.

SUGGESTED READING

Kalichman L, Cole R, Kim DH, et al. Spinal stenosis prevalence and association with symptoms: the Framingham Study. *Spine J.* 2009;9(7):545–550.

Matsunaga S, Sakou T, Morizono Y, et al. Natural history of degenerative spondylolisthesis. Pathogenesis and natural course of the slippage. *Spine.* 1990;15(11):1204–1210.

McTimoney CA, Micheli LJ. Current evaluation and management of spondylosis and spondylolisthesis. *Curr Sports Med Rep.* 2003;2:41–46.

Niggemann P, Kuchta J, Grosskurth D, et al. Spondylolysis and isthmic spondylolisthesis: impact of vertebral hypoplasia on the use of the Meyerding classification. *Br J Radiol.* 2012;85(1012):358–362.

Wiltse LL, Neuman DH, MacNab I. Classification of spondylosis and spondylolisthesis. *Clin Orthop.* 1976;117:23–29.

■ SCOLIOSIS: BASIC CONCEPTS

KEY FACTS

■ Scoliosis may be idiopathic, congenital, or acquired (Table 2-7).

■ Idiopathic scoliosis may be infantile (≤3 years), juvenile (3 years to puberty), or adolescent (puberty and older).

Infantile	Occurs in males more than in females
	Left thoracic curve most common
	Curves less than 30 degrees may resolve
Juvenile	Occurs in females more than in males
	Right thoracic curve most common
	Progression of curves more common than in infantile type
Adolescent	Frequently detected on school physical examination
	Occurs in females more than in males
	Curves tend to progress during growth spurts
	Curves less than 30 degrees tend not to progress at skeletal maturity

■ Congenital scoliosis is commonly the result of vertebral anomalies. Other organ anomalies are common as well.

■ The increased use of instrumentation in adult degenerative spine disease had led to an increased incidence of iatrogenic deformity (proximal junctional kyphosis, flat back syndrome, etc.).

■ Sagittal balance is the most important prognostic factor after surgical correction.

■ Pelvic incidence is a compensatory angulation of the pelvis in response to changes in lumbar lordosis in an attempt to keep the head oriented over the pelvic axis.

■ Pelvic incidence = sacral slope + pelvic tilt.

■ Pelvic incidence–lumbar lordosis mismatch >20 degrees is a reliable indicator of impaired sagittal balance.

Table 2-7   SCOLIOSIS

Idiopathic
  Infantile
  Juvenile
  Adolescent

Congenital
  Hemivertebrae
  Wedge vertebrae
  Unilateral bar
  Bilateral bar (block vertebrae)
  Neuromuscular development
    Myelodysplasia
    Diastematomyelia
    Meningocele
  Extraskeletal development
    Rib fusions
    Myositis ossificans progressiva
  Neuromuscular
    Syringomyelia
    Myopathies

Skeletal dysplasia

Trauma

Metabolic bone disease

Neoplasms

■ SCOLIOSIS: IMAGING

KEY FACTS

■ Routine radiographs: Imaging of scoliosis is accomplished primarily with radiographs. Standing full-length spine AP and lateral views are needed for curve evaluation and measurement. Lateral bending views are used to evaluate flexibility of curves. Flexible (nonrigid) curves correct with bending to the convex side. Rigid curves do not correct.

■ CT or MRI may be needed to evaluate certain neural or osseous anomalies. CT is important for surgical planning in order to better characterize pedicle morphology for screw placement.

■ Curve measurement: Lippman–Cobb method. Lines are drawn along the endplates (or pedicles if the endplate is indistinct) of the upper and lower most vertebrae that have maximally tilted endplates to the concavity of the curve. With larger curves, the points where the lines cross measure the angle L. For smaller curves, perpendicular lines are drawn to the end lines, and the angle s is formed by these lines (Fig. 2-43). Regardless of which method is used to calculate the angle L = angle s.

■ Rotation: The degree of rotation is important for selecting the type and length of spinal instrumentation. The apex vertebra is selected, and the position of the spinous process is used to grade rotation from 1 to 4 (+ concave side, − convex side).

■ Treatment: Treatment varies with the extent of curve, degree of rotation, and surgical preference. Anterior, posterior, or combined instrumentation may be required. Treatment goals include (1) achieving solid fusion, (2) preventing curve progression, (3) improving cosmetic appearance, and (4) reducing or preventing back pain and functional impairment.

■ Complications of instrumentation
  ● Loss of correction
  ● Rod fracture
  ● Cable rupture
  ● Hook displacement
  ● Screw pullout
  ● Pseudoarthrosis
  ● Neurologic
  ● Infection
  ● Myofascial pain syndrome

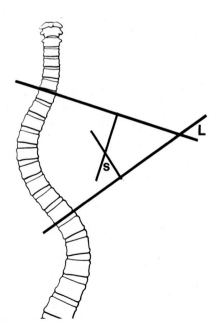

FIGURE 2-43. Lippman–Cobb measurement. Lines are configured along the endplate or pedicles of the upper and lower vertebrae maximally directed to the concave side. Where these cross measures angles for large curves (*L*). Perpendicular lines are drawn to the endplate lines for smaller curves (*s*). Angle *L* = angle *s*.

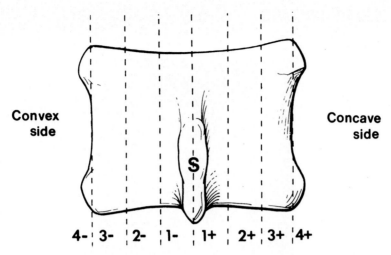

FIGURE 2-44. Rotational measurement. Neutral is spinous process midline (S). Positive is rotation of the spinous process to the concave side and negative to the convex side graded 1 to 4.

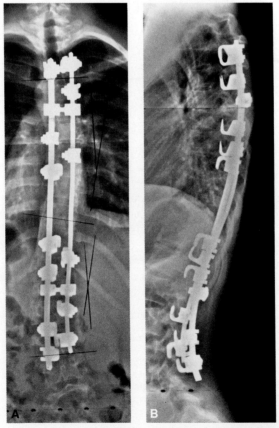

FIGURE 2-45. Standing anteroposterior (AP) **(A)** and lateral **(B)** radiographs after reduction with rods and hooks.

(continued)

▪ SCOLIOSIS: IMAGING *(Continued)*

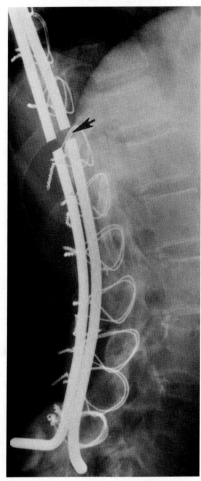

FIGURE 2-46. Lateral radiograph with fractured Luque rods *(arrow)* after treatment with rods and sublaminar wires.

SUGGESTED READING

Busch CH, Kalen V. Three-dimensional computed tomography in assessment of congenital scoliosis. *Skeletal Radiol.* 1999;28:632–637.

Everett CR, Patel RK. A systematic literature review of nonsurgical treatment in adult scoliosis. *Spine.* 2007;32(19, suppl):S130–S134.

Helenius I, Remes V, Yrjonen T, et al. Harrington and Cotrel-Dubousset instrumentation in adolescent idiopathic scoliosis. *J Bone Joint Surg.* 2003;85A:2303–2309.

McAlister WH, Shackelford GD. Measurement of spinal curvatures. *Radiol Clin North Am.* 1975;13:113–121.

Rose PS, Bridwell KH, Lenke LG, et al. Role of pelvic incidence, thoracic kyphosis, and patient factors on sagittal plane correction following pedicle subtraction osteotomy. *Spine.* 2009;34:785–791.

Yadla S, Maltenfort MG, Ratliff JK, et al. Adult scoliosis surgery outcomes: a systematic review. *Neurosurg Focus.* 2010;28:E3.

■ DEGENERATIVE DISC DISEASE

KEY FACTS

■ Disc degeneration (intervertebral osteochondrosis) is a normal sequela of aging and appears to have a hereditary component.

■ Chronic axial loading predisposes to accelerated degenerative changes.

■ Loss of disc height (water and elasticity) or extension of disc material into adjacent vertebral endplates (Schmorl node) or through the annulus fibrosis may occur.

■ Nuclear trial sign is an abnormal curvilinear endplate change suggestive of a migratory path of the herniated disc fragment. Reported only in the thoracic spine.

■ Traction on the vertebral margins results in osteophyte formation. Unlike the cervical spine, thoracolumbar osteophytes rarely cause neural element compromise unless associated with a chronic disc protrusion/herniation.

■ Biomechanical changes cause facet degeneration in many patients. Compensatory ligamentous hypertrophy occurs as a support mechanism to facet degeneration. The combination of disc and facet disease may lead to spinal canal narrowing (spinal stenosis), neural foraminal narrowing, and/or lateral recess narrowing.

■ Disc degeneration at multiple levels may be the result of calcium pyrophosphate dihydrate deposition or ochronosis.

■ Image features
  ● Radiographic: Loss of disc space height, asymmetric in many cases. Calcification or vacuum disc phenomenon, osteophyte formation, loss of normal lordosis, subluxation if facet degeneration present.
  ● MRI: Loss of disc height and abnormal signal intensity caused by decreased water and cellularity.
  ● Endplate changes:
    ❖ Type I: Decreased signal intensity on T1-weighted sequences and increased signal intensity on T2-weighted sequences consistent with marrow edema: early phase.
    ❖ Type II: Increased signal on T1-weighted sequences compared with normal marrow and slight increase on isointense with marrow on T2-weighted sequences consistent with fat infiltration in the marrow: subacute phase.
    ❖ Type III: End-stage degenerative disease with decreased signal on T1- and T2-weighted sequences consistent with sclerosis: chronic phase.
    ❖ Types I, II, and III changes can be seen in combination.

(continued)

■ DEGENERATIVE DISC DISEASE   *(Continued)*

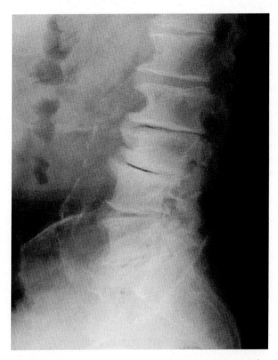

FIGURE 2-47. Lateral radiograph of the lumbar spine demonstrates prominent osteophytes and vacuum disc phenomenon at L2–L5 levels. There is loss of the lumbar lordotic curve.

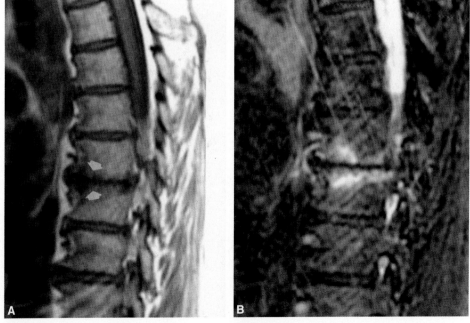

FIGURE 2-48. Type I endplate changes. Sagittal T1 **(A)** and T2 **(B)** magnetic resonance (MR) demonstrate decreased signal relative to marrow on T1 **(A)** and increased signal on T2 **(B)** MR.

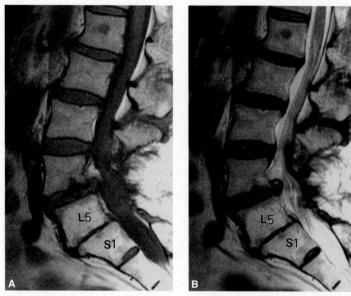

FIGURE 2-49. Type II endplate changes. Sagittal T1 **(A)** and T2 **(B)** magnetic resonance (MR) demonstrate increased signal relative to marrow on both T1- and T2-weighted sequences.

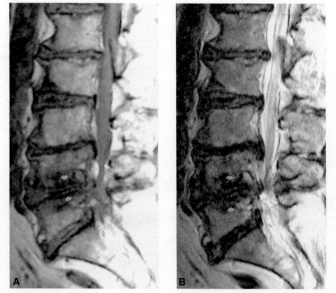

FIGURE 2-50. Type III endplate changes. Decreased signal (*arrows*) seen on both T1 **(A)** and T2 **(B)** magnetic resonance (MR).

SUGGESTED READING

Adams MA, Roughley PJ. What is intervertebral disc degeneration, and what causes it? *Spine (Phila Pa 1976)*. 2006;31:2151–2161.

Modic MT, Steinberg PM, Ross JS, et al. Degenerative disc disease: assessment of changes in vertebral marrow with MR imaging. *Radiology*. 1988;166:193–199.

■ DISC HERNIATION

KEY FACTS

■ Disc herniations may occur in the lumbar, thoracic, and cervical regions. They result from annular defects with herniation of nucleus pulposus.

■ Disc herniation may be central or to the right or left of midline. Herniations to the right or left frequently compress the traversing and/or exiting nerve roots.

■ Terminology (Fig. 2-51)

- Normal disc: No disc material extends beyond the periphery of vertebral endplates.
- Symmetric bulging disc: Symmetric circumferential extension of the disc annulus beyond the edges of the vertebral endplates.
- Asymmetric bulging disc: Extension of *greater* than 25% of the circumference of the disc annulus beyond the edges of the vertebral endplates.
- Disc protrusion: Extension of *less* than 25% of the circumference of the disc material beyond the edges of the vertebral endplates. The greatest dimension of the displaced disc material is *less* than the base of displaced disc material, when measured in the same plane.
- Disc extrusion: The greatest dimension of the displaced disc material is *greater* than the base of displaced disc material, when measured in the same plane.
- Disc sequestration: An extrusion that is no longer connected to the parent disc. The sequestered fragment can migrate several disc levels superiorly or inferiorly.

■ Imaging is usually accomplished with MR. Myelography or CT myelography may also be useful.

■ The natural history of disc herniations is >80% resolve spontaneously within 6 to 8 weeks.

■ Surgery is reserved for unresolved herniations with intractable pain, or those that cause myelopathy or motor impairment.

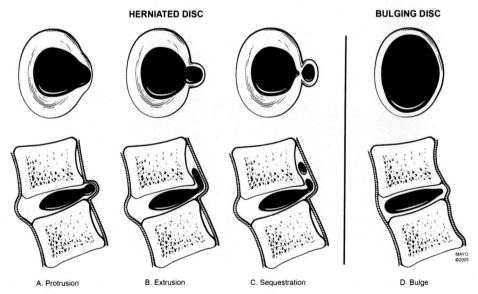

FIGURE 2-51. Disc bulge, protrusion, extrusion, and sequestration based on consensus terminology. (From Witte RJ, Lane JI, Miller GM, et al. Spine. In: Berquist TH, ed. *MRI of the Musculoskeletal System.* 5th ed. Philadelphia: Lippincott Williams & Wilkins; 2006:121–202.)

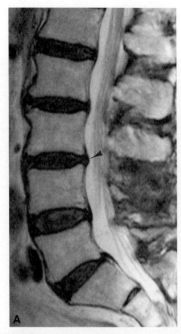
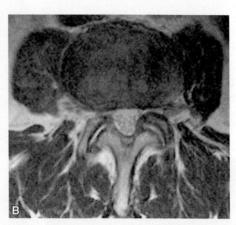

FIGURE 2-52. Lumbar disc bulge at L3–L4. Sagittal T1 **(A)** and axial T2 **(B)** magnetic resonance (MR) demonstrate broad-based bulging of the posterior annulus (*arrowhead*). The normal disc contour at L3–L4 would be slightly concave.

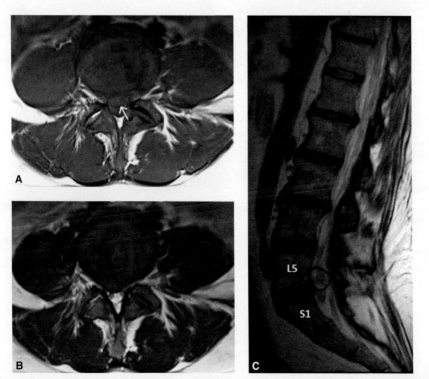

FIGURE 2-53. Lumbar disc protrusion. Axial T1 **(A)**, axial T2 **(B)**, and sagittal T1 **(C)** magnetic resonance (MR) show an L4 -L5 focal right paracentral disc protrusion flattening the left ventral aspect of the thecal sac (Protrusion marked by arrow in Figure A).

(continued)

■ DISC HERNIATION *(Continued)*

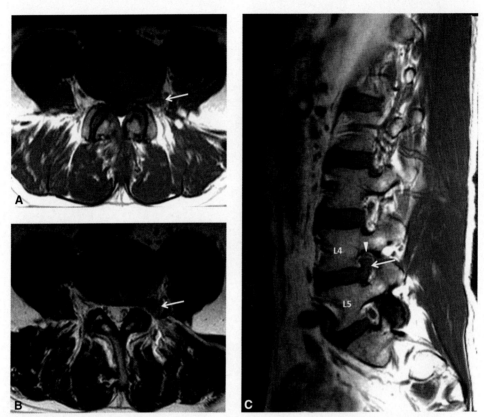

FIGURE 2-54. Lumbar disc extrusion. Axial T1 **(A)**, axial T2 **(B)**, and sagittal T1 **(C)** magnetic resonance (MR) show L4–L5 disc extrusion within the left neural foramina (*arrows*) causing superior displacement and compression of the exiting L4 nerve roots/dorsal root ganglia (*arrowhead* in **C**).

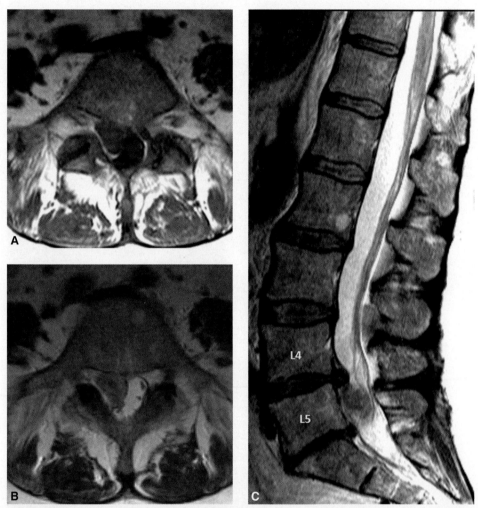

FIGURE 2-55. Lumbar disc sequestration. Axial T1 **(A)** and axial T2 **(B)** magnetic resonance (MR) demonstrate disc material in the right lateral recess of L5. Sagittal T2 **(C)** MR shows the large disc fragment posterior to the L5 vertebral body separate from the parent L4–L5 disc.

(continued)

■ DISC HERNIATION *(Continued)*

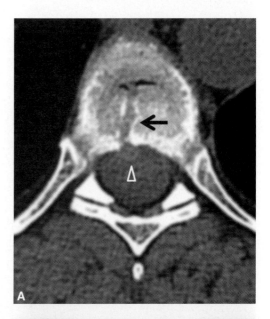

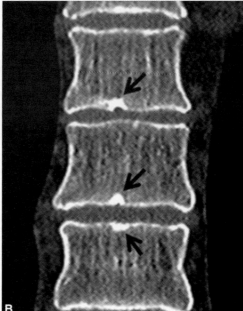

FIGURE 2-56. Nuclear trial sign. Axial **(A)** and coronal **(B)** computed tomography (CT): a focal thoracic disc herniation (*arrow head*) associated with an abnormal curvilinear corticated lucency within the endplate (*black arrow*) suggestive of the migratory path taken by the herniated disc fragment. Also seen at adjacent level on the coronal image, this sign for unknown reasons is limited to thoracic spine.

SUGGESTED READING

Fardon DF, Williams AL, Dohring EJ, et al. Lumbar disc nomenclature: version 2.0. *Spine J.* 2014;14(11):2525–2545.

Jenkins JR, Whittemore AR, Bradley WE. Anatomic basis of vertebrogenic pain and autonomic syndrome associated with lumbar disc extrusion. *Am J Neuroradiol.* 1989;10:219–231.

Weishaupt D, Zanetti M, Hodler J, et al. MR imaging of the lumbar spine. Prevalence of intervertebral disc extrusion and sequestration, nerve root compression, endplate abnormalities and osteoarthritis of the facet joints in asymptomatic volunteers. *Radiology.* 1998;209:661–666.

■ SYNOVIAL CYSTS

KEY FACTS

- ■ Synovial cysts typically arise from the facet joints and are associated with degenerative disease.
- ■ Patients present with compressive symptoms similar to disc herniation or spinal stenosis.
- ■ Simple cysts are well defined, with low signal intensity on T1-weighted and high signal intensity on T2-weighted sequences. Signal intensity may vary if calcification, hemorrhage, or air is present in the cyst.
- ■ Cysts are most common in the lumbar spine at L4–L5 and L5–S1.
- ■ Conservative treatment options include foraminal injections of steroid, or attempt at percutaneous fluoroscopy guided rupture.
- ■ Recurrent synovial cysts after surgical excision indicate instability and warrant evaluation for a fusion procedure.

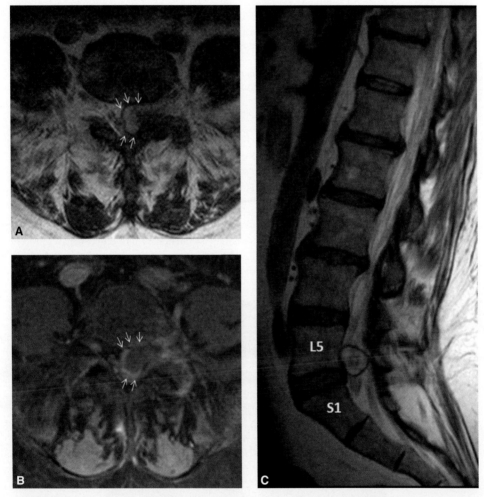

FIGURE 2-57. Synovial cyst. **(A–C)** Axial T2, axial postcontrast T1, and sagittal T2 magnetic resonance (MR). A large synovial cyst arising from the markedly degenerated left L5–S1 facet and compressing the dural sac. Note the cyst wall (*arrows* in **B**) enhancement following intravenous (IV) contrast.

SUGGESTED READING

Krauss WE, Atkinson JLD, Miller GM. Juxtafacet cysts of the cervical spine. *Neurosurgery.* 1998;43:1363–1368.

Silbergleit R, Geborski S, Brunberg J, et al. Lumbar synovial cysts. Correlation of myelographic CT, MR, and pathologic finding. *Am J Neuroradiol.* 1990;11:777–779.

▪ INFECTION (INFECTIOUS DISCOSPONDYLITIS OR SPONDYLODISCITIS)

KEY FACTS

- ▪ Spinal infections may occur by hematogenous spread, usually arterial, although the Batson venous plexus can be a route. Infectious discospondylitis or rarely isolated vertebral osteomyelitis without discitis accounts for 4% to 7% of all cases of osteomyelitis.
- ▪ The source of infection often is unknown, although common sources include cutaneous, genitourinary, and respiratory systems. Infection can also be transmitted during intervention or by spread from adjacent soft tissues.
- ▪ Most common in men 50 to 70 years old. The lumbar spine is involved most often.
- ▪ Patients present with pain and history of recent primary infection or surgical procedure. *Staphylococcus aureus* is the most common organism.
- ▪ Tuberculous spondylitis most often involves the thoracic spine. Disc spaces are preserved for a longer time compared with pyogenic infections. Paraspinal abscesses are common.
- ▪ Intravenous drug users are at high risk for development of epidural abscess without discospondylitis.
- ▪ Image features
  - ● Routine radiographs: Progressive loss of disc height with endplate irregularity. Later, bone sclerosis may occur with pyogenic or tuberculous infections. It is uncommon for infection to occur in a vacuum disc. Soft tissue swelling.
  - ● CT: Defines bone loss earlier and provides method to monitor needle aspiration to isolate organisms.
  - ● MRI: Intervertebral disc fluid signal (T1-hypointense and T2-hyperintense) and enhancement, extensive marrow edema and enhancement with indistinct endplates of adjacent vertebral bodies and abnormal paraspinal/epidural soft tissue are highly consistent findings of discitis-osteomyelitis. Peripheral contrast enhancement with central fluid signal = abscess. Solid heterogeneous enhancement = phlegmon. Distinction between Type 1 degenerative changes from osteomyelitis can be occasionally challenging. Unlike Type I discogenic change, where the edema involves immediate subchondral marrow with relative well-defined zone of transition with the healthy marrow, the marrow edema of discitis-osteomyelitis is usually diffuse with ill-defined margin. Correlation with clinical history, cell count, sedimentation rate, and C-reactive protein is important.

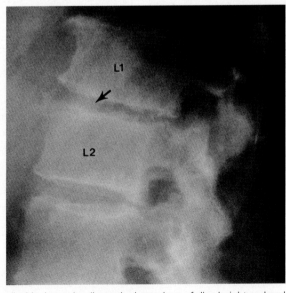

FIGURE 2-58. Early discitis. Lateral radiograph shows loss of disc height and early endplate irregularity at L1–L2 (*arrow*). Note the normal disc below.

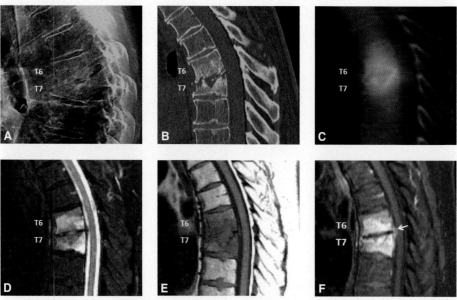

FIGURE 2-59. Late discitis-osteomyelitis. **(A–F)** Lateral radiograph, sagittal computed tomography (CT), nuclear medicine bone scan, sagittal T2 magnetic resonance (MR), sagittal precontrast T1 MR, and postcontrast T1 MR: T6–T7 loss of disc height, severe endplate and subchondral bone destruction, diffuse marrow edema and enhancement with small amount of epidural phlegmon (*arrow*). Also note abnormal increased radiotracer uptake and normal adjacent discs. Disc biopsy cultures grew mycobacterium avium complex.

(continued)

■ INFECTION (INFECTIOUS DISCOSPONDYLITIS OR SPONDYLODISCITIS) *(Continued)*

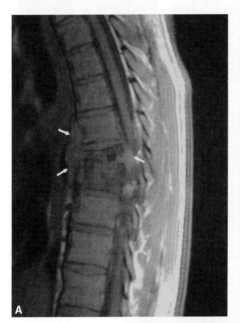
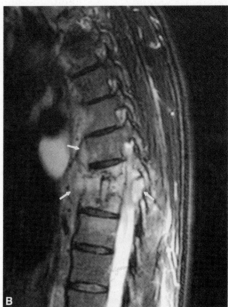
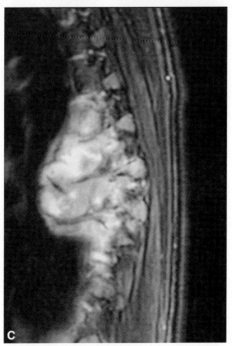

FIGURE 2-60. Tuberculous spondylitis in the thoracic spine: Sagittal T1-weighted **(A)** and T2-weighted **(B)** images demonstrate disc space loss and vertebral compression with paravertebral soft tissue extension *(arrows)*. Off-axis sagittal image **(C)** shows a large multiloculated paraspinal abscess.

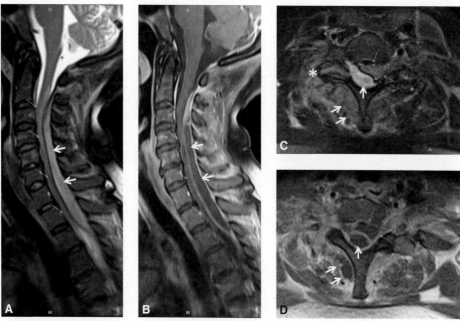

FIGURE 2-61. Epidural abscess. **(A–D)** Sagittal T2, sagittal postcontrast T1, axial T2, and axial postcontrast T1 magnetic resonance (MR) obtained with fat suppression: A large right dorsolateral epidural fluid collection within the cervical spinal canal with enhancement of the wall (*arrows*) causes severe left anterior displacement and compression of the spinal cord (*thin arrow* on axial images). The source of abscess is septic right facet joint (*asterisk*) that demonstrates effusion and periarticular edema. Also note abscess abutting the spinous process (*double arrow* on axial images).

SUGGESTED READING

Hong SH, Choi JY, Lee JW, et al. MR imaging assessment of the spine: infection or an imitation? *Radiographics.* 2009;29(2):599–612.

Jung NY, Jee WH, Ha KY, et al. Discrimination of tuberculous spondylitis from pyogenic spondylitis on MRI. *Am J Roentgenol.* 2004;182:1405–1410.

Stabler A, Reiser MF. Imaging of spinal infections. *Radiol Clin North Am.* 2001;39:115–135.

Sundaram VK, Doshi A. Infections of the spine: a review of clinical and imaging findings. *Appl Radiol.* 2016;45(8):10–20.

■ ARTHROPATHIES

KEY FACTS

■ Arthropathies in the spine involve the vertebral bodies, facet joints, and disc spaces.

■ Arthropathies cause four types of "phytes."

● Syndesmophyte: Vertical ossification bridging the vertebrae. Seen with ankylosing spondylitis, reactive arthritis, psoriatic arthritis, and inflammatory bowel disease.

● Marginal osteophyte: Horizontal bone extending from the vertebral endplate. Seen with trauma and degenerative disc disease.

● Nonmarginal osteophyte: Bone extension that is several millimeters away from the endplate.

● Paraspinal osteophyte: Ossification of the soft tissues surrounding the vertebrae. Seen with diffuse idiopathic skeletal hyperostosis (DISH).

● Small marginal or nonmarginal osteophytes with normal disc spaces are seen with spondylosis deformans.

● Ankylosing spondylitis results in ankylosis with smooth symmetric syndesmophytes.

● Reactive arthritis and psoriatic spondylitis cause asymmetric prominent syndesmophytes. Psoriatic spine involvement is more common than reactive arthritis.

● DISH has normal disc spaces with ligament and tendon ossification. Diagnosis is made when four or more contiguous vertebrae are involved.

● Rheumatoid arthritis most commonly involves the upper cervical spine. Inflammation may erode the odontoid (14% to 35%). Instability at C1–C2 may cause cord compression and basilar invagination.

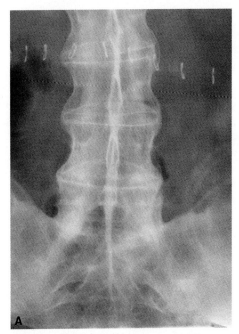 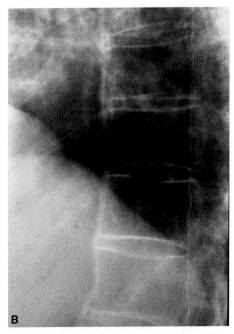

FIGURE 2-62. Ankylosing spondylitis. **(A)** Anteroposterior (AP) radiograph or the lumbar spine and sacroiliac joints. Note the smooth symmetric syndesmophytes. **(B)** Lateral radiograph of the lower thoracic spine shows smooth ossification of the anterior longitudinal ligament.

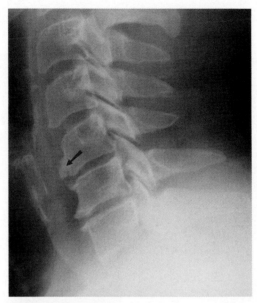

FIGURE 2-63. Lateral radiograph of the cervical spine demonstrates marginal osteophytes at C6–C7 and a nonmarginal osteophyte at C5 (*arrow*).

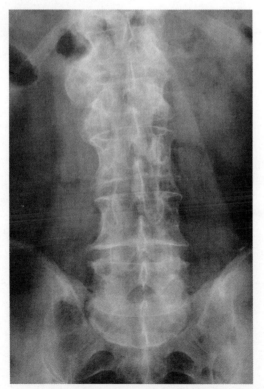

FIGURE 2-64. Psoriatic arthritis: anteroposterior (AP) radiograph of the lumbar spine demonstrates prominent asymmetric upper lumbar osteophytes. There is also asymmetric sacroiliac joint involvement.

(continued)

■ ARTHROPATHIES *(Continued)*

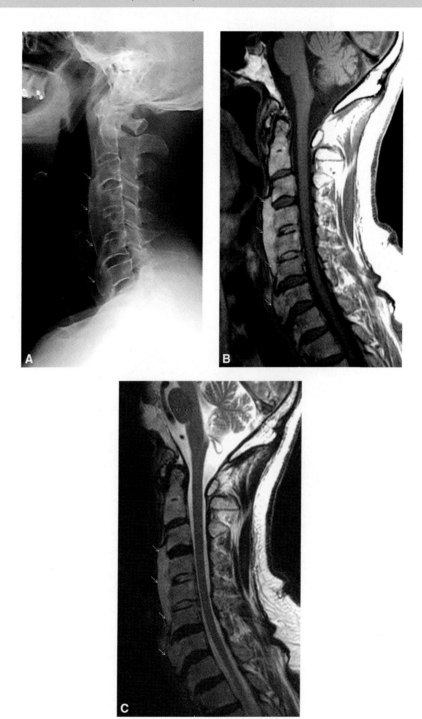

FIGURE 2-65. Diffuse idiopathic skeletal hyperostosis (DISH). **(A–C)** Lateral radiograph, sagittal T1 and T2 magnetic resonance (MR) of the cervical spine with prominent flowing anterior (anterior longitudinal ligament) ossification (*arrows*) over at least four contiguous vertebrae with well-preserved disc spaces.

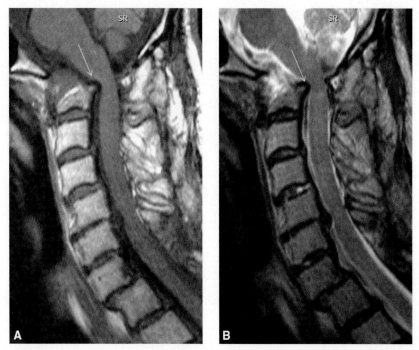

FIGURE 2-66. Rheumatoid arthritis (RA). Several diseases entities including RA can lead to formation of pannus, severe erosion, and/or fracture of the odontoid process with resultant compromise of the spinal canal. **(A, B)** Sagittal T1 and T2 magnetic resonance (MR) show severe erosion of the odontoid with upward migration and impingement of the cervicomedullary junction against the arch of C1 (*arrow*).

SUGGESTED READING

Arnbak B, Leboeuf-Yde C, Jensen TS. A systematic critical review on MRI in spondyloarthritis. *Arthritis Res Ther.* 2012;14(2):R55. doi:10.1186/ar3768.

Brower AC. *Arthritis in Black and White.* 2nd ed. Philadelphia: WB Saunders; 1997:175–191.

Canella C, Schau B, Ribeiro E, et al. MRI in seronegative spondyloarthritis: imaging features and differential diagnosis in the spine and sacroiliac joints. *Am J Roentgenol.* 2013;200(1):149–157.

■ TUMORS AND TUMORLIKE CONDITIONS: BONE LESIONS

KEY FACTS

- The spine is a common site for metastasis and multiple myeloma.
- Most metastases involve the thoracic spine. They are usually multiple and may be epidural or intradural.
- Patients with primary or metastatic bone lesions generally present with pain.
- Vertebral hemangiomas are the most common benign neoplasms of the vertebra.
  - Usually small and asymptomatic, these are incidentally detected due to characteristic MRI features.
  - Occasionally if locally aggressive with extravertebral extension, they become symptomatic due to pathologic fracture, spinal cord, or nerve/root compression. Hypervascular and most commonly involve thoracic spine.
- Imaging approaches
  - Routine radiographs: AP and lateral radiographs of the symptomatic site or skeletal survey for suspected myeloma or metastasis. Lesions may be lytic, blastic, or mixed, depending on the primary.
  - Radionuclide scans: Screening for metastatic disease. May be false-negative in myeloma or with aggressive metastatic lesions.
  - CT: Excellent for isolated lesions to demonstrate bone involvement and tumor matrix.
  - MRI: Metastatic screening can be accomplished with whole body imaging. Primary lesions are examined using T1-weighted and T2-weighted sequences in two image planes. Lesions enhance with gadolinium administration.
- Decompressive surgery for metastatic lesions is indicated in cases of epidural compression causing myelopathy.
- Both chordomas and benign notochordal cell tumors (BNCTs) originate from notochordal remnants and may be mistaken for each other because of the alarming similar hyperintense appearance on T2-weighted MRI. However, the following imaging characteristics can help differentiate these two conditions. Chordomas show variable degree of osteolysis, enhancement, bone expansion, intra and extraosseous components, and soft tissue mass. On the contrary, BNCTs are nondestructive, nonexpansile mildly sclerotic lesions that remain intraosseous and do not show enhance. Often small (<1 cm in size) BNCT can occupy the entire vertebral body. Some literature suggests that these two entities might be related and supports the idea that BNCT might progress to chordoma.

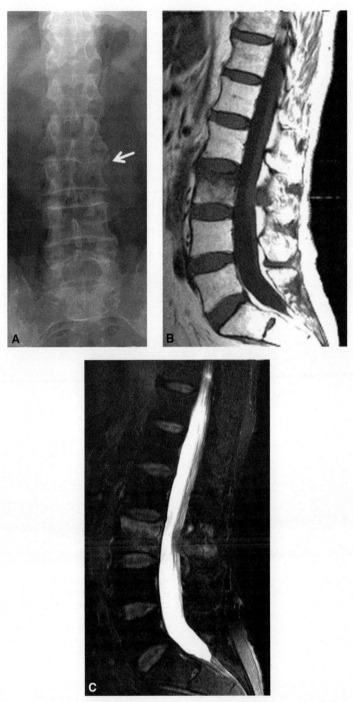

FIGURE 2-67. Vertebral metastasis. **(A–C)** Anteroposterior (AP) radiograph, sagittal T1, and fat-suppressed T2 magnetic resonance (MR) of lumbar spine. Lung cancer metastasis destroying the left L3 vertebral pedicle (*arrow*). Also note mild pathologic collapse of the ipsilateral superior L3 endplate and diffuse hyperintense T1 bone marrow appearance due to fat infiltration secondary to prior radiation therapy.

(continued)

■ TUMORS AND TUMORLIKE CONDITIONS: BONE LESIONS *(Continued)*

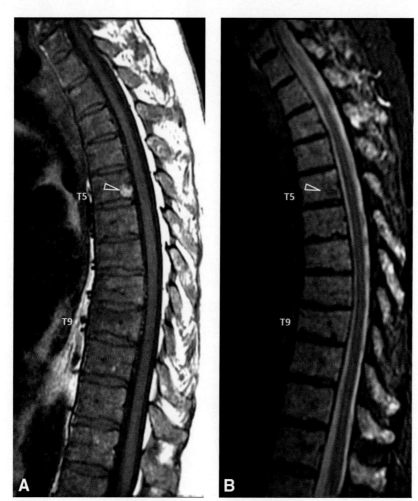

FIGURE 2-68. Multiple myeloma. **(A, B)** Sagittal T1 and fat-suppressed T2 magnetic resonance (MR) of the lumbar spine in a patient with multiple myeloma show diffuse abnormal marrow infiltration with heterogeneously hypointense T1 and hyperintense T2 signal. Other marrow infiltrative disorders such as leukemia, lymphoma, or metastasis can have similar appearance. The normal marrow is hyperintense to the intervertebral disc on T1-weighted imaging and hypo- to isointense to muscle on T2-weighted imaging. There is mild pathologic fracture collapse of the T9 vertebral body. Also note an incidental small typical hemangioma of the T5 vertebral body with characteristic bright T1 signal that suppresses—becomes dark on fat suppression due to the presence of fat (*arrow head*).

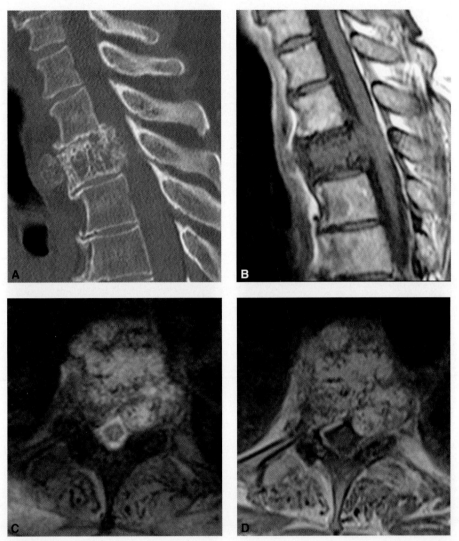

FIGURE 2-69. Aggressive vertebral hemangioma. **(A–D)** Sagittal computed tomography (CT), sagittal T1, axial T2, and postcontrast T1 magnetic resonance (MR). Diffuse lobulated expansion of a thoracic vertebral body by abnormal soft tissue. Note classic "corduroy cloth" appearance due to thickened weight bearing vertical bony trabeculae, hyperdense on CT, and hypointense on magnetic resonance imaging (MRI) ("polka dotted" appearance on axial CT—not shown). There is diffuse enhancement of the lesion with encroachment upon the spinal canal. Aggressive hemangiomas often lack fat which is characteristic for a typical hemangioma.

(continued)

■ TUMORS AND TUMORLIKE CONDITIONS: BONE LESIONS *(Continued)*

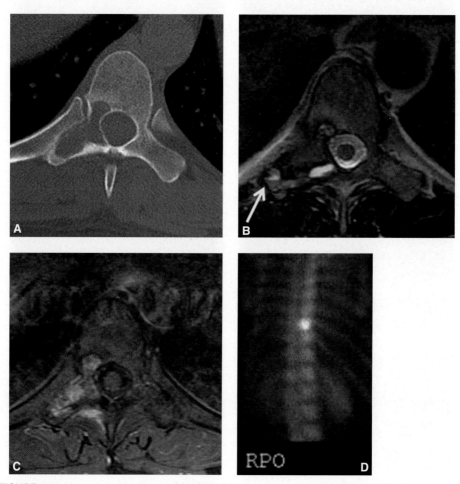

FIGURE 2-70. Aneurysmal bone cyst. **(A–D)** Axial computed tomography (CT), axial T2, fat-suppressed postcontrast T1 magnetic resonance (MR), and nuclear medicine bone scan. A thoracic right transverse process demonstrates a well-defined slightly expansile osteolytic lesion on CT with a characteristic blood-fluid level on T2-weighted image (*arrow* in **B**). Also note nonspecific heterogenous enhancement and increased radiotracer uptake.

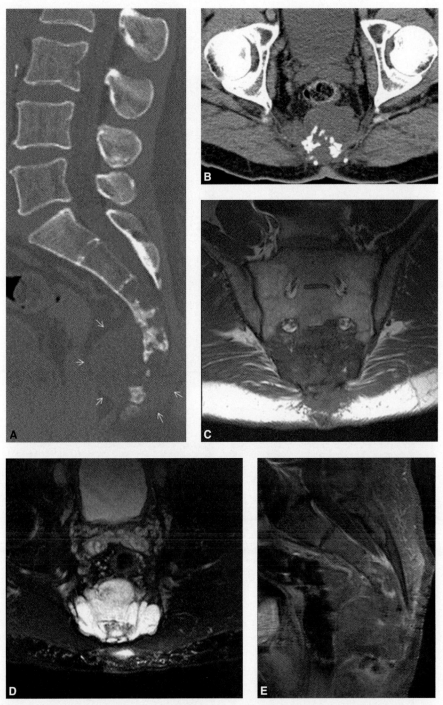

FIGURE 2-71. Sacrococcygeal chordoma. **(A, B)** Sagittal bone window and axial soft tissue window computed tomography (CT). Centrally located lytic lesion destroying the lower sacrum with sclerosis, calcifications, and expansile soft tissue mass (*arrows*). **(C–E)** Coronal noncontrast T1, axial T2, and sagittal contrast-enhanced T1 magnetic resonance (MR) demonstrate tumor extension into the sacral spinal canal and characteristic high T2 signal.

(continued)

■ TUMORS AND TUMORLIKE CONDITIONS: BONE LESIONS *(Continued)*

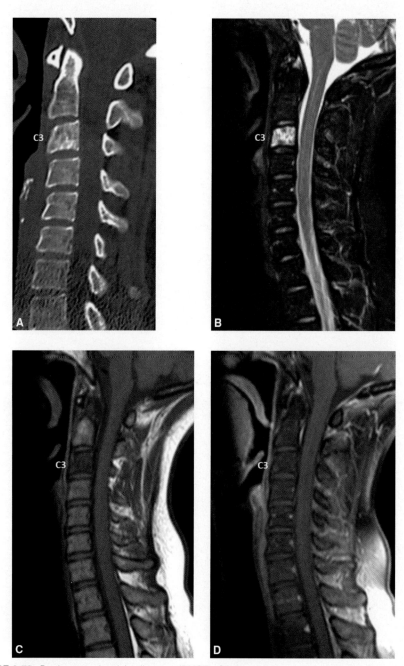

FIGURE 2-72. Benign notochordal cell tumor (BNCT). C3 vertebral body demonstrates heterogenous sclerotic pattern with slight trabecular accentuation **(A)**, fairly homogenous high T2 **(B)** and low T1 marrow signal **(C)** with no postcontrast T1 enhancement **(D)**. The vertebral body morphology is well preserved without evidence for extraosseous extension, expansion, or osteolysis.

SUGGESTED READING

Kim YS, Han IH, Lee IS, et al. Imaging findings of solitary spinal bony lesions and the differential diagnosis of benign and malignant lesions. *J Korean Neurosurg Soc.* 2012;52(2):126–132. doi:10.3340/jkns.2012.52.2.126.

Rodallec MH, Feydy A, Larousserie F, et al. Diagnostic imaging of solitary tumors of the spine: what to do and say. *Radiographics.* 2008;28(4):1019–1041.

Unni KK. *Dahlin's Bone Tumors: General Aspects and Data on 11,087 Cases.* 5th ed. Philadelphia: Lippincott-Raven; 1996.

Yamaguchi T, Iwata J, Sugihara S, et al. Distinguishing benign notochordal cell tumors from vertebral chordoma. *Skeletal Radiol.* 2008; 37:291–299.

■ TUMORS AND TUMORLIKE CONDITIONS: SOFT TISSUE MASSES

KEY FACTS

■ Soft tissue masses may reside in the paraspinal soft tissues (including the retroperitoneum) or spinal canal. The latter are categorized as extradural, intradural extramedullary, or intramedullary. Table 2-8 summarizes common tumors in these locations.

■ Paraspinal tumors
   ● 17.2% of desmoid tumors involve the back.
   ● Nineteen percent of liposarcomas occur in the retroperitoneum.
   ● Leiomyosarcomas account for 5% to 10% of sarcomas. In women, 66% involve the retroperitoneum or vena cava.
   ● Neuroblastoma is the third most common tumor in children; 50% occur before age 2 years.

■ Extradural tumors
   ● Metastasis—most involve the thoracic region. Lung and breast are most common.
   ● Soft tissue sarcomas in the paraspinal region may invade the extradural space.

■ Intradural extramedullary tumors
   ● Meningiomas and nerve sheath tumors (schwannoma and neurofibroma) are most common.
   ● Meningiomas—most common in thoracic region. Occurs more in females than in males. May be posterior or anterior to the cord.
   ● Nerve sheath tumors—no site or sex predilection. Can be multiple. Seventy percent intradural extramedullary, 15% extradural, and 15% both intra and extradural component that remodels and enlarges the neural foramen (dumbbell lesions). Rarely intramedullary in location. Imaging appearance of schwannoma and neurofibroma is often indistinguishable. Intradural location, cystic changes, and hemorrhage favor schwannoma. Extradural location, hyperintense rind, and hypointense collagenous center on T2-weighted imaging ("target sign") favor neurofibroma.

■ Intradural intramedullary tumors
   ● Ependymoma: Most common, 62% of intramedullary lesions. Myxopapillary variant is commonly found in the conus and filum terminale. Typically occurs in patients 30 to 60 years old, with no sex predilection. May contain blood products.
   ● Astrocytoma: Second most common tumor. Most common cord tumor in children. There is greater predilection for upper cord and becomes less common caudally. Rare to find in filum terminale.
   ● Hemangioblastomas rare benign tumors representing 1.6% to 6.4% of spinal tumors. Two-thirds of spinal hemangioblastomas are sporadic, and the remainder are associated with von Hippel–Lindau disease.

■ Metastasis can involve all the three compartments.

■ Tumorlike lesions include:
   ● Extradural: Lipomatosis, hematoma, and pseudomeningoceles
   ● Intradural extramedullary: Dural arteriovenous fistula
   ● Intramedullary: Cavernous malformations, hematoma, and abscess

Table 2-8   SOFT TISSUE TUMORS

Paraspinal	Intradural Extramedullary
Lipoma	Meningioma
Desmoid tumors	Neurolemmoma
Lymphangiomas	Neurofibroma
Liposarcoma	Lipoma
Leiomyosarcoma	Intradural cysts
Rhabdomyosarcoma	Metastasis
Neuroblastoma (50% <2 years of age)	
Paraganglioma	
Extradural Tumors	**Intradural Intramedullary**
Metastasis	Ependymoma
Lymphoma	Astrocytoma
Paraspinal sarcomas	Hemangioblastoma
	Metastasis (uncommon)

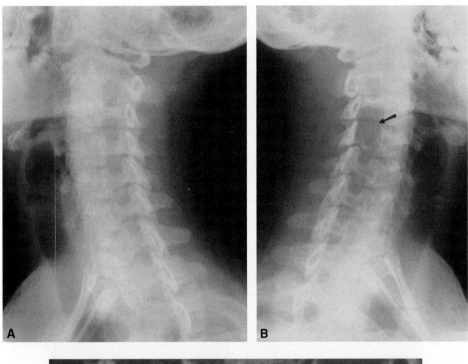

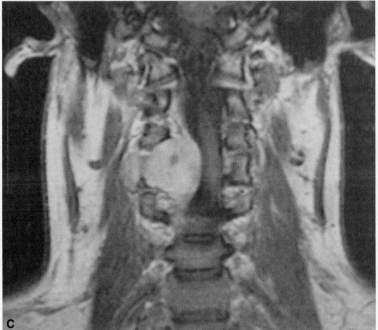

FIGURE 2-73. Nerve sheath tumor. Oblique radiographs of the cervical spine show normal foramina in **(A)** and marked expansion in **(B)** (*arrow*). Coronal magnetic resonance (MR) image **(C)** demonstrates a large presumed neurofibroma extending through the foramen and displacing the cord.

(continued)

■ TUMORS AND TUMORLIKE CONDITIONS: SOFT TISSUE MASSES *(Continued)*

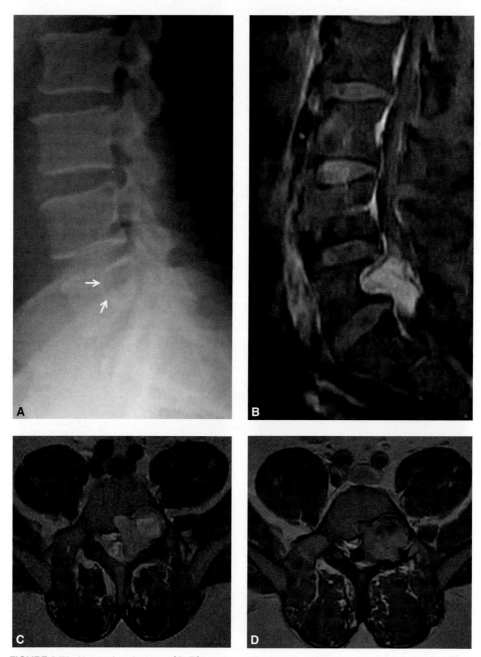

FIGURE 2-74. Nerve sheath tumor. **(A–D)** Lumbar spine lateral radiograph, postcontrast sagittal T1, axial T2, and postcontrast T1 magnetic resonance (MR). Well-corticated lucent lesion completely eroding the L5 pedicle (*arrows*) and scalloping the L5 vertebral body from a lobulated variable T2 signal intensity, heterogeneously enhancing dumbbell-shaped extradural mass.

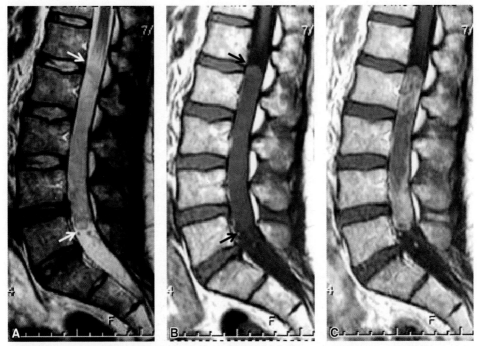

FIGURE 2-75. Myxopapillary Ependymoma. **(A–C)** Sagittal T2, pre- and postcontrast T1 magnetic resonance (MR). Inferior to the conus is a large well-defined intradural mass occupying the entire thecal sac from L2–L5 level (*between arrows*). The mass has hyperintense T2 and isointense T1 signal, and enhances heterogeneously. Small lesions demonstrate solid enhancement, while larger lesions have variable enhancement because of the presence of hemorrhage.

SUGGESTED READING

Beall DP, Googe DJ, Emery RL, et al. Extramedullary intradural spinal tumors: a pictorial review. *Curr Probl Diagn Radiol.* 2007;36(5):185–198.

Chu BC, Terae S, Hida K, et al. MR findings in spinal hemangioblastoma: correlation with symptoms and with angiographic and surgical findings. *Am J Neuroradiol.* 2001;22:206–217.

Lowe GM. Magnetic resonance imaging of intramedullary spinal cord tumors. *J Neurooncol.* 2000;47:195–210.

Smith AB, Soderlund KA, Rushing EJ, et al. Radiologic-pathologic correlation of pediatric and adolescent spinal neoplasms: part 1, intramedullary spinal neoplasms. *Am J Roentgenol.* 2012;198:34–43.

Soderlund KA, Smith AB, Rushing EJ, et al. Radiologic-pathologic correlation of pediatric and adolescent spinal neoplasms: part 2, intradural extramedullary spinal neoplasms. *Am J Roentgenol.* 2012;198(1):44–51.

Witte RJ, Lane JI, Miller GM, et al. Spine. In: Berquist TH, ed. *MRI of the Musculoskeletal System.* 5th ed. Philadelphia: Lippincott Williams & Wilkins; 2006:121–202.

■ INFLAMMATORY CONDITIONS OF SPINAL CORD AND NERVE ROOTS

KEY FACTS

- ■ Spinal cord:
  - ● Multiple sclerosis
    - ❖ Small poorly marginated patchy hyperintense T2 lesions (demyelination plaques) usually eccentric, commonly involving the posterolateral cord
    - ❖ Incomplete rim of enhancement, if seen, is characteristic of demyelination
    - ❖ Oligoclonal bands in the cerebrospinal fluid (CSF) seen in >90% of cases
  - ● Idiopathic transverse myelitis
    - ❖ T2-weighted hyperintensity involving most of the axial cord spanning more than one vertebral body segment, with or without cord swelling and/or enhancement
    - ❖ Lesion is central and uniform compared with the patchy peripheral lesion of multiple sclerosis
    - ❖ Cerebrospinal fluid pleocytosis and elevated IgG index, usually elevated white blood cells
  - ● Neuromyelitis optica spectrum disorder (NMOSD) or
    - ❖ Inflammatory disease that can affect the optic nerves, spinal cord, brain stem, and cerebral hemispheres
    - ❖ Transverse myelitis concurrent or subsequent to optic neuritis—traditional neuromyelitis optica (NMO)
    - ❖ Seventy percent patients have AQP4 antibody: Neuromyelitis optica immunoglobulin G (NMO-IgG)—antibody directed against aquaporin-4 water channel on astrocyte footplate
    - ❖ MRI: At least three contiguous segments of longitudinally extensive transverse myelitis (abnormal intramedullary hyperintense T2 lesion) or spinal cord atrophy in patients with history compatible with acute myelitis
  - ● Acute disseminated encephalomyelitis (ADEM)
    - ❖ Poorly marginated T2-weighted hyperintensities of two or three vertebral bodies in length; usually do not show contrast enhancement
    - ❖ Can be monophasic, recurrent (second attack involving the same areas >3 months from the first attack), or multiphasic (second event in a different area)
    - ❖ Twenty-five percent patients with ADEM are subsequently diagnosed with multiple sclerosis
- ■ Nerve
    - ❖ Acute inflammatory demyelinating polyneuropathy/Guillain–Barré syndrome: Commonly presents as rapidly progressing ascending flaccid paralysis; MRI shows enhancement with or without mild thickening of the cauda equina and other spinal nerve roots—ventral root enhancement > dorsal roots
    - ❖ Chronic inflammatory demyelinating polyneuropathy: Slowly progressive both proximal and distal musculature weakness; thickening and enhancement of nerve roots, brachial and lumbosacral plexus, and peripheral nerves; denervation changes within supplied muscles—edema in subacute phase and fatty atrophy is chronic phase

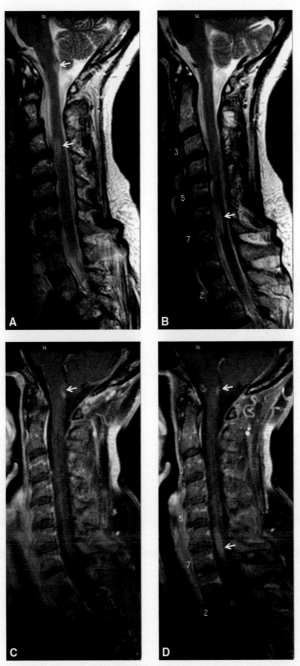

FIGURE 2-76. Multiple sclerosis (MS). **(A, B)** Sagittal T2 and postcontrast T1 **(C, D)** magnetic resonance (MR). Typical multifocal eccentric intramedullary hyperintense T2 plaques of demyelination (*arrows*). Note caudal dorsal medullary obex and C6-enhancing active plaques and a quiescent nonenhancing chronic C3 plaque. Contrary to MS, spinal cord involvement in ADEM is confluent.

(continued)

■ INFLAMMATORY CONDITIONS OF SPINAL CORD AND NERVE ROOTS *(Continued)*

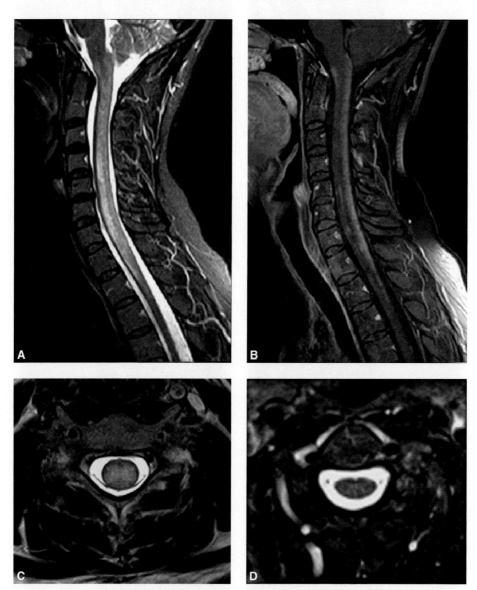

FIGURE 2-77. Neuromyelitis optica spectrum disorder (NMOSD). **(A–C)** Sagittal T2, sagittal postcontrast T1, and axial T2 magnetic resonance (MR). Longitudinally extensive—over four to seven segments, holocord (entire transverse diameter) involvement by abnormal hyperintense T2 signal with spinal cord swelling and heterogenous enhancement. Contrast enhancement is often inconsistent. **(D)** Axial T2 MR one year later shows resolution of intramedullary signal with spinal cord atrophy. Patient was positive for AQP4 antibodies and was diagnosed as NMOSD. Note that transverse myelitis due to other etiologies will have similar appearance.

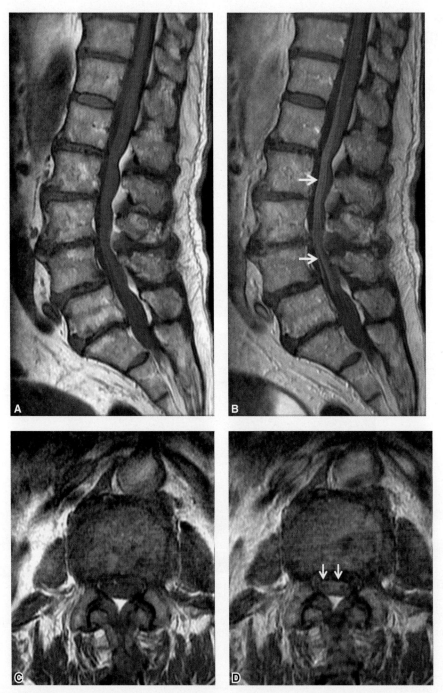

FIGURE 2-78. Acute inflammatory demyelinating polyneuropathy (AIDP). **(A–D)** Sagittal pre- and postcontrast, and axial pre- and postcontrast T1 magnetic resonance (MR). Diffuse contrast enhancement and mild thickening of anterior spinal nerve roots (*arrows*) in a patient with Guillain–Barré syndrome. Less often posterior nerve root enhancement can also be seen.

(continued)

■ INFLAMMATORY CONDITIONS OF SPINAL CORD AND NERVE ROOTS   *(Continued)*

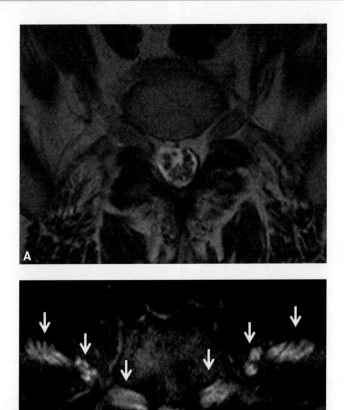

FIGURE 2-79. Chronic inflammatory demyelinating polyneuropathy (CIDP). **(A, B)** Nonfat-suppressed and fat-suppressed axial T2 magnetic resonance (MR). Note diffuse thickening of the cauda equina roots without clumping within the thecal sac. Marked thickening of the lumbar nerves and lumbar plexus (arrows) resembling "onion bulbs"—best appreciated on the fat-suppressed T2-weighted image. The thickened nerves usually enhance due to breakdown of the blood-brain barrier (not shown).

SUGGESTED READING

Li HF, Ji XJ. The diagnostic, prognostic, and differential value of enhanced MR imaging in Guillain–Barré syndrome. *Am J Neuroradiol.* 2011;32(7):E140.

Vallat JM, Sommer C, Magy L. Chronic inflammatory demyelinating polyradiculoneuropathy: diagnostic and therapeutic challenges for a treatable condition. *Lancet Neurol.* 2010;9(4):402–412.

Wingerchuk DM, Banwell B, Bennett JL, et al. International consensus diagnostic criteria for neuromyelitis optica spectrum disorders. *Neurology.* 2015;85(2):177–189.

■ MISCELLANEOUS CONDITIONS

KEY FACTS

■ Spinal dural arteriovenous fistula
- Most common vascular malformation of the spinal cord; most commonly affect elderly men; typically found in the thoracolumbar region.
- Ateriorvenous (AV) shunt is between radiculomeningeal artery enters a radicular vein, located inside the dura along the spinal nerve root.
- Shunt causes increased venous pressure, venous back congestion with impaired venous drainage of the spinal cord, and the clinical findings of progressive myelopathy.
- MRI: Spinal cord edema seen as centrally located abnormal intramedullary signal (T1 hypointense and T2 hyperintense) over multiple segments; perimedullary dilated and serpiginious veins seen as flow voids on the T2-weighted images usually pronounced on the dorsal surface; chronic venous congestion with a breakdown of the blood–spinal cord barrier can lead to diffuse enhancement within the spinal cord.

■ Dorsal thoracic arachnoid web
- Thickened arachnoid septation or "web" over the dorsal cord surface results in focal deformity and anterior displacement of the spinal cord. Sometimes with syringomyelia, it is believed to be due to altered CSF flow dynamics due to the web.
- MRI: Often diagnosed incidentally and indirectly, when thoracic cord is seen focally deformed and displaced anteriorly with widened dorsal CSF column (scalpel sign). Web often not seen on routine T2 sequences and even with CT myelogram. Obtain high resolution 3D heavily T2-weighted sequence (CISS or T2 SPACE) with sagittal and/or coronal reconstructions for direct visualization of the web. Syrinx may be seen above and/or below the web.

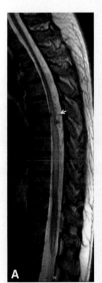 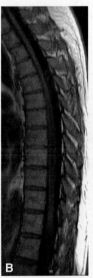 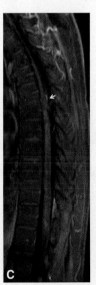 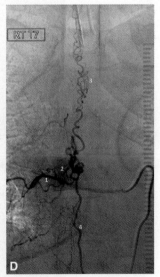

FIGURE 2-80. Spinal dural arteriovenous fistula (SDAVF). **(A–D)** Sagittal T2, pre- and postcontrast T1 magnetic resonance (MR), and spinal angiogram. Magnetic resonance imaging (MRI) shows edema of the thoracic spinal cord, perimedullary dilated veins (*arrows*), and enhancement characteristic for SDAVF. The arteriovenous (AV) shunt occurs along the spinal nerve root between radiculomeningeal artery and radicular vein. Increased spinal venous pressure from arterial shunting causes impaired normal spinal venous drainage, venous congestion, and cord edema, which leads to progressive myelopathy. Angiogram shows dilated the fistula at T7 (1: segmental artery, 2: fistula, 3: dilated perimedullary veins, 4: draining vein).

(continued)

■ **MISCELLANEOUS CONDITIONS** *(Continued)*

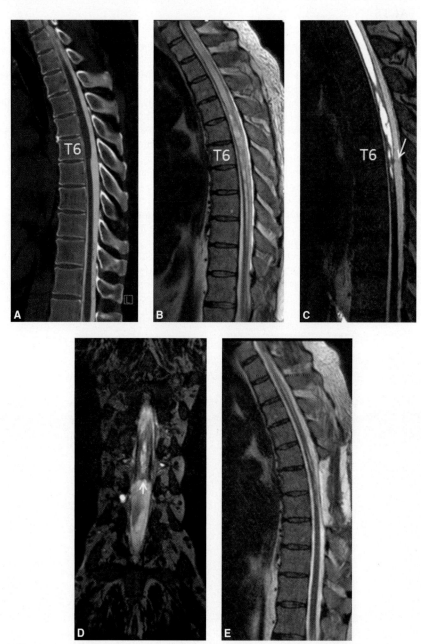

FIGURE 2-81. Dorsal arachnoid web. **(A, B)** Sagittal T2 magnetic resonance (MR) and computed tomography (CT) myelogram demonstrate diffuse thoracic syrinx, focal anterior displacement, and deformity of the spinal cord with widening of the posterior CSF column—"scalpel sign." **(C, D)** Sagittal and coronal reconstructions of high resolution heavily T2-weighted SPACE sequence demonstrate the dorsal arachnoid web (*arrows*). **(E)** Postoperative magnetic resonance imaging (MRI) following resection of the web shows resolution of the syrinx.

SUGGESTED READING

Krings T, Geibprasert S. Spinal dural arteriovenous fistulas. *Am J Neuroradiol.* 2009;30:639–648.

Reardon MA, Raghavan P, Carpenter-Bailey K, et al. Dorsal thoracic arachnoid web and the "scalpel sign": a distinct clinical-radiologic entity. *Am J Neuroradiol.* 2013;34(5):1104–1110.

■ CONGENITAL ANOMALIES

KEY FACTS

- Congenital spinal disorders include a spectrum of abnormalities.
  - Spinal dysraphism
  - Sacral anomalies
  - Caudal regression
  - Vertebral anomalies
  - Congenital scoliosis (Scoliosis; Basic Concepts)
  - Chiari malformation
  - Certain conditions may be diagnosed radiographically. MRI is the technique of choice for non-invasive evaluation of patients with suspected anomalies

■ CONGENITAL ANOMALIES: SPINAL DYSRAPHISM

KEY FACTS

- Spinal dysraphism is a general term for incomplete midline fusion of osseous and neural structures.
- Spina bifida is failure of vertebral fusion that may be occult or obvious, with skin defect and exposed neural elements.
  - Spina bifida occulta: No obvious skin defect. Isolated posterior element fusion failure. More severe forms may have spinal lipoma, diastematomyelia tethered cord (72% associated with lipoma), or thickening of the filum terminale.
  - Spina bifida aperta: Associated with meningocele, myelocele, meningomyelocele, and myelocystocele.
  - Normal conus should not extend below the L3 interspace. The adult position (above the L2 interspace) is achieved at several months of age.
  - Normal filum terminale is 2 mm or less in thickness.

■ **CONGENITAL ANOMALIES: SPINAL DYSRAPHISM**   *(Continued)*

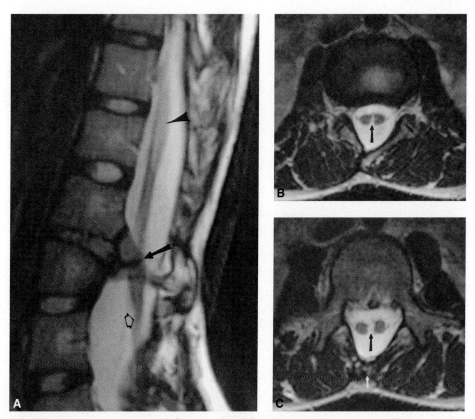

FIGURE 2-82. Diastematomyelia. **(A)** Sagittal. **(B, C)** Axial T2 magnetic resonance (MR) demonstrates diastematomyelia (*arrow*) with splitting of the cord at L2–L3. There is associated tethered cord with the tip (*open arrow*) at the conus at L4. There is also syringohydromyelia at T12–L1 (*arrowhead*) and spina bifida occulta at L5 (*white arrow*).

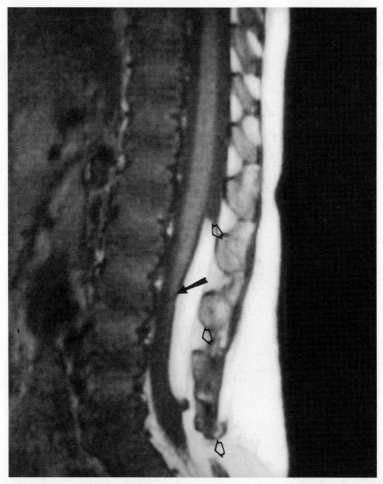

FIGURE 2-83. Tethered cord with lipoma in a 14-month-old child. Sagittal T1 magnetic resonance (MR) shows the conus as the L3 interspace (*arrow*) and an intraspinal lipoma (*open arrows*) that communicates with the subcutaneous fat.

SUGGESTED READING

Rufener RL, Ibrahim M, Raybaud CA. Congenital spine and spinal cord malformations—pictorial review. *Am J Roentgenol*. 2010;194:S26–S37.

Tortori-Donati P, Rossi A, Cama A. Spinal dysraphism: a review of neuroradiological features with embryological correlations and proposal for a new classification. *Neuroradiology*. 2000;42(7):471–491.

■ CONGENITAL ANOMALIES: CAUDAL REGRESSION SYNDROME

KEY FACTS

■ Caudal regression syndrome includes a spectrum of disorders from minimal coccygeal absence to severe absence of the distal spinal column, with anal atresia and malformed genitalia.
■ Tethered cord, meningocele, myelocele, and meningomyelocele may be associated.
■ MRI is the technique of choice to evaluate the spectrum of abnormalities.

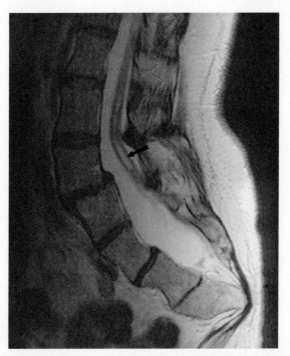

FIGURE 2-84. Sacral agenesis. Sagittal T2 magnetic resonance (MR) shows sacral and coccygeal agenesis with a tethered cord at L3–L4 and central syringohydromyelia (*arrow*).

SUGGESTED READING

Barkovich AJ, Raghavan N, Chuang S, et al. The wedge-shaped conus terminus: A radiographic sign of caudal regression. *Am J Neuroradiol.* 1989;10:1223–1231.

Boruah DK, Dhingani DD, Achar S, et al. Magnetic resonance imaging analysis of caudal regression syndrome and concomitant anomalies in pediatric patients. *J Clin Imaging Sci.* 2016;6:36.

Rossi A, Biancheri R, Cama A, et al. Imaging in spine and spinal cord malformations. *Eur J Radiol.* 2004;50(2):177–200.

■ CONGENITAL ANOMALIES: CHIARI MALFORMATION

KEY FACTS

- ■ Chiari malformation is a complex congenital disorder of the hindbrain.
- ■ There are three categories of Chiari malformation.
  - ● Type I: Adult type. Inferior displacement of cerebellar tonsils and sometimes the inferior vermis through the foramen magnum. Syringomyelia may occur because of cerebrospinal fluid flow obstruction. (By convention, tonsillar ectopia should be more than 5 mm inferior to a line drawn from the basion to the opisthion.) Associated with Klippel–Feil anomalies.
  - ● Type II: Also known as Arnold–Chiari malformation childhood. Posterior fossa is small, with displacement of tonsils, medulla, and vermis through an enlarged foramen magnum. The cervicomedullary junction may appear kinked. Meningocele or meningomyelocele and hydrocephalus are nearly always associated.
  - ● Type III: More severe. Displacement of entire cerebellum into upper cervical or occipital encephalocele.
- ■ Phase-contrast MR imaging is used to evaluate the effect of tonsilar ectopia on CSF flow in order to assess its possible clinical importance.
- ■ The presence of a syrinx often indicates longstanding tonsilar compression.
- ■ The surgical management of Chiari I malformations is widely different between surgeons and institutions. The current evidence shows good outcomes for patients with >5 mm of tonsilar ectopia and tussive headaches.

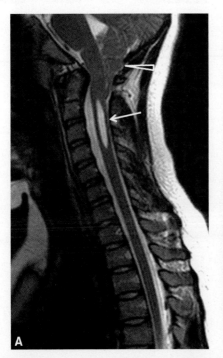 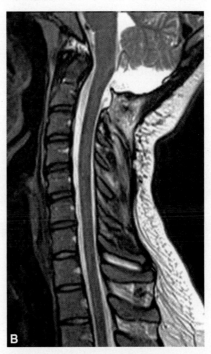

FIGURE 2-85. Type I Chiari malformation. **(A)** Sagittal T2 magnetic resonance (MR) shows cerebellar tonsils below the foramen magnum (*arrowhead*), complete loss of cerebrospinal fluid (CSF) cistern of foramen magnum and upper cervical syrinx (*arrow*). **(B)** Postoperative MR following decompression surgery shows opening up of foramen magnum and resolution of the syrinx.

(continued)

■ CONGENITAL ANOMALIES: CHIARI MALFORMATION *(Continued)*

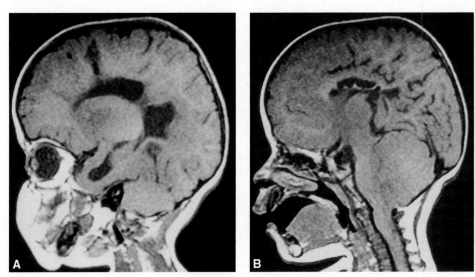

FIGURE 2-86. Type II Chiari malformation in a 14-month-old child. **(A, B)** Sagittal T1 magnetic resonance (MR) demonstrates hydrocephalus with a small posterior fossa and downward herniation of the cerebellum and medulla.

SUGGESTED READING

Geerdink N, van der Vliet T, Rotteveel J, et al. Essential features of Chiari II malformation in MR imaging: an interobserver reliability study—part 1. *Child's Nerv Syst.* 2012;28(7):977-985. doi:10.1007/s00381-012-1761-5.

Hofkes SK, Iskandar BJ, Turski PA, et al. Differentiation between symptomatic Chiari I malformation and asymptomatic tonsilar ectopia by using cerebrospinal fluid flow imaging: initial estimate of imaging accuracy. *Radiology.* 2007;245(2):532–540.

Rozenfeld M, Frim DM, Katzman GL, et al. MRI findings after surgery for Chiari malformation Type I. *Am J Roentgenol.* 2015;205(5):1086–1093.

Stevenson KL. Chiari Type II malformation: past, present, and future. *Neurosurg Focus.* 2004;16(2):5.

■ CONGENITAL ANOMALIES: SEGMENTATION ANOMALIES

KEY FACTS

■ Segmentation anomalies of the vertebrae include hemivertebra, block vertebrae, and butterfly vertebrae. Scoliosis may result.

■ Vertebral body anomalies are detected on routine radiographs. MRI may be required to exclude other spinal anomalies.

■ Bertolotti syndrome is a rare presentation of radiculopathy and/or back pain secondary to a false articulation of the transverse process of a sacralized L5 vertebra with the sacral ala.

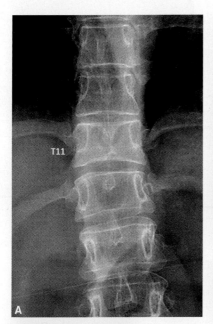

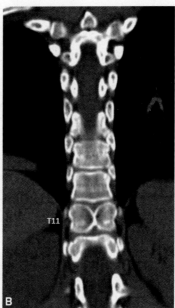

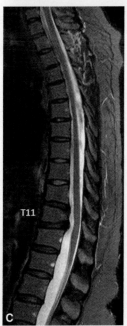

FIGURE 2-87. Butterfly vertebra. **(A)** Anteroposterior (AP) radiograph of the spine shows a butterfly vertebra at T11. **(B)** Coronal computed tomography (CT) image shows failure of fusion of the lateral halves of T11 vertebral body due to persistent notochordal tissue with some bony bridging. **(C)** Sagittal T2 magnetic resonance (MR) shows characteristic posterior wedging of the vertebral body in the median plane.

(continued)

■ CONGENITAL ANOMALIES: SEGMENTATION ANOMALIES (Continued)

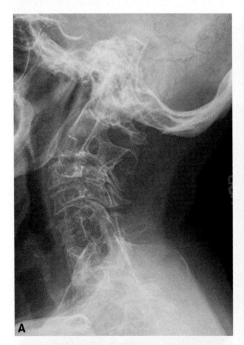

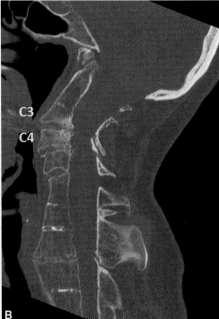

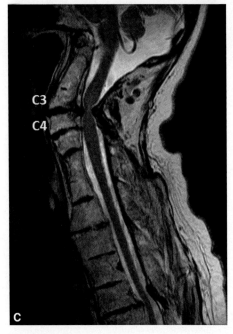

FIGURE 2-88. Klippel–Feil and platybasia. **(A–C)** Lateral radiograph, sagittal computed tomography (CT), and T2 magnetic resonance (MR) of the cervical spine show failure of segmentation of C2–C3, C6–T1, and T2–T4 vertebrae, respectively. Also note abnormal obtuseness of basal angle due to platybasia and severe spinal canal stenosis from accelerated degenerative changes at normally segmented C3–C4 level.

SUGGESTED READING

Kumar R, Guinto FC Jr, Madewell JE, et al. The vertebral body: radiographic configurations in various congenital and acquired disorders. *Radiographics.* 1988;8(3):455–485.

Nokes SR, Murtagh FR, Jones JD III, et al. Childhood scoliosis: MR imaging. *Radiology.* 1987;164:791–797.

Quinlan JF, Duke D, Eustace S. Bertolotti's syndrome. A cause of back pain in young people. *Bone Joint J.* 2006;88(9):1183–1136.

CHAPTER

3

Pelvis, Hips, and Thighs

Daniel E. Wessell, Jeffrey J. Peterson, and Thomas H. Berquist

■ TRAUMA: PELVIC FRACTURES—MINOR

KEY FACTS

- Mechanism of injury—fall or minor trauma
- Usually older age group
- Fractures of individual bones or single break in pelvic ring
- Minor fractures account for 25% of pelvic fractures
- Common minor fractures
  - Avulsion fractures (Fig. 3-1)
    - ❖ Traumatic and apophyseal in adolescents
    - ❖ Pathologic in the older age group
  - Ischial fractures
  - Pubic rami fractures
  - Transverse sacral fractures (up to 70% missed on routine radiographs)
- Complications—pain, rarely significant complications compared with complex fractures

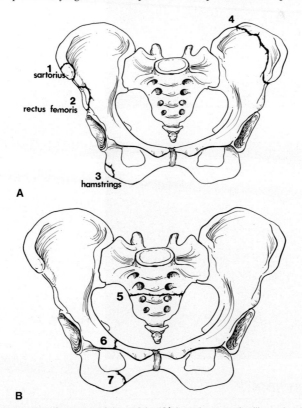

FIGURE 3-1. Common minor fractures of the pelvis. **(A)** Anterior superior iliac spine (1), anterior inferior iliac spine (2), ischial tuberosity (3), and iliac wing (4); 1 to 3 are avulsion injuries with muscles labeled. **(B)** Transverse sacral fracture (5) and isolated pubic rami fractures (6 and 7).

(continued)

■ TRAUMA: PELVIC FRACTURES—MINOR *(Continued)*

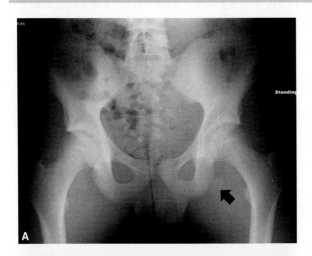

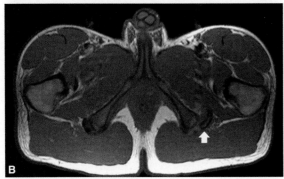

FIGURE 3-2. **(A)** Anteroposterior (AP) radiograph of the pelvis demonstrating a left ischial tuberosity avulsion fracture (*black arrow*). **(B)** Axial T1-weighted magnetic resonance (MR) image of the same patient redemonstrates the fracture (*white arrow*).

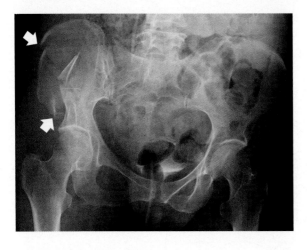

FIGURE 3-3. Anteroposterior (AP) pelvis radiograph demonstrating an isolated comminuted right iliac wing fracture (*white arrows*).

SUGGESTED READING

Bui-Mansfield LT, Chew FS, Lenchik L, et al. Nontraumatic avulsions of the pelvis. *Am J Roentgenol.* 2002;178:423–427.
Singer G, Eberl R, Wegmann H, et al. Diagnosis and treatment of apophyseal injuries of the pelvis in adolescents. *Semin Musculoskelet Radiol.* 2014;18(5):498–504.
Young JWR, Resnick C. Fractures of the pelvis: current concepts in classification. *Am J Roentgenol.* 1990;155:1169–1175.

■ TRAUMA: PELVIC FRACTURES—SINGLE BREAK IN PELVIC RING

KEY FACTS

- Mechanism of injury—minor trauma
- Usually nondisplaced pubic rami fractures involving one side
- Account for approximately one-third of pelvic fractures
- Complications—pain, local hematoma
- Magnetic resonance (MR) may detect unsuspected posterior ring injuries

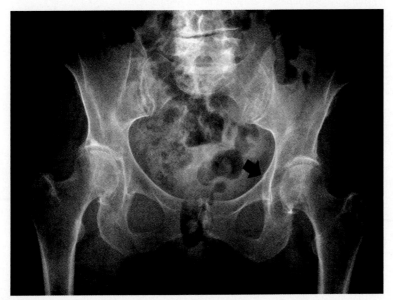

FIGURE 3-4. Anteroposterior (AP) pelvis radiograph demonstrating minimally displaced left superior and inferior pelvic rami fractures (*black arrows*) resulting in a single break in the pelvic ring.

SUGGESTED READING

Berquist TH. *Imaging of Orthopedic Trauma*. 2nd ed. New York: Raven Press; 1992:207–310.

Cosker TDA, Ghandour A, Gupta SK, et al. Pelvic ramus fractures in the elderly: 50 patients studied with MRI. *Acta Orthop*. 2005;76:513–516.

Mucha P, Farnell MB. Analysis of pelvic fracture management. *J Trauma*. 1984;24:379–386.

■ TRAUMA: PELVIC FRACTURES—COMPLEX

KEY FACTS

- Mechanism of injury—high-velocity trauma, such as a motor vehicle accident
  - Lateral compression (41% to 72% of cases)
  - Anteroposterior (AP) compression (15% to 25% of cases)
  - Vertical shearing injuries (6% of cases)
  - Combined mechanisms (14% of cases)
- Two or more breaks in the pelvic ring
- Occur in younger age group (52% are less than 30 years of age)
- Complications may be severe[*]

Hemorrhage	71%
Other associated fractures	65%
Genitourinary	22%
Neural injury	21%
Head injury	11%
Chest injury	11%
Abdomen injury	11%

- Additional imaging, specifically computed tomography (CT), is usually required to define extent of injury

[*]Total > 100% result from multiple complications.

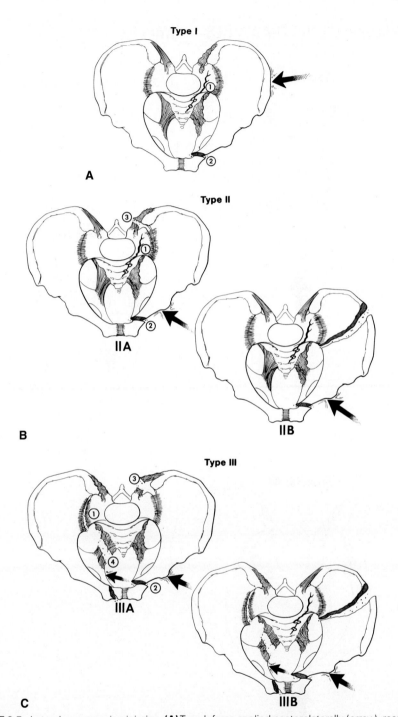

FIGURE 3-5. Lateral compression injuries. **(A)** Type I: force applied posterolaterally (*arrow*), resulting in a crush injury to the sacrum, ilium, and sacroiliac joint (*1*) and oblique or horizontal pubic rami fractures (*2*). **(B)** Type II: force directed anterolaterally (*arrow*), resulting in diastasis of the sacroiliac joint (*1* and *3*) (Type IIA) or iliac wing fracture (Type IIB) plus oblique or horizontal pubic rami fractures (*2*). **(C)** Type III: force applied anterolaterally (*arrow*) with oblique or horizontal pubic rami fractures (*2*) and involvement of both sacroiliac joints and ligaments (*1, 3,* and *4*) (Type IIIA) or sacroiliac joints and ipsilateral iliac wing fracture (Type IIIB).

(continued)

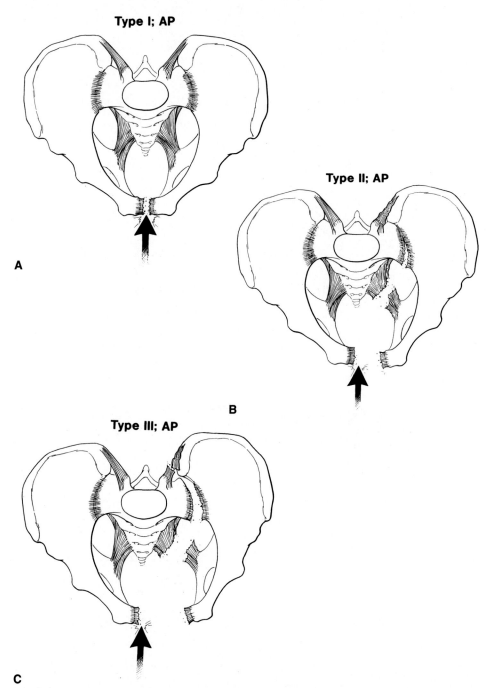

FIGURE 3-6. Anteroposterior (AP) compression injuries. **(A)** Type I AP compression injury with vertical pubic rami fractures. Sacroiliac joints are normal. Note the elevated bladder resulting from a large pelvic hematoma. **(B)** Type II: wider diastasis of the pubic symphysis or vertical pubic rami fractures with disruption of the anterior sacroiliac ligaments. **(C)** Type III: wider diastasis of the pubic symphysis or displaced vertical pubic rami fractures with disruption of both the anterior and posterior sacroiliac ligaments. **(D)** AP compression injury with vertical pubic rami fractures. Sacroiliac joints are normal. Note the elevated bladder resulting from a large pelvic hematoma (Type I). **(E)** AP pelvis radiograph demonstrating a Type II AP compression injury with diastasis of the pubic symphysis, and widening of the anterior right sacroiliac joint (*white arrow*).

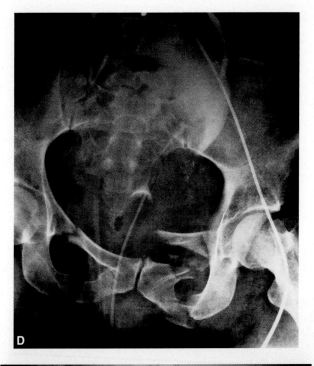

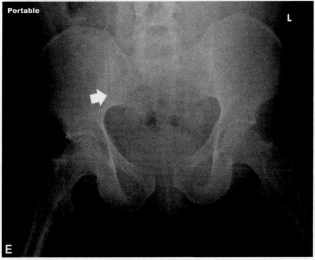

FIGURE 3-6. (*continued*)

(*continued*)

■ TRAUMA: PELVIC FRACTURES—COMPLEX *(Continued)*

Vertical Shear

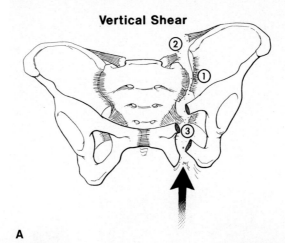

A

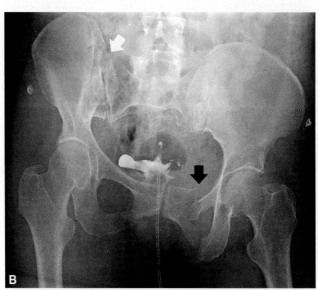

B

FIGURE 3-7. Vertical shearing injury. **(A)** Force is applied vertically (*arrow*) with vertical pubic rami fractures (*3*) or step-off at the pubic symphysis and disruption of the anterior and posterior sacroiliac ligaments (*1* and *2*). **(B)** Anteroposterior (AP) pelvis radiograph demonstrating widening and step-off of the right sacroiliac joint (*white arrow*) and vertically displaced left pelvic rami fractures (*black arrow*). Contrast and catheter in bladder from computed tomography (CT) cystogram to evaluate for bladder injury.

SUGGESTED READING

Failinger S, McGarrity PL. Unstable fractures of the pelvic ring. *J Bone Joint Surg.* 1992;74A:781–791.

Khurana B, Sheehan SE, Sodickson AD, et al. Pelvic ring fractures: what the orthopedic surgeon wants to know. *Radiographics.* 2014;34(5):1317–1333.

Young JWR, Resnick C. Fractures of the pelvis: current concepts and classification. *Am J Roentgenol.* 1990;155: 1169–1175.

■ TRAUMA: ACETABULAR FRACTURES—SIMPLE

KEY FACTS

- Mechanism of injury—lower extremity trauma with force directed to the femoral head.
- Fractures involve posterior acetabulum if hip flexed. Posterior dislocation may occur.
- Transverse and anterior fractures occur with lateral blow to greater trochanter.
- AP and Judet views may detect injury. CT with coronal and sagittal reformatting is useful to evaluate and characterize subtle fractures and the joint space involvement.
- Complications—minor, or arthrosis in later years.

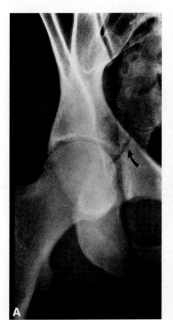 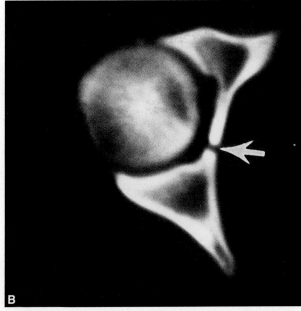

FIGURE 3-8. (A) Judet view of the hip demonstrating a nondisplaced central acetabular fracture (*curved arrow*). **(B)** Computed tomography (CT) image demonstrating an uncomplicated central acetabular fracture (*arrow*).

SUGGESTED READING

Durkee NJ, Jacobson J, Jamadar D, et al. Classification of common acetabular fractures: radiographic and CT appearances. *Am J Roentgenol.* 2006;187:915–925.
Letournel E. Acetabular fracture classification and management. *Clin Orthop.* 1980;151:81–106.

▪ TRAUMA: ACETABULAR FRACTURES—COMPLEX

KEY FACTS

▪ Multiple fracture classification systems have been proposed.

▪ Two-column, transverse with posterior wall involvement, and posterior wall fractures account for 66% of acetabular fractures. "T" and transverse fractures are the next two most common injury patterns. These five patterns account for 90% of acetabular fractures.

▪ Definition of extent of articular and anterior and posterior column involvement is critical for treatment planning.

▪ CT with reformatting in sagittal and coronal planes, or three-dimensional volume rendering, or shaded surface display is essential.

▪ Complications are similar to complex pelvic fractures (see section on Pelvic Fractures—Complex).

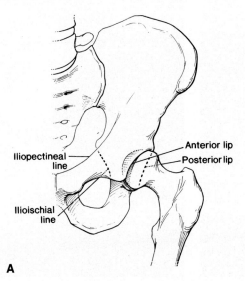

A

FIGURE 3-9. (A) Acetabular margins and the anterior (iliopectineal) and posterior (ilioischial) columns. **(B, C)** Three-dimensional shaded surface displays computed tomography (CT) images of the pelvis with electronic subtraction of the right femur demonstrating the anterior (*A*) and posterior columns (*P*). Images are obtained with 45-degree right posterior obliquity **(B)** and left posterior obliquity **(C)** like the Judet radiographic views of the pelvis.

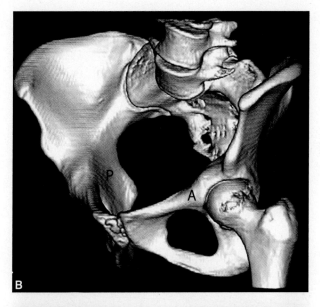

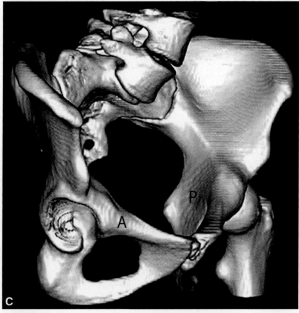

FIGURE 3-9. (continued)

(continued)

■ TRAUMA: ACETABULAR FRACTURES—COMPLEX *(Continued)*

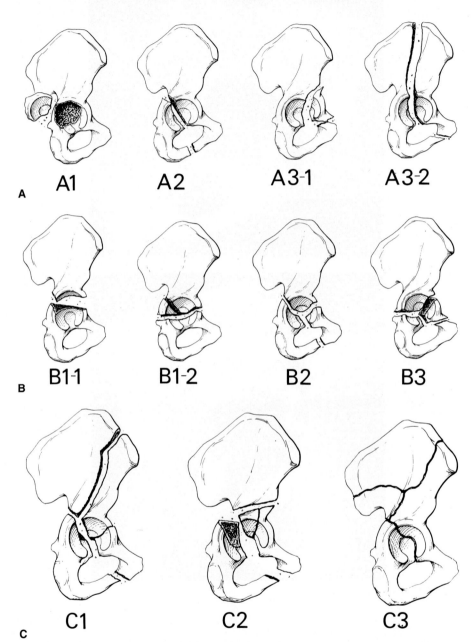

FIGURE 3-10. Fracture patterns (AO classification). **(A)** Type A: A1, posterior wall fracture; A2, posterior column fracture; A3-1, anterior wall fracture; A3-2, anterior column fracture. **(B)** Type B1-1, transverse fracture; Type B1-2, transverse with posterior wall fracture; Type B2, fracture; Type B3, anterior column with posterior transverse fracture. **(C)** Type C1, both columns with fracture extending to the iliac crest; Type C2, both columns extending to anterior inferior iliac spine; Type C3, both columns with extension to sacroiliac joint. Types A1, B1-1, B1-2, B-2, and C1 are the most common.

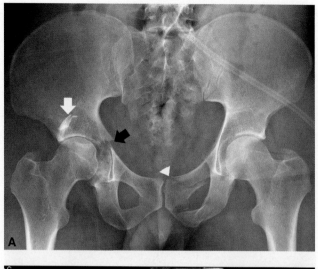

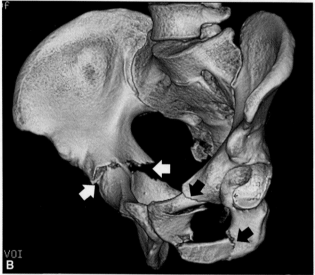

FIGURE 3-11. Complex acetabular fracture. **(A)** Anteroposterior (AP) pelvis radiograph shows a displaced right transverse acetabular fracture (*black arrow*), a displaced right posterior wall fracture (*white arrow*), and left superior and inferior pelvic rami fractures (*white arrowhead*). **(B, C)** Three-dimensional shaded surface displays computed tomography (CT) images of the fractures. The right posterior oblique view **(B)** demonstrates the transverse acetabular fracture (*white arrows*) and the pelvic rami fractures (*black arrows*). The posterior view **(C)** demonstrates the transverse acetabular fracture (*white arrow*) and the posterior wall fracture (*black arrow*).

(continued)

■ TRAUMA: ACETABULAR FRACTURES—COMPLEX *(Continued)*

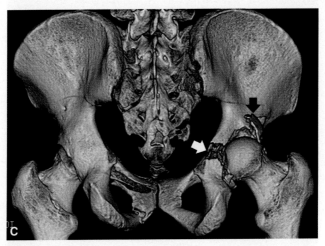

FIGURE 3-11 *(continued)*

SUGGESTED READING

Brandser E, Marsh JL. Acetabular fractures: easier classification with a systematic approach. *Am J Roentgenol.* 1998;171:1217–1228.
Saks BJ. Normal acetabular anatomy for acetabular fracture assessment: CT and plain film correlation. *Radiology.* 1986;159:139–145.
Scheinfeld MH, Dym AA, Spektor M, et al. Acetabular fractures: what radiologists should know and how 3D CT can aid classification. *Radiographics.* 2015;35:555–577.

■ TRAUMA: FRACTURE/DISLOCATION—DISLOCATION OF THE HIP

KEY FACTS

- Hip dislocations account for 5% of all skeletal dislocations.
- Mechanism of injury—high-velocity trauma, usually in young adults
  - Posterior dislocations—10 times more common than anterior. Compressive force to foot or knee with hip flexed. Posterior acetabular fractures are common.
  - Anterior dislocations—forced abduction and external rotation. Femoral head and anterior acetabular fractures are common.
- Up to 75% have multiple other injuries.
- Most complete dislocations are obvious on the AP view of pelvis or involved hip.
- CT is useful for complete evaluation of the joint space and associated fractures, especially after reduction.

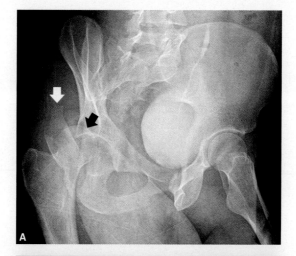

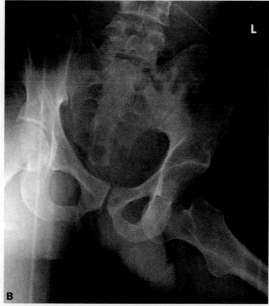

FIGURE 3-12. (A) Left posterior oblique (Judet) radiograph demonstrates posterior dislocation of the right femoral head (*black arrow*) and a posterior wall acetabular fracture (*white arrow*). **(B)** Anteroposterior (AP) pelvic radiograph demonstrates an anterior dislocation of the left femoral head.

(continued)

■ TRAUMA: FRACTURE/DISLOCATION—DISLOCATION OF THE HIP   *(Continued)*

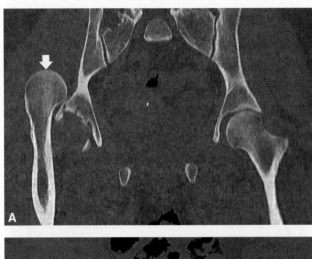

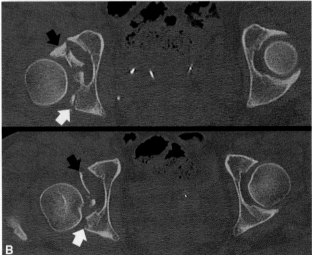

FIGURE 3-13. (A) Coronal multiplanar reformat computed tomography (CT) image of a posterior dislocation. Note the posterosuperior position of the femoral head (*white arrow*), which is typical. **(B)** Two axial CT images after attempted reduction of the posterior dislocation shown in **(A)**. Multiple intra-articular fragments (*black arrows*) from the posterior wall fracture (*white arrows*) are preventing reduction.

SUGGESTED READING

Pfeifer K, Leslie M, Menn K et al. Imaging findings of anterior hip dislocations. *Skeletal Radiol.* 2017; doi:10.1007/s00256-017-2605-x

Richardson P, Young JWR, Porter D. CT detection of cortical fracture of the femoral head associated with posterior dislocation of the hip. *Am J Roentgenol.* 1990;155:93–94.

Rosenthal RE, Coher WL. Fracture dislocations of the hip: an epidemiologic review. *J Trauma* 1979;19:572–581.

■ TRAUMA: FEMORAL NECK FRACTURES

KEY FACTS

- Occur in the elderly and in females more than in males
- Mechanism of injury—minimal trauma or fall
- Garden classification
  - Type I: incomplete involving lateral cortex
  - Type II: complete, but undisplaced
  - Type III: partially displaced
  - Type IV: completely displaced
  - Some prefer undisplaced (Types I and II) and displaced (Types III and IV)
- Imaging of subtle undisplaced fractures may require magnetic resonance imaging (MRI) for detection. Displaced fractures usually are obvious on routine radiographs
- Complications
  - Mortality: 10% to 20% in the first 30 days after injury and surgery
  - Mortality: approximately 30% first year after injury
  - Avascular necrosis (AVN) is common with displaced fractures
- Treatment—pin undisplaced and endoprostheses used for displaced fractures because of high incidence of AVN

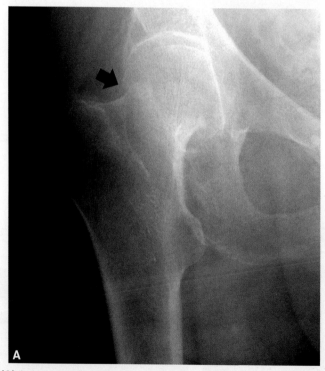

FIGURE 3-14. (A) Anteroposterior (AP) right hip radiograph demonstrates an impacted femoral neck fracture (*black arrows*) with cortical disruption and trabecular compression laterally. **(B)** Treated by percutaneous pinning.

(continued)

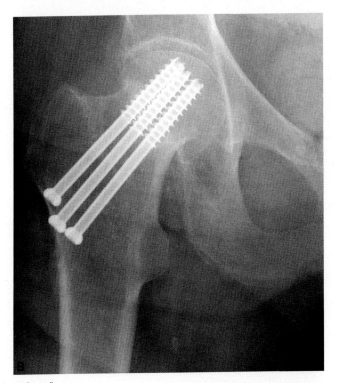

FIGURE 3-14 *(continued)*

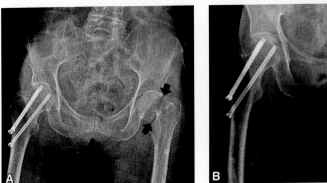 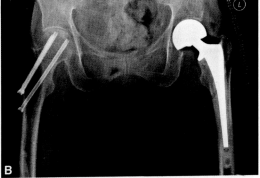

FIGURE 3-15. (A) Displaced femoral neck fracture (*black arrows*). **(B)** Treated with bipolar hemiarthroplasty. Note the prior right femoral neck fracture treated by percutaneous pinning.

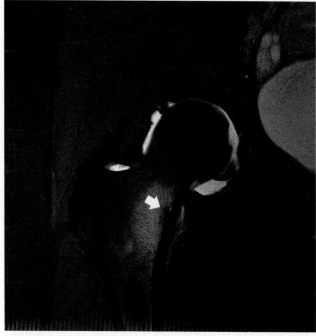

FIGURE 3-16. Femoral neck stress fracture. Coronal fast spin-echo, T2-weighted fat-suppressed image demonstrates edema with a central linear low-intensity fracture line (*arrow*).

SUGGESTED READING

Berquist TH. *Imaging Atlas of Orthopedic Appliances and Prostheses.* New York: Raven Press; 1995:217–352.

Garden RS. Stability and union of subcapital fractures of the femur. *J Bone Joint Surg.* 1964;64B:630–712.

Morgan CG, Wenn RT, Sikand M, et al. Early mortality after hip fracture: is delay before surgery important. *J Bone Joint Surg.* 2005;87A:483–490.

Sheehan SE, Shyu JY, Weaver MJ, et al. Proximal femoral fractures: what the orthopedic surgeon wants to know *Radiographics.* 2015;35:1563–1584.

■ TRAUMA: TROCHANTERIC FRACTURES

KEY FACTS

■ Three types of fracture: avulsion, intertrochanteric, and subtrochanteric
■ Intertrochanteric fractures
  ● Most common in elderly because of falls
  ● Extracapsular; comminution of fracture with detachment of trochanters common
  ● Significant mortality (18% to 30%) in year of injury
■ Subtrochanteric fractures
  ● More common in younger patients with high-velocity trauma
  ● Can be associated with chronic bisphosphonate treatment
  ● Reduction more difficult to maintain than intertrochanteric fractures
■ Avulsion fractures
  ● Caused by abrupt muscle contraction (Fig. 3-17)
  ● Occur in active athletes
  ● Greater trochanteric avulsions also seen in elderly patients
■ Routine radiographs usually are diagnostic

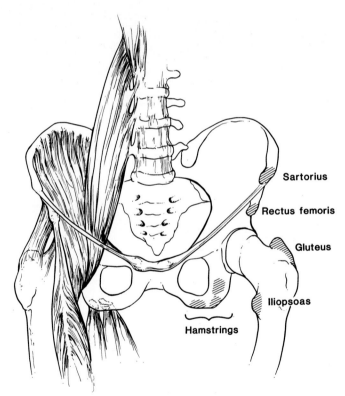

FIGURE 3-17. Sites for avulsion fractures in the pelvis and hips with muscle origins labeled.

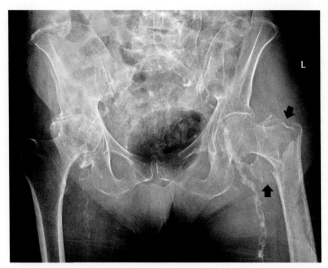

FIGURE 3-18. Anteroposterior (AP) pelvic radiograph of a comminuted intertrochanteric femur fracture (*black arrows*) angular deformity (coxa vara deformity).

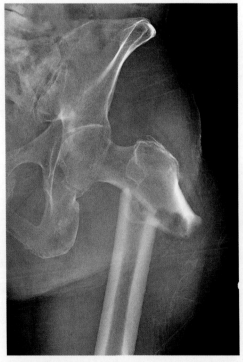

FIGURE 3-19. Anteroposterior (AP) hip radiograph of a subtrochanteric femur fracture with overriding and marked angulation of the fragments (coxa vara deformity). Soft tissue swelling lateral to the fracture is secondary to a hematoma.

SUGGESTED READING

Jensen JS. Classification of trochanteric fractures. *Acta Orthop Scand.* 1980;51:803–810.

Lorich DG, Geller DS, Nelson JH. Osteoporotic pertrochanteric hip fractures. *J Bone Joint Surg.* 2004;86A:398–410.

Porrino JA Jr, Kohl CA, Taljanovic M, et al. Diagnosis of proximal femoral insufficiency fractures in patients receiving bisphosphonate therapy. *Am J Roentgenol.* 2010;194:1061–1064.

■ TRAUMA: INSUFFICIENCY FRACTURES

KEY FACTS

■ Insufficiency fractures occur because of normal stress on bone with abnormal elastic resistance.

■ Insufficiency fractures most commonly involve the sacrum, pubic rami, and supra-acetabular regions and femoral necks.

■ Most insufficiency fractures occur in elderly osteopenic patients or patients on steroid therapy.

■ Patients present with back, hip, or groin pain.

■ Image features
  ● Radiographs: Bone sclerosis or condensation, typically linear.
  ● Radionuclide scans: Increased tracer in area of fracture. Bilateral sacral fractures give "H" appearance (Honda sign).
  ● MRI: Marrow edema pattern with or without visible fracture line.
  ● CT: Fracture lines clearly defined.

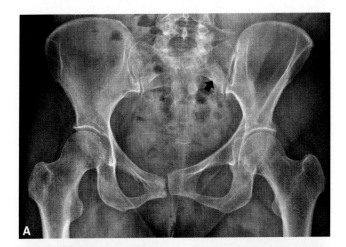

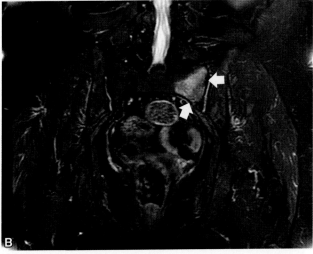

FIGURE 3-20. (A) Anteroposterior (AP) pelvis radiograph demonstrates subtle bone condensation in the left sacral ala (*black arrow*) caused by a sacral insufficiency fracture. **(B)** Coronal Short Tau Inversion Recovery (STIR) magnetic resonance (MR) image demonstrates marrow edema at the site of the fracture (*white arrows*).

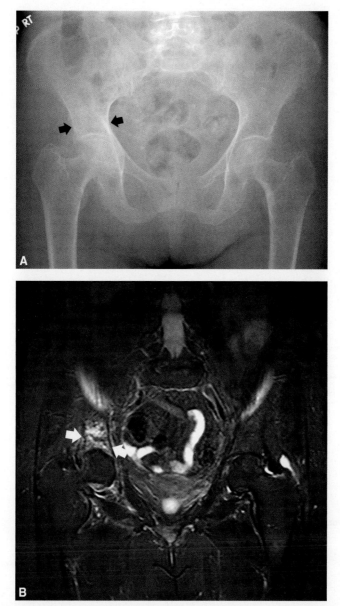

FIGURE 3-21. (A) Anteroposterior (AP) pelvis radiograph with subtle bone condensation in the right acetabulum (*black arrows*) caused by an acetabular insufficiency fracture. **(B)** Coronal STIR magnetic resonance (MR) image demonstrates a fracture line (*white arrows*) and adjacent marrow edema.

SUGGESTED READING

Cabarrus MC, Ambekar A, Lu Y, et al. MRI and CT of insufficiency fractures of the pelvis and the proximal femur. *Am J Roentgenol.* 2008;191:995–1001.

Pek WCG, Khong PL, Yur Y, et al. Imaging of pelvic insufficiency fractures. *Radiographics.* 1996;16:335–348.

■ TRAUMA: SOFT TISSUE TRAUMA

KEY FACTS

■ Soft tissue injuries to the pelvis, hips, and thighs may include
  ● Muscle/tendon injuries
  ● Ligament injuries
  ● Neurovascular injuries
  ● Acetabular labral tears
  ● Bursitis
  ● Snapping tendon syndromes
  ● Greater trochanteric pain syndrome
■ Imaging approaches vary with suspected clinical condition

Condition	Imaging Approach
Muscle/tendon injury	MRI
Ligament injury	MRI or MR arthrography of the hip for intra-articular hip pathology
Neurovascular injury	MRI
Acetabular labral tears	MR arthrography of the hip
Bursitis	Ultrasound or MRI
Snapping tendon syndrome	Tendon injection with motion studies, ultrasound

MR, magnetic resonance; MRI, magnetic resonance imaging.

SUGGESTED READING

Cvtanic O, Henzie G, Skezas DS, et al. MRI diagnosis of tears in the abductor tendons (gluteus medius and gluteus minimus). *Am J Roentgenol.* 2004;182:137–143.

Czermy C, Hofmann S, Nenhold A, et al. Lesions of the acetabular labrum: accuracy of MR imaging and MR arthrography in detection and staging. *Radiology.* 1999;220:225–230.

DeSmet AA, Fisher DR, Heiner JP, et al. Magnetic resonance imaging of muscle tears. *Skeletal Radiol.* 1990;19:283–286.

Khan W, Zoga AC, Meyers WC. Magnetic resonance imaging of athletic pubalgia and the sports hernia: current understanding and practice. *Magn Reson Imaging Clin N Am.* 2013;21:97–110.

Lonner JH, Van Kleunen JP. Spontaneous rupture of the gluteus medius and minimus tendons. *Am J Orthop.* 2002;31:579–581.

Rubin DA. Imaging diagnosis and prognostication of hamstring injuries. *Am J Roentgenol.* 2012;199:525–533.

■ TRAUMA: SOFT TISSUE TRAUMA—MUSCLE/TENDON TEARS

KEY FACTS

- Muscle/tendon tears are common in athletes and patients engaged in exercise programs.
- Underlying disorders (diabetes mellitus, steroid therapy, connective tissue diseases, and renal failure) may also lead to myotendinous injuries.
- Categories of injury
  - Grade 1 strain: a few fibers torn
  - Grade 2 strain: approximately 50% of fibers torn
  - Grade 3 strain: complete tear
  - Hematoma
  - Myositis ossificans
- Muscles involved include the hamstrings, adductors, gluteal, iliopsoas, and abdominal muscles.
- Radiographs or CT is useful for avulsion injuries or myositis ossificans.
- MRI is superior for the detection and staging of injuries.

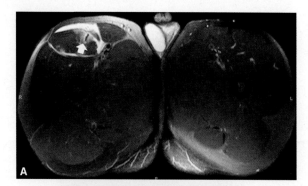

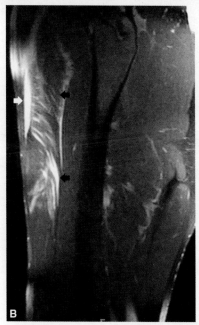

FIGURE 3-22. Axial **(A)** and sagittal **(B)** T2-weighted fat-suppressed images of a Grade 2 strain of the rectus femoris. **(A)** The muscle edema is centered at the myotendinous junction (*white arrow*). **(B)** Feathery edema extends through the muscle fibers (*black arrows*) with a small anterior hematoma (*white arrow*).

(continued)

■ TRAUMA: SOFT TISSUE TRAUMA—MUSCLE/TENDON TEARS   *(Continued)*

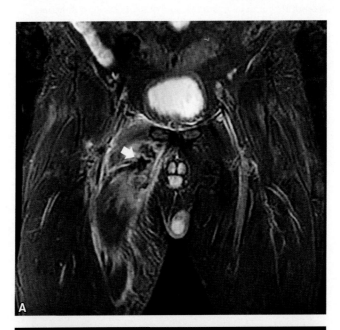

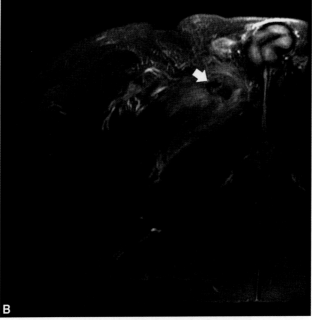

FIGURE 3-23. Coronal **(A)** and axial **(B)** T2-weighted fat-suppressed images of an adductor tendon tear (*white arrows*) with surrounding muscle edema.

SUGGESTED READING

DeSmet AA, Fisher DR, Heiner JP, et al. Magnetic resonance imaging of muscle tears. *Skeletal Radiol.* 1990;19:283–286.

Douis H, Gillett M, James S. Imaging in the diagnosis, prognostication, and management of lower limb muscle injury. *Semin Musculoskelet Radiol.* 2011;15:27–41.

Koulouris G, Connell D. Evaluation of the hamstring muscle complex following acute injury. *Skeletal Radiol.* 2003;32:582–589.

■ TRAUMA: SOFT TISSUE TRAUMA—BURSITIS

KEY FACTS

- There are 20 synovial-lined bursae about the hip.
- Bursitis from chronic tendon friction most commonly involves the trochanteric, iliopsoas, ischiogluteal, and obturator externus bursae.
- The iliopsoas bursa communicates with the hip joint in 15% to 20% of patients. Bursitis is common in patients with rheumatoid arthritis, osteoarthritis (50%), gout, infection, and prior joint arthroplasty.
- Imaging of bursitis can be accomplished with ultrasound, CT, MRI, or direct contrast injection.
- Combined anesthetic and steroid injections can be used for therapy.

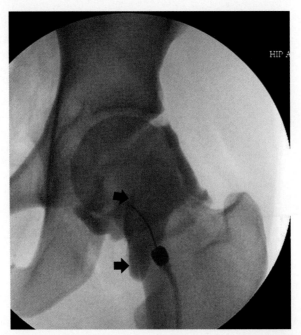

FIGURE 3-24. Hip arthrogram/injection with filling of the iliopsoas bursa (*black arrows*).

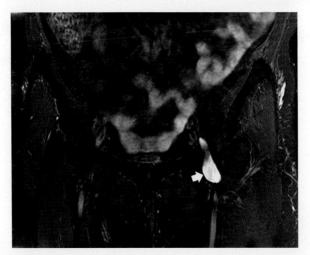

FIGURE 3-25. Coronal T2-weighted fat-suppressed image demonstrating an enlarged iliopsoas bursa (*white arrow*).

(continued)

■ TRAUMA: SOFT TISSUE TRAUMA—BURSITIS *(Continued)*

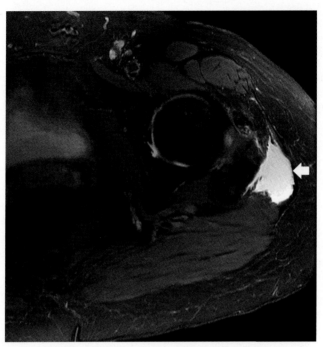

FIGURE 3-26. Axial T2-weighted fat-suppressed image of a distended trochanteric bursa (*white arrow*).

SUGGESTED READING

Bencardino JT, Palmer WE. Imaging of hip disorders in athletes. *Radiol Clin North Am.* 2002;40:267–287.

Gaetke-Udager K, Girish G, Kaza RK, et al. MR imaging of the pelvis: a guide to incidental musculoskeletal findings for abdominal radiologists. *Abdom Imaging.* 2014;39:776–796.

Robinson P, White LM, Agur A, et al. Obturator externus bursa: anatomic origin and MR imaging features of pathologic involvement. *Radiology.* 2003;228:230–234.

Wunderholdinger P, Bremer C, Schellenberger E, et al. Imaging features of iliopsoas bursitis. *Eur Radiol.* 2002;12:409–415.

■ TRAUMA: SOFT TISSUE TRAUMA—GREATER TROCHANTERIC PAIN SYNDROME

KEY FACTS

- ■ Greater trochanteric pain syndrome is common in middle-aged or elderly females, runners, and individuals engaged in step aerobics.
- ■ Pain is caused by bursitis or tearing of the gluteus medius and minimus tendons.
- ■ These tendons are analogous to the rotator cuff with an avascular zone near the trochanteric attachments.
- ■ Pain is exacerbated by lying on the affected side or stair climbing.
- ■ Differential diagnosis: Bursitis, fibromyalgia, iliotibial band syndrome, abductor tendonitis.
- ■ Radiographs show trochanteric enthesophytes in 50% of patients. Enthesophytes may cause impingement.
- ■ MRI demonstrates bursitis in 85% of patients and partial or complete tendon tears with muscle atrophy.
- ■ Treatment is conservative with therapeutic injections. Tendon tears may require surgical repair.

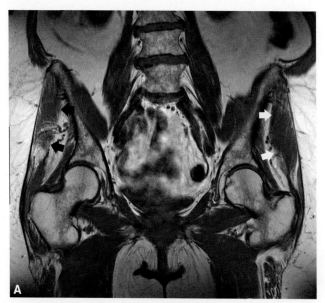

FIGURE 3-27. (A) Coronal T1-weighted image shows right gluteus medius atrophy (*black arrows*) in comparison to the left (*white arrows*). **(B)** T2-weighted fat-suppressed image shows a high-grade tear in the right gluteus medius tendon (*white arrow*).

(continued)

■ TRAUMA: SOFT TISSUE TRAUMA—GREATER TROCHANTERIC PAIN SYNDROME *(Continued)*

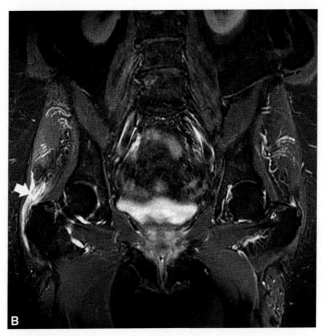

FIGURE 3-27 *(continued)*

SUGGESTED READING

Bird PA, Oakley SP, Shnier R, et al. Prospective evaluation of magnetic resonance imaging and physical examination findings in patients with greater trochanteric pain syndrome. *Arthritis Rheum.* 2001;44:2138–2145.

Kingzett-Taylor A, Tirovan PFJ, Feller J, et al. Tendinosis and tears of the gluteus medius and minimus muscles as a cause of hip pain: MR imaging findings. *Am J Roentgenol.* 1999;173:1123–1126.

Klauser AS, Martinoli C, Tagliafico A, et al. Greater trochanteric pain syndrome. *Semin Musculoskelet Radiol.* 2013;17:43–48.

■ TRAUMA: SOFT TISSUE TRAUMA—ACETABULAR LABRAL TEARS

KEY FACTS

■ The labrum attaches to the acetabular margin posteriorly, superiorly, and anteriorly. Inferiorly, it merges with the transverse ligament.

■ The labrum is triangular (69%), round (19%), or flat (12.5%).

■ Signal intensity is normally low, but internal signal intensity increases with age. Size and shape may also vary from left to right.

■ Labral detachments and tears occur. Lesions are most common in the superior and anterior quadrants.

■ Labral tears, especially detachments, may be associated with paralabral cysts.

■ MR arthrography is the technique of choice for labral evaluation.

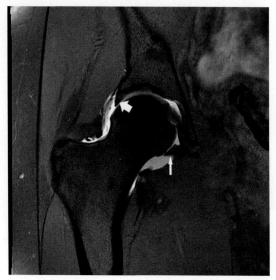

FIGURE 3-28. Coronal T1-weighted fat-suppressed magnetic resonance (MR) arthrogram image demonstrating the normal triangular shape of the superior labrum (*thick white arrow*) and the transverse ligament inferiorly (*thin white arrow*).

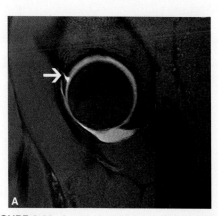
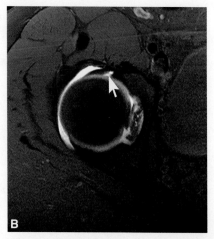

FIGURE 3-29. Acetabular labral tear. **(A)** Sagittal and **(B)** axial T1-weighted fat-suppressed magnetic resonance (MR) arthrogram images demonstrating an anterior acetabular labral tear (*white arrows*).

(continued)

■ TRAUMA: SOFT TISSUE TRAUMA—ACETABULAR LABRAL TEARS *(Continued)*

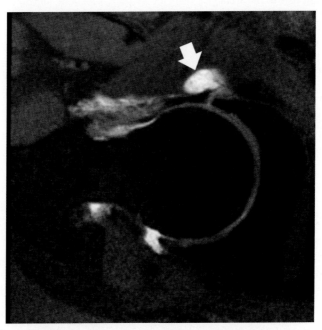

FIGURE 3-30. Small field-of-view oblique axial T1-weighted fat-suppressed magnetic resonance (MR) arthrogram image with anterior labral tear and paralabral cyst (*white arrow*).

SUGGESTED READING

Andingoz U, Ozturk MH. MR imaging of the acetabular labrum: a comparative study of both hips in 180 asymptomatic volunteers. *Eur Radiol.* 2001;11:567–574.

Naraghi A, White LM. MRI of labral and chondral lesions of the hip. *Am J Roentgenol.* 2015;205:479–490.

Petersilge CA. MR arthrography for evaluation of the acetabular labrum. *Skeletal Radiol.* 2001;30:423–430.

■ TRAUMA: SOFT TISSUE TRAUMA—FEMOROACETABULAR IMPINGEMENT

KEY FACTS

■ There are two types of femoroacetabular impingement.
  ● Cam type: Abnormal morphology of anterior head–neck junction (i.e., decreased femoral head–neck offset). Alpha angles greater than 55 degrees associated with impingement. Typically seen in young adult males. May have associated anterosuperior cartilage or labral pathology.
  ● Pincer type: Femoral head–neck junction contacts the acetabular rim because of acetabular overcoverage (e.g., coxa profunda or acetabular retroversion). Typically seen in somewhat older females. Associated with anterior labral tears/degeneration and posterior cartilage pathology.
■ Femoroacetabular impingement leads to early degenerative arthritis.
■ MR arthrography is the imaging technique of choice.

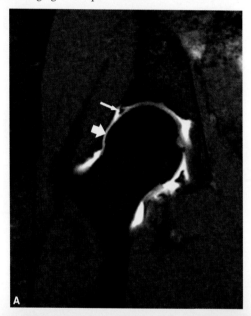

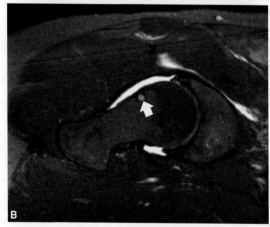

FIGURE 3-31. (A) Coronal T1-weighted fat-suppressed magnetic resonance (MR) arthrogram image demonstrates a bony prominence at the lateral head–neck junction (*thick white arrow*) causing impingement and a superior labral tear (*thin white arrow*). **(B)** An oblique axial T2-weighted fat-suppressed MR arthrogram image demonstrates decreased anterior femoral head–neck offset with a small subjacent synovial herniation pit (*white arrow*).

(continued)

■ TRAUMA: SOFT TISSUE TRAUMA—FEMOROACETABULAR IMPINGEMENT *(Continued)*

SUGGESTED READING

Kassarjian A, Yoon LS, Belzile E, et al. Triad of MR arthrographic findings in patients with cam-type femoroacetabular impingement. *Radiology.* 2005;236:588–592.

Riley GM, McWalter EJ, Stevens KJ, et al. MRI of the hip for the evaluation of femoroacetabular impingement; past, present, and future. *J Magn Reson Imaging.* 2015;41:558–572.

Siebenrock KA, Schoeniger R, Ganz R. Anterior femoroacetabular impingement due to acetabular retroversion. *J Bone Joint Surg.* 2003;85A:278–286.

■ OSTEONECROSIS

KEY FACTS

- Osteonecrosis is the general term for death or necrosis of bone and marrow elements.
  - AVN—epiphyseal or subchondral necrosis
  - Infarct—metaphyseal or diaphyseal necrosis
- Cause
  - Trauma
  - Corticosteroids
  - Sickle cell disease
  - Alcoholism

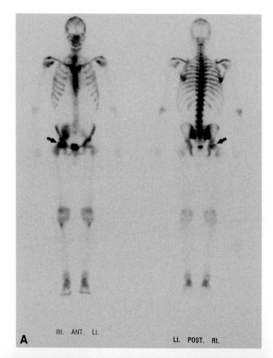

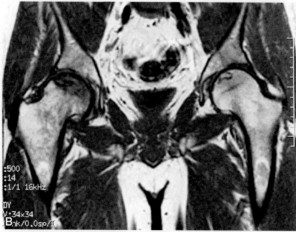

FIGURE 3-32. **(A)** Whole-body bone scan shows increased radiotracer uptake in the right femoral head (*black arrows*). **(B)** Coronal T1-weighted magnetic resonance (MR) image shows a bilateral femoral head avascular necrosis (AVN). Marrow edema on the right (i.e., replacement of the normal marrow fat on the T1-weighted image) is consistent with acute or acute-on-chronic AVN. AVN on the left appears chronic.

(continued)

■ OSTEONECROSIS   *(Continued)*

SUGGESTED READING

Jones JP Jr. Etiology and pathogenesis of osteonecrosis. *Semin Arthroplasty.* 1991;2:160–168.

Mitchell DG, Rao VM, Dalinka MK, et al. Femoral head avascular necrosis: correlation of MR imaging, radiographic staging, radionuclide imaging, and clinical findings. *Radiology.* 1987;162:709–715.

Murphey MD, Foreman KL, Klassen-Fischer MK, et al. From the radiologic pathology archives imaging of osteonecrosis: radiologic-pathologic correlation. *Radiographics.* 2014;34:1003–1028.

■ OSTEONECROSIS: AVASCULAR NECROSIS

KEY FACTS

- Early detection is critical to optimize treatment and preserve joint function.
- MRI is the imaging technique of choice, although radiographs and radionuclide scans are also useful (Table 3-1). MRI technique should assess articular and weight-bearing involvement. Sagittal and coronal imaging is especially helpful.
- The extent of articular involvement is useful for prognosis. Less than 45% of weight-bearing involvement has a good prognosis. Greater than 45% of weight-bearing involvement carries a poor prognosis, with articular collapse common (Fig. 3-33F).
- Early stages (Table 3-1) of AVN may be treated with core decompression with or without bone grafting (Stages I and II). More advanced disease (Stages III and IV) usually requires resurfacing, bipolar implants, or total joint arthroplasty.

Table 3-1   STAGES OF AVASCULAR NECROSIS

Stage	Clinical Features	Radiographs	MRI Features
0	No symptoms	Normal	Normal or uniform edema pattern ($\downarrow$ signal T1WI, $\uparrow$ T2WI)
I	May have pain	Usually normal	Same as Stage 0
II	Pain, stiffness	Mixed lucency and sclerosis in subchondral bone	Geographic zone of demarcation
III	Stiffness, groin, and knee pain	Crescent sign with cortical collapse, joint space preserved	Same as Stage II with articular collapse
IV	Severe limp and pain	Stage III plus joint space narrowing	Same as Stage III plus joint space narrowing

MRI, magnetic resonance imaging; T1WI, T1-weighted image; T2WI, T2-weighted image.

(continued)

■ **OSTEONECROSIS: AVASCULAR NECROSIS** *(Continued)*

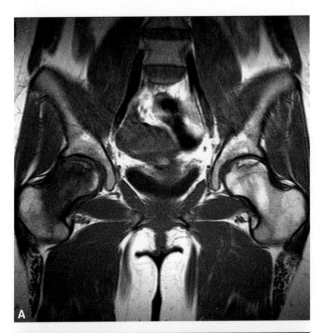

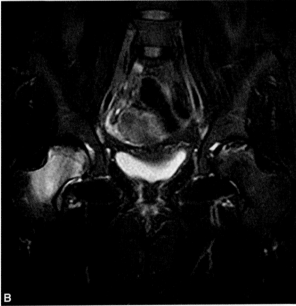

FIGURE 3-33. Magnetic resonance imaging (MRI) of avascular necrosis (AVN) (multiple examples). **(A)** Coronal T1-weighted and coronal STIR images **(B)** demonstrate bilateral AVN with greater articular involvement on the right than on the left. On the right, there is early subchondral collapse and extensive marrow edema. **(C)** Sagittal T1-weighted image in a different patient demonstrates extensive involvement of the femoral head articular surface without collapse. In yet another patient, an oblique coronal T1-weighted image **(D)** and an oblique coronal Spoiled gradient recalled (SPGR) fat-suppressed postcontrast image **(E)** show enhancement at the margin of the necrotic bone (caused by revascularization). In the final example patient, a coronal T1-weighted image **(F)** demonstrates a simple method to approximate the weight-bearing surface involvement. Angle *A* (*white lines*) is formed by lines from the center of the femoral head to the weight-bearing margins of the acetabulum. Angle *N* (*black lines*) is formed by lines from the necrotic margins to the center of the femoral head. *N*/*A* × 100% = % of weight-bearing involvement. In this case, 41°/72° × 100 = 57%, indicating a poorer prognosis.

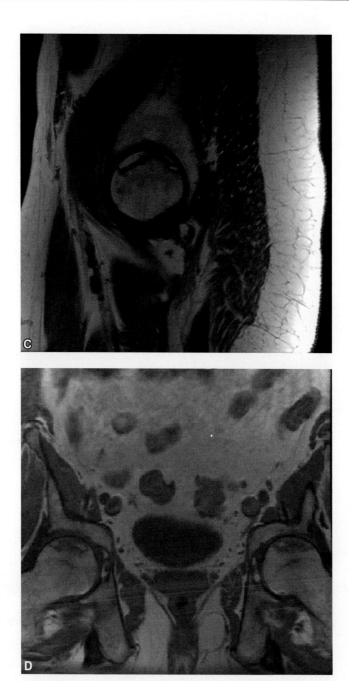

FIGURE 3-33 *(continued)*

(continued)

■ OSTEONECROSIS: AVASCULAR NECROSIS *(Continued)*

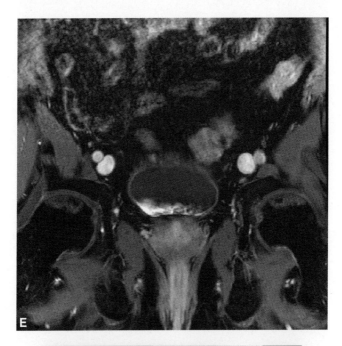

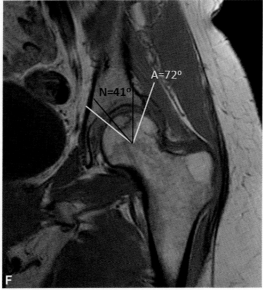

FIGURE 3-33 *(continued)*

SUGGESTED READING

Ficat RF. Treatment of avascular necrosis of the femoral head. *Hip.* 1983;2:279–295.

Karantanas AH, Drakonaki EE. The role of MR imaging in avascular necrosis of the femoral head. *Semin Musculoskelet Radiol.* 2011;15:281–300.

Koo KH, Kim R. Quantifying the extent of osteonecrosis of the femoral head. A method using MRI. *J Bone Joint Surg.* 1995;77B:825–830.

Liebermann JR, Berry DJ, Mont MA, et al. Osteonecrosis of the hip: management in the 21st century. *J Bone Joint Surg.* 2002;84A:834–853.

■ OSTEONECROSIS: BONE INFARCTS

KEY FACTS

■ Patients may be asymptomatic or present with pain.
■ Location (metaphyseal or diaphyseal) differs from AVN (subchondral).
■ Cause is similar (see section on Osteonecrosis) to AVN.
■ Radiographs demonstrate serpentine peripheral ossification at the necrotic margins.
■ MR images show a clear zone of demarcation on T1- and T2-weighted images.
■ Malignant degeneration, although rare, can occur.

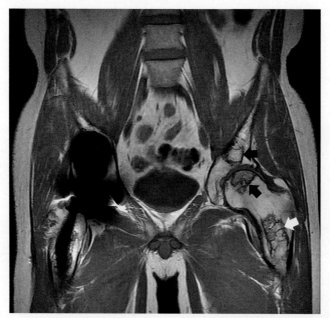

FIGURE 3-34. Coronal T1-weighted magnetic resonance imaging (MRI) showing avascular necrosis (AVN) of the left femoral head and acetabulum (*black arrows*) and an infarct in the trochanteric region (*white arrow*). Metal susceptibility artifact is seen on the right from a total hip arthroplasty.

SUGGESTED READING

Berquist TH. *MRI of the Musculoskeletal System.* 6th ed. Philadelphia: Lippincott Williams & Wilkins; 2013:204–318.
Stacy GS, Lo R, Montag A. Infarct-associated bone sarcomas: multimodality imaging findings. *Am J Roentgenol.* 2015;205:W432–W441.

■ BONE MARROW EDEMA

KEY FACTS

■ Marrow edema pattern or transient bone marrow edema may be the earliest feature of AVN, or resolve with no sequelae.

■ Radiographs demonstrate osteopenia within 8 weeks after onset of symptoms. There is increased uptake on radionuclide scans.

■ MR images show decreased signal intensity on T1-weighted images and increased signal intensity on T2-weighted fat-suppressed images involving the femoral head and neck. Lack of progression on MRI over a 6- to 12-week period is typical. Subchondral low signal intensity on T2-weighted or contrast-enhanced images suggests progression or a nontransient process.

■ Other diagnoses must be excluded.
  ● Early AVN
  ● Transient osteoporosis of the hip
  ● Infection
  ● Neoplasm

■ Conservative treatment is usually preferred unless subchondral changes are identified.

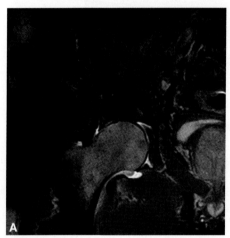 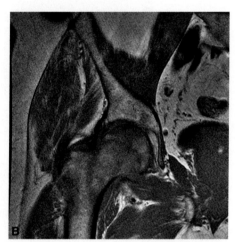

FIGURE 3-35. Transient marrow edema. Coronal T2-weighted fat-suppressed image **(A)** demonstrating high signal intensity and coronal T1-weighted image **(B)** showing low signal intensity in the right femoral head and neck caused by transient marrow edema.

SUGGESTED READING

Hayes CW, Conway WF, Daniel WW. MR imaging of bone marrow edema pattern: transient osteoporosis, transient bone marrow edema, or osteonecrosis. *Radiographics.* 1993;13:1001–1011.

Korompilias AV, Karantanas AH, Lykissas MG, et al. Bone marrow edema syndrome. *Skeletal Radiol.* 2009;38:425–436.

Van de Berg BC, Malghen JJ, Lecouret FE, et al. Idiopathic bone marrow edema lesions in the femoral head: predictive value of MR image findings. *Radiology.* 1999;212:527–535.

■ TRANSIENT OSTEOPOROSIS OF THE HIP

KEY FACTS

■ One of several conditions that presents with pain and bone marrow edema pattern (Figs. 3-33, 3-35, and 3-36).
■ Cause is unknown. Males outnumber females in the ratio 3:1; most are middle aged. Females are often affected in the third trimester of pregnancy.
■ Three clinical phases
  ● Pain, limp; lasts approximately 1 month
  ● Symptoms ease; osteopenia seen on radiographs; lasts approximately 2 months
  ● Symptoms regress; last approximately 3 months
■ Differential diagnosis includes
  ● Reflex sympathetic dystrophy
  ● Bone marrow edema
  ● AVN
  ● Infection
■ Image features
  ● Radiographs: Osteopenia in femoral head and neck after 4 to 6 weeks
  ● Radionuclide scans: Increased uptake in femoral head and neck
  ● MR images: Increased signal on T2-weighted fat-suppressed images and decreased signal on T1-weighted images in the femoral head and neck. Joint effusions are common.

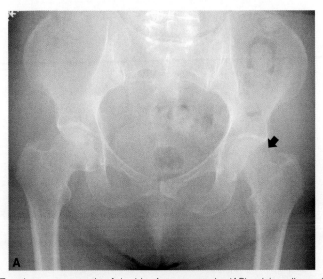

FIGURE 3-36. Transient osteoporosis of the hip. Anteroposterior (AP) pelvis radiographs **(A, B)** showing osteoporosis in the left hip (*black arrow* in **A**) during the symptomatic phase and return to normal **(B)** approximately 6 months later. Coronal T1-weighted magnetic resonance (MR) images **(C, D)** in the same patient, showing marrow edema in the left hip during the symptomatic phase **(C)** and return to normal **(D)** approximately 6 months later.

(continued)

■ TRANSIENT OSTEOPOROSIS OF THE HIP   *(Continued)*

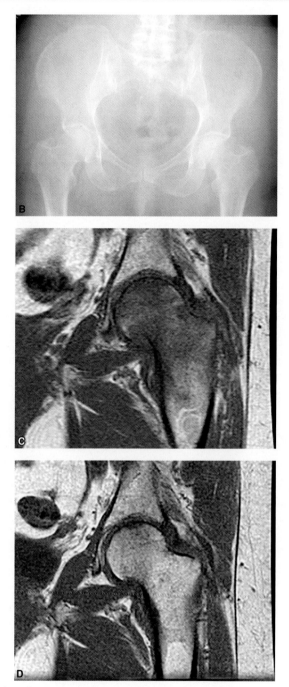

FIGURE 3-36 *(continued)*

SUGGESTED READING

Guerra JJ, Steinberg MR. Distinguishing transient osteonecrosis from avascular necrosis of the hip. *J Bone Joint Surg.* 1995;77A:616–624.

Vande Berg BC, Lecouvet FE, Koutaissoff S, et al. Bone marrow edema of the femoral head and transient osteoporosis of the hip. *Eur J Radiol.* 2008;67:68–77.

■ NEOPLASMS

KEY FACTS

■ Metastatic disease is common in the pelvis and hips.

■ Primary bone and soft tissue tumors common in the pelvic region are summarized in Table 3-2. Specific image features of neoplasms are noted in Chapter 10.

■ Routine radiographs are most useful for predicting the nature (benign vs. malignant) of osseous neoplasms.

■ MRI is most useful for characterizing soft tissue tumors and staging of bone and soft tissue tumors (Table 3-3).

■ CT is useful for evaluating calcifications, tumor matrix, thin cortical bone, and osteoid osteomas (Fig. 3-37).

Table 3-2   COMMON OSSEOUS NEOPLASM IN THE PELVIS, HIPS, AND UPPER FEMURS

Bone Tumors	
Malignant	**Benign**
Chordoma (sacrum)	Osteoid osteoma
Ewing sarcoma	Chondroblastoma
Chondrosarcoma	Giant cell tumor
Fibrosarcoma	Osteochondroma
Myeloma	Chondroma
Osteosarcoma	
Lymphoma	

Table 3-3   COMMON SOFT TISSUE TUMORS OF THE PELVIS, HIPS, AND THIGHS

Malignant	**Benign**
Liposarcoma	Lipoma
Alveolar sarcoma	Myxoma
Synovial sarcoma	Hemangioma
Epithelioid sarcoma	Benign nerve sheath tumors
Malignant fibrous histiocytoma	Desmoid tumors[a]
Fibrosarcoma	

[a]Aggressive lesions with high recurrence rate.

(continued)

■ **NEOPLASMS**   *(Continued)*

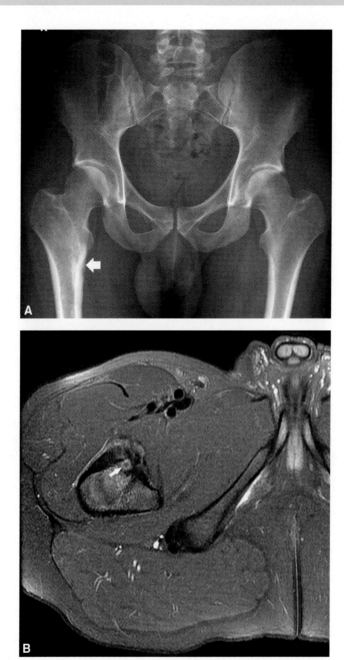

FIGURE 3-37. Osteoid osteoma. **(A)** Anteroposterior (AP) pelvis radiograph demonstrating cortical thickening/periosteal reaction of the right proximal femur medial cortex (*white arrow*). **(B)** Axial T2-weighted fat-suppressed magnetic resonance (MR) image of the nidus of the osteoid osteoma (*white arrow*) with adjacent marrow edema and cortical thickening anteriorly. **(C)** Axial computed tomography (CT) image more clearly demonstrating the nidus of the osteoid osteoma (*black arrow*). **(D)** Axial CT image with radiofrequency ablation treatment needle placed across the nidus of the osteoid osteoma.

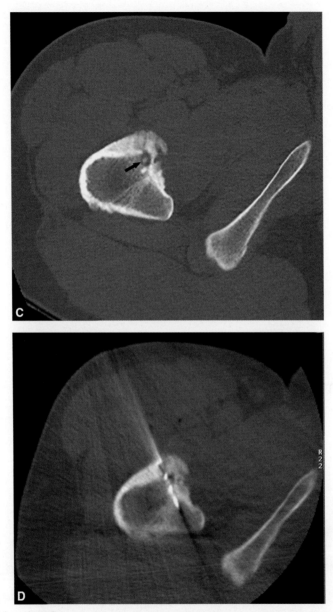

FIGURE 3-37 (*continued*)

(continued)

■ NEOPLASMS *(Continued)*

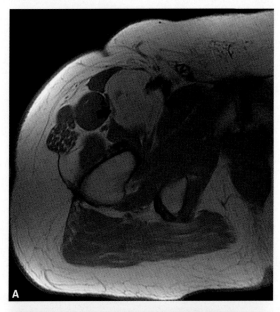

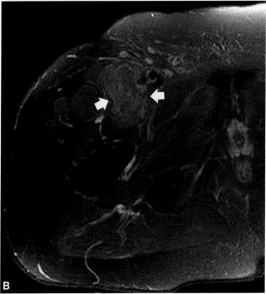

FIGURE 3-38. Atypical lipomatous tumor. Axial T1-weighted **(A)** and T2-weighted **(B)** fat-suppressed images demonstrate a fatty mass that is high signal intensity on T1-weighted images (*black arrows*) and low signal intensity on T2-weighted images (*white arrows*). No high-signal-intensity nodules or thick separations are seen on the T2-weighted images.

SUGGESTED READING

Bancroft LW, Peterson JJ, Kransdorf MJ. MR imaging of tumors and tumor-like lesions of the hip. *Magn Reson Imaging Clin N Am.* 2005;13:757–774.

Berquist TH. MRI of musculoskeletal neoplasms. *Clin Orthop.* 1989;244:101–118.

Goldblum JR, Folpe AL, Weiss SW. *Enzinger and Weiss's Soft Tissue Tumors.* 6th ed. Philidelphia: Elsevier; 2014.

Kransdorf MJ, Murphey MD. Imaging of soft-tissue musculoskeletal masses: fundamental concepts. *RadioGraphics.* 2016;36:1931–1948.

Rajiah P, Ilaslan H, Sundaram M. Imaging of sarcomas of pelvic bones. *Semin Ultrasound CT MR.* 2011;32:433–441.

Unni KK, Inwards CY. *Dahlin's Bone Tumors: General Aspects and Data on 11,087 Cases.* 6th ed. Philadelphia: Lippincott Williams & Wilkins; 2010.

■ ARTHROPATHIES

KEY FACTS

- ■ Arthropathies may affect the hips, sacroiliac joints, bursae, and soft tissue attachments about the joints (see Chapter 13).
- ■ Multiple local and systemic disorders may involve the articular structures of the pelvis and hips.

Systemic	Local
Rheumatoid arthritis	Posttraumatic arthritis
Seronegative spondyloarthropathies (Reactive arthritis ankylosing spondylitis, psoriatic arthritis)	Infection
	Synovial chondromatosis
Juvenile chronic arthritis	Pigmented villonodular synovitis
Connective tissue diseases	Paget disease
Collagen vascular diseases	Crystalline arthropathies

■ ARTHROPATHIES: THE HIP

KEY FACTS

- Joint space evaluation is a critical radiographic criterion for evaluating arthropathies.
- Joint space narrowing may be medial, axial, or superolateral (Fig. 3-39).
  - Superolateral—common with degenerative arthritis
  - Medial—posttraumatic
  - Axial—inflammatory arthropathies, that is, rheumatoid arthritis
- Osteophyte formation, bone repair or sclerosis, osteopenia, protrusio acetabuli, cystic changes, calcification, and enthesopathy are useful differentiating features.
- Key features of common arthropathies are as follows:

Condition	Image Features
Rheumatoid arthritis	Bilateral symmetric axial joint space narrowing
	Osteopenia
	Small erosions
	Cystic changes
	Protrusio acetabuli
	No osteophytes
Ankylosing spondylitis	Bilateral symmetric axial narrowing
	Osteopenia
	Ankylosis
Calcium pyrophosphate dihydrate deposition disease	Bilateral asymmetric axial narrowing
	Cartilage calcification
	Degenerative disease with multiple subchondral cysts and osteophytes
Synovial chondromatosis	Joint space normal or widened early scalloping at head–neck junction
	Joint ossifications
	Confirm with conventional or MR arthrography
Pigmented villonodular synovitis	Joint space normal or widened early erosive changes
	Increased soft tissue density or masses
	MRI confirms diagnosis
Septic arthritis	Osteopenia
	Uniform rapid joint space narrowing with pyogenic infections
	Gradual joint space narrowing with tuberculosis or atypical mycobacterial infections

MR, magnetic resonance; MRI, magnetic resonance imaging.

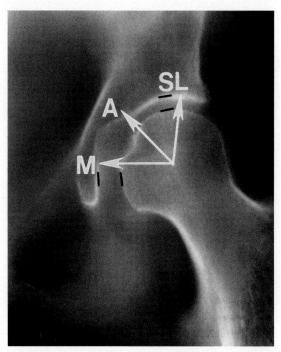

FIGURE 3-39. Normal anteroposterior (AP) view of the hip with joint spaces marked (*black lines*). Narrowing may occur medially (*M*), axially (*A*), or superolaterally (*SL*).

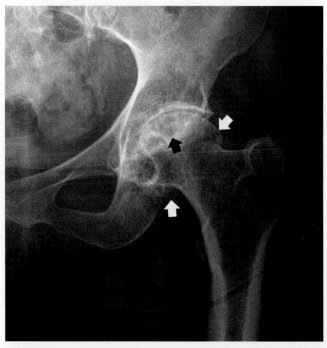

FIGURE 3-40. Osteoarthritis. Anteroposterior (AP) radiograph of the left hip shows superolateral joint space narrowing, marginal osteophytes (*white arrows*), and a subchondral geode (*black arrow*). There is bone sclerosis in the femoral head and acetabulum.

(continued)

■ ARTHROPATHIES: THE HIP (Continued)

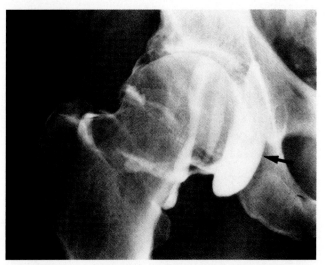

FIGURE 3-41. Osteoarthritis. Anteroposterior (AP) arthrogram shows superolateral joint space narrowing with a large communicating iliopsoas bursa (*arrow*).

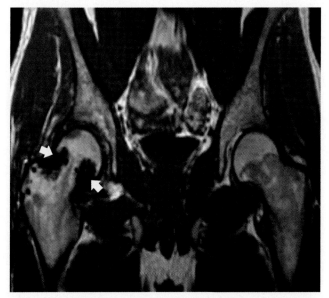

FIGURE 3-42. Pigmented villonodular synovitis. Coronal T1-weighted image demonstrates erosions (*arrows*) of the head–neck junction with lobulated low signal intensity in the capsule.

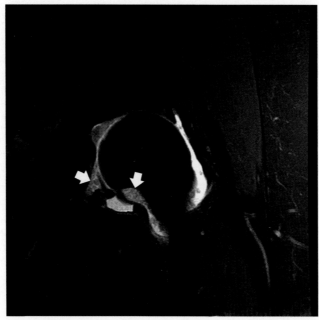

FIGURE 3-43. Synovial chondromatosis. Coronal T2-weighted fat-suppressed magnetic resonance (MR) image demonstrates a high-signal-intensity joint effusion with small low-signal-intensity structures throughout the joint (*arrows*).

SUGGESTED READING

Brower AC, Flemming DJ. *Arthritis in Black and White*. 3rd ed. Philadelphia: Elsevier Saunders; 2012:93–108.
Resnick D. Patterns of migration of the femoral head in osteoarthritis of the hip. Roentgenographic-pathologic correlation and comparison with rheumatoid arthritis. *Am J Roentgenol* 1975;124:62–74.

■ ARTHROPATHIES: SACROILIAC JOINTS

KEY FACTS

- Sacroiliac joint consists of a true synovial joint (anterior inferior 50% to 67% of joint) and ligamentous attachments.
- Joint space abnormalities include (generalization with overlap)
  - Widening and irregularity—infection, inflammatory arthropathies, subchondral resorption with hyperparathyroidism, renal osteodystrophy
  - Narrowing—osteoarthritis, rheumatoid arthritis
  - Erosions—inflammatory arthropathies
  - Sclerosis—osteoarthritis, calcium pyrophosphate deposition disease
  - Ankylosis—spondyloarthropathies
- Distribution is a useful diagnostic criterion.

Condition	Features
Ankylosing spondylitis	Bilateral symmetric irregularity or ankylosis
Psoriatic arthritis	Bilateral asymmetric erosions or ankylosis
Reactive arthritis	Bilateral asymmetric with erosions or ankylosis
Inflammatory bowel	Bilateral symmetric involvement disease
Rheumatoid arthritis	Bilateral symmetric joint space narrowing
Infection	Unilateral erosions

- Routine radiographs usually are diagnostic. CT and/or MRI are useful in selected cases.

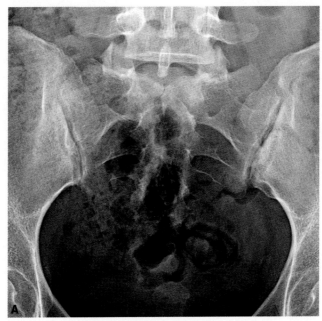

FIGURE 3-44. (A) Normal sacroiliac joints. **(B)** Bilateral sacroiliac ankylosis and spine changes of ankylosing spondylitis (fusion of the visualized spinous processes).

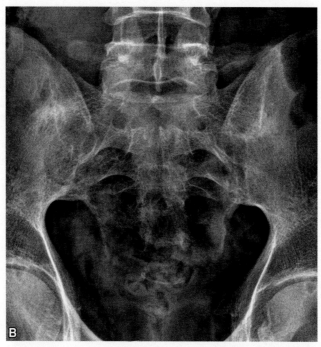

FIGURE 3-44 *(continued)*

SUGGESTED READING

Braunstein EM, Martel W, Moidel R. Ankylosing spondylitis in men and women: a clinical and radiologic comparison. *Radiology.* 1982;144:91–94.

Brower AC. *Arthritis in Black and White.* 2nd ed. Philadelphia: WB Saunders; 1997:155–174.

Brower AC, Flemming DJ. *Arthritis in Black and White.* 3rd ed. Philadelphia: Elsevier Saunders; 2012:138–154.

Navallas M, Ares J, Beltrán B, et al. Sacroiliitis associated with axial spondyloarthropathy: new concepts and latest trends. *RadioGraphics.* 2013;33:933–956.

■ INFECTION

KEY FACTS

■ Infections may involve the osseous structures, articulations, or soft tissues of the pelvis, hips, and thighs.
■ Osteomyelitis may be hematogenous, posttraumatic, or postsurgical, or attributable to extension from adjacent soft tissue infection.
■ Joint space infections may result from adjacent osteomyelitis, previous surgery, or invasive procedures.
■ Soft tissue infections usually are the result of puncture wounds, previous trauma, or surgical procedures.
■ Imaging of the suspected infection varies with the site and clinical features.
  ● Radiographs: Significant bone loss or cartilage loss is required before radiographs are positive.
  ● Radionuclide scans are sensitive but not specific, and there is less differentiation between bone and soft tissue.
  ● MRI is the technique of choice for early detection of bone, joint, or soft tissue infection.
  ● Needle aspiration or bone biopsy may be required to isolate organisms.

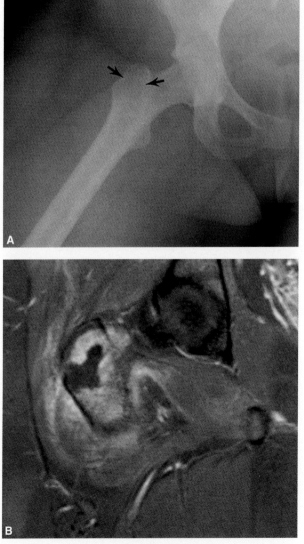

FIGURE 3-45. Greater trochanteric abscess. **(A)** Oblique radiograph shows a lucent area in the greater trochanter (*arrows*). **(B)** Coronal T1-weighted fat-suppressed image after gadolinium enhancement demonstrates an irregular lesion with peripheral enhancement.

SUGGESTED READING

Christian S, Kraas J, Conway WF. Musculoskeletal infections. *Semin Roentgenol.* 2007;42:92–101.

Gold RH, Hawkins RA, Katz RD. Bacterial osteomyelitis findings on plain radiographs, CT, MR, and scintigraphy. *Am J Roentgenol.* 1991;157:365–370.

Hayeri MR, Ziai P, Shehata ML, et al. Soft-tissue infections and their imaging mimics: from cellulitis to necrotizing fasciitis. *RadioGraphics.* 2016;36;1888–1910.

Resnick D. Osteomyelitis, septic arthritis, and soft-tissue infections: mechanisms and situations. In: Resnick D, ed. *Diagnosis of Bone and Joint Disorders.* Philadelphia: WB Saunders; 2002:2377–2480.

■ PEDIATRIC HIP DISORDERS: LEGG–CALVÉ–PERTHES DISEASE

KEY FACTS

■ Legg–Calvé–Perthes disease is an ischemic disorder of the femoral head commonly seen in males aged 3 to 12 years.
■ Most patients present between 5 and 8 years of age; 15% are bilateral.
■ Patients present with pain and Trendelenburg gait.
■ Radiographic features (AP and frog-leg oblique views)
   ● Initial features include a small capital femoral epiphysis and joint space widening. Lucent or necrotic areas may be evident in the epiphysis on frog-leg views. MRI may be confirmatory at this stage.
   ● Collapse of the femoral head and fragmentation occur in the next stage.
   ● Reparative stage with return to normal bone density.
   ● Remodeling of the femoral head and neck.
■ MRI
   ● Useful for early evaluation of unossified or partially ossified epiphysis.
   ● Physeal involvement more easily assessed.
   ● Preoperative evaluation of femoral head position and acetabular coverage.
■ Classifications systems
   ● Catterall classification based on extent of femoral head involvement on AP radiographs:
      Group I: ≤25% of femoral head involved
      Group II: 25% to 50% of femoral head involved
      Group III: 50% to 75% of femoral head involved
      Group IV: 100% of femoral head involved
   ● Herring classification based on radiographic height of epiphysis
      Group A: normal height
      Group B: 50% of normal height
      Group C: less than 50% of normal height
■ Treatment
   ● Most do well with conservative therapy.
   ● Surgical or nonsurgical repositioning of the femoral head using braces or femoral or acetabular osteotomies.

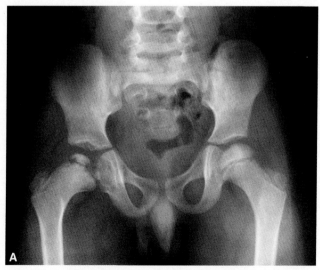

FIGURE 3-46. Legg–Calvé–Perthes disease. **(A)** Radiograph shows the right capital epiphysis is 100% involved (Catterall Group IV) with greater than 50% loss of height (Herring Group C). **(B)** Several years later, the epiphysis is still flat and irregular. Fat planes (*arrows*) are displaced because of a joint effusion. **(C)** Four years later, the physis is closed with flattening and widening of the femoral head and neck on the right.

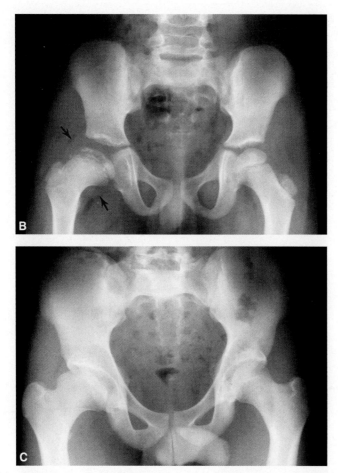

FIGURE 3-46 (continued)

(continued)

■ **PEDIATRIC HIP DISORDERS: LEGG–CALVÉ–PERTHES DISEASE** *(Continued)*

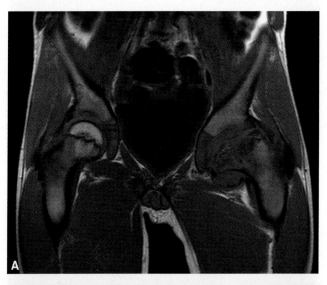

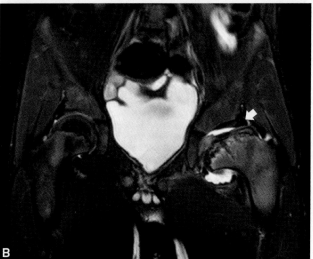

FIGURE 3-47. Coronal T1- **(A)** and T2- **(B)** weighted images of a child with Legg–Calvé–Perthes disease on the left. There is an effusion on the left and central necrosis of the epiphysis. Note the enlarged superior labrum (*arrow* in **B**) and the broad femoral head and neck compared with the right.

SUGGESTED READING

Catterall A. Legg–Calvé–Perthes disease. RSNA Instructional Course Lecture. Chicago, Illinois, 1989;9:19–22.

Dillman JR, Hernandez RJ. MRI of Legg–Calvé–Perthes disease. *Am J Roentgenol.* 2009;193:1394–1407.

Hochbergs P, Echewall G, Egund N, et al. Femoral head shape in Legg–Calvé–Perthes disease. Correlation between conventional radiography, arthrography, and MR imaging. *Acta Radiol.* 1994;35:545–548.

Weishaupt D, Exner GU, Hilfiker PR, et al. Dynamic MR imaging of the hip in Legg–Calvé–Perthes disease: comparison with arthrography. *Am J Roentgenol.* 2000;174:1635–1637.

■ PEDIATRIC HIP DISORDERS: DEVELOPMENTAL DYSPLASIA OF THE HIP

KEY FACTS

■ Developmental dysplasia of the hip is more common in females than in males (5:1 to 9:1, respectively) and is more common in whites than in African Americans. Up to 33% of cases are bilateral.

■ Cause is related to ligament laxity, intrauterine position, high levels of maternal estrogen, and hereditary considerations.

■ Joint laxity in newborns is common, so diagnosis is difficult before 2 to 4 weeks of age.
  ● Early detection and reduction can result in normal development in 95% of cases.

■ Imaging approaches
  ● Ultrasound—to access clinically suspected subluxation/dislocation. Ultrasound is most useful until femoral head ossifies at 6 months (normal ossification: 2 to 6 months in females and 3 to 7 months in males). Evaluate femoral head size and position, acetabular roof, and joint stability.
  ● Radiographs (AP and frog-leg obliques)—smaller femoral ossification center, superolateral displacement of femur. Acetabular angle: normal 28 degrees at birth decreasing to 22 ± 5 degrees by 1 year. Angle is increased in dysplastic hips (Fig. 3-48A). Shenton line forms a smooth arc along the superior pubic ramus and femoral neck in the normal hip. The arc is interrupted in dysplastic hips (Fig. 3-48A). Features become more obvious with age. Perkin line is perpendicular to Hilgenreiner line (line through triradiate cartilage). This divides the hip into quadrants. The femoral head or medial metaphyseal beak should lie in the inferior medial quadrant (Fig. 3-48B).
  ● MRI—useful for identification of unossified femoral head, labrum, and acetabular structures. Complications such as AVN can be identified.

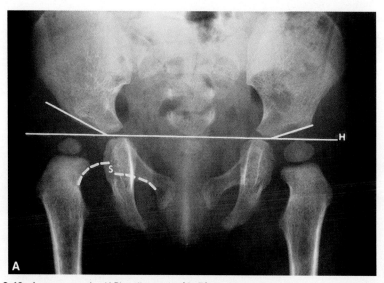

FIGURE 3-48. Anteroposterior (AP) radiographs **(A, B)** demonstrating developmental dysplasia on the right. The acetabular angle (*line* along acetabulum to Hilgenreiner line [*H*]) is increased, and the hip is displaced superolaterally with interruption of Shenton line (*S*) (*broken white lines*). The femoral head should lie in the inferomedial (*im*) quadrant. Four quadrants (im, inferomedial; il, inferolateral; sl, superolateral; sm, superomedial) are formed by a line (Perkins line) at the acetabular margin perpendicular to Hilgenreiner line. The femoral head is out of the im quadrant in **(B)**.

(continued)

■ PEDIATRIC HIP DISORDERS: DEVELOPMENTAL DYSPLASIA OF THE HIP   *(Continued)*

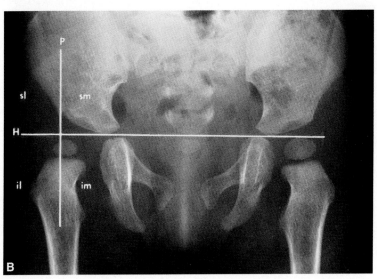

FIGURE 3-48 *(continued)*

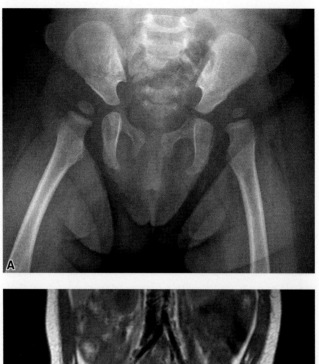

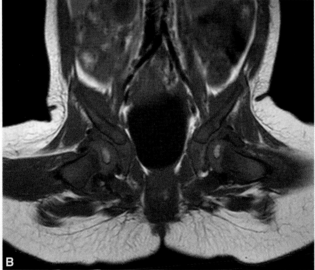

FIGURE 3-49. Anteroposterior (AP) pelvis radiograph **(A)** of a 1-year-old demonstrating bilateral developmental hip dysplasia with dislocation of the femoral heads. Oblique coronal T1-weighted magnetic resonance (MR) image **(B)** in the frog-leg position (patient in a Spica cast) shows relocation of both femoral heads.

(continued)

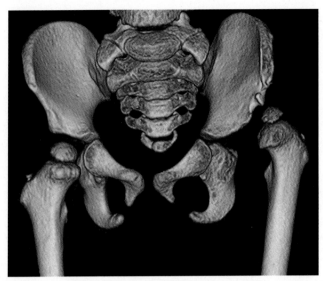

FIGURE 3-50. Three-dimensional shaded surface displays computed tomography (CT) image demonstrating left developmental hip dysplasia with shallow acetabular roof and posterior superior dislocation of the femoral head.

SUGGESTED READING

Hubbard AM, Dormans JP. Evaluation of developmental dysplasia, Perthe's disease, and neuromuscular dysplasia of the hip before and after surgery: an imaging update. *Am J Roentgenol.* 1995;164:1062–1073.

Keller MS, Nijs EL. The role of radiographs and US in developmental dysplasia of the hip: how good are they? *Pediatr Radiol.* 2009;39:S211–S215.

Weinstein SL, Mubarak SJ, Wenger DR. Developmental hip dysplasia and dislocation. *J Bone Joint Surg.* 2003;85A:2024–2035.

■ PEDIATRIC HIP DISORDERS: SLIPPED CAPITAL FEMORAL EPIPHYSIS

KEY FACTS

- Slipped capital femoral epiphysis (SCFE) is the most common adolescent hip disorder. It frequently leads to early osteoarthritis.
- SCFE is twice as common in males as in females.
- Males present at ages 10 to 17 years (most common 13 to 14 years), and females present at 8 to 15 years (most common 11 to 12 years). African Americans are affected more commonly than whites.
- The condition is bilateral in 23% to 81%.
- Patients present with pain and a limp.
- Classification of SCFE is based on clinical and radiographic criteria:
  - Preslip: Weakness with thigh or knee pain. Radiographs show slight physeal widening.
  - Acute: Slip of capital epiphysis is mild, moderate, or severe, depending on displacement.
  - Chronic: Displaced femoral head with remodeling and degenerative joint disease.
- Imaging evaluation
- Radiographs
  - Posterior displacement is most common initially (99%).
  - Medial displacement occurs commonly.
  - Signs of slipped epiphysis include
    - ✧ Osteopenia
    - ✧ Irregular or widened physis
    - ✧ A line drawn along the lateral femoral neck should intersect the capital epiphysis so that one-sixth of the head lies lateral to the line on an AP radiograph.
    - ✧ Femoral head should be symmetrically positioned to the metaphysis on the frog-leg view.
- CT/MRI
  - Useful for early physeal changes and articular anatomy in selected cases.
- Treatment—pin fixation
- Complications—osteoarthritis, chondrolysis, and AVN

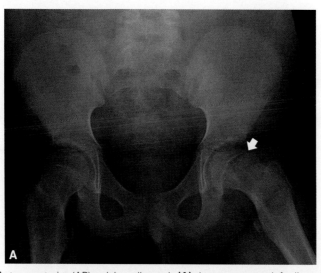

FIGURE 3-51. Anteroposterior (AP) pelvic radiograph **(A)** demonstrates a left slipped capital femoral epiphysis (SCFE, *white arrow*). The frog-leg view of the left hip **(B)** better demonstrates the severity (*black arrow*) of the SCFE. Follow-up frog-leg view **(C)** after pinning in place.

(continued)

■ PEDIATRIC HIP DISORDERS: SLIPPED CAPITAL FEMORAL EPIPHYSIS *(Continued)*

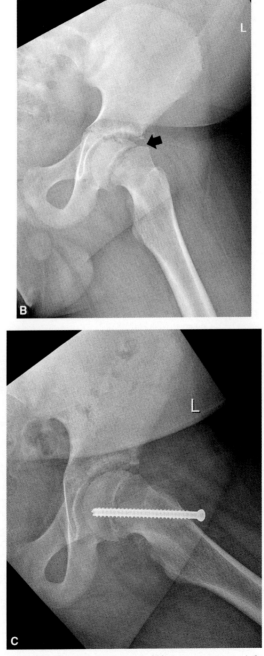

FIGURE 3-51. Anteroposterior (AP) pelvic radiograph **(A)** demonstrates a left slipped capital femoral epiphysis (SCFE, *white arrow*). The frog-leg view of the left hip **(B)** better demonstrates the severity (*black arrow*) of the SCFE. Follow-up frog-leg view **(C)** after pinning in place.

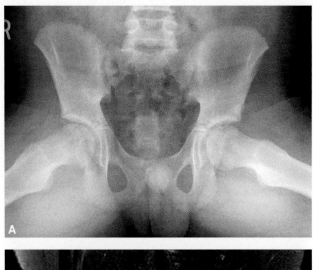

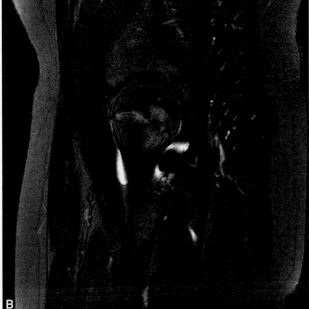

FIGURE 3-52. Anteroposterior (AP) bilateral frog-leg lateral radiograph **(A)** demonstrating a right slipped capital epiphysis. Sagittal T2-weighted fat-suppressed magnetic resonance (MR) image **(B)** of the same patient demonstrates widening of the physis anteriorly with periphyseal edema and slight posterior angulation of the femoral head.

SUGGESTED READING

Boles CA, El-Khoury GY. Slipped capital femoral epiphysis. *Radiographics.* 1997;17:809–823.

Futami T, Suzuki S, Seto Y, et al. Sequential magnetic resonance imaging in slipped capital femoral epiphysis: assessment of preslip of the contralateral hip. *J Pediatr Orthop.* 2001;10:298–303.

Jarrett DY, Matheney T, Kleinman PK. Imaging SCFE: diagnosis, treatment and complications. *Pediatr Radiol.* 2013;43:S71–S82.

Umans H, Lieblings MS, Moy L, et al. Slipped capital femoral epiphysis: a physeal lesion diagnosed by MRI with radiographic and CT correlation. *Skeletal Radiol.* 1998;27:139–144.

■ PEDIATRIC HIP DISORDERS: ROTATIONAL/ORIENTATION ABNORMALITIES—COXA VARA AND COXA VALGA

KEY FACTS

■ The normal angle between the femoral neck and shaft is 150 degrees at birth. The angle decreases to 120 to 135 degrees in adults.

■ Coxa vara is reduced at neck–shaft angle.
  ● Congenital because of abnormal limb position. Minimal progression after birth.
  ● Acquired from trauma, tumors, dysplasias, and osteopenia.
  ● Acquired coxa vara is bilateral in 50% of cases. Changes lead to minimal leg-length discrepancy.

■ Coxa valga is an increased neck–shaft angle.
  ● Usually the result of neuromuscular disorders (i.e., polio, cerebral palsy)

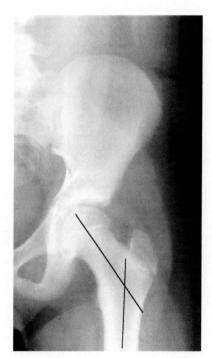

FIGURE 3-53. Normal femoral neck angle (*lines*) seen on anteroposterior (AP) radiograph.

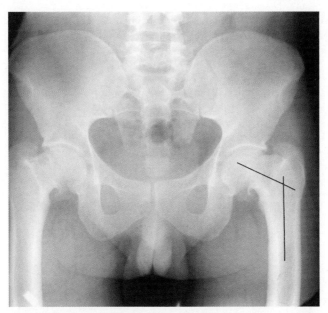

FIGURE 3-54. Coxa vara. Anteroposterior (AP) view of the hips in a patient with healed slipped capital femoral epiphyses showing a decreased femoral neck angle (*lines*).

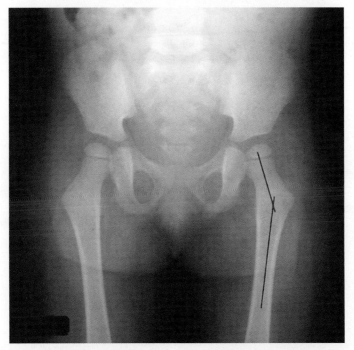

FIGURE 3-55. Coxa valga. Child with thalassemia and increased femoral neck angle (*lines*).

(continued)

■ PEDIATRIC HIP DISORDERS: ROTATIONAL/ORIENTATION ABNORMALITIES—FEMORAL ANTEVERSION

KEY FACTS

■ Femoral anteversion is the angle formed between a line drawn along the axis of the femoral neck and distal condylar orientation.

■ Femoral anteversion is 32 degrees at birth and decreases to 16 degrees at age 16 years and older.

■ An increased angle is seen in children with hip dysplasia and cerebral palsy.

■ Retroversion or a decreased angle may lead to SCFE.

■ Imaging can be accomplished using selected CT or MRI of the femoral head and neck and femoral condyles.

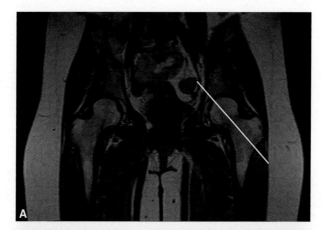

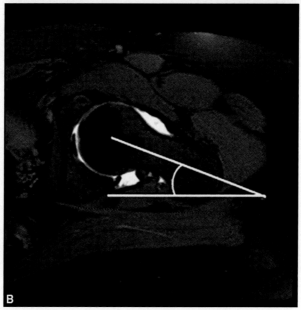

FIGURE 3-56. Femoral anteversion measurement. **(A)** Coronal magnetic resonance (MR) image demonstrating angle of acquisition (*line*) of oblique axial image in **(B)**. Oblique axial MR image **(B)** of the left hip with line through the central axis of the neck and horizontal line forming an angle. **(C)** Axial image of the knee. A line is drawn along the posterior condyles, and an angle is formed with a horizontal line. The angle in **(C)** is added to the angle in **(B)** to find the angle between the femoral neck and the posterior condylar line of the knee (i.e., the femoral anteversion).

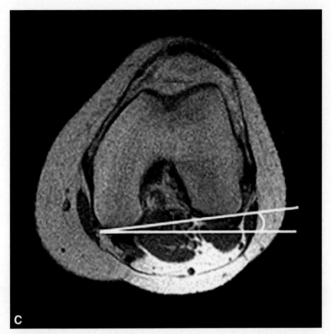

FIGURE 3-56 *(continued)*

SUGGESTED READING

Jarrett DY, Oliveira AM, Zou KH, et al. Technical innovation. Axial oblique CT to assess femoral anteversion. *Am J Roentgenol.* 2010;194:1230–1233.

Sutter R, Dietrich TJ, Zingg PO, et al. Assessment of femoral antetorsion with MRI: comparison of oblique measurements to standard transverse measurements. *Am J Roentgenol.* 2015;205:130–135.

Tomozak RJ, Guenther DP, Rieber A, et al. MR imaging measurement of the femoral anteversion angle as a new technique. Comparison with CT in children and adults. *Am J Roentgenol* 1997;168:791–794.

Knee

Thomas Magee, Jeffrey J. Peterson, and Thomas H. Berquist

■ SKELETAL TRAUMA: OSTEOCHONDRAL FRACTURES

KEY FACTS

- Fractures involving the joint surface result from direct blows or shearing forces.
- Fractures may be subtle, requiring computed tomography (CT) or magnetic resonance imaging (MRI) for detection.
- Osteochondral patellar fractures are commonly associated with dislocation.
- Associated soft tissue injury is common.

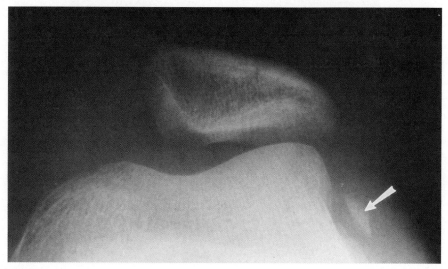

FIGURE 4-1. Patellar view demonstrates subluxation after reduction of a patellar dislocation. There is a displaced osteochondral fragment (*arrow*) laterally.

SUGGESTED READING

Capps GW, Hayes CW. Easily missed injuries about the knee. *Radiographics.* 1994;14:1191–1210.

Dezell PB, Schils JP, Recht MP. Subtle fractures about the knee: innocuous-appearing yet indicative of internal derangement. *Am J Roentgenol.* 1996;167:699–703.

■ SKELETAL TRAUMA: PATELLAR FRACTURES

KEY FACTS

- Patellar fractures account for 1% of all skeletal fractures.
- The mechanism of injury is direct trauma (motor vehicle accidents 28% and falls 68%) or indirect trauma (4%), such as quadriceps contraction.
- Types of patellar fracture: Transverse or oblique 34%; comminuted 16%; longitudinal 28%; apical or basal 28%.
- A bipartite patella most commonly involves the upper outer quadrant. It is usually often bilateral and should not be confused with a fracture.
- Routine radiographs (anteroposterior [AP], lateral, and patellar views) are usually diagnostic.
- Treatment includes reduction with internal fixation for displaced fractures. Fractures with less than 2 to 3 mm of displacement and articular surface congruency can be treated conservatively (casting). Badly comminuted fractures may require partial or complete patellectomy.
- Complications
  - Osteoarthritis
  - Nonunion

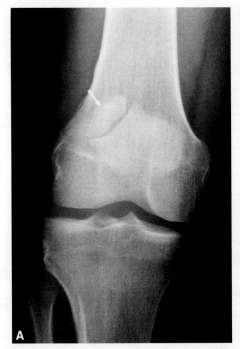 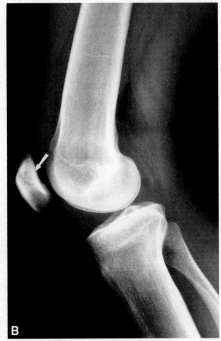

FIGURE 4-2. Anteroposterior (AP) **(A)** and lateral **(B)** radiographs of a bipartite patella (*arrow*).

(continued)

■ SKELETAL TRAUMA: PATELLAR FRACTURES *(Continued)*

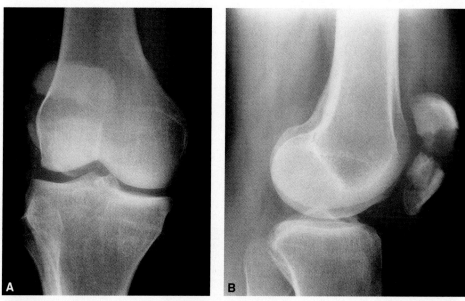

FIGURE 4-3. Anteroposterior (AP) **(A)** and lateral **(B)** radiographs of a comminuted displaced patellar fracture.

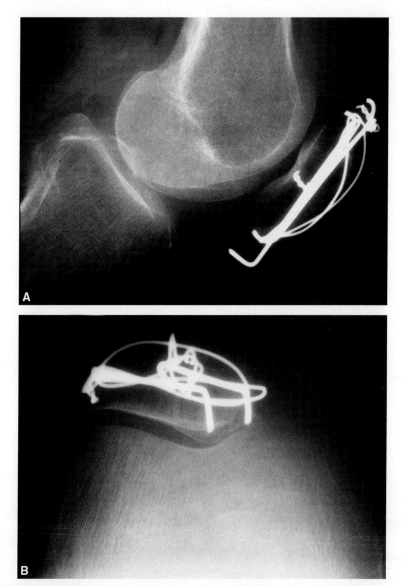

FIGURE 4-4. Lateral **(A)** and patellar **(B)** views after reduction with K-wires and tension band. The articular surface is reduced.

SUGGESTED READING

Bostrom A. Fracture of the patella. *Acta Orthop Scand Suppl.* 1972;143:1–80.
Walker CW, Moore TE. Imaging of skeletal and soft tissue injuries in and around the knee. *Radiol Clin North Am.* 1997;35(3):631–653.

▪ SKELETAL TRAUMA: SUPRACONDYLAR FRACTURES

KEY FACTS

▪ Supracondylar fractures involve the distal 9 cm of the femur. Fractures of the distal femur account for 7% of all femoral fractures. Open injuries account for 5% to 10%.

▪ Intra-articular extension is common. These complex fractures are difficult to manage.

▪ Associated tibial plateau fractures are common.

▪ Mechanisms of injury include minor trauma to the flexed knee in elderly patients and high-velocity forces applied to the anterolateral, lateral, or medial aspect of the knee.

▪ Routine radiographs (AP and lateral) are diagnostic.

▪ Treatment may be conservative (casting or traction) or operative to reduce and achieve restoration of the joint and leg length.

▪ Complications:

Early	Late
Vascular injury	Infection
Infection	Nonunion
1% of closed	Malunion
20% of open	Osteoarthritis
Failed reduction	

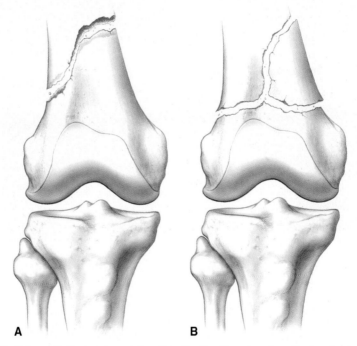

A   **B**

FIGURE 4-5. Orthopedic Trauma Association Classification. Type A: extra-articular, simple **(A)** or comminuted **(B)**. Type B: partial articular, one condyle involved **(C)**. Type C: complete articular, both condyles involved with "Y" pattern **(D)** or severely comminuted **(E)**.

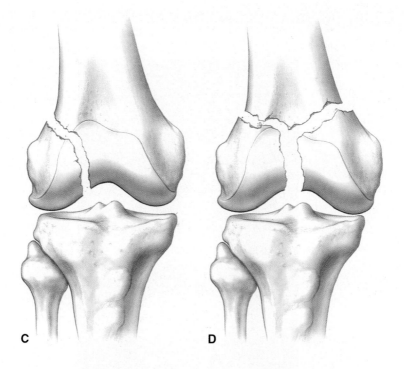

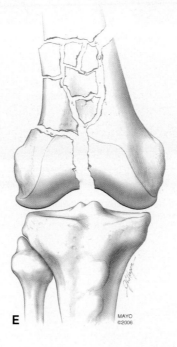

FIGURE 4-5. (*continued*)

(*continued*)

■ SKELETAL TRAUMA: SUPRACONDYLAR FRACTURES *(Continued)*

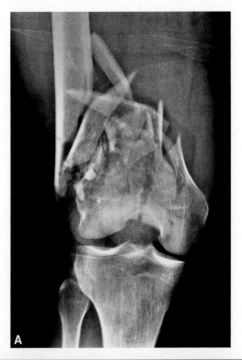

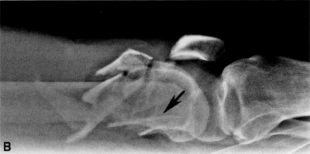

FIGURE 4-6. Anteroposterior (AP) **(A)** and lateral **(B)** radiographs of a severely comminuted complete articular fracture. Note the loss of length and posterior rotation (*arrow*) of the distal fragment in **(B)**.

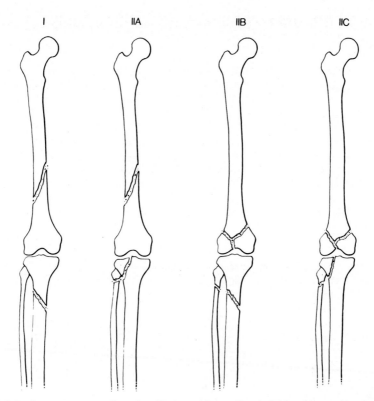

FIGURE 4-7. Ipsilateral fractures of the tibia, fibula, and femur. Type I: tibial and femoral fractures without knee involvement (71% of cases). Type IIA: femoral fracture with tibial articular involvement (16.5% of cases). Type IIB: femoral articular involvement and proximal tibia and fibular fractures. Type IIC: both articular surfaces involved (8% of cases).

SUGGESTED READING

Fraser RD, Hunter GA, Waddle JP. Ipsilateral fractures of the femur and tibia. *J Bone Joint Surg.* 1978;60B:510–515.

O'Brien P, Meek RN, Blachut PA, et al. Fractures of the distal femur. In: Bucholz RW, Heckman JD, eds. *Rockwood and Green's Fractures in Adults.* 5th ed. Philadelphia: Lippincott Williams & Wilkins; 2001:1731–1773.

Orthopedic Trauma Association Committee on Coding and Classifications. Fractures and dislocations compendium. *J Orthop Trauma* 1996;10(suppl):41–45.

■ SKELETAL TRAUMA: PROXIMAL TIBIAL FRACTURES

KEY FACTS

- Proximal tibial fractures may be extra-articular or articular (tibial plateau or condylar fractures).
- Tibial plateau (condyle) fractures account for 1% of all fractures and 8% of fractures in the elderly. The majority (55% to 70%) of plateau fractures involve the lateral plateau. Isolated medial plateau factures occur in 10% to 23% of cases, and medial and lateral fractures occur in 10% to 30% of cases.
- Mechanism of injury is motor vehicle accidents (54%) or falls (46%) leading to vertical compression (T and Y fractures) varus and valgus forces (medial and lateral plateau fractures, respectively).
- Ligament and meniscal injuries are common with varus, valgus, or twisting forces.
- AP and lateral radiographs are usually diagnostic for displaced fractures.
- CT and MRI are frequently indicated to evaluate fragment position, articular surface congruity, and associated soft tissue injury.
- Management is based on four key factors: degree of articular depression, degree of fragment separation, degree of comminution, and extent of soft tissue injury.
- Depression of 4 to 8 mm and separation of fragments 4 mm or more generally indicate a need for internal fixation.
- Complications include infection, nonunion, and arthropathy.
- Ipsilateral, femoral, and tibial condylar fractures are not uncommon and have the following significant associated injuries:
  - Abdominal and chest injuries 20%
  - Open injury to leg 60%
  - Neurovascular injury 7%

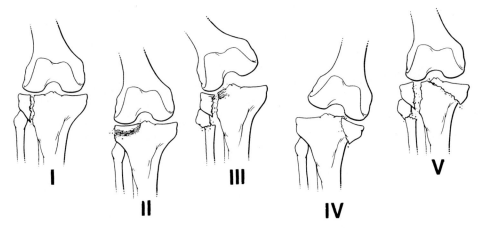

FIGURE 4-8. Hohl classification of tibial plateau fractures: I, undisplaced fracture (24%); II, central depression (26%); III, split compression, usually with fibular fracture (29%); IV, total condylar depression (11%); V, comminuted bicondylar fractures (10%).

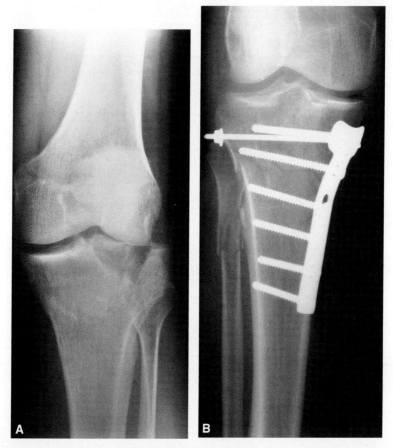

FIGURE 4-9. A: Tibial plateau fracture with splitting and separation laterally. **B:** Tibial plateau fracture reduced with buttress plate and screws to restore joint congruency.

(continued)

■ SKELETAL TRAUMA: PROXIMAL TIBIAL FRACTURES   *(Continued)*

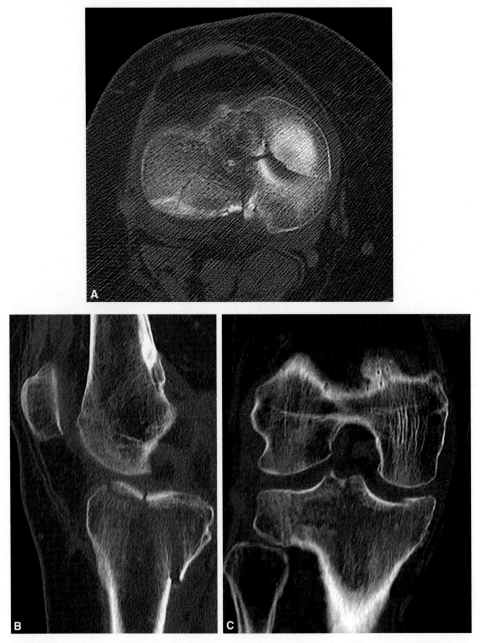

FIGURE 4-10. Computed tomography (CT) images in the axial **(A)**, sagittal **(B)**, and coronal **(C)** planes demonstrate a minimally depressed fracture with minimal articular displacement.

SUGGESTED READING

Hohl M. Tibial condylar fractures. *J Bone Joint Surg.* 1967;49A:1455–1467.

Walker CW, Moore TE. Imaging of skeletal and soft tissue injuries in and around the knee. *Radiol Clin North Am.* 1997;35(3):631–653.

■ SKELETAL TRAUMA: MISCELLANEOUS FRACTURES

KEY FACTS

- Other tibial and femoral fractures include avulsion fractures, tibial spine fractures, tuberosity fractures, physeal fractures, stress fractures, and bone bruises.
- Subtle osseous injury may be initially detected by the presence of a lipohemarthrosis on cross-table lateral radiographs.
- Physeal fractures about the knee account for only 0.5% to 3% of physeal injuries. Femoral physeal fractures are more common because of the ligament support of the knee. Most injuries are Salter–Harris Types I and IV.
- The Segond fracture is an avulsion injury at the insertion of the anterolateral ligament (ALL) on the upper lateral tibia. Anterior cruciate ligament (ACL) tears are associated with 75% to 100% of cases.
- Stress fractures of the tibia and femur are subtle early radiographically. MRI has replaced radionuclide scans for more effective and specific early diagnosis.
- Bone bruises are usually not evident on radiographs, but easily detected with MRI. Associated meniscal and/or ligament injuries are common and also easily appreciated on magnetic resonance (MR) images.

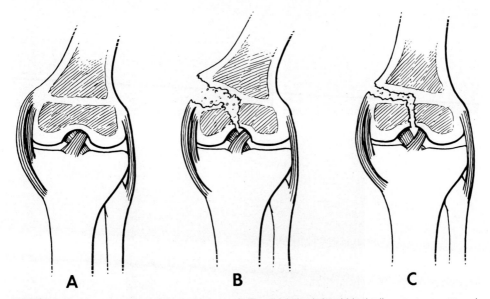

FIGURE 4-11. Ligament support about the knee. **A:** The tibial physis is within the ligament support, and the femoral physis is proximal resulting in greater risk for fracture **(B, C)**.

(continued)

▪ SKELETAL TRAUMA: MISCELLANEOUS FRACTURES *(Continued)*

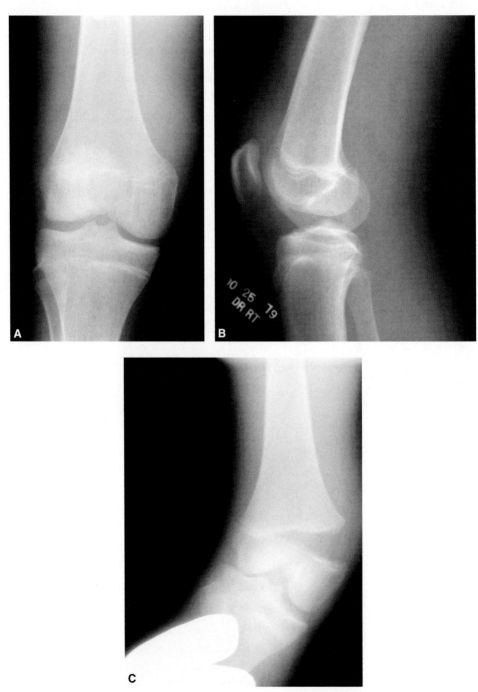

FIGURE 4-12. Anteroposterior (AP) **(A)**, lateral **(B)**, and stress views **(C)** of a Salter–Harris Type III femoral fracture.

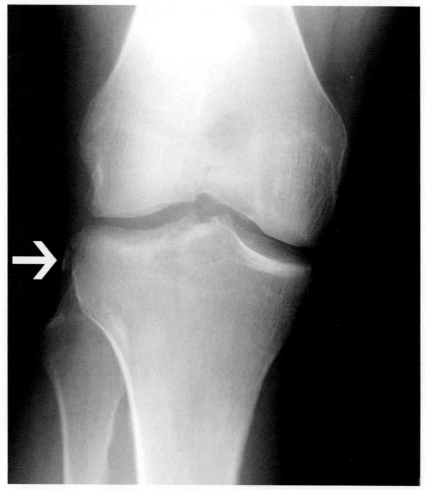

FIGURE 4-13. Anteroposterior (AP) radiograph of a Segond fracture (*arrow*).

(continued)

▪ SKELETAL TRAUMA: MISCELLANEOUS FRACTURES   *(Continued)*

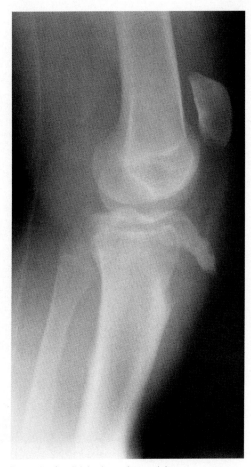

FIGURE 4-14. Lateral radiograph of a tibial tuberosity avulsion.

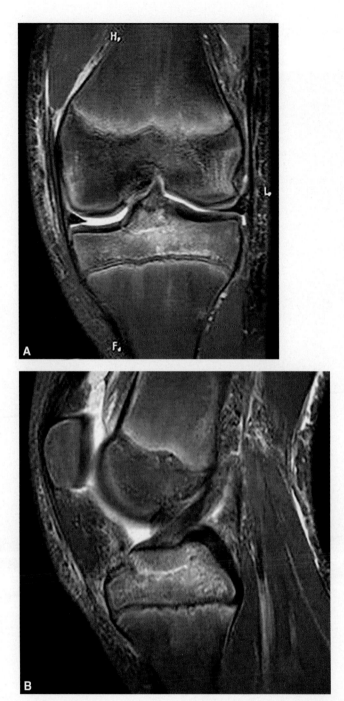

FIGURE 4-15. Tibial spine–anterior cruciate ligament (ACL) avulsion. Fluid sensitive coronal **(A)** and sagittal **(B)** magnetic resonance (MR) images demonstrate the ACL avulsion fracture at its attachment upon the tibial spine.

(continued)

■ SKELETAL TRAUMA: MISCELLANEOUS FRACTURES   *(Continued)*

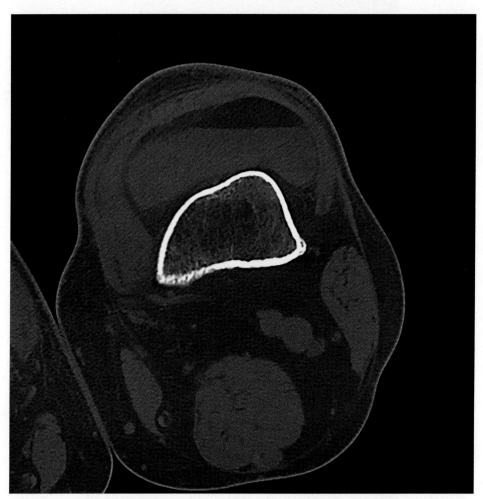

FIGURE 4-16. Axial computed tomography (CT) demonstrates a lipohemarthrosis indicating an intra-articular fracture.

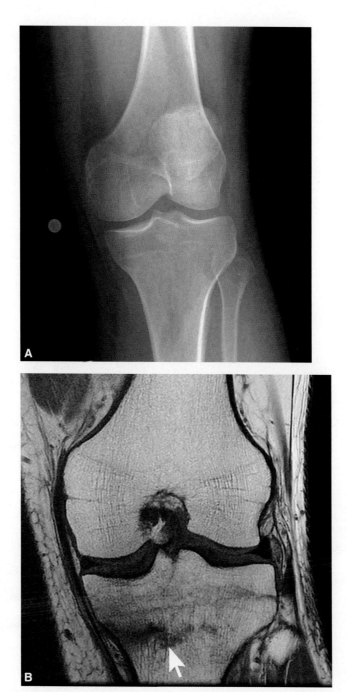

FIGURE 4-17. A: Anteroposterior (AP) radiograph is normal. **B:** Coronal T1-weighted image clearly demonstrates the stress fracture (*arrow*).

(continued)

■ SKELETAL TRAUMA: MISCELLANEOUS FRACTURES *(Continued)*

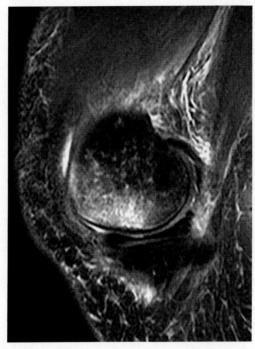

FIGURE 4-18. Bone contusion involving the medial femoral condyle clearly demonstrated on the sagittal T2-weighted magnetic resonance (MR) image resulting from varus injury.

SUGGESTED READING

Claes S, Luyckx T, Vereecke E, et al. The Segond fracture: a bony injury of the anterolateral ligament of the knee. *Arthroscopy.* 2014;30(11):1475–1482.

Dezell PB, Schils JP, Recht MP. Subtle fractures about the knee: innocuous-appearing yet indicative of internal derangement. *Am J Roentgenol.* 1996;167:699–703.

■ MENISCAL LESIONS: MENISCAL TEARS

KEY FACTS

■ Meniscal tears are the most common cause of knee pain and instability.

■ Patients present with pain, locking, or "giving way."

■ Tears may be the result of acute trauma or repetitive trauma with progressive degeneration.

■ The lateral meniscus is C-shaped and less firmly attached to the capsule (separated posteriorly by popliteus tendon sheath). The medial meniscus is more firmly attached, and the posterior horn is larger (see Fig. 4-19).

■ MRI has replaced other imaging techniques for diagnosis of meniscal tears. Tears are most easily identified on spin-echo proton density images. Conventional spin-echo sequences are 93% sensitive compared with 80% for fast spin-echo sequences. Sagittal, coronal, and axial image planes should all be evaluated to properly characterize the type of tear.

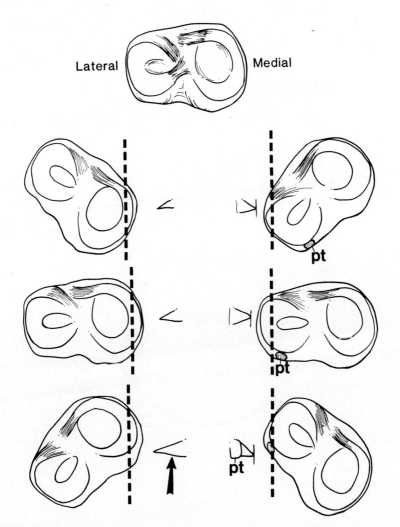

FIGURE 4-19. Meniscal appearance (medial and lateral) with the knee in different degrees of rotation. Note the posterior horn of the medial meniscus (*arrow*) is larger. The popliteus tendon (*pt*) sheath separates the lateral meniscus from the capsule posteriorly.

(continued)

■ MENISCAL LESIONS: MENISCAL TEARS *(Continued)*

- Meniscal tears are described by configuration and location. The posterior horn is most commonly involved.
- MR criteria for classifying meniscal tears have been clearly defined (see Fig. 4-21).
- Treatment depends on the location (peripheral vs. central) and type of tear. Peripheral tears may heal or be repaired as in the vascular zone. Displaced fragments may be removed arthroscopically.

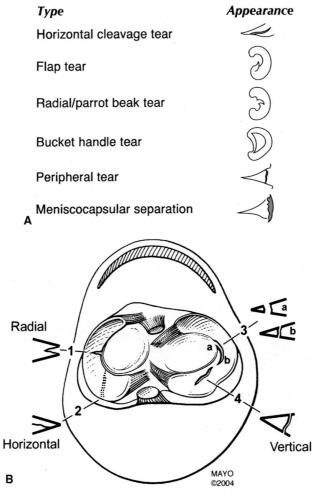

FIGURE 4-20. A: Types and appearances of meniscal tears. **B:** Meniscal tears seen in the axial and coronal planes.

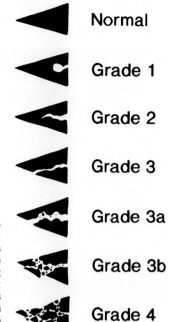

Normal

Grade 1

Grade 2

Grade 3

Grade 3a

Grade 3b

Grade 4

FIGURE 4-21. Magnetic resonance (MR) classification of meniscal tears. Normal low signal intensity. Grade 1: globular increased signal intensity that does not communicate with the articular surface. Grade 2: linear increased signal intensity that does not communicate with the articular surface. Grade 3: linear increased signal intensity that communicates with the articular surface, a true tear. Grades 3a and b: more extensive articular involvement. Grade 4: complex tears with distortion of the meniscus.

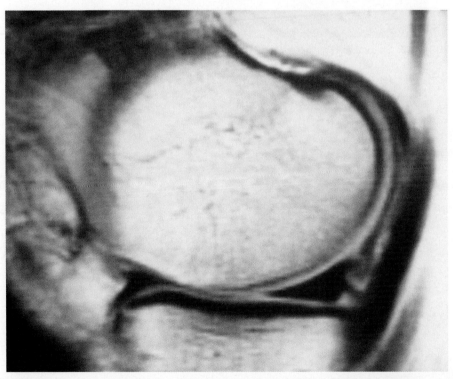

FIGURE 4-22. Sagittal proton density–weighted image of a normal low-intensity meniscus.

(continued)

■ MENISCAL LESIONS: MENISCAL TEARS *(Continued)*

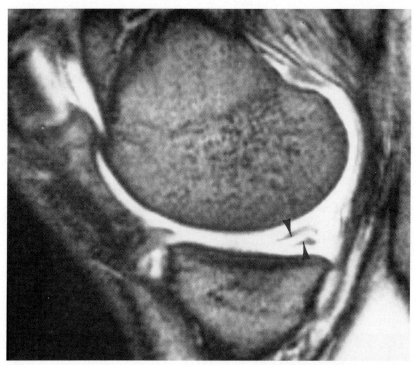

FIGURE 4-23. Gradient echo sagittal image of a linear tear (*arrowheads*) in the posterior medial meniscus.

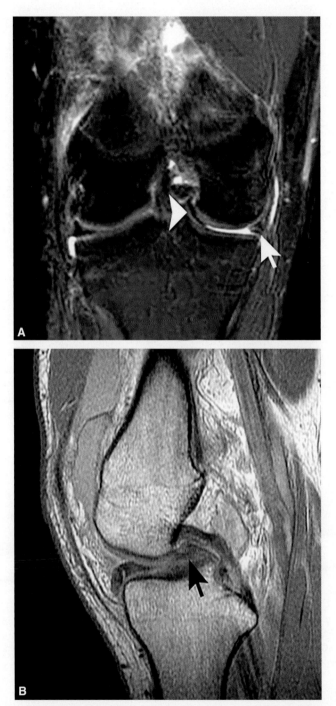

FIGURE 4-24. Coronal fat-suppressed T2-weighted image **(A)** of a bucket-handle tear of the medial meniscus. Note truncated meniscus (*arrow*) and displaced fragment (*arrowhead*). Sagital proton density image **(B)** shows the "double posterior cruciate ligament" (PCL) sign (*arrow*).

(continued)

■ MENISCAL LESIONS: MENISCAL TEARS (Continued)

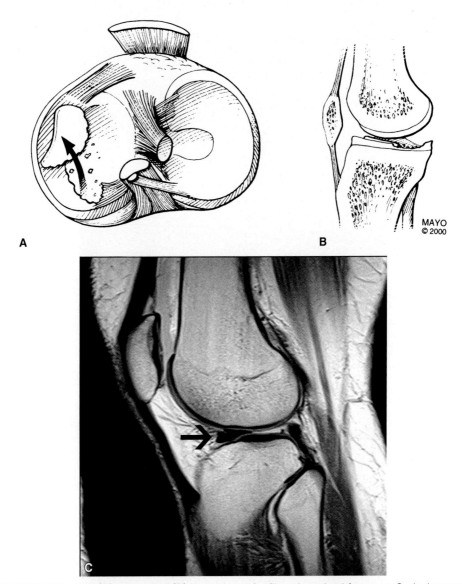

FIGURE 4-25. Axial **(A)** and sagittal **(B)** illustrations of a flipped meniscal fragment. Sagittal proton density image **(C)** demonstrates a small posterior meniscal remnant and a large flipped meniscal fragment anteriorly (*arrow*).

SUGGESTED READING

Blackman GB, Majors NM, Helms CA. Comparison of fast spin-echo versus conventional spin-echo MRI for evaluation of meniscal tears. *Am J Roentgenol.* 2005;184:1740–1743.

Crues JV III, Murk J, Levy TL, et al. Meniscal tears of the knee: accuracy of MR imaging. *Radiology.* 1987;164:445–448.

De Smet AA. How I diagnose meniscal tears on knee MRI. *Am J Roentgenol.* 2012;199(3):481–499.

Lance V, Heilmeier UR, Joseph GB, et al. MR imaging characteristics and clinical symptoms related to displaced meniscal flap tears. *Skeletal Radiol.* 2015;44(3):375–384.

Magee T. Three-Tesla MR imaging of the knee. *Radiol Clin North Am.* 2007;45(6):1055–1062.

Nguyen JC, De Smet AA, Graf BK, et al. MR imaging-based diagnosis and classification of meniscal tears. *Radiographics.* 2014;34(4):981–999.

■ MENISCAL LESIONS: POSTOPERATIVE MENISCUS

KEY FACTS

- Menisci may be partially or completely resected or repaired.
- Image features applied to diagnosis of meniscal tears (increased signal intensity extending to the articular surface and displaced fragments) can be applied after repair.
- Intra-articular gadolinium may improve accuracy for evaluating the postoperative meniscus. Intra-articular gadolinium is 92% accurate for detection of retear.
- Arthroscopy is most useful in complex or equivocal cases.

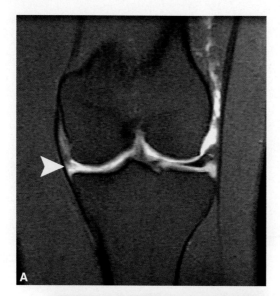

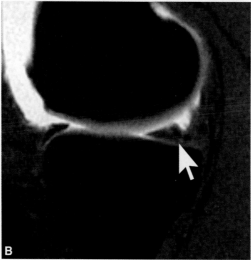

FIGURE 4-26. A: Coronal image from a magnetic resonance (MR) arthrogram shows changes in a near-complete meniscectomy of the body of the medial meniscus (*arrowhead*). **B:** Sagittal image from an MR arthrogram shows changes in a prior meniscal repair (*arrow*) with no contrast extending into the meniscus to suggest retear. **C:** Sagittal image from an MR arthrogram shows changes in a prior partial meniscectomy with abnormal contrast extending into the substance of the medial meniscal remnant compatible with retear (*arrow*).

(continued)

■ **MENISCAL LESIONS: POSTOPERATIVE MENISCUS** *(Continued)*

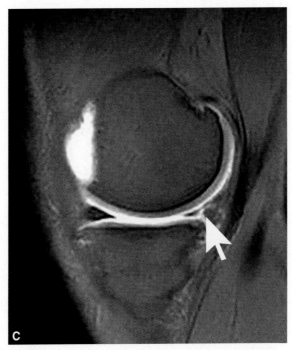

FIGURE 4-26. *(continued)*

SUGGESTED READING

Davis KW, Tuite MJ. MR imaging of the postoperative meniscus of the knee. *Semin Musculoskelet Radiol.* 2002;6(1):35–45.

Lum PS, Schweitzer ME, Bhatea M, et al. Repeat tear of postoperative meniscus: Potential MR imaging signs. *Radiology.* 1999;210:183–188.

Magee TH. Accuracy of 3-Tesla MR and MR arthrography in diagnosis of meniscal retear in the post-operative knee. *Skeletal Radiol.* 2014;43(8):1057–1064.

Sciulli RL, Boutin RD, Brown RR, et al. Evaluation of the postoperative meniscus of the knee: a study comparing conventional arthrography, conventional MR imaging, MR arthrography with iodinated contrast material, and MR arthrography with gadolinium-based contrast material. *Skeletal Radiol.* 1999;28(9):508–514.

■ MENISCAL LESIONS: MENISCAL CYSTS

KEY FACTS

■ Meniscal cysts are reported in 1% of patients undergoing meniscectomy.
■ They are most common anterolaterally but can occur medially.
■ Meniscal tears are usually present and may be the basis for cyst formation.
■ Patients present with tenderness and joint-line swelling.
■ Meniscal cysts can be diagnosed with arthrography, but MRI is preferred.
■ Treatment requires decompression of the cyst and meniscal repair.
■ MR features include
  ● Well-defined high signal intensity lesion adjacent to or partially including the meniscus on T2-weighted sequences.
  ● Cysts may be septated (47%) and up to 5 cm in size.
■ Ganglion cysts and cruciate ligament cysts may be confused with meniscal cysts.

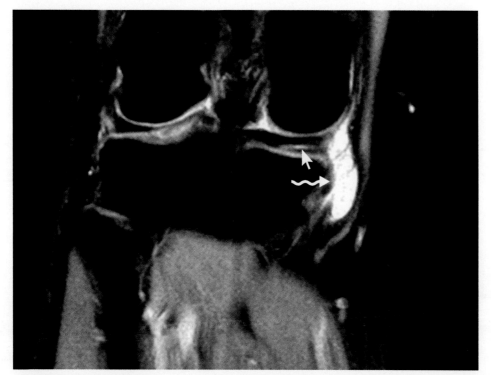

FIGURE 4-27. Meniscal cyst (*curved arrow*) seen on a sagittal T2-weighted image arising from a tear of the medial meniscus (*arrow*).

SUGGESTED READING

Anderson JJ, Connor GF, Helms CA. New observations on meniscal cysts. *Skeletal Radiol.* 2010;39(12):1187–1191.
Burk DL, Dalinka MK, Kanal E, et al. Meniscal and ganglion cysts of the knee: MR evaluation. *Am J Roentgenol.* 1988;150:331–336.
Campbell SE, Sanders TG, Morrison WB. MR imaging of meniscal cysts: incidence, location, and clinical significance. *Am J Roentgenol.* 2001;177:409–413.
De Smet AA, Graf BK, del Rio AM. Association of parameniscal cysts with underlying meniscal tears as identified on MRI and arthroscopy. *Am J Roentgenol.* 2011;196(2):W180–W186.

■ MENISCAL LESIONS: DISCOID MENISCI

KEY FACTS

- Discoid menisci are reported in 1.5% to 15.5% of lateral and 0.1% to 0.3% of medial menisci.
- Discoid menisci are broad and disk shaped, and more prone to meniscal tears. Meniscal tears are more difficult to evaluate with discoid menisci because of degeneration and the high incidence of multiple tears.
- The transverse diameter of a normal meniscus is 10 to 11 mm. A discoid meniscus projects farther into the joint and therefore appears larger on coronal and sagittal MR images (visible on three or more 4-mm–thick sagittal images).

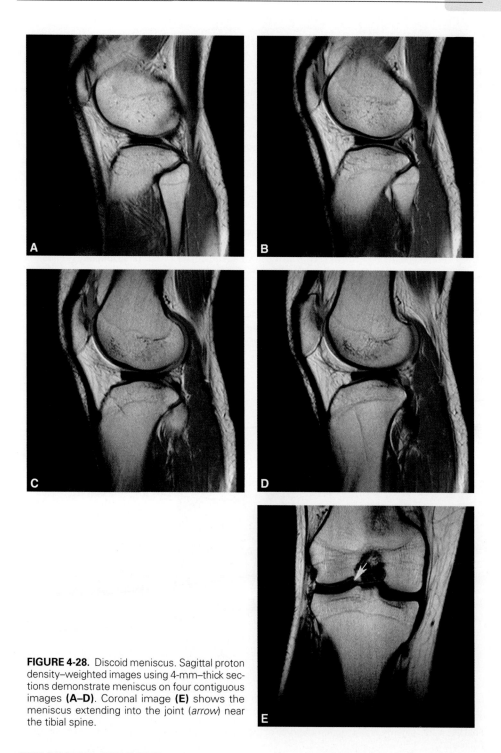

FIGURE 4-28. Discoid meniscus. Sagittal proton density–weighted images using 4-mm–thick sections demonstrate meniscus on four contiguous images **(A–D)**. Coronal image **(E)** shows the meniscus extending into the joint (*arrow*) near the tibial spine.

SUGGESTED READING

Ryu KN, Kim IS, Kun EJ, et al. MR imaging of tears of discoid menisci. *Am J Roentgenol* 1998;171:963–967.

Samoto N, Kozuma M, Tokuhisa T, et al. Diagnosis of discoid lateral meniscus of the knee on MR imaging. *Magn Reson Imaging.* 2002;20(1):59–64.

■ LIGAMENT AND TENDON INJURIES: BASIC CONCEPTS

KEY FACTS

- ■ Complete evaluation of the ligaments, tendons, and capsule is difficult with conventional techniques, including CT and arthrography.
- ■ MRI offers the ability to evaluate all supporting structures of the knee.
- ■ Key anatomic structures for image evaluation include
  - ● ACL: oblique course with anteromedial and posterolateral bands. Extends from the lateral femoral condyle to the tibial plateau.
  - ● Posterior cruciate ligament (PCL): thicker than ACL. Extends from medial femoral condyle to posterior intercondylar region of the tibia.
  - ● Medial collateral ligament (MCL): three layers. The first layer is composed of fascia covering the quadriceps, the second layer includes the MCL, and the third layer is the capsular ligament. The MCL extends from the medial femoral condyle to attach on the tibia approximately 5 cm below the joint line.
  - ● Lateral collateral ligament (LCL): also known as the fibular collateral ligament. Extends from lateral femoral condyle to the fibular head. Separate from capsule.
  - ● Quadriceps tendon: formed by four muscles of quadriceps group, resulting in layers until it attaches to the patella.
  - ● Patellar tendon: extends from the patella to the tibial tuberosity.
  - ● Popliteus tendon: extends from the lateral femoral condyle passing between the lateral meniscus and capsule to join the muscle origin on the posterior tibia.

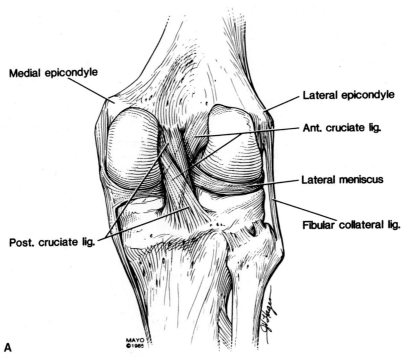

A

FIGURE 4-29. Ligament and tendon anatomy of the knee seen from posterior **(A)**, lateral **(B)**, and axial **(C)** planes.

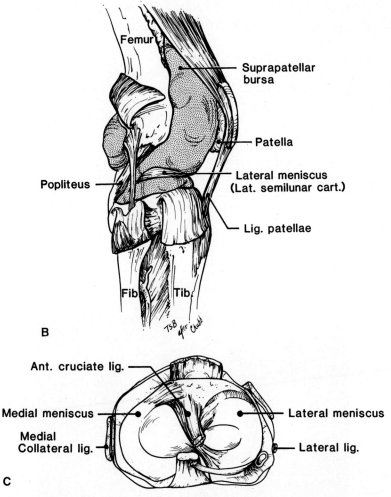

FIGURE 4-29. *(continued)*

SUGGESTED READING

Berquist TH. *MRI of the Musculoskeletal System.* 5th ed. Philadelphia: Lippincott Williams & Wilkins; 2006:303–429.

■ LIGAMENT AND TENDON INJURIES: ANTERIOR CRUCIATE LIGAMENT—ACUTE (PRIMARY FEATURES)

KEY FACTS

- ACL is the most frequently injured ligament.
- Up to 70% have associated injuries of the meniscus (usually posteromedial) and MCL (O'Donoghue's triad: ACL tear, MCL tear, and medial meniscal tear).
- Patients usually describe a twisting injury and a loud pop, and they are unable to bear weight on the injured knee.
- MRI is the most effective imaging technique for evaluating the cruciate ligaments and associated injuries. T2-weighted sequences are most useful. Sagittal, coronal, and axial images should all be evaluated.
- Primary features of acute ACL tears:
  - Acute—complete tear
    - ❖ Discontinuity with increased signal intensity between segments or at tibial or femoral attachment
    - ❖ Flat or horizontal distal segment with high signal intensity near femoral attachment
    - ❖ Complete absence of ligament with high signal intensity in the midjoint space
    - ❖ Wavy ligament
  - Acute—incomplete tear
  - Increased signal intensity (T2-weighted sequence) with thickening and normal course

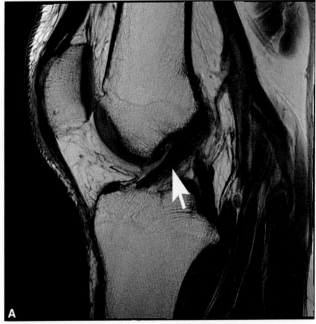

FIGURE 4-30. A: Sagittal proton density–weighted image demonstrates the normal low signal intensity of the anterior cruciate ligament (ACL) (*arrow*). **B:** Acute ACL tear. Sagittal T2-weighted image demonstrates an ACL tear (*arrow*). There is a joint effusion (*curved arrow*) that is almost always present with an acute injury. Coronal fast spin-echo T2-weighted image **(C)** shows no visualized ACL (*arrow*) and an associated medial collateral ligament (MCL) tear (*arrowhead*).

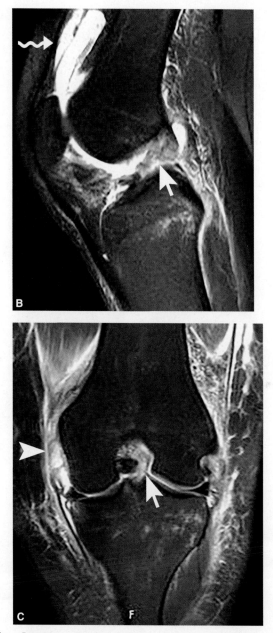

FIGURE 4-30. *(continued)*

SUGGESTED READING

Kijowski R, Sanogo ML, Lee KS, et al. Short-term clinical importance of osseous injuries diagnosed at MR imaging in patients with anterior cruciate ligament tear. *Radiology.* 2012;264(2):531–541.

Naraghi A, White LM. MR imaging of cruciate ligaments. *Magn Reson Imaging Clin N Am.* 2014;22(4):557–580.

■ LIGAMENT AND TENDON INJURIES: ANTERIOR CRUCIATE LIGAMENT—ACUTE (SECONDARY FEATURES)

KEY FACTS

■ Numerous secondary signs have been described to improve accuracy and fully evaluate ACL injuries:
  - Joint effusion
  - Angulation of PCL—acute angle in upper PCL forming "?"
  - Abnormal PCL angle—normal 113 to 114 degrees; less than 105 degrees 86% specific for ACL tear
  - Anterior subluxation
  - Bone bruise—lateral compartment 97% specific
  - Segond fractures (see Fig. 4-13)
  - Deep femoral notch (>1.5 mm)
  - MCL tear
  - Meniscal tears

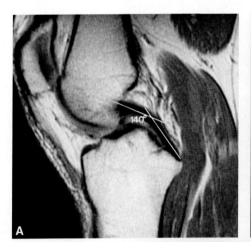
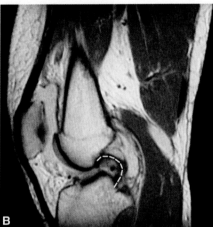
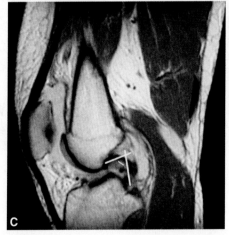

FIGURE 4-31. A: Normal posterior cruciate ligament (PCL) with an angle (*lines*) of 140 degrees. Normal greater than 113 to 114 degrees. **B:** Anterior cruciate ligament (ACL) tear with hooked PCL (*broken line*). **C:** ACL tear with hooked PCL and angle (*lines*) of less than 90 degrees.

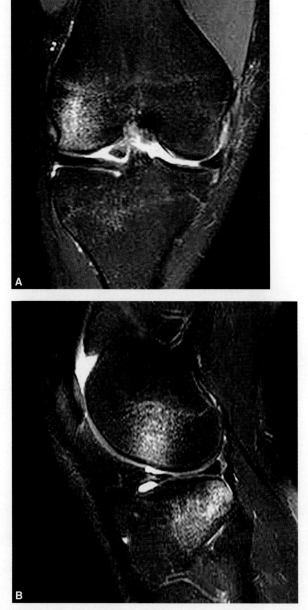

FIGURE 4-32. Coronal **(A)** and sagittal **(B)** T2-weighted images of a lateral compartment bone contusions in a patient with an anterior cruciate ligament (ACL) tear.

SUGGESTED READING

Brandser EA, Riley MA, Berbaum KS, et al. MR imaging of anterior cruciate ligament injury: independent value of primary and secondary signs. *Am J Roentgenol.* 1996;167(1):121–126.

Tung GA, Davis LM, Wiggins ME, et al. Tears of the anterior cruciate ligament: primary and secondary signs at MR imaging. *Radiology.* 1993;188(3):661–667.

■ LIGAMENT AND TENDON INJURIES: ANTERIOR CRUCIATE LIGAMENT—CHRONIC TEARS

KEY FACTS

- ■ Chronic ACL injuries are usually partial tears, or overlooked or untreated tears.
- ■ Patients present with instability. A small joint effusion may be present, when symptoms are active. Large effusions seen with acute tears are unusual.
- ■ MR image features include
  - ● Small or no joint effusion
  - ● Ligament laxity, thickening, and intermediate signal intensity on T2-weighted images
  - ● Ligament atrophy

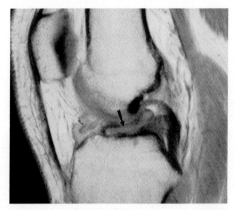

FIGURE 4-33. Old partial anterior cruciate ligament (ACL) tear with intermediate signal intensity and horizontal distal remnant (*arrow*). There is no joint effusion.

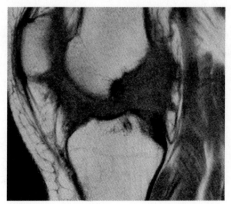

FIGURE 4-34. Sagittal T1-weighted images with thickening and intermediate signal intensity in the region of the anterior cruciate ligament (ACL), but no visible fibers. There is no joint effusion, and the femur is shifted posteriorly on the tibia.

SUGGESTED READING

Umans H, Winpfheimer O, Havamati N, et al. Diagnosis of partial tears of the anterior cruciate ligament of the knee: value of MR imaging. *Am J Roentgenol.* 1995;165:893–897.

■ LIGAMENT AND TENDON INJURIES: POSTERIOR CRUCIATE LIGAMENT

KEY FACTS

- PCL is thicker and more easily included on a single sagittal section.
- Most PCL tears involve the midsubstance; 19% are proximal and the remainder are distal.
- PCL tears are less common than ACL tears. Both ligaments may be torn simultaneously.
- MR features of PCL tears are the same as described for ACL tears.

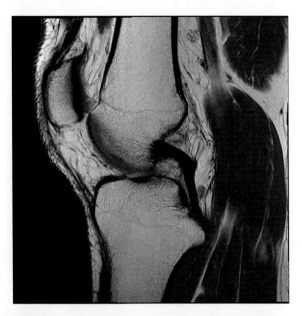

FIGURE 4-35. Sagittal proton density–weighted image demonstrates a normal posterior cruciate ligament (PCL).

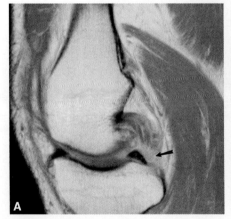
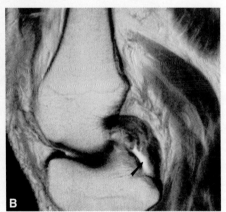

FIGURE 4-36. Posterior cruciate ligament (PCL) tear. Sagittal proton density–weighted **(A)** and T2-weighted **(B)** images demonstrate thickening and increased signal intensity in the PCL with avulsion from the tibial attachment (*arrow*).

SUGGESTED READING

Naraghi A, White LM. MR imaging of cruciate ligaments. *Magn Reson Imaging Clin N Am.* 2014;22(4):557–580. doi:10.1016/j.mric.2014.07.003.

Sonin AH, Fitzgerald SW, Friedman H, et al. Posterior cruciate ligament injury: MR imaging diagnosis and patterns of injury. *Radiology.* 1994;190(2):455–458.

■ LIGAMENT AND TENDON INJURIES: MEDIAL AND LATERAL COLLATERAL LIGAMENTS

KEY FACTS

■ MCL injuries are far more common than LCL injuries. MCL injuries are usually the result of valgus stress, whereas lateral injuries are the result of varus stress or internal torsion injuries.

■ MCL injuries are commonly associated with capsular and meniscal injury. Tears of the ACL are evident in 30%.

■ O'Donoghue's triad (ACL, MCL, and meniscal tears) is a common injury pattern.

■ Associated bone bruises are common.

■ MR imaging using conventional or fast spin-echo T2- or T2-weighted images in the axial and coronal planes allows detection and classification of collateral ligament injuries.

■ Image features are similar to those described for ACL tears.

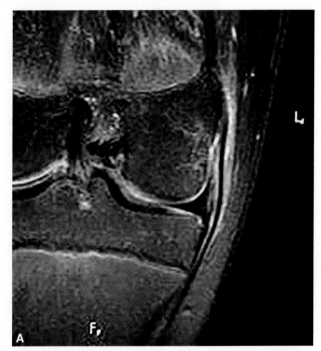

FIGURE 4-37. Coronal magnetic resonance (MR) images show Grade 1 **(A)**, Grade 2 **(B)**, and Grade 3 **(C)** injuries of the medial collateral ligament of the knee.

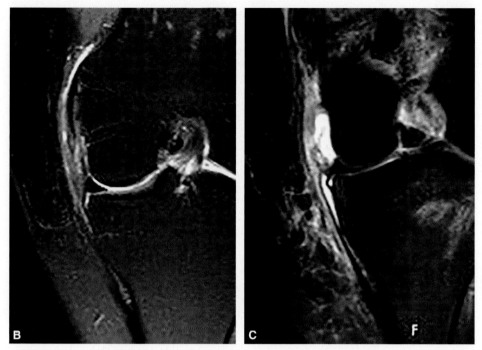

FIGURE 4-37. *(continued)*

SUGGESTED READING

Schweitzer ME, Tran D, Deely DM, et al. Medial collateral ligament injuries: evaluation of multiple signs, prevalence and location of associated bone bruises, and assessment with MR imaging. *Radiology.* 1995;194(3):825–829.

▪ LIGAMENT AND TENDON INJURIES: QUADRICEPS TENDON

KEY FACTS

▪ The quadriceps tendon is formed by slips of four muscles (rectus femoris, vastus lateralis, intermedius, and medialis), resulting in a layered appearance on axial and sagittal MR images.

▪ Quadriceps rupture may be the result of acute or repetitive trauma.

▪ Quadriceps tears are more common in elderly patients with rheumatoid arthritis, systemic lupus erythematosus, or metabolic disease.

▪ Most tears occur just above the patella.

▪ MR images in the sagittal and axial planes using T2-weighted sequences show thickening and increased signal intensity for partial tears and separation with fluid (increased signal) between segments with complete tears. The patella may be inferiorly displaced.

▪ Ultrasound may also be used to evaluate the quadriceps tendon.

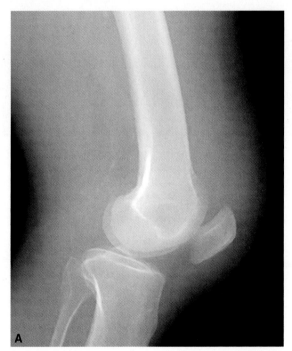

FIGURE 4-38. Lateral radiograph **(A)** shows soft tissue swelling in the region of the distal quadriceps tendon and anterior and inferior tilting of the patella. Sagittal T1-weighted magnetic resonance (MR) image **(B)** demonstrates a complete quadriceps tear at the patellar attachment (*arrow*).

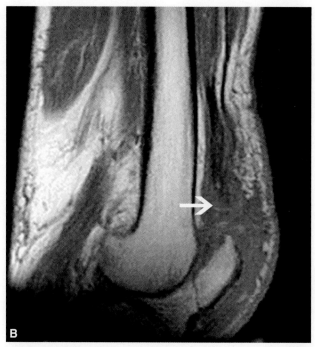

FIGURE 4-38. *(continued)*

SUGGESTED READING

Staeubli HU, Bollmann C, Kreutz R, et al. Quantification of intact quadriceps tendon, quadriceps tendon insertion and suprapatellar fat pad: MR arthrography, anatomy, and cryosection in the sagittal plane. *Am J Roentgenol.* 1999;173:691–698.

Yu JS, Petersilge C, Sartoris DJ, et al. MR imaging of injuries of the extensor mechanism. *Radiographics.* 1994;14:541–551.

▪ LIGAMENT AND TENDON INJURIES: PATELLAR TENDON

KEY FACTS

- Patellar tendon injuries include tendinitis, tendinosis, tendon tears, and chronic overuse syndromes.
- Patellar tendon tears may be partial or complete. Signal intensity changes on MR images are similar to those for ACL tears.
- Jumper's knee—tendinosis caused by repetitive microtrauma in athletes involved in running and jumping sports. There is increased risk for tendon rupture.
- Imaging of patellar tendon abnormalities is accomplished most easily with conventional or fast spin-echo T2-weighted images in the axial and sagittal planes.
- Ultrasound may also be used to evaluate the patellar tendon.

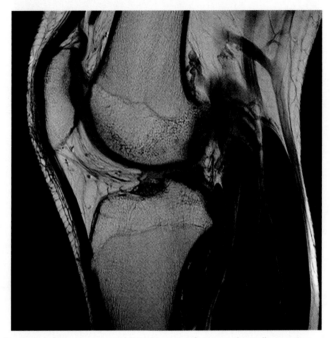

FIGURE 4-39. Sagittal proton density–weighted image of a normal patellar tendon.

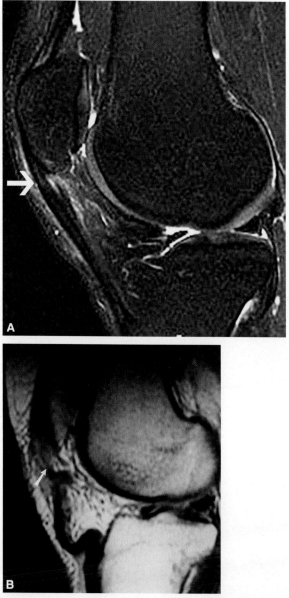

FIGURE 4-40. Patellar tendon disorders. **A:** Sagittal T2-weighted image shows thickening and increased signal intensity at the patellar attachment (*arrow*) resulting from "jumper's knee." **B:** Sagittal T1-weighted image demonstrates a complete tear of the tendon (*arrow*) with a wavy appearance distally.

SUGGESTED READING

Hodgson RJ, O'Connor PJ, Grainger AJ. Tendon and ligament imaging. *Br J Radiol.* 2012;85(1016):1157–1172.
Yu JS, Petersilge C, Sortores DJ, et al. MR imaging of injuries of the extensor mechanism. *Radiographics.* 1994;14:541–551.

▪ LIGAMENT AND TENDON RECONSTRUCTION

KEY FACTS

- ▪ Ligament and tendon reconstruction can be accomplished using tendon grafts, allografts, or synthetic materials.
- ▪ Routine radiographs and MRI are important to evaluate results and potential complications.
- ▪ Complications include
  - ● Improper tunnel position
  - ● Hardware failure
  - ● Bone plug fracture
  - ● Patellar fracture (stress riser from donor site)
  - ● Graft (tendon) failure
  - ● Graft impingement
  - ● Anterior arthrofibrosis (cyclops lesion)
  - ● Postoperative infection
- ▪ Routine radiographs should include AP, patellar, notch, and cross-table lateral views. The latter is obtained with the knee extended to evaluate graft impingement.
- ▪ MR images are obtained using routine knee protocols, except sagittal images should be obtained with the knee extended to evaluate for impingement.

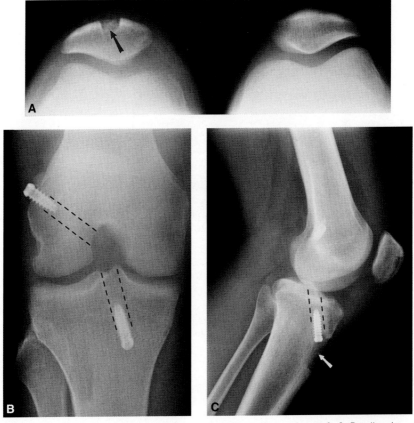

FIGURE 4-41. Anterior cruciate ligament (ACL) repair with patellar tendon graft. **A:** Patellar view shows bone donor site (*arrow*). **B:** Notch view shows interference screws fixing the bone plugs. Graft tunnel positions (*broken lines*). **C:** Lateral view demonstrates the tibial tunnel (*broken lines*) and tuberosity donor sight (*arrow*). **D:** Cross-table lateral with extension shows the tibial tunnel (*arrows*) in proper position posterior to intercondylar roof (*white line*).

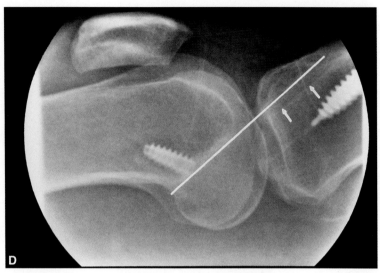

FIGURE 4-41. *(continued)*

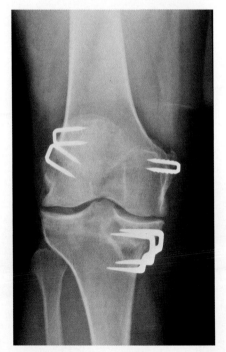

FIGURE 4-42. Anteroposterior (AP) radiograph after anterior cruciate ligament (ACL) and medial collateral ligament (MCL) repairs. Staples fix the ends of the tendon grafts.

(continued)

■ **LIGAMENT AND TENDON RECONSTRUCTION**   *(Continued)*

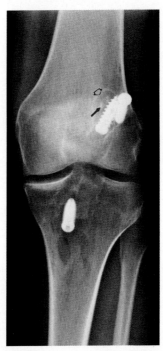

FIGURE 4-43. Anteroposterior (AP) radiograph after anterior cruciate ligament (ACL) repair with fracture of the bone plug (*arrow*) and lucency about the screws (*open arrow*) caused by loosening.

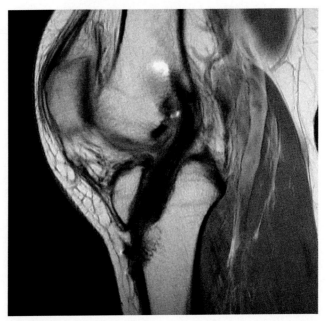

FIGURE 4-44. Sagittal magnetic resonance (MR) image of an intact anterior cruciate ligament (ACL) reconstruction. Note normal low signal intensity of the tendon. There is some artifact from the screws.

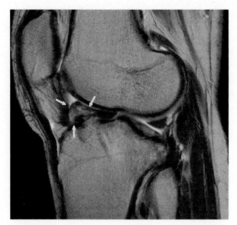

FIGURE 4-45. Sagittal T2-weighted image demonstrates a large "cyclops" lesion (*arrows*) in the anterior fat.

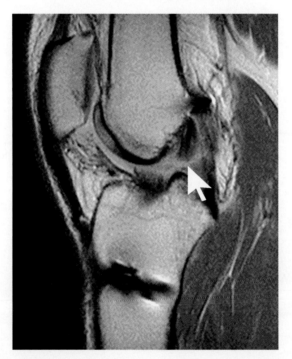

FIGURE 4-46. Sagittal T1-weighted image after anterior cruciate ligament (ACL) reconstruction shows complete disruption of the graft (*arrow*).

SUGGESTED READING

Naraghi AM, Gupta S, Jacks LM, et al. Anterior cruciate ligament reconstruction: MR imaging signs of anterior knee laxity in the presence of an intact graft. *Radiology*. 2012;263(3):802–810.

Naraghi A, White LM. MR imaging of cruciate ligaments. *Magn Reson Imaging Clin N Am*. 2014;22(4):557–580.

Sanders TG. Imaging of the postoperative knee. *Semin Musculoskelet Radiol*. 2011;15(4):383–407.

White LM, Kramer J, Recht MP. MR imaging evaluation of the postoperative knee: ligaments, menisci, and articular cartilage. *Skeletal Radiol*. 2005;34:431–452.

■ PLICAE

KEY FACTS

■ Plicae are embryonic synovial remnants that may be present in asymptomatic knees.

■ Plicae are noted in approximately 20% of patients.

■ The three most common plicae are suprapatellar, mediopatellar, and infrapatellar.

- Suprapatellar plica—remnant separating suprapatellar bursa from medial and lateral compartments.
- Mediopatellar plica—extends from above the patella to insert on the synovium of the infrapatellar fat pad. This plica is most often symptomatic.
- Infrapatellar plica—courses along the upper margin of the ACL

■ Chronic inflammation causes thickening of the plicae, which results in pain and snapping.

■ Similar symptoms may be found with loose bodies, patellar tracking disorders, meniscal tears, and jumper's knee.

■ Plicae are evaluated most easily on axial and sagittal T2-weighted MR images.

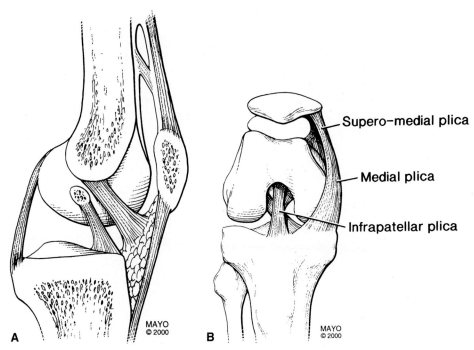

FIGURE 4-47. Plicae of the knee in the sagittal **(A)** and frontal plane with the knee flexed **(B)**.

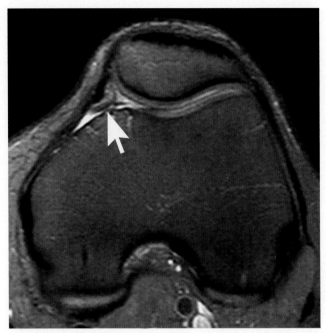

FIGURE 4-48. Axial T2-weighted images show a medial patellar plica (*arrow*).

SUGGESTED READING

Boles CA, Butler J, Lee JA, et al. Magnetic resonance characteristics of medial plica of the knee: correlation with arthroscopic resection. *J Comput Assist Tomogr.* 2004;28(3):397–401.

García-Valtuille R, Abascal F, Cerezal L, et al. Anatomy and MR imaging appearances of synovial plicae of the knee. *Radiographics.* 2002;22(4):775–784.

Kosarek FJ, Helms CA. The MR appearance of the infrapatellar plica. *Am J Roentgenol.* 1999;172(2):481–484.

■ PATELLAR DISORDERS: PATELLOFEMORAL RELATIONSHIPS

KEY FACTS

■ Patellar configuration and articular relationship to the femoral condyles are important when evaluating tracking disorders and patellofemoral pain syndromes.

■ Patellar configurations were described by Wiberg: Type I, medial and lateral facets are equal; Type II, lateral facet larger than medial (most common); and Type III, small medial facet and hypoplastic medial femoral condyle.

■ On a lateral radiograph taken with 30 degrees of flexion, the ratio of patellar tendon length to patellar height should be 1.02 ± 0.13.

■ On patellar views or axial MR images, the sulcus angle formed by lines along the femoral condyle should be 138 to 142 degrees. An increased angle is seen with dysplasias and leads to subluxation.

■ The patella should normally be at or just medial to the medial articular margin line, which is drawn perpendicular to a line along the condylar margins.

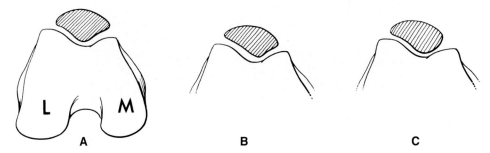

FIGURE 4-49. Wiberg patellar configurations. **A:** Medial and lateral facets equal in size: Type I. **B:** Lateral facet larger than medial: Type II. **C:** Small medial facet with dysplastic condyle: Type III.

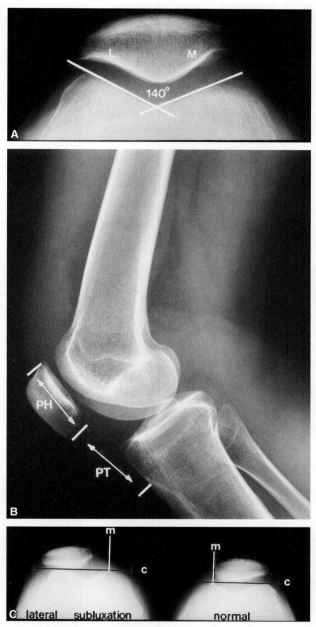

FIGURE 4-50. Normal radiographic relationships. **A:** Sulcus angle formed by lines along the femoral condyles is normally 138 to 142 degrees. **B:** Lateral radiograph with the knee flexed 30 degrees. The patellar tendon (PT) length over the patellar height (PH) = 1.02 ± 0.13. **C:** The medial patellar edge should be at or just medial to a line (*m*) perpendicular to a line (*c*) along the condylar margins.

SUGGESTED READING

Laurin CA, Dussault R, Levesquelt P. The tangential x-ray investigation of the patellofemoral joint. *Clin Orthop.* 1979;144:16–26.

■ PATELLAR DISORDERS: PATELLAR TRACKING AND INSTABILITY

KEY FACTS

■ Position of the patella in relation to the condyles of the femur varies with position, so flexion and extension studies are required.

■ Conditions include

- Lateral subluxation—lateral translation of the patella, so the facet extends beyond the articular margin of the condyles
- Excessive lateral pressure syndrome—lateral facet joint narrowed or patella tilted without subluxation
- Medial subluxation—medial translation of the patella, so the facet extends beyond the medial condyle
- Lateral–medial subluxation—patella starts in lateral subluxation and shifts to medial during knee flexion
- Dislocation—complete loss of articular interfaces

■ Imaging can be accomplished with axial patellar radiographs in differing degrees of flexion, or using fast CT or MR techniques to image the patellofemoral relationships through flexion and extension.

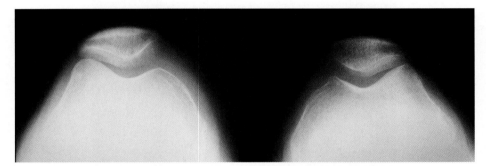

FIGURE 4-51. Patellar views of both knees show lateral tilt without subluxation because of lateral pressure syndrome.

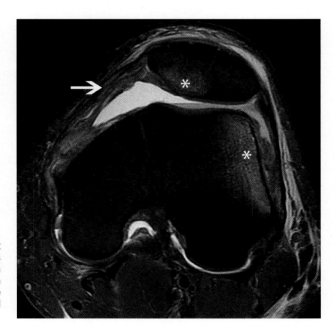

FIGURE 4-52. Axial T2-weighted fat suppressed image demonstrates evidence of a prior lateral dislocation with a tear of the medial retinaculum (*arrow*) and bone contusions in the medial patella and lateral femoral condyle (*asterisks*).

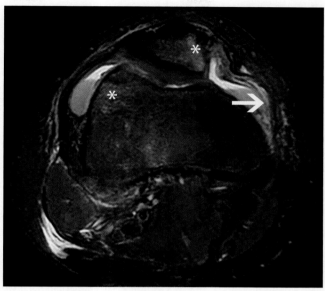

FIGURE 4-53. Axial T2-weighted magnetic resonance (MR) images after patellar dislocation with fluid–fluid levels indicative of hemarthrosis. A medial retinacular tear (*arrow*) and bone contusions in the medial patella and lateral femoral condyle are depicted (*asterisks*).

SUGGESTED READING

Diederichs G, Issever AS, Scheffler S. MR imaging of patellar instability: injury patterns and assessment of risk factors. *Radiographics*. 2010;30(4):961–981.

Dietrich TJ, Fucentese SF, Pfirrmann CW. Imaging of individual anatomical risk factors for patellar instability. *Semin Musculoskelet Radiol*. 2016;20(1):65–73.

■ PATELLAR DISORDERS: CHONDROMALACIA PATELLA

KEY FACTS

- Patellar articular damage may result from subluxation, fracture, or repetitive microtrauma.
- Chondromalacia affects older males and younger females more often than young males. It more often involves the lateral facet and mid and lower patella.
- MRI with or without gadolinium provides a method to more accurately image articular changes in the patella.
- MRI features correlate with arthroscopic findings in chondromalacia (Table 4-1).
- Routine radiographs are normal until changes in bone occur in late stages of chondromalacia. MR images in the axial and sagittal planes are most useful. Numerous pulse sequences have been used to study articular cartilage. We prefer a fat-suppressed proton density–weighted fast spin-echo or double-echo steady-state sequences.

Table 4-1 ARTHROSCOPIC AND MAGNETIC RESONANCE CLASSIFICATION OF CHONDROMALACIA PATELLAE

Arthroscopic Classification	MRI Classification and Image Features
Grade 1: Softening of cartilage	Grade1: Normal contour $\pm$ signal intensity
Grade 2: Blister-like swelling	Grade 2: Focal areas of swelling/blistering with surface $\uparrow$ signal intensity or focal thinning with fluid extending into the defect measuring <50% of the depth of the cartilage
Grade 3: Surface irregularity and areas of thinning	Grade 3: Irregularity with focal thinning and fluid extending into the defect measuring >50% of the depth of the cartilage
Grade 4: Ulceration and bone exposed	Grade 4: Areas of bone exposure

MRI, magnetic resonance imaging.

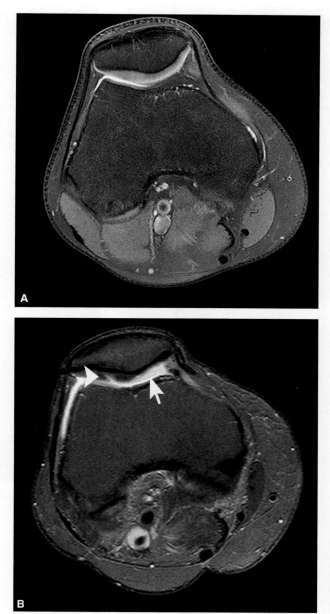

FIGURE 4-54. Normal articular cartilage (*arrows*) seen on proton density fat-suppressed proton density images **(A)**. Patellar chondromalacia seen on fat-suppressed fast spin-echo image **(B)** with diffuse Grade III chondromalacia involving the medial facet of the patella (*arrow*) and a focal chondral flap tear involving the lateral facet of the patella (*arrowhead*).

SUGGESTED READING

Rose PM, Demlow TA, Szumowski J, et al. Chondromalacia patellae: fat-suppressed MR imaging. *Radiology.* 1994;193:437–440.

■ LOOSE BODIES

KEY FACTS

- ■ Loose bodies may develop in patients after fracture or meniscal tears, or in patients with osteochondromatosis, synovial chondromatosis, or osteochondritis dissecans.
- ■ Loose bodies may be osseous, cartilaginous, fibrous, or a combination, depending on the etiology.
- ■ Calcified or ossified bodies can be identified on routine radiographs. Fibrous or cartilaginous lesions require MRI, arthrography, or arthroscopy for detection.
- ■ Technically, a loose body should move in the joint and not be attached to an intra-articular structure.
- ■ In the knee, loose bodies are located most commonly in the intercondylar region, near the tibial attachment of the ACL, or posteriorly above and below the joint line.

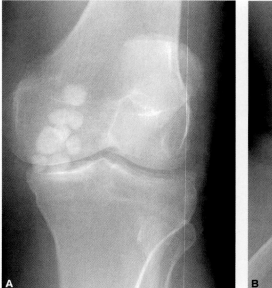 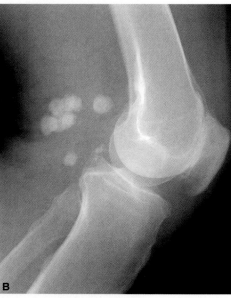

FIGURE 4-55. Anteroposterior (AP) **(A)** and lateral **(B)** radiographs of an ossified loose body posteriorly. Axial **(C)** fat-suppressed proton density magnetic resonance (MR) images demonstrate the loose bodies in a popliteal cyst.

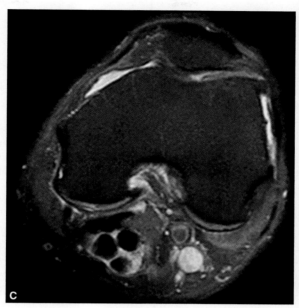

FIGURE 4-55. (*continued*)

SUGGESTED READING

Brossmann J, Preidler KW, Daener B, et al. Imaging of osseous and cartilaginous intra-articular bodies of the knee: comparison with MR imaging, and MR arthrography with CT and CT arthrography in cadavers. *Radiology.* 1996;200:509–517.

■ OSTEOCHONDRITIS DISSECANS

KEY FACTS

- Osteochondritis dissecans is a disease of teenagers. Average age of onset usually is 15 years. Males outnumber females in the ratio 3:1.
- Lesions in the knee most often involve the lateral aspect of the medial femoral condyle, but other regions, such as the patella, may also be involved. The condition is bilateral in 25%.
- Cause is repetitive trauma and/or ischemia.
- Detection of osteochondritis dissecans is generally possible with routine radiographs. The notch view is particularly useful for femoral condyle lesions. Appropriate classification of lesions requires conventional or CT arthrography, MRI, or MR arthrography (Table 4-2).
- T2-weighted MR images are 97% sensitive and 100% specific. A high–signal-intensity line around the lesion indicates instability.
- Unstable lesions may require surgical or arthroscopic treatment. Stable or minimally symptomatic lesions are treated conservatively.

Table 4-2 OSTEOCHONDRITIS DISSECANS

	Histologic and MR Features	
Grade	**Arthroscopic Features**	**MR Features**
Grade 0	Normal	Normal
Grade 1	Focal softening, fissuring	Cartilage intact, signal intensity abnormal in bone and cartilage
Grade 2	Defect in cartilage	Breach in cartilage
Grade 3	Fragment partially detached	Thin rim of abnormal signal intensity around fragment
Grade 4	Displaced fragment or loose in joint	Mixed signal intensity with fragment loose or displaced

MR, magnetic resonance.

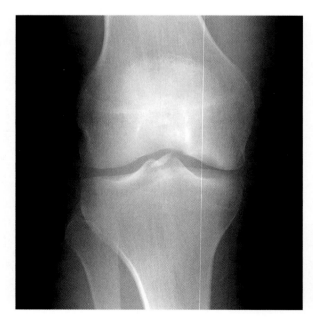

FIGURE 4-56. Anteroposterior (AP) radiograph depicting the characteristic appearance and location of osteochondritis dissecans involving the medial femoral condyle. Note the small unstable loose fragment now displaced into the intercondylar notch.

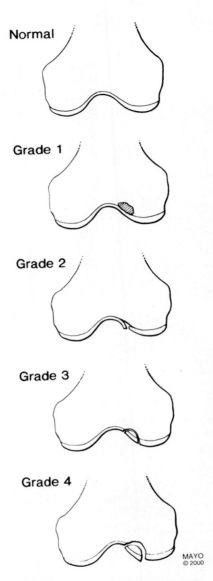

FIGURE 4-57. Magnetic resonance (MR) features of osteochondritis dissecans. Grade 1 = abnormal signal intensity, Grade 2 = linear defect in the cartilage, Grade 3 = abnormal signal intensity ($\uparrow$T2-weighted image and $\downarrow$T1-weighted image) around the fragment, Grade 4 = fragment has abnormal signal intensity surrounding it, and it may be loose.

(continued)

■ OSTEOCHONDRITIS DISSECANS *(Continued)*

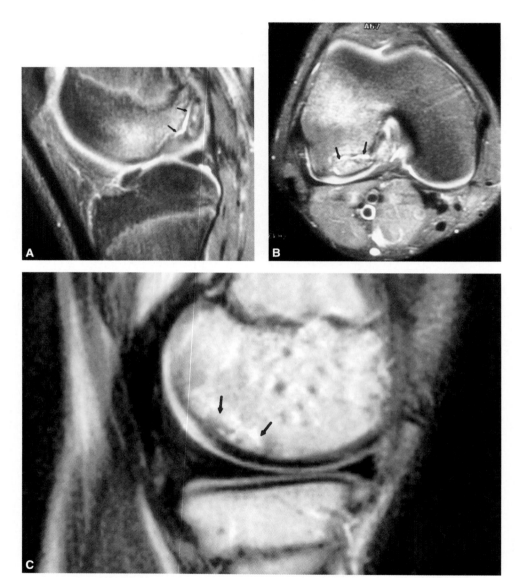

FIGURE 4-58. Magnetic resonance (MR) images of osteochondritis dissecans in two different patients. T2-weighted sagittal **(A)** and axial **(B)** images show a large defect with high-intensity fluid (*arrows*) separating the fragment from the condyle. This is an unstable lesion. **C:** Sagittal T2-weighted image in a different patient shows abnormal signal intensity (*arrows*), no fluid line around the lesion, and intact cartilage. This is a stable lesion.

SUGGESTED READING

DeSmet AA, Ilahi O, Graf BK. Reassessment of MR criteria for osteochondritis dissecans of the knee and ankle. *Skeletal Radiol.* 1996;25:159–163.

Ellermann JM, Donald B, Rohr S, et al. Magnetic resonance imaging of osteochondritis dissecans: validation study for the ICRS classification system. *Acad Radiol.* 2016;23(6):724–729.

Zbojniewicz AM, Stringer KF, Laor T, et al. Juvenile osteochondritis dissecans: correlation between histopathology and MRI. *Am J Roentgenol.* 2015;205(1):W114–W123.

■ OSTEONECROSIS

KEY FACTS

■ Osteonecrosis (bone death) in the knee may involve the epiphysis (avascular necrosis) or diaphysis and metaphysis (bone infarct).

■ Most cases are the result of systemic diseases, bone marrow disorders, or steroid therapy.

■ Spontaneous osteonecrosis of the knee is a condition affecting the weight-bearing surface of the femoral condyle (usually medial) that occurs in elderly or middle-aged patients, especially women.

■ Features of spontaneous osteonecrosis:
  - Pain, tenderness
  - Involves weight-bearing surface, unlike osteochondritis dissecans
  - Cause is likely related to subchondral insufficiency fracture
  - Leads to degenerative arthritis, loose bodies

■ Image features
  - Radiographs: osteonecrosis—subchondral sclerosis, fracture, articular collapse; infarction—peripheral calcification
  - Radionuclide scans: increased tracer
  - MRI: osteonecrosis—geographic zone of demarcation, bone marrow edema, articular collapse; infarction—serpiginous zone demarcating the margins of infarction

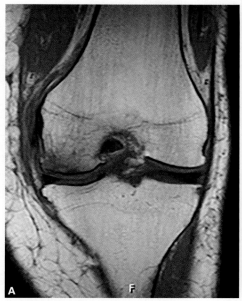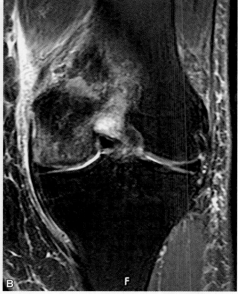

FIGURE 4-59. Spontaneous osteonecrosis. Coronal T1-weighted **(A)** and coronal T2-weighted **(B)** images of the knee show a subchondral fracture and early collapse of the medial femoral condyle.

(continued)

■ OSTEONECROSIS *(Continued)*

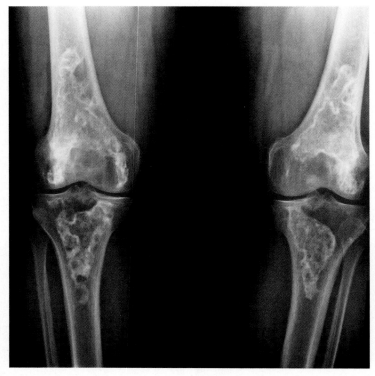

FIGURE 4-60. Standing view of the knees demonstrates bilateral bone infarcts with dense ossification or calcification along the margins.

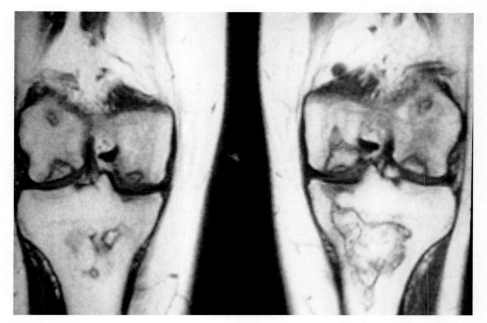

FIGURE 4-61. Coronal T1-weighted image of the knees with avascular necrosis in both femoral condyles and tibial and femoral bone infarcts.

SUGGESTED READING

Kattapuram TM, Kattapuram SV. Spontaneous osteonecrosis of the knee. *Eur J Radiol*. 2008;67(1):42–48. doi:10.1016/j.ejrad.2008.01.055.

Ramnath RR, Kattapuram SV. MR appearance of SONK-like subchondral abnormalities in the adult knee: SONK redefined. *Skeletal Radiol*. 2004;33(10):575–581.

Yamamoto T, Bullough PG. Spontaneous osteonecrosis of the knee: the result of subchondral insufficiency fracture. *J Bone Joint Surg*. 2000;82A:858–869.

■ OSTEOCHONDROSES

KEY FACTS

- Osteochondroses include a variety of disorders involving epiphyseal or apophyseal centers of the immature skeleton.
- Osteochondroses about the knee include Osgood–Schlatter disease, Blount disease, and Sinding–Larsen–Johansson disease.
- Osgood–Schlatter disease
    - Tibial tuberosity affected in 11 to 15 year olds.
    - Males outnumber females in the ratio 2:1; bilateral in 25%.
    - Patients present with local pain and swelling.
    - Radiographs show swelling and fragmentation of the tuberosity.
    - Diagnosis is clinical, and other imaging studies are usually not indicated.
- Blount disease
    - Growth disturbance of the medial tibial epiphysis
    - Infantile—appears in first year after birth
    - Adolescent—appears at ages 8 to 15 years
    - Radiographs show fragmentation of the epiphysis, and deformity and depression of the metaphysis
- Sinding–Larsen–Johansson disease
    - Tenderness and swelling over lower patella
    - Appears in 10 to 14 year olds
    - Radiographs show fragmentation of the lower pole of the patella

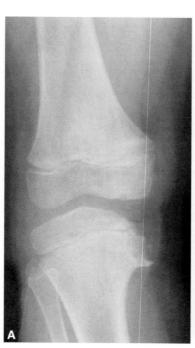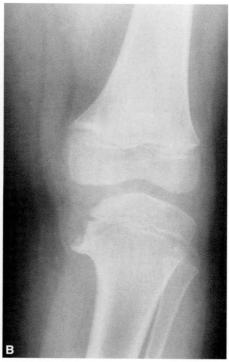

FIGURE 4-62. Blount disease. Anteroposterior (AP) radiographs of both knees **(A, B)** show metaphyseal and epiphyseal deformities medially with genu varum deformities of the knees.

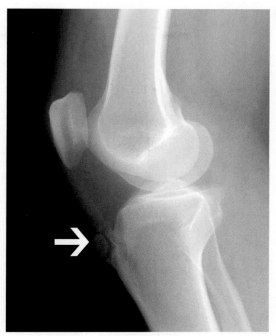

FIGURE 4-63. Osgood–Schlatter disease. Lateral radiograph demonstrates swelling and fragmentation (*arrow*) of the tibial tuberosity.

SUGGESTED READING

Craig JG, van Holsbeeck M, Zaltz I. The utility of MR in assessing Blount disease. *Skeletal Radiol.* 2002;31:208–213.
Resnick D. Osteochondrosis. In: Resnick D, ed. *Bone and Joint Imaging.* 2nd ed. Philadelphia: WB Saunders; 1996:960–978.

■ ARTHROPATHIES

KEY FACTS

■ Numerous arthropathies can involve the knee. The most common are primary osteoarthritis followed by calcium pyrophosphate deposition disease.

■ Arthropathies may involve one or all compartments. Distribution and involvement of one or both knees are useful for radiographic diagnosis.

■ The condition and image features of common arthropathies of the knee are summarized as follows:

Condition	Radiographic Features
Osteoarthritis	Primarily medial and patellofemoral involvement Joint space narrowing, osteophytes, increased bone density
CPPD	Joint space narrowing Bone sclerosis Chondrocalcinosis
Rheumatoid arthritis	Bilateral, symmetrical uniform joint space narrowing Osteopenia Marginal erosions Cystic changes
Psoriatic arthritis	Bilateral asymmetric involvement No osteopenia Bone proliferation
Reiter arthritis	Bilateral asymmetric No osteopenia Bone proliferation
Ankylosing spondylitis	Knee involvement uncommon Early erosions and bone sclerosis lead to ankylosis
Juvenile chronic arthritis	Unilateral with tricompartmental involvement Overgrowth of epiphysis and patella Looks similar to hemophilia
Hemophilia	Overgrowth of epiphysis and wide notch Square patella More cysts compared with juvenile chronic arthritis
Septic arthritis	Unilateral Aggressive weight-bearing cartilage loss
Pigmented villonodular synovitis	Knee most common joint involved Joint space narrows early Cystic changes Increased soft tissue density or mass-like structures about the joint Unilateral

CPPD, calcium pyrophosphate deposition disease.

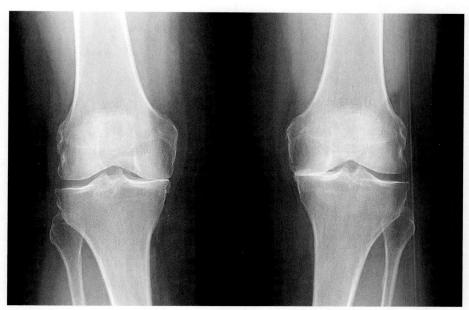

FIGURE 4-64. Standing view of the knees shows bilateral medial compartment narrowing caused by osteoarthritis.

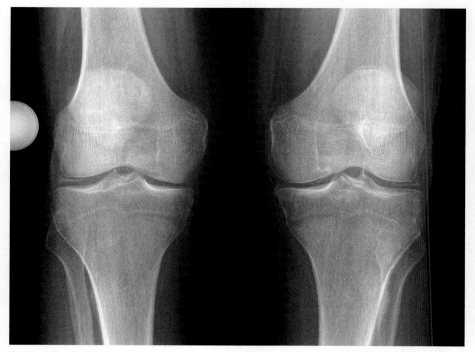

FIGURE 4-65. Calcium pyrophosphate deposition disease. Standing anteroposterior (AP) view of the knees shows cartilage calcification and degenerative joint changes.

(continued)

■ ARTHROPATHIES *(Continued)*

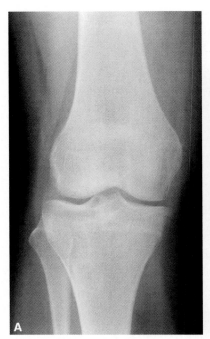
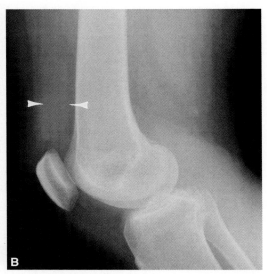

FIGURE 4-66. Rheumatoid arthritis. Anteroposterior (AP) **(A)** and lateral **(B)** radiographs demonstrate a joint effusion (*arrowheads*) with slight joint space narrowing. There are no erosions.

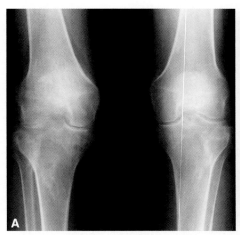
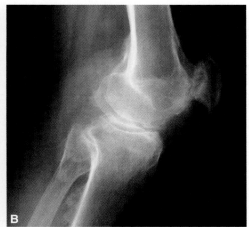

FIGURE 4-67. Reactive arthritis. Standing anteroposterior (AP) **(A)** and lateral **(B)** views of the knee demonstrate bilateral arthropathy with bone proliferation or whiskering at the ligament and tendon attachments.

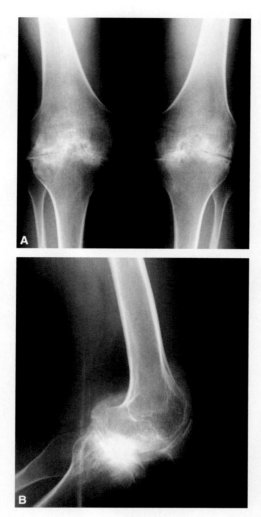

FIGURE 4-68. Hemophilic arthropathy. Standing **(A)** and lateral **(B)** views show the loss of joint space, wide notches, osteopenia, epiphyseal deformity, and squaring of the patella.

(continued)

■ ARTHROPATHIES *(Continued)*

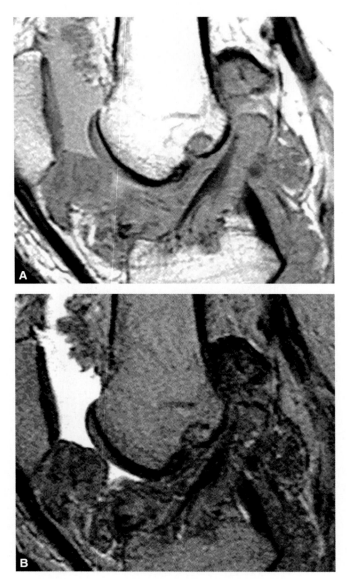

FIGURE 4-69. Pigmented villonodular synovitis. Sagittal proton density–weighted **(A)** and T2-weighted **(B)** images demonstrate extensive synovial proliferation with areas of low signal intensity caused by hemosiderin deposition.

SUGGESTED READING

Brower AC. *Arthritis in Black and White.* 2nd ed. Philadelphia: WB Saunders; 1997.

■ NEOPLASMS: BONE TUMORS AND TUMORLIKE CONDITIONS

KEY FACTS

■ Primary and metastatic neoplasms and other tumorlike conditions are common about the knee (Table 4-3).

■ Approximately 50% of osteosarcomas occur in the knee.

■ Sixty percent of Ewing sarcomas involve the knee or pelvis.

■ Thirty-two percent of chondroblastomas and more than 50% of giant cell tumors occur in the knee.

■ Patellar tumors are rare (0.06% of all tumors).

■ Skeletal lesions are characterized most easily on routine radiographs. CT and MRI are useful for staging. Radionuclide scans are useful for localizing subtle lesions.

Table 4-3 PRIMARY SKELETAL NEOPLASMS OF THE KNEE

Lesion	Total/No. in Knee/% in Knee
Malignant	
Osteosarcoma	1,649/795/48
Fibrosarcoma	255/80/31
Chondrosarcoma	895/143/16
Ewing sarcoma	512/71/14
Lymphoma	694/75/11
Benign	
Giant cell tumor	568/282/50
Chondromyxoid fibroma	45/17/38
Osteochondroma	872/325/37
Chondroblastoma	119/44/37
Aneurysmal bone cyst	289/68/24
Chondroma	290/44/15
Osteoid osteoma	331/41/12

(continued)

■ NEOPLASMS: BONE TUMORS AND TUMORLIKE CONDITIONS *(Continued)*

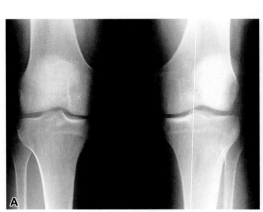

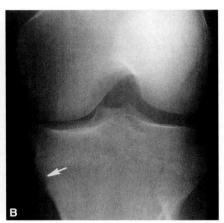

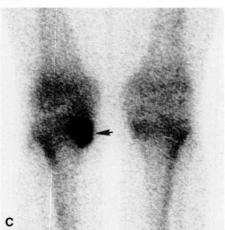

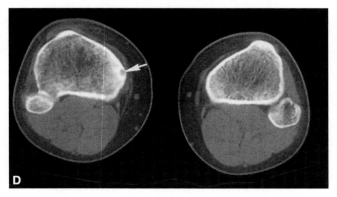

FIGURE 4-70. Osteoid osteoma. Anteroposterior (AP) standing **(A)** and notch **(B)** views of the right knee show a questionable tibial defect (*arrow*). **C:** Radionuclide bone scan is positive (*arrow*) in this region. **D:** Computed tomography (CT) image clearly defines the osteoid osteoma (*arrow*).

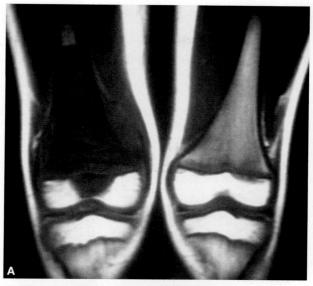

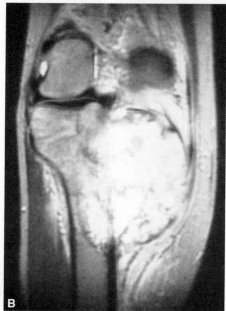

FIGURE 4-71. Osteosarcoma. **A:** Coronal T1-weighted image demonstrates low signal intensity tumor involving the distal femur and extending into the epiphysis on the right. **B:** T2-weighted image in a different patient shows the extent of soft tissue involvement.

SUGGESTED READING

Kransdorf M, Berquist TH. Musculoskeletal neoplasms. In: Berquist TH, ed. *MRI of the Musculoskeletal System*. 5th ed. Philadelphia: Lippincott Williams & Wilkins; 2006:802–915.

Unni KK. *Dahlin's Bone Tumors: General Aspects and Data on 11,087 Cases*. Philadelphia: WB Saunders; 1996.

■ NEOPLASMS: SOFT TISSUE TUMORS AND MASSES

KEY FACTS

■ Soft tissue masses about the knee may be true neoplasms or cysts, such as popliteal cysts or ganglion cysts. Ganglion cysts may also involve the cruciate ligaments and are likely posttraumatic.

■ Posterior soft tissue lesions are common and include popliteal cysts, meniscal cysts, ganglion cysts, popliteal varices, popliteal artery aneurysms, and hemangiomas.

■ Popliteal cysts communicate with the joint and are seen in less than 5% of MRI studies.

■ MRI is the technique of choice for detection and characterization of soft tissue masses.
  ● Benign: typically homogeneous. Increased intensity on T2-weighted images and decreased intensity on T1-weighted images. Well-defined margins.
  ● Malignant: typically inhomogeneous. Best appreciated on T2-weighted images. Poorly defined margins. May encase neurovascular structures.

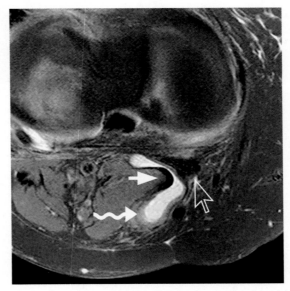

FIGURE 4-72. Popliteal cyst. Fat-suppressed fast spin-echo proton density axial image shows a well-defined fluid signal intensity popliteal cyst (*wavy arrow*) arising from the knee joint extending between the medial head of the gastrocnemius (*arrow*) and the semimembranosus (*open arrow*).

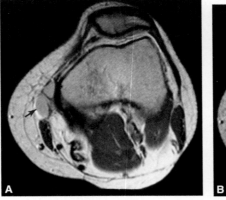 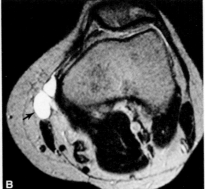

FIGURE 4-73. Axial proton density–weighted **(A)** and T2-weighted **(B)** images of a septated ganglion cyst medially (*arrow*).

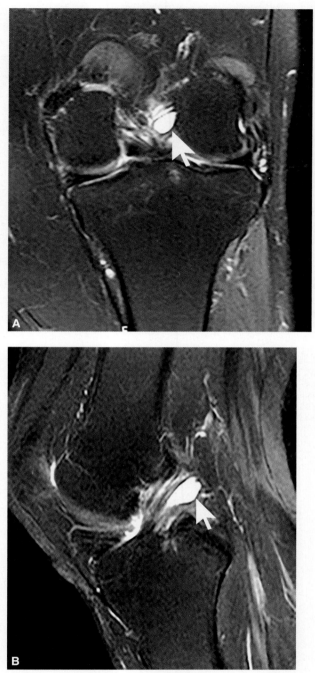

FIGURE 4-74. Coronal T2-weighted **(A)** and sagittal T2-weighted **(B)** images demonstrate an anterior cruciate ligament (ACL) ganglion (*arrow*).

(continued)

■ NEOPLASMS: SOFT TISSUE TUMORS AND MASSES *(Continued)*

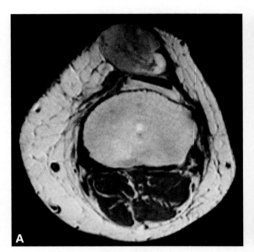 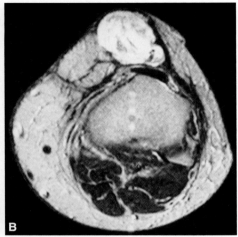

FIGURE 4-75. Undifferentiated pleomorphic sarcoma. Axial proton density–weighted **(A)** and T2-weighted **(B)** images show an irregular, inhomogeneous mass anterior to the patella.

SUGGESTED READING

Hwang S, Panicek DM. The evolution of musculoskeletal tumor imaging. *Radiol Clin North Am.* 2009;47(3):435–453.

Kransdorf M, Berquist TH. Musculoskeletal neoplasms. In: Berquist TH, ed. *MRI of the Musculoskeletal System.* 5th ed. Philadelphia: Lippincott Williams & Wilkins; 2006:802–915.

Kransdorf MJ, Bridges MD. Current developments and recent advances in musculoskeletal tumor imaging. *Semin Musculoskelet Radiol.* 2013;17(2):145–155.

■ CHRONIC OVERUSE/MISCELLANEOUS CONDITIONS: BURSITIS

KEY FACTS

- There are numerous bursae about the knee that may become inflamed and symptomatic (Table 4-4).
- Patients present with local pain and tenderness. Other injuries (ligament or menisci) must be excluded.
- Inflamed distended bursae appear as fluid-filled masses on ultrasound, CT, and MR images.
- Aspiration, therapeutic injections, or resection may be required.

Table 4-4   BURSAE ABOUT THE KNEE

Anterior	
Prepatellar	Between patella and skin
Retropatellar	Between patellar tendon and tibia
Pretibial	Between tibial tuberosity and skin
Suprapatellar[a]	Between quadriceps and femur
Lateral	
Gastrocnemius	Between lateral head of gastrocnemius and joint capsule
Fibular	Between fibular collateral ligament and biceps tendon
Fibular popliteal	Between fibular collateral ligament and popliteus tendon
Popliteal[a]	Between popliteus tendon and lateral femoral condyle
Medial	
Gastrocnemius[a]	Between medial head of gastrocnemius and capsule
Pes anserine	Between tibial collateral ligament and gracilis, sartorius, and semitendinosus tendons
Semimembranosus-tibial collateral ligament	Between semimembranosus tendon and medial collateral ligament

[a] Communicates with the joint.

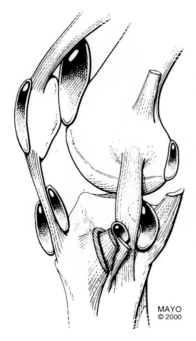

MAYO
© 2000

FIGURE 4-76. Bursae about the knee.

(continued)

■ CHRONIC OVERUSE/MISCELLANEOUS CONDITIONS: BURSITIS *(Continued)*

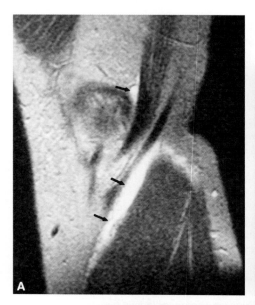
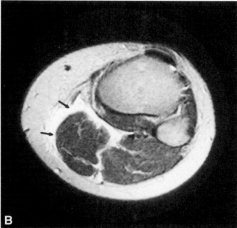
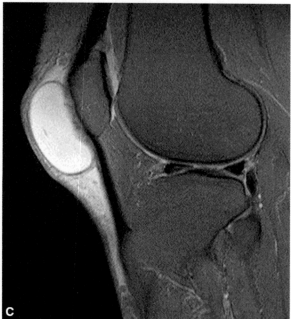

FIGURE 4-77. Pes anserine and prepatellar bursitis. Sagittal **(A)** and axial **(B)** T2-weighted images demonstrate high signal intensity *(arrows)* along the medial tendons. Sagittal fluid-sensitive sequence **(C)** in a different patient depicts marked prepatellar bursitis.

SUGGESTED READING

Forbes JR, Nelius CA, Janzen DL. Acute pes anserine bursitis: MR imaging. *Radiology.* 1995;194:525–527.

■ CHRONIC OVERUSE/MISCELLANEOUS CONDITIONS: ILIOTIBIAL BAND SYNDROME

KEY FACTS

- The iliotibial band extends from the greater trochanter to insert on the supracondylar tubercle of the femur.
- Iliotibial band syndrome is common in long-distance runners, cyclists, and football players.
- The syndrome is caused by friction of the band over the femur and underlying soft tissues.
- Differential diagnoses include lateral meniscal tears, LCL injuries, and lateral hamstring strains.
- Imaging is accomplished using ultrasound or MRI. A poorly defined fluid collection and thickening of the iliotibial band are the most common findings.

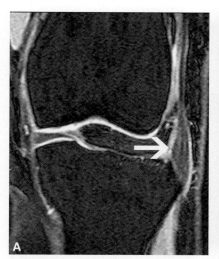 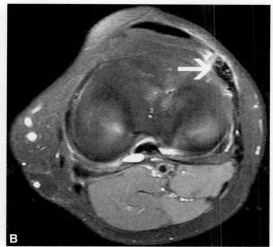

FIGURE 4-78. Iliotibial band syndrome. Coronal **(A)** and axial **(B)** magnetic resonance (MR) images demonstrate thickening of the distal iliotibial band with surrounding edema (*arrows*).

SUGGESTED READING

Muhle C, Ahn JM, Yeh L, et al. Iliotibial band friction syndrome: MR imaging findings in 16 patients and MR arthrographic study of six cadaveric knees. *Radiology.* 1999;212(1):103–110.
Murphy BJ, Hechtman KS, Uribe JW, et al. Iliotibial band friction syndrome: MR image findings. *Radiology.* 1992;185:569–571.
O'Keeffe SA, Hogan BA, Eustace SJ, et al. Overuse injuries of the knee. *Magn Reson Imaging Clin N Am.* 2009;17(4):725–739.

■ CHRONIC OVERUSE/MISCELLANEOUS CONDITIONS: MUSCLE TEARS

KEY FACTS

- Ligament and tendon tears are more common than muscle injuries in the knee. Most muscle tears occur in the calf and thigh.
- Tears in the popliteus, plantaris, and quadriceps can occur in the knee.
- The plantaris is a small muscle arising from the lateral femoral condyle. The tendon courses between the gastrocnemius and the soleus. Tears are common in athletes, especially tennis players. Differential diagnoses include gastrocnemius tears and deep vein thrombosis.
- Popliteal muscle tears involve the body of the muscle. Bone bruises (33%) and tears of the ACL (17%) and PCL (29%) are commonly associated.
- Muscle tears can be graded using axial and coronal or sagittal MR images.
  - Grade 1 strain: A few torn fibers are seen as an area of high signal intensity on T2-weighted or short-T1 inversion recovery images.
  - Grade 2 strain: Approximately 50% of the fibers are torn.
  - Grade 3 strain: There is a complete tear.

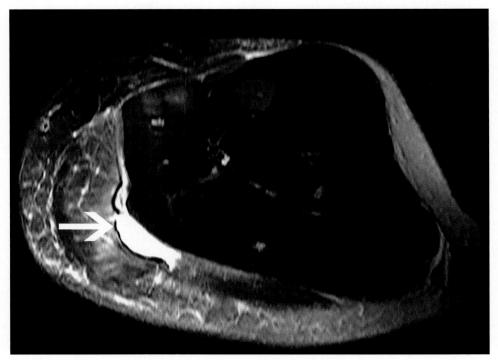

FIGURE 4-79. Plantaris tear. Axial T2-weighted magnetic resonance (MR) image shows fluid (*arrow*) between the soleus and the gastrocnemius. The tendon of the plantaris is absent.

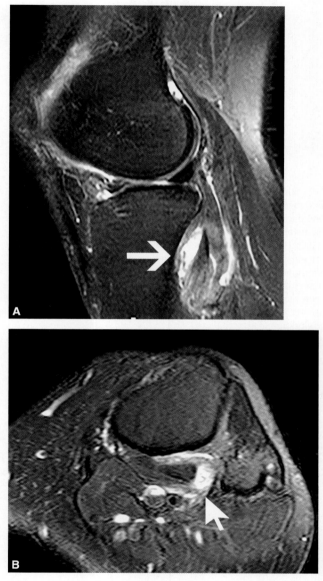

FIGURE 4-80. Popliteus muscle tear. Sagittal **(A)** and axial **(B)** T2-weighted images demonstrate increased signal intensity and hemorrhage along the popliteus muscle compatible with tear (*arrow*).

SUGGESTED READING

Brown TR, Quinn SF, Wensel JP, et al. Diagnoses of popliteus injuries with MR imaging. *Skeletal Radiol.* 1995;24:511–514.
O'Keeffe SA, Hogan BA, Eustace SJ, et al. Overuse injuries of the knee. *Magn Reson Imaging Clin N Am.* 2009;17(4):725–739.

Foot, Ankle, and Calf

Joseph M. Bestic, Jeffrey J. Peterson, Thomas H. Berquist

■ FRACTURES/DISLOCATIONS: ANKLE FRACTURES—PEDIATRIC

KEY FACTS

- Image features of ankle fractures depend on age (growth plate development), relationship of ligaments to epiphyses, and mechanism of injury.
- Metaphyseal and diaphyseal fractures are frequently incomplete.
- Fractures of the distal tibia and fibula frequently involve the growth plate.
- Fracture of the distal tibial physis is the second most common growth plate injury.
- The Salter–Harris classification is frequently used for growth plate fractures:
  - Type I: Separation of epiphysis, fracture confined to growth plate (6%)
  - Type II: Fracture through growth plate extending into the metaphysis (75%)
  - Type III: Fracture through growth plate extending through epiphysis (8%)
  - Type IV: Extends from articular surface of epiphysis through growth plate and metaphysis (10%)
  - Type V: Compression of growth plate (1%)
  - Complications are more significant with Types III to V

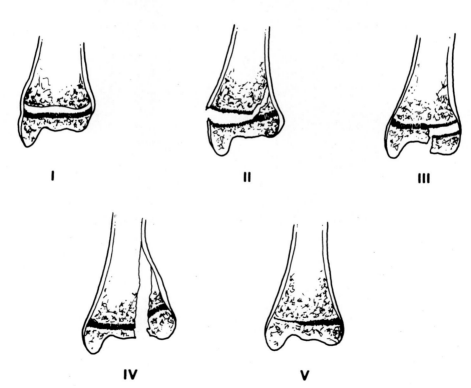

FIGURE 5-1. The five Salter–Harris fracture patterns.

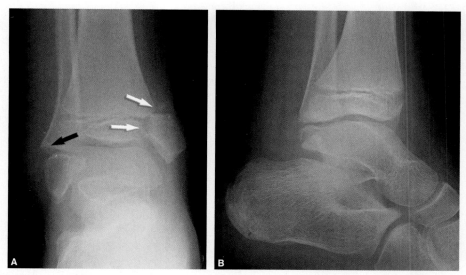

FIGURE 5-2. Anteroposterior (AP) **(A)** and lateral **(B)** radiographs demonstrate marked swelling with a Salter–Harris Type IV (*white arrows*) tibial fracture and Type II fibular fracture (*black arrow*) as the result of an inversion injury.

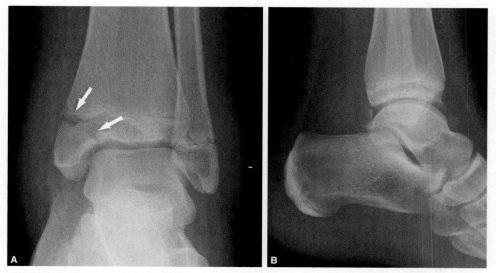

FIGURE 5-3. Anteroposterior (AP) **(A)** and lateral **(B)** radiographs of an eversion injury with opening of the tibial physis and a Salter–Harris Type III fracture (*white arrows*).

SUGGESTED READING

Blackburn EW, Aronsson DD, Rubright JH, et al. Ankle fractures in children. *J Bone Joint Surg Am*. 2012;94(13):1234–1244.
Rogers LF. Radiology of epiphyseal injuries. *Radiology*. 1970;96:289–299.
Wuerz TH, Gurd DP. Pediatric physeal ankle fracture. *J Am Acad Orthop Surg*. 2013;21(4):234–244.

■ FRACTURES/DISLOCATIONS: ANKLE FRACTURES— PEDIATRIC: TRIPLANE FRACTURE

KEY FACTS

- ■ Triplane fractures are the result of external rotation forces, and account for 6% of physeal fractures.
- ■ The fracture consists of three fragments instead of two seen with most growth plate fractures.
- ■ Fracture fragments include (1) anterior lateral tibial epiphysis (Salter–Harris Type III); (2) remainder of the tibial epiphysis with metaphyseal attachment (looks like Salter–Harris Type II); and (3) tibial metaphysis.
- ■ Complication rates are similar to those for a Salter–Harris Type IV fracture.
- ■ Computed tomography (CT) may be required to properly characterize the injury.

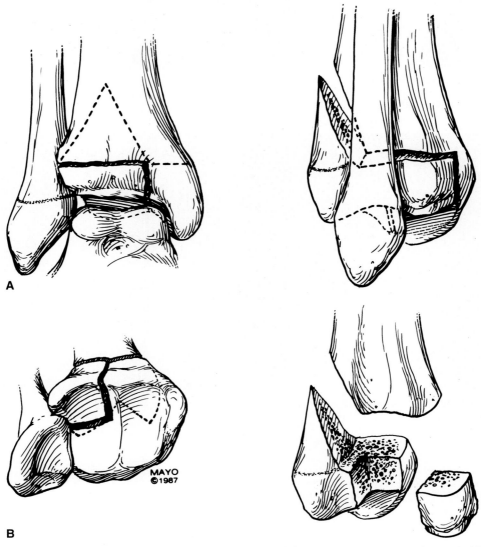

FIGURE 5-4. Triplane fracture seen from the front and side **(A)** and from the articular surface and with fragments separated **(B)**.

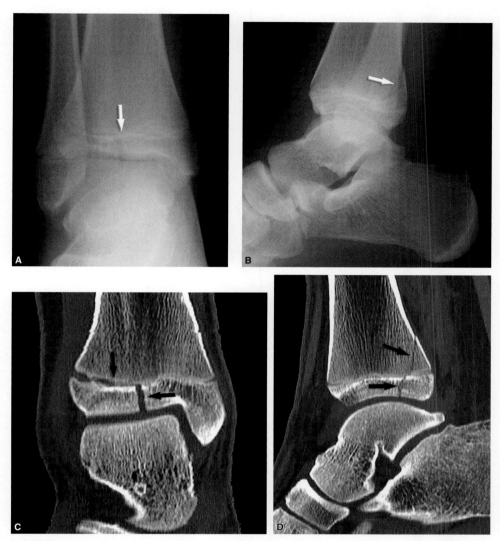

FIGURE 5-5. Anteroposterior (AP) **(A)** and lateral **(B)** radiographs demonstrate a triplane fracture (*white arrows*). Coronal **(C)** and sagittal **(D)** reformatted computed tomography (CT) images define the fractures (*black arrows*) and degree of displacement.

SUGGESTED READING

Cone RO III, Nguyen V, Flournoyr JG, et al. Triplane fracture of the distal tibial epiphysis: radiologic and CT studies. *Radiology*. 1984;153:763–767.

Schnetzler KA, Hoernschemeyer D. The pediatric triplane ankle fracture. *J Am Acad Orthop Surg*. 2007;15(12):738–747.

■ FRACTURES/DISLOCATIONS: ANKLE FRACTURES—PEDIATRIC: JUVENILE TILLAUX

KEY FACTS

- Distal tibial epiphysis fuses from medial to lateral, placing the lateral physis at risk in adolescents.
- Distal tibial physis fuses at approximately age 15 in females and age 17 in males.
- Juvenile Tillaux fracture is a Salter–Harris Type III fracture of the lateral tibial physis.
- The fracture is displaced by the distal tibiofibular ligament when the foot is externally rotated.

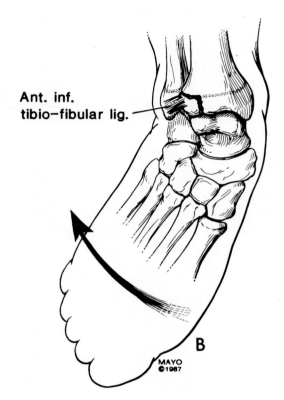

FIGURE 5-6. Mechanism of injury for juvenile Tillaux fractures.

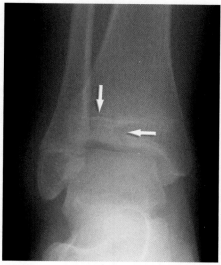

FIGURE 5-7. Anteroposterior (AP) radiograph shows a Salter–Harris III fracture—juvenile Tillaux fracture (*white arrows*).

SUGGESTED READING

Horn BD, Crisci K, Krug M, et al. Radiologic evaluation of juvenile Tillaux fractures of the distal tibia. *J Pediatr Orthop.* 2001;21(2):162–164.

Mann DC, Rajmaira S. Distribution of physeal and nonphyseal fractures in 2,650 long bone fractures in children aged 10 to 16 years. *J Pediatr Orthop.* 1990;10:713–716.

■ FRACTURES/DISLOCATIONS: ANKLE FRACTURES— PEDIATRIC COMPLICATIONS

KEY FACTS

- Fractures not involving the growth plate generally heal without sequelae.
- Growth plate fractures may heal with premature or asymmetric closure. Complications vary with Salter–Harris fracture type.
- Low risk (6.7% complications): Types I and II fibular fractures; Types I, III, and IV tibial fractures with less than 2 mm of displacement.
- High risk (32% complications): Types III and IV tibial fractures with more than 2 mm of displacement; juvenile Tillaux fractures, triplane fractures, comminuted epiphyseal fractures, and Type V fractures.
- Complications include leg length discrepancy, rotational deformity, malunion, nonunion, and avascular necrosis.
- Routine radiographs are usually adequate to define complications. CT or magnetic resonance imaging (MRI) may be required to assess growth plate involvement.

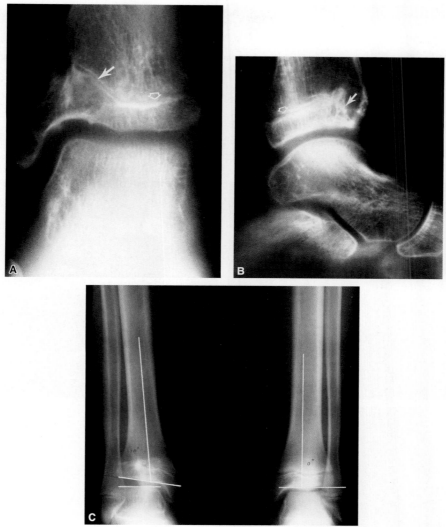

FIGURE 5-8. Prior Salter–Harris IV fracture of the distal tibia. Anteroposterior (AP) **(A)** and lateral **(B)** radiographs demonstrate premature closure and angular deformity of the anteromedial growth plate (*arrow*). The physis remains open laterally and posteriorly (*open arrow*). Standing radiographs **(C)** in a different patient with an old physeal fracture on the right and leg length discrepancy and angular deformity of the articular surface (*lines*).

SUGGESTED READING

Blackburn EW, Aronsson DD, Rubright JH, et al. Ankle fractures in children. *J Bone Joint Surg Am.* 2012;94(13):1234–1244.
Spiegel PG, Cooperman DR, Laros GS. Epiphyseal fractures of the distal ends of the tibia and fibula. *J Bone Joint Surg.* 1978;60A:1046–1050.

■ FRACTURES/DISLOCATIONS: ANKLE FRACTURES—ADULT

KEY FACTS

- The mechanism of injury for ankle fractures is rarely pure inversion (supination) or eversion (pronation). Abduction, adduction, lateral rotation, and axial loading forces are usually associated.
- Fracture patterns, specifically the location and appearance of the fibular fracture and talar shift in the ankle mortise, can allow definition of the mechanism of injury and ligament involvement in more than 90% of cases.
- Anteroposterior (AP), lateral, and mortise views are usually adequate for diagnosis.
- The lateral view is particularly useful to define joint effusions. An effusion should raise the question of subtle osteochondral injury, which may require CT or MRI for further evaluation.

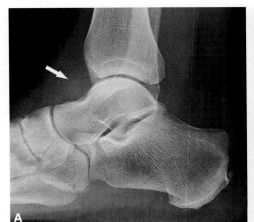
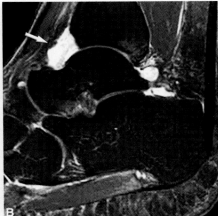
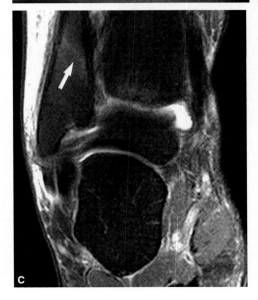

FIGURE 5-9. (A) Joint effusion (white *arrow*) seen on the lateral radiograph. Sagittal fat-suppressed proton density image **(B)** demonstrates a large effusion (white *arrow*). Coronal fat-suppressed proton density image **(C)** reveals an oblique, nondisplaced distal fibular fracture (white *arrow*), which was not evident radiographically.

SUGGESTED READING

Arimoto HR, Forrester DM. Classification of ankle fractures: an algorithm. *AJR Am J Roentgenol.* 1980;135:1057–1063.
Michelson JD. Fractures about the ankle. *J Bone Joint Surg Am.* 1995;77:142.

■ FRACTURES/DISLOCATIONS: ANKLE ADULT— SUPINATION–ADDUCTION INJURIES

KEY FACTS

■ Supination–adduction injuries (inversion) cause traction laterally, resulting in ligament injury or a transverse lateral malleolar fracture below the ankle joint (Stage I). When force continues, a medial impaction (steep oblique) fracture of the medial malleolus occurs (Stage II) (Fig. 5-10).

■ Supination–adduction injuries account for approximately 20% of ankle fractures.

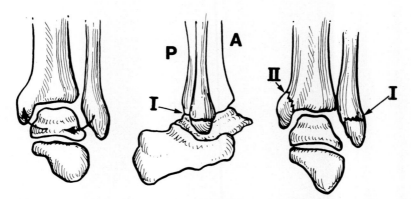

FIGURE 5-10. Inversion (supination)–adduction injury. The forces cause a transverse fracture below the joint line (Stage I) or ligament tear. With continued stress, a steep oblique fracture of the medial malleolus occurs (Stage II).

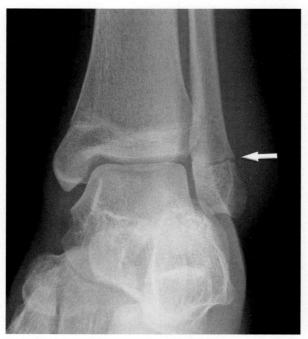

FIGURE 5-11. Supination–adduction injury with a transverse fracture of the lateral malleolus (*white arrow*) below the level of the ankle joint.

(continued)

■ FRACTURES/DISLOCATIONS: ANKLE ADULT—SUPINATION–ADDUCTION INJURIES *(Continued)*

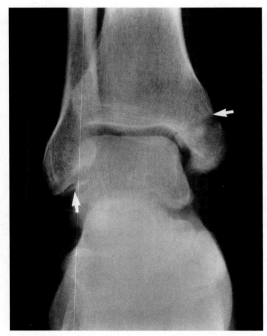

FIGURE 5-12. Supination–adduction Stage II injury with an oblique fracture (*arrow*) of the medial malleolus and avulsed fragments from the lateral malleolus (*arrow*).

SUGGESTED READING

Funk, JR. Ankle injury mechanisms: lessons learned from cadaveric studies. *Clin Anat.* 2011;24(3):350–361.

Lauge-Hansen N. Fractures of the ankle. II. Combined experimental-surgical and experimental-roentgenologic investigations. *Arch Surg.* 1950;60:957–985.

Okanobo H, Khurana B, Sheehan S, et al. Simplified diagnostic algorithm for Lauge-Hansen classification of ankle injuries. *Radiographics.* 2012;32(2):E71–E84.

■ FRACTURES/DISLOCATIONS: ANKLE ADULT— SUPINATION LATERAL ROTATION INJURIES

KEY FACTS

■ Supination lateral rotation injuries cause medial tension, with the talus causing posterior displacement of the lateral malleolus.

■ The anterior distal tibiofibular ligament is injured (Stage I). If force continues, a spiral fracture of the lateral malleolus occurs just above the joint (best seen on the lateral view). This Stage II injury is the most common ankle fracture. With continued force, a posterior tibial fracture or distal tibiofibular ligament tear occurs (Stage III), and eventually a transverse medial malleolar or medial (deltoid) ligament injury occurs (Stage IV) (Fig. 5-13).

■ Supination lateral rotation injuries account for 55% to 58% of ankle fractures.

■ All supination or inversion injuries account for 75% to 78% of ankle fractures.

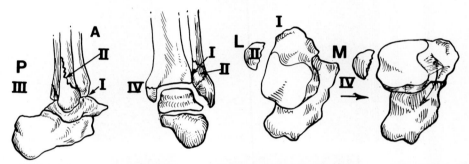

FIGURE 5-13. Supination lateral rotation injuries. The talus causes posterior fibular displacement with disruption of the anterior distal tibiofibular ligament (Stage I). If force continues, a spiral fracture of the fibula occurs just above the joint line (best seen on the lateral view) (Stage II). Continued force results in a posterior tibial fracture or tear in the posterior distal tibiofibular ligament (Stage III) and, finally, a transverse medial malleolar fracture or deltoid ligament tear (Stage IV).

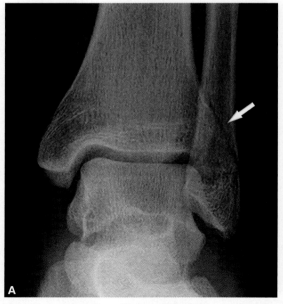

FIGURE 5-14. Supination lateral rotation Stage II injury. Anteroposterior (AP) **(A)**, mortise **(B)**, and lateral **(C)** radiographs. The fracture is clearly demonstrated only on the AP and lateral views (*white arrows*).

(continued)

■ FRACTURES/DISLOCATIONS: ANKLE ADULT— SUPINATION LATERAL ROTATION INJURIES *(Continued)*

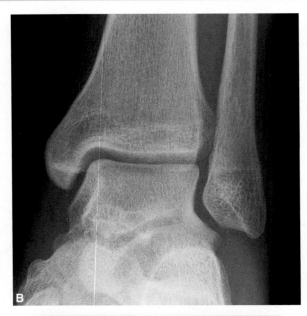

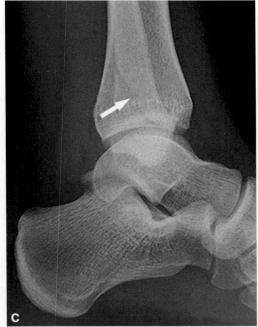

FIGURE 5-14. *(continued)*

SUGGESTED READING

Berquist TH. *Radiology of the Foot and Ankle*, 2nd ed. Philadelphia: Lippincott Williams & Wilkins; 2000:171–280.

Funk, JR. Ankle injury mechanisms: lessons learned from cadaveric studies. *Clin Anat.* 2011;24(3):350–361.

Okanobo H, Khurana B, Sheehan S, et al. Simplified diagnostic algorithm for Lauge-Hansen classification of ankle injuries. *Radiographics.* 2012;32(2):E71–E84.

■ FRACTURES/DISLOCATIONS: ANKLE ADULT— PRONATION–ABDUCTION INJURIES

KEY FACTS

■ Pronation–abduction (eversion) injuries result from medial tension leading to deltoid ligament injury or a transverse medial malleolar fracture (Stage I). Continued force results in tears of the anterior and posterior distal tibiofibular ligaments or a posterior tibial fracture (Stage II) followed by an oblique lateral malleolar fracture near the joint level (best seen on AP view) (Stage III) (Fig. 5-15).

■ When displaced, internal fixation is necessary to reduce the ankle mortise.

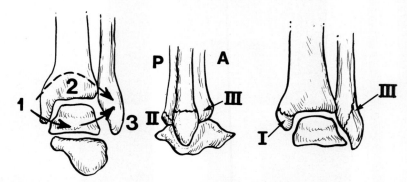

FIGURE 5-15. Pronation (eversion)–abduction injuries. Medial tension causes a transverse malleolar fracture or deltoid ligament tear (Stage I). Continued force results in disruption of the distal anterior and posterior tibiofibular ligaments or a posterior tibial fracture (Stage II) followed by an oblique fibular fracture near the joint line best seen on the anteroposterior (AP) radiograph (Stage III).

(continued)

■ FRACTURES/DISLOCATIONS: ANKLE ADULT— PRONATION–ABDUCTION INJURIES *(Continued)*

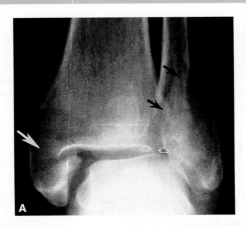

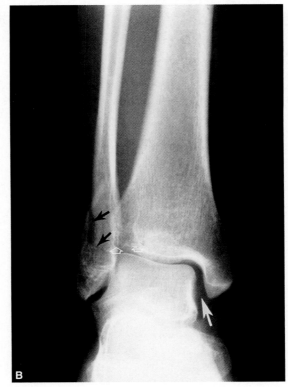

FIGURE 5-16. Pronation–abduction Stage III injuries. **(A)** There is a transverse medial malleolar fracture (*white arrow*), tibiofibular ligament tears with separation of the tibia and fibula (*open arrows*), and an oblique fibular fracture (*black arrows*). **(B)** Widening of the medial ankle mortise (*white arrow*) caused by a ligament tear with increased tibiofibular distance (*open arrows*) and oblique fibular fracture (*black arrows*).

SUGGESTED READING

Arimoto HR, Forrester DM. Classification of ankle fractures: an algorithm. *AJR Am J Roentgenol.* 1980;135:1057–1063.

Funk, JR. Ankle injury mechanisms: lessons learned from cadaveric studies. *Clin Anat.* 2011;24(3):350–361.

Okanobo H, Khurana B, Sheehan S, et al. Simplified diagnostic algorithm for Lauge-Hansen classification of ankle injuries. *Radiographics.* 2012;32(2):E71–E84.

■ FRACTURES/DISLOCATIONS: ANKLE ADULT— PRONATION LATERAL ROTATION INJURIES

KEY FACTS

- ■ Pronation lateral rotation injuries cause medial tension as the talus rotates laterally.
- ■ The medical malleolus (low transverse fracture) or medial ligaments are injured initially (Stage I). As force continues, the anterior tibiofibular and interosseous membranes are torn (Stage II), followed by a high fibular fracture (more than 5 to 6 cm above the joint) (Stage III). Posterior tibial avulsion or distal tibiofibular ligament tears occur with continued force (Stage IV) (Fig. 5-17).
- ■ Pronation injuries account for 22% to 25% of ankle fractures.
- ■ Treatment of these fractures usually requires internal fixation of the fibular fracture and screw fixation of the medial malleolus.

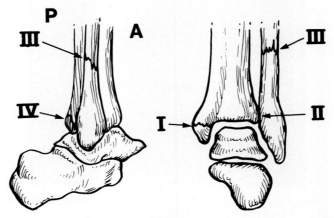

FIGURE 5-17. Pronation lateral rotation injuries. Medial tension results in a low transverse medial malleolar fracture or deltoid ligament tear (Stage I), followed by tearing of the distal anterior tibiofibular ligament and interosseous membrane (Stage II). With continued force, a high (>6 cm) fibular fracture occurs (Stage III) followed by a posterior distal tibiofibular ligament tear or avulsion fracture (Stage IV).

(continued)

■ FRACTURES/DISLOCATIONS: ANKLE ADULT—PRONATION LATERAL ROTATION INJURIES *(Continued)*

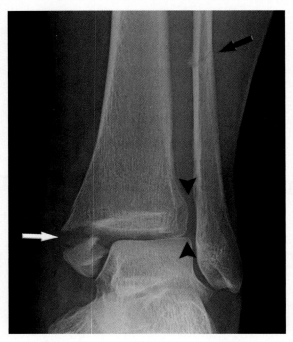

FIGURE 5-18. Pronation lateral rotation Stage IV injury with a transverse medial malleolar fracture (*white arrow*), disruption of the tibiofibular and interosseous ligaments (black *arrowheads*), and a high fibular fracture (*black arrow*).

SUGGESTED READING

Arimoto HR, Forrester DM. Classification of ankle fractures: an algorithm. *AJR Am J Roentgenol*. 1980;135:1057–1063.

Funk, JR. Ankle injury mechanisms: lessons learned from cadaveric studies. *Clin Anat*. 2011;24(3):350–361.

Okanobo H, Khurana B, Sheehan S, et al. Simplified diagnostic algorithm for Lauge-Hansen classification of ankle injuries. *Radiographics*. 2012;32(2):E71–E84.

■ FRACTURES/DISLOCATIONS: ANKLE ADULT— PLAFOND FRACTURES (PILON)

KEY FACTS

- ■ Plafond fractures do not fit neatly into other fracture classifications. Tibial plafond fractures account for less than 10% of lower extremity fractures.
- ■ Fractures are the result of axial loading; 72% occur in patients less than 50 years of age.
- ■ Up to 20% of plafond fractures are open, resulting in increased incidence of infection.
- ■ Treatment of these fractures is difficult, because the articular surface needs to be anatomically reduced.
- ■ CT and MRI may be required to clearly demonstrate the extent of injury for surgical treatment planning.

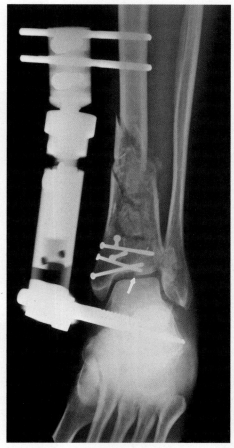

FIGURE 5-19. Mortise view of a tibial plafond fracture reduced with external fixateur and tibial screws. Note the residual articular deformity (*arrow*).

SUGGESTED READING

Bonar SK, Marsh JL. Tibial plafond fractures: changing principles of treatment. *J Am Acad Orthop Surg*. 1994;2:297–304.
Ovadia DN, Beals RK. Fractures of the tibial plafond. *J Bone Joint Surg*. 1986;68A:543–551.
Topliss CJ, Jackson M, Atkins RM. Anatomy of pilon fractures of the distal tibia. *J Bone Joint Surg Br*. 2005;87(5): 692–697.

■ FRACTURES/DISLOCATIONS: ANKLE ADULT—COMPLICATIONS

KEY FACTS

■ Complications resulting from ankle fractures may be related to injury or treatment.
■ Loss of reduction occurs more commonly with closed techniques (casting) than internal fixation.
■ Degenerative arthritis is the most common long-term complication, occurring in 30% to 40% of cases.
■ Complications are summarized as follows:
  ● Loss of reduction (up to 26% treated by casting alone)
  ● Osteoarthritis
  ● Chronic instability
  ● Loss of motion
  ● Nonunion
  ● Malunion
  ● Reflex sympathetic dystrophy
  ● Infection
  ● Adhesive capsulitis
  ● Tendon rupture
  ● Neurovascular injury

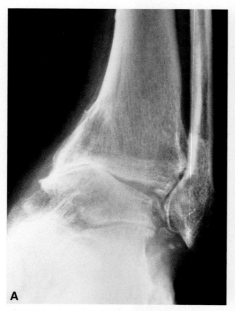 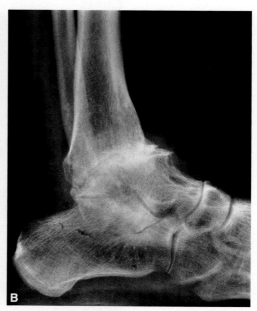

FIGURE 5-20. Anteroposterior (AP) **(A)** and lateral **(B)** radiographs demonstrate severe posttraumatic arthritis with osseous fragments in the joint and marked tibiotalar joint asymmetry.

SUGGESTED READING

Chen SH, Wu PH, Lee YS. Long-term results of pilon fractures. *Arch Orthop Trauma Surg.* 2007;127(1):55–60.
Pettrone FA, Gail M, Pee D, et al. Quantitative criteria for prediction of results of displaced fracture of the ankle. *J Bone Joint Surg.* 1983;65A:667–677.

■ FRACTURES/DISLOCATIONS: TALAR FRACTURES—TALAR NECK

KEY FACTS

- Fractures of the talar neck are common in adults and rare in children.
- Talar neck fractures account for 6% of foot and ankle injuries and 30% of talar fractures.
- The mechanism of injury is abrupt dorsiflexion of the foot during a fall or motor vehicle accident.
- Talar neck fractures may be undisplaced or displaced. The latter are associated with subtalar subluxation/dislocation.
- Displaced fractures usually require internal fixation.
- Complications include avascular necrosis (usually evident by 6 to 8 weeks), osteoarthritis (97%), and malunion or nonunion (15%).

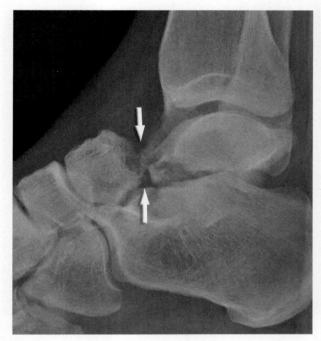

FIGURE 5-21. Lateral radiograph of the foot shows a comminuted talar neck fracture (*arrows*).

(continued)

■ FRACTURES/DISLOCATIONS: TALAR FRACTURES—
TALAR NECK   *(Continued)*

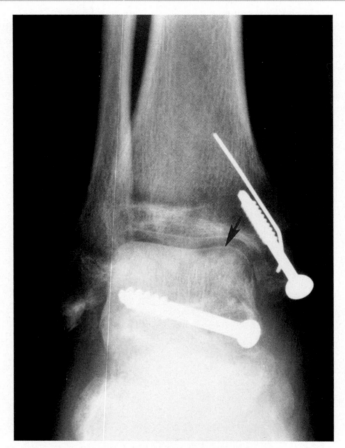

FIGURE 5-22. Hawkins sign. Anteroposterior (AP) radiograph after fixation of talar neck and medial malleolar fractures. The lateral talus is sclerotic, indicating loss of flow. There is normal subchondral osteopenia (*arrow*) medially.

SUGGESTED READING

Daniels TR, Smith JW. Talar neck fractures (review). *Foot Ankle*. 1993;14:225–234.

Hawkins LG. Fractures of the neck of the talus. *J Bone Joint Surg*. 1970;52A:991–1002.

Melenevsky Y, Mackey RA, Abrahams RB, et al. Talar fractures and dislocations: a radiologist's guide to timely diagnosis and classification. *RadioGraphics*. 2015;35(3):765–779.

■ FRACTURES/DISLOCATIONS: TALAR FRACTURES—BODY, HEAD, PROCESS FRACTURES

KEY FACTS

■ Fractures of the talar body and posterior or lateral processes are uncommon in adults and rare in children.

■ Most fractures are the result of significant falls or motor vehicle accidents with axial compression.

■ Lateral talar process fractures ("snowboarder's fracture") are easily missed on radiographs (40% are overlooked initially).

■ CT is important to detect and manage talar body and process fractures.

■ Treatment is anatomic reduction, which requires internal fixation for displaced fractures.

■ Complications are the same as with talar neck fractures. Malunion and avascular necrosis occur in 16%.

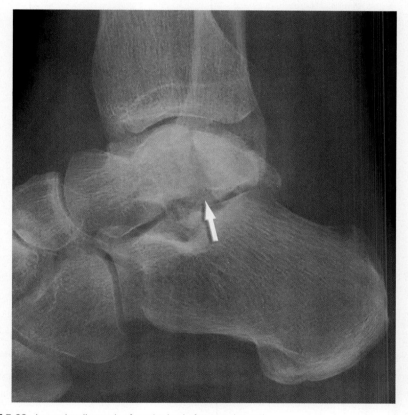

FIGURE 5-23. Lateral radiograph of a talar body fracture (*arrow*).

(continued)

■ FRACTURES/DISLOCATIONS: TALAR FRACTURES— BODY, HEAD, PROCESS FRACTURES *(Continued)*

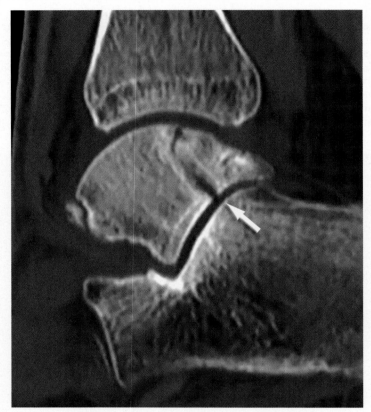

FIGURE 5-24. Sagittal computed tomography (CT) image demonstrates talar body fracture (*arrow*) entering the posterior subtalar joint.

SUGGESTED READING

Boack DH, Manegold S. Peripheral talar fractures. *Injury.* 2004;35(S2):B23–B25.

Melenevsky Y, Mackey RA, Abrahams RB, et al. Talar fractures and dislocations: a radiologist's guide to timely diagnosis and classification. *RadioGraphics.* 2015;35(3):765–779.

Sneppen O, Christensen SB, Krogsoe O, et al. Fracture of the body of the talus. *Acta Orthop Scand.* 1977;48:317–324.

■ FRACTURES/DISLOCATIONS: TALAR FRACTURES— TALAR DOME FRACTURES

KEY FACTS

- Most common talar fracture.
- Talar dome fractures are difficult to detect (50% missed), and prognosis is more guarded compared with nonarticular chip or avulsion fractures.
- Fractures are most common in adults. Only 8% occur in patients less than 16 years of age.
- Acute lesions are most often lateral. Ten percent involve both the lateral and medial talar dome.
- CT or MRI is important for detection, localization, and measurement of lesion size and displacement.
- Displaced lesions should be resected or arthroscopically removed.
- Arthrosis is the most common complication (50%).

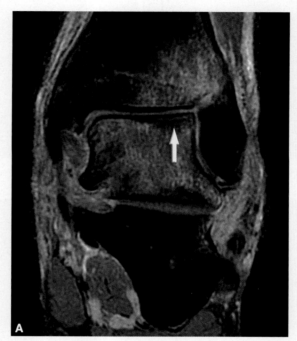

FIGURE 5-25. Coronal **(A)** and sagittal fat-suppressed T2-weighted **(B)** images demonstrate marrow edema and a subtle nondisplaced talar dome fracture (*arrows*).

(continued)

■ FRACTURES/DISLOCATIONS: TALAR FRACTURES— TALAR DOME FRACTURES (Continued)

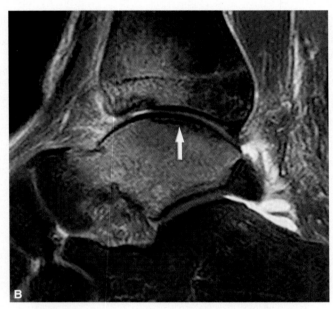

FIGURE 5-25. (continued)

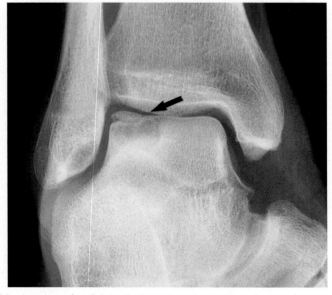

FIGURE 5-26. Mortise view of a slightly displaced lateral talar dome fracture fragment (arrow).

SUGGESTED READING

Clark TWI, Janzen DL, Kendall H, et al. Detection of radiographically occult ankle fractures following acute trauma: positive predictive value of ankle effusion. *AJR Am J Roentgenol.* 1995;164:1185–1189.

Melenevsky Y, Mackey RA, Abrahams RB, et al. Talar fractures and dislocations: a radiologist's guide to timely diagnosis and classification. *RadioGraphics.* 2015;35(3):765–779.

■ FRACTURES/DISLOCATIONS: TALAR AND SUBTALAR DISLOCATIONS

KEY FACTS

- The majority of eversion and inversion motion occurs in the subtalar joint.
- Talar dislocations account for only 1% of all dislocations.
- Fifteen percent of talar injuries are caused by dislocation.
- Subtalar dislocations may be medial (56%), lateral (34%), posterior (6%), or anterior (4%).
- Associated talar or calcaneal fractures occur in 75% of lateral and 45% of medial dislocations.
- Total dislocation is rare. There is a high incidence of infection, which may require talectomy. Avascular necrosis is also common.
- Postreduction CT with coronal and sagittal reformatting is essential to assess reduction and detect associated fractures.

(continued)

■ FRACTURES/DISLOCATIONS: TALAR AND SUBTALAR DISLOCATIONS *(Continued)*

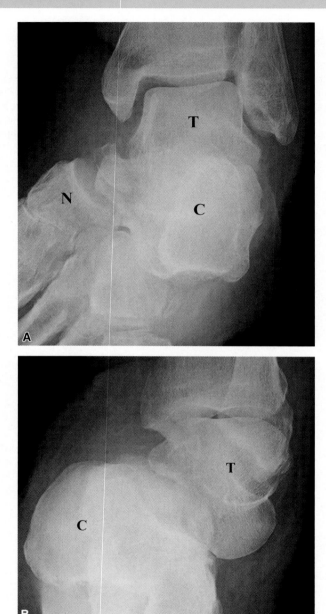

FIGURE 5-27. Subtalar and talonavicular dislocation. **(A)** Anteroposterior (AP) view of the ankle shows the talus (*T*), calcaneus (*C*), and navicular (*N*). The calcaneus is rotated under the talus. **(B)** Oblique view shows the talus lateral to the calcaneus.

SUGGESTED READING

Detenbeck LC, Kelly PJ. Total dislocation of the talus. *J Bone Joint Surg.* 1969;51A: 283–288.
Melenevsky Y, Mackey RA, Abrahams RB, et al. Talar fractures and dislocations: a radiologist's guide to timely diagnosis and classification. *RadioGraphics.* 2015;35(3):765–779.

■ FRACTURES/DISLOCATIONS: CALCANEAL FRACTURES—INTRA-ARTICULAR

KEY FACTS

- ■ The calcaneus is the most commonly fractured bone in the adult foot, accounting for 60% of foot fractures, but only 2% of all skeletal fractures.
- ■ Calcaneal fractures in children account for only 5% of foot fractures.
- ■ Pediatric fractures are usually extra-articular (63%), whereas adult fractures are usually intra-articular (70% to 75%).
- ■ Most adult fractures are the result of axial loading resulting from falls or motor vehicle accidents. Ten percent are bilateral. Associated vertebral fractures occur in 10%.
- ■ CT with coronal and sagittal reformatting is required to classify the injury and assess articular involvement and fracture complexity.
- ■ Treatment goals are to reestablish articular alignment, calcaneal width, and the posterior facet (Böhler's angle).
- ■ Complications include
  - Prolonged pain and disability
  - Lower extremity fractures (20%–46%)
  - Soft tissue injury
  - Neurovascular injury

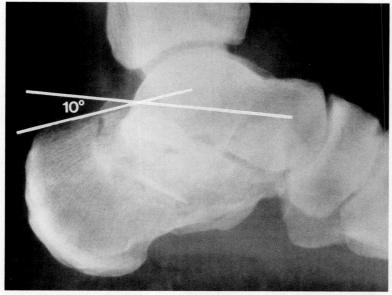

FIGURE 5-28. Lateral radiograph in a patient with a comminuted calcaneal fracture. Böhler's angle measures 10 degrees.

(continued)

■ FRACTURES/DISLOCATIONS: CALCANEAL FRACTURES— INTRA-ARTICULAR   *(Continued)*

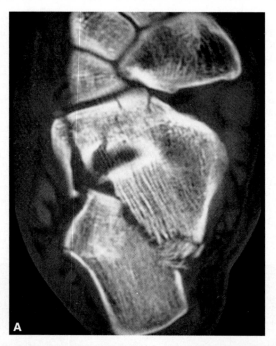

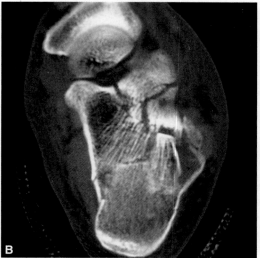

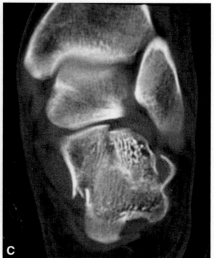

FIGURE 5-29. Comminuted intra-articular calcaneal fracture. Axial **(A, B)** and coronal **(C)** computed tomography (CT) images clearly show fragment position and articular involvement.

SUGGESTED READING

Badillo K, Pacheco JA, Padua SO, et al. Multidetector CT evaluation of calcaneal fractures. *Radiographics.* 2011;31(1): 81–92.

Crosby LA, Fitzgibbons I. Computerized tomographic scanning of acute intra-articular fractures of the calcaneus. *J Bone Joint Surg.* 1990;72A:852–859.

Daftary A, Haims AH, Baumgartner MR. Fractures of the calcaneus: a review with emphasis on CT. *Radiographics.* 2005;25:1215–1226.

■ FRACTURES/DISLOCATIONS: CALCANEAL FRACTURES—EXTRA-ARTICULAR

KEY FACTS

- Extra-articular fractures account for 25% of calcaneal fractures. This includes all fractures that do not involve the posterior facet.
- Mechanism of injury: twisting, compression, or avulsion forces.
- Certain fractures may present as ankle sprains: anterior calcaneal process, peroneal tubercle, lateral calcaneal process, sustentaculum tali, calcaneal tuberosity, and medial calcaneal process fractures.
- CT is frequently required to detect the injury and exclude intra-articular involvement.

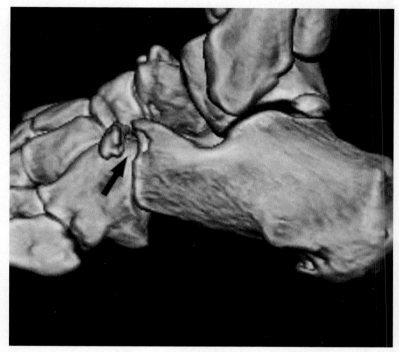

FIGURE 5-30. Computed tomography (CT) shaded surface display rendering of the hind foot demonstrates an anterior calcaneal process fracture (*arrow*).

(continued)

■ FRACTURES/DISLOCATIONS: CALCANEAL FRACTURES— EXTRA-ARTICULAR   *(Continued)*

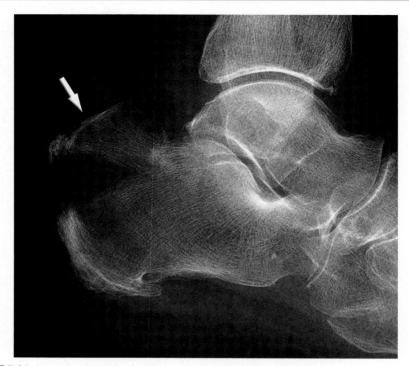

FIGURE 5-31. Lateral radiograph of a calcaneal tuberosity avulsion fracture (*arrow*).

SUGGESTED READING

Badillo K, Pacheco JA, Padua SO, et al. Multidetector CT evaluation of calcaneal fractures. *Radiographics*. 2011;31 (1): 81–92.
Gilheany MF. Injury to the anterior process of the calcaneous. *Foot*. 2002;12:142–149.

■ FRACTURES/DISLOCATIONS: MIDFOOT INJURIES

KEY FACTS

- ■ The midfoot consists of the lesser tarsal bones (navicular, cuboid, and three cuneiforms) and tarsometatarsal (Lisfranc) joints.
- ■ Injuries may be the result of medial (30%), longitudinal (41%), lateral (17%), or plantar (4%) forces, and crush injuries (5%).
- ■ Isolated tarsal fractures are uncommon.

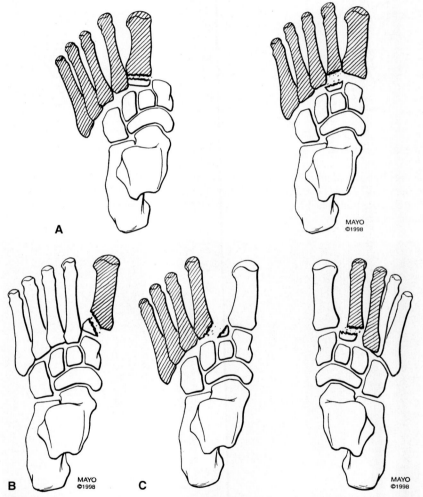

FIGURE 5-32. Patterns of Lisfranc fracture/dislocations. **(A)** Type A—total incongruity. **(B)** Type B—partial incongruity. **(C)** Lateral dislocation. **(D)** Type C or divergent with total displacement **(A)** and partial displacement **(B)**.

(continued)

■ FRACTURES/DISLOCATIONS: MIDFOOT INJURIES *(Continued)*

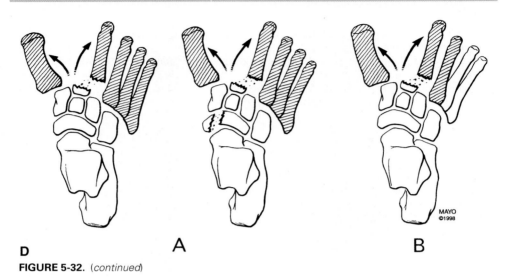

D   **A**   **B**

FIGURE 5-32. *(continued)*

■ Tarsometatarsal fracture/dislocations are Lisfranc injuries (1% of all fracture/dislocations). The mechanism of injury is forced plantar flexion of the forefoot. CT with reformatting is essential to define the extent of injury. Magnetic resonance (MR) may be able to depict subtle injuries of the Lisfranc ligament.

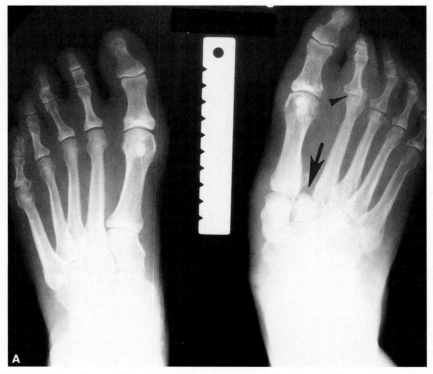

FIGURE 5-33. Lisfranc fracture/dislocation. **(A)** Anteroposterior (AP) radiograph shows a fracture/dislocation (*arrow*) at the tarsometatarsal joints. There is also a dislocation (*arrowhead*) of the second metatarsophalangeal (MTP) joint. Computed tomography (CT) images in the axial **(B)**, sagittal and coronal **(C, D)** planes demonstrate widening of the 1–2 metatarsal bases (*arrow*) with multiple osteochondral fractures (*arrowheads*).

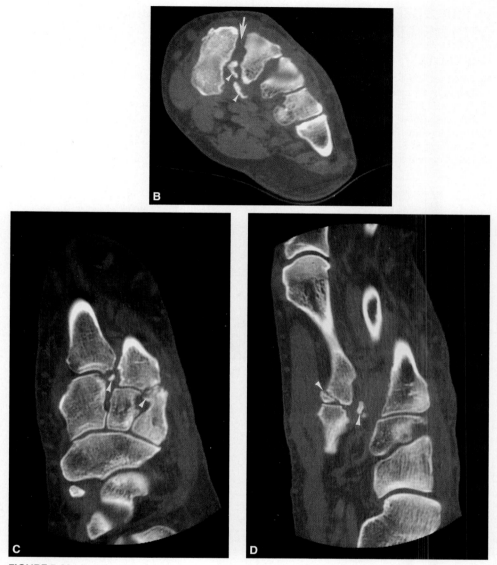

FIGURE 5-33. (continued)

SUGGESTED READING

Karasick D. Fracture and dislocation of the foot. *Semin Roentgenol.* 1994;29:152–175.

Makawana NK, Van Lefland MR. Injuries of the midfoot. *Curr Orthop.* 2005;19:231–242.

Siddiqui NA, Galizia MS, Almusa E, et al. Evaluation of the tarsometatarsal joint using conventional radiography, CT, and MR imaging. *RadioGraphics.* 2014;34:514–531.

■ FRACTURES/DISLOCATIONS: FOREFOOT INJURIES—FIFTH METATARSAL FRACTURES

KEY FACTS

- Fractures of the fifth metatarsal base are common in children and adults.
- Fractures are categorized as proximal or distal.
- Proximal fractures are divided into three zones (Fig. 5-34). Zone 1—avulsion fractures; Zone 2—Jones fractures caused by forefoot adduction; Zone 3—typically athletic stress fractures.
- Distal fractures (Dancer's fracture) are usually the result of a direct blow.
- Treatment of fractures in Zone 1 and distal fractures is conservative. Fractures in Zones 2 and 3 may require internal fixation.

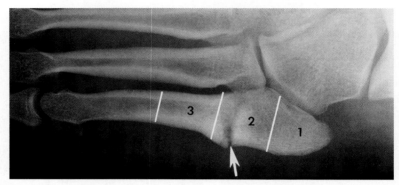

FIGURE 5-34. Oblique radiograph demonstrates the three zones of the proximal fifth metatarsal. There is an ununited Jones fracture (*arrow*) in Zone 2.

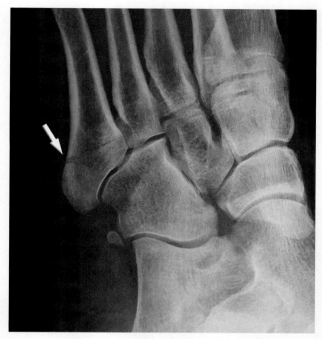

FIGURE 5-35. Subtle nondisplaced avulsion fracture of the fifth metatarsal base in Zone 1 (*arrow*).

SUGGESTED READING

Chuckpaiwong B, Queen RM, Easley ME, et al. Distinguishing Jones and proximal diaphyseal fractures of the fifth metatarsal. *Clin Orthop Relat Res*. 2008;466(8): 1966–1970.

Ekrol I, Court-Brown CM. Fractures of the base of the fifth metatarsal. *Foot*. 2004;14:96–98.

Theodorou DJ, Theodorou SJ, Kakitubata Y, et al. Fractures of the fifth metatarsal base: anatomic and imaging evidence of pathogenesis of avulsion of the plantar aponeurosis and short peroneal tendon. *Radiology*. 2003;226:857–865.

■ FRACTURES/DISLOCATIONS: FOREFOOT INJURIES— METATARSOPHALANGEAL FRACTURE/DISLOCATIONS

KEY FACTS

- Isolated fractures of the first metatarsal are rare.
- Proximal metatarsal fractures are often associated with midfoot fracture/dislocations.
- Distal metatarsal fractures are usually related to a blow from a heavy object.
- Phalangeal fractures are the most common forefoot injury. Jamming or dropping a heavy object results in fracture.
- Dislocations of the metatarsophalangeal (MTP) and interphalangeal joints may occur as isolated events or be associated with fractures.
  - The first MTP and proximal interphalangeal joints are most commonly dislocated.

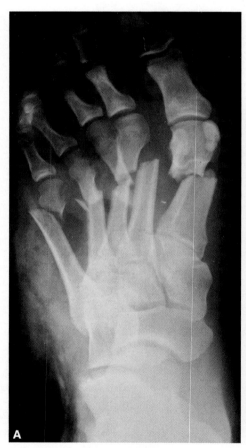
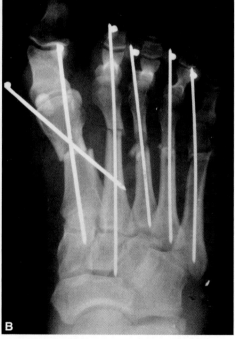

FIGURE 5-36. Crush injury. **(A)** Anteroposterior (AP) radiograph demonstrates complex comminuted metatarsal fractures. **(B)** Fractures were reduced using K-wire fixation.

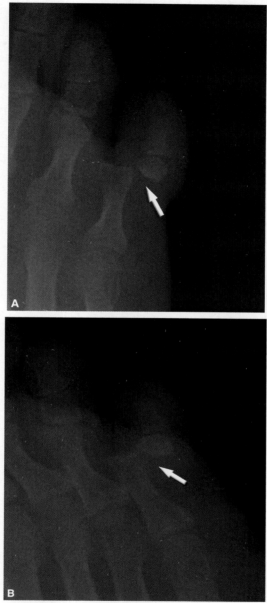

FIGURE 5-37. Dislocation. Anteroposterior (AP) **(A)** and oblique **(B)** radiographs demonstrate lateral dislocation at the fifth proximal interphalangeal joint (*arrow*).

SUGGESTED READING

Karasick D. Fractures and dislocations of the foot. *Semin Roentgenol*. 1994;29:152–175.
Mizel MS, Yodlowski ML. Disorders of the lesser metatarsophalangeal joints. *J Am Acad Orthop Surg*. 1995;3:166–173.

■ FRACTURES/DISLOCATIONS: STRESS FRACTURES

KEY FACTS

- Most stress fractures are fatigue fractures caused by repetitive stress or muscle tension on normal bone.
- Stress fractures commonly occur in military recruits or civilians engaged in a new activity such as running.
- More than 80% of stress fractures involve the tibia, fibula, metatarsals, and calcaneus.
- Table 5-1 summarizes the location and cause of stress fractures.
- Early detection may be difficult with routine radiographs. MRI provides the most specific early diagnosis.

Table 5-1 STRESS FRACTURES

Location	Cause
Metatarsals	Marching
	Running
	Ballet
	Prior surgery
	Rheumatoid arthritis
Tarsals	Long-distance running
Calcaneus	Jumping
	Running
Sesamoids	Marching
	Standing
	Skiing
	Cycling
Distal tibia	Running
Distal fibula	Running
	Parachute jumping

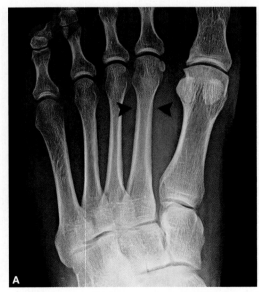

FIGURE 5-38. Metatarsal stress fracture. **(A)** Anteroposterior (AP) radiograph obtained at time of initial presentation shows no evidence of suspected second metatarsal stress fracture (*black arrowheads*). **(B)** Coronal T2-weighted image of the foot with fat suppression obtained after 1 month of continued symptoms reveals a nondisplaced fracture involving the distal shaft of the second metatarsal (*white arrow*). **(C)** Follow-up radiograph obtained approximately 1 month after magnetic resonance imaging (MRI) demonstrates a healing second metatarsal stress fracture (*black arrow*).

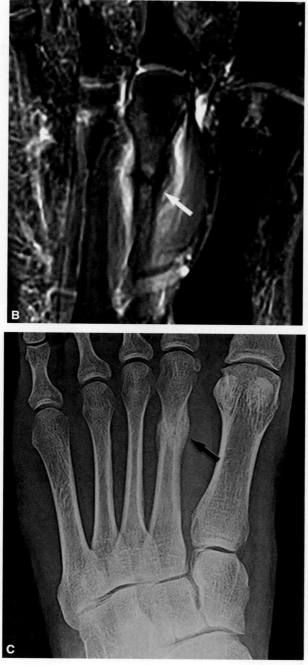

FIGURE 5-38. *(continued)*

(continued)

■ FRACTURES/DISLOCATIONS: STRESS FRACTURES *(Continued)*

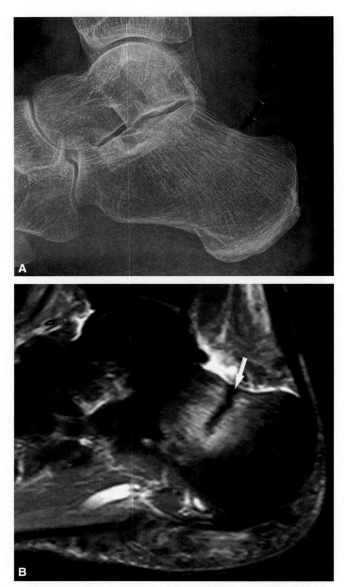

FIGURE 5-39. Calcaneal stress fracture. **(A)** Lateral radiograph shows subtle region of sclerosis in the dorsal aspect of the posterior calcaneus (*black arrow*). **(B)** Sagittal T2-weighted image with fat suppression demonstrates a calcaneal stress fracture (*white arrow*) with surrounding edema.

SUGGESTED READING

Berger FH, de Jonge MC, Maas M. Stress fractures in the lower extremity. The importance of increasing awareness amongst radiologists. *Eur J Radiol.* 2007;62:16–26.
Daffner RH. Stress fractures. *Skel Radiol.* 1987;2:221–229.

■ SOFT TISSUE TRAUMA/OVERUSE SYNDROMES: LIGAMENT INJURIES

KEY FACTS

■ Ligament support for the ankle includes the distal tibiofibular (anterior and posterior) and interosseous ligaments. Medially, the deltoid ligament expands as it extends from the medial malleolus to insert on the talus and calcaneus. There are three lateral ligaments: anterior talofibular, calcaneofibular, and posterior talofibular.

■ Injury to the lateral ligaments is most common. However, medial ligament injuries and syndesmotic sprains also occur.

■ Imaging approaches are important to classify the extent of injury. Table 5-2 defines imaging techniques and features of ligament injury.

■ Complete tears (i.e., two lateral ligaments) are more likely to be treated by operative intervention.

Table 5-2   IMAGING OF ANKLE LIGAMENT INJURIES

Technique	Features of Ligament Tears
Stress Views	
AP	Tibiotalar shift >2 mm compared with normal side
Varus/Valgus	Joint opening (talar tilt) >5 degrees compared with normal side
Arthrography	Calcaneofibular tear-contrast fills peroneal tendon sheaths. Syndesmotic tear-contrast extends beyond recess. Medial tear-contrast extravasates medially
Tenography	Contrast enters ankle joint from peroneal tendon sheath
MRI	↑ Signal intensity and thickening with partial tears on T2-weighted sequences
	↑ Signal intensity with segments separated in complete tears on T2-weighted sequences

AP, anteroposterior; MRI, magnetic resonance imaging.

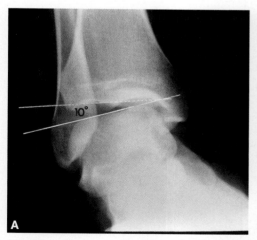 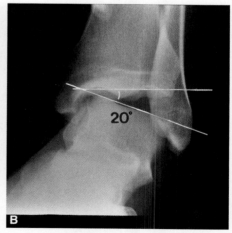

FIGURE 5-40. Stress views. Normal ankle **(A)** and injured ankle **(B)** show that the joint laterally on the injured side is 10 degrees greater than the normal side because of tears in the calcaneofibular and anterior talofibular ligaments.

(continued)

■ SOFT TISSUE TRAUMA/OVERUSE SYNDROMES: LIGAMENT INJURIES   *(Continued)*

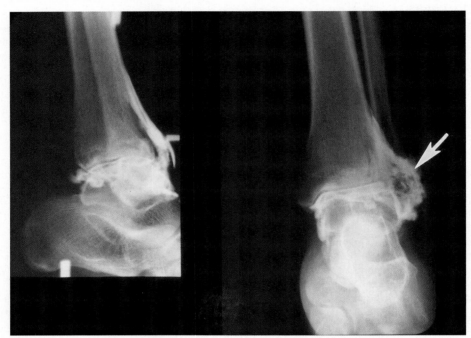

FIGURE 5-41. Arthrogram of the left ankle shows contrast anteriorly (*arrow*) because of an anterior talofibular ligament tear. The peroneal tendon sheaths do not fill, indicating the calcaneofibular ligament is intact.

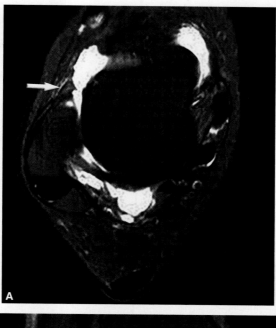

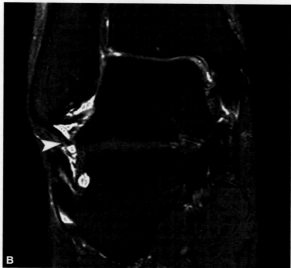

FIGURE 5-42. (A) Axial T2-weighted magnetic resonance (MR) image with fat suppression shows a joint effusion with a torn anterior talofibular ligament (*white arrow*). **(B)** Coronal T2-weighted MR image with fat suppression shows a torn calcaneofibular ligament (*white arrowhead*).

SUGGESTED READING

Berquist TH. *Imaging of Orthopedic Trauma,* 2nd ed. New York: Raven Press; 1992.

Perrich KD, Goodwin DW, Hecht PJ, et al. Ankle ligaments on MRI: appearance of normal and injured ligaments. *AJR Am J Roentgenol.* 2009;193(3):687–695.

■ SOFT TISSUE TRAUMA/OVERUSE SYNDROMES: PERONEAL TENDON INJURIES

KEY FACTS

- Peroneal tendon subluxation
  - Uncommon
  - Cause—chronic ankle sprains, retinacular laxity, shallow fibular grooves
  - Image features—fibular flake fractures, subluxation on tenograms or MRI with motion studies. Dynamic ultrasound can be very useful.
- Peroneal tendon rupture
  - Uncommon.
  - Patients present with instability.
  - Tears may be degenerative, partial, or complete.
  - Peroneus brevis tears are longitudinal and associated with subluxation.
  - Image features—increased signal and thickening of the tendon with partial tears; increased signal with segment separation with complete tears.
- Tenosynovitis and stenosing tenosynovitis
  - Common.
  - Associated with repetitive trauma, previous fracture, and subluxation.
  - Image features—fluid in tendon sheath on fluid-sensitive MR images; narrowing of the tendon sheath with stenosing tenosynovitis on MRI or tenogram.
- Treatment is conservative for partial tears and surgical repair for complete tears.

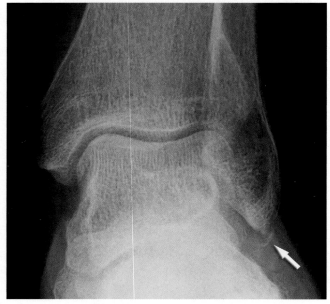

FIGURE 5-43. Anteroposterior (AP) radiograph demonstrates a flake fracture (*arrow*) caused by peroneal tendon dislocation.

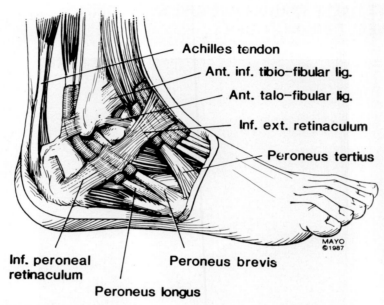

FIGURE 5-44. Peroneal tendon anatomy.

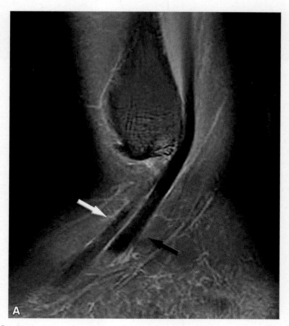

FIGURE 5-45. (A) Sagittal proton density–weighted image with fat suppression of the normal low signal intensity peroneus brevis (*white arrow*) and peroneus longus (*black arrow*) tendons. **(B)** Sagittal proton density–weighted image with fat suppression shows a ruptured peroneus brevis tendon with proximal retraction (*white arrowhead*). Note only the peroneus longus tendon is visualized distally (*black arrow*). There is a fluid-filled gap along the expected course of the peroneus brevis tendon (*white arrow*).

(continued)

■ SOFT TISSUE TRAUMA/OVERUSE SYNDROMES: PERONEAL TENDON INJURIES   *(Continued)*

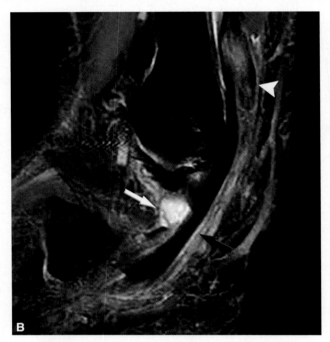

FIGURE 5-45. *(continued)*

SUGGESTED READING

DiGiovanni BF, Fraga CJ, Cohen BE, et al. Associated injuries found in chronic lateral ankle instability. *Foot Ankle Int.* 2000;21:809–815.

Khoury NJ, El-Khoury GY, Saltzman CL, et al. Peroneus, longus, and brevis tendon tears: MR imaging evaluation. *Radiology.* 1996;200:833–841.

Tjin A, Ton ER, Schweitzer ME, et al. MR imaging of peroneal tendon disorders. *AJR Am J Roentgenol.* 1997;168:135–140.

Wang XT, Rosenberg ZS, Mechlin MB, et al. Normal variants and diseases of the peroneal tendons and superior peroneal retinaculum: MR imaging features. *RadioGraphics.* 2005; 25:587–602.

■ SOFT TISSUE TRAUMA/OVERUSE SYNDROMES: ACHILLES TENDON

KEY FACTS

- ■ The Achilles tendon is the largest and strongest tendon of the foot and ankle. There is no tendon sheath.
- ■ Disorders include tendinosis and partial and complete tendon tears.
- ■ There are four categories of tendinosis based on their histology.
  - ● Hypoxic fibromatosis: most common, occurs in the critical zone (2–6 cm above the insertion). Low signal intensity and thickening on MR images.
  - ● Myxoid degeneration: second most common form of tendinosis. Thickening with slight increased signal intensity on T2-weighted MR images.
  - ● Lipoid degeneration: occurs in older patients.
  - ● Calcific/ossific degeneration: 3% of tendinosis cases. Calcification or ossification in the tendon on radiographs.
- ■ Patients with tendon tears present with pain, local swelling, and inability to rise up on their toes.
- ■ Diagnosis is clinically missed in 25%.
- ■ Differential diagnoses include muscle tear and deep venous thromboses.
- ■ Imaging can be accomplished with ultrasound or MRI. Axial and longitudinal ultrasound or axial and sagittal T2-weighted MR images are obtained.
- ■ Treatment is cast immobilization for incomplete tears and surgical repair for complete tears.

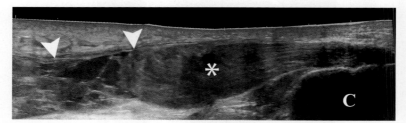

FIGURE 5-46. Ultrasound of Achilles tendon tear. Longitudinal image of a left Achilles tendon rupture with heterogeneous fluid-filled gap (*arrowheads*). Note markedly thickened, tendinopathic distal Achilles tendon (*asterisk*), which can be followed to its insertion on the calcaneous (*C*).

(continued)

■ SOFT TISSUE TRAUMA/OVERUSE SYNDROMES: ACHILLES TENDON *(Continued)*

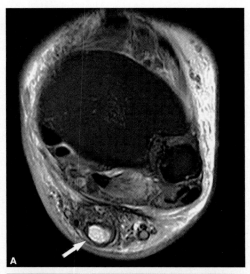

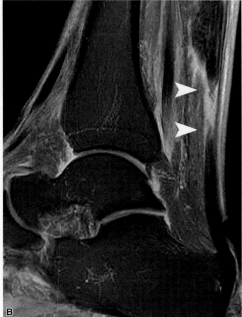

FIGURE 5-47. Magnetic resonance imaging (MRI) of Achilles rupture. **(A)** Axial T2-weighted MR image with fat suppression shows a fluid-filled gap *(arrow)* at level of Achilles tendon rupture. **(B)** Sagittal proton density–weighted image with fat suppression demonstrates distraction of Achilles tendon fibers at site of rupture with an intervening fluid-filled gap *(arrowheads)*.

SUGGESTED READING

Pierre-Jerome C, Moncayo V, Terk MR. MRI of the Achilles tendon: a comprehensive review of the anatomy, biomechanics, and imaging of overuse tendinopathies. *Acta Radiol*. 2010;51:438–454.
Schweitzer ME, Karasick D. MR imaging of disorders of the Achilles tendon. *AJR Am J Roentgenol*. 2000;175:613–625.
Tuite MJ. MR imaging of the tendons of the foot and ankle. *Semin Musculoskeletal Radiol*. 2002;6:119–131.

■ SOFT TISSUE TRAUMA/OVERUSE SYNDROMES: MEDIAL TENDON INJURIES

KEY FACTS

- ■ From anterior to posterior, the medial tendons include the tibialis posterior, flexor digitorum longus, and flexor hallucis longus.
- ■ Abnormalities in the medial tendons include degeneration, partial and complete tears, and subluxation or dislocation.
- ■ Tibialis posterior tendon disorders are most common. Patients are usually middle-aged or older females with ankle pain, instability, and foot deformities.
- ■ More than 50% have abnormalities on routine radiographs.

Feature	Incidence
↓ Calcaneal inclination	50%
↑ Lateral talometatarsal angle	47%
↑ Anterior talocalcaneal angle	43%
Medial swelling	27%
Accessory navicular	17%

- ■ There are three types of accessory navicular. Type I: oval, embedded in tendon. Type II: triangular with fibrocartilaginous synchondrosis. Type III: cornuate and incompletely incorporated into the navicular. Types II and III: associated with posterior tibial tendon dysfunction.
- ■ Flexor digitorum longus and flexor hallucis longus tenosynovitis occur and may be seen in ballet dancers and soccer players. Rupture of these tendons is uncommon.
- ■ MRI is the technique of choice. Axial and sagittal T2-weighted images define the type and extent of injury.

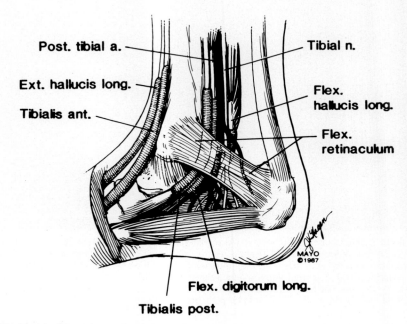

FIGURE 5-48. Medial tendon and tarsal tunnel anatomy.

(continued)

■ SOFT TISSUE TRAUMA/OVERUSE SYNDROMES: MEDIAL TENDON INJURIES   *(Continued)*

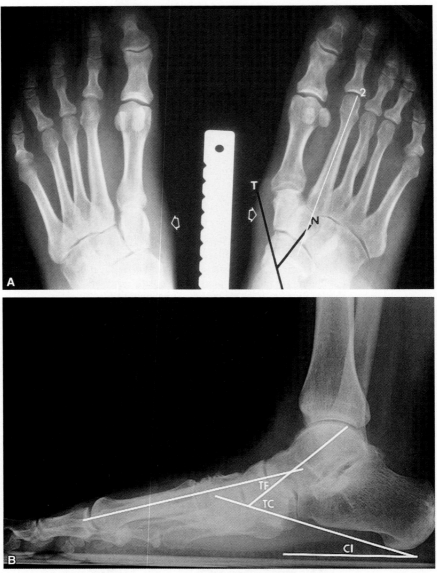

FIGURE 5-49. Standing anteroposterior (AP) **(A)** and lateral **(B)** radiographs of the foot in an elderly female with posterior tibial tendon tears. **(A)** There is medial soft tissue swelling (*open arrows*) bilaterally. The foot is pronated with the talar axis (*T*) projecting medially, and the navicular (*N*) is rotated laterally. The second metatarsal axis (*2*) is medial to the talocalcaneal angle. **(B)** The calcaneal inclination (*CI*) angle is reduced to 11 degrees. The talus is plantar flexed, increasing the talocalcaneal (*TC*) angle to 60 degrees. The talar first metatarsal angle (*TF*) should be zero, but in this case it is –28 degrees.

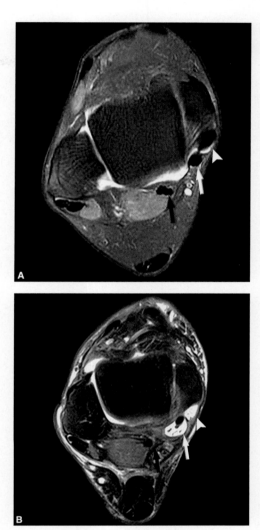

FIGURE 5-50. Magnetic resonance imaging (MRI) of a posterior tibial tendon tear. **(A)** Axial proton density–weighted image with fat suppression shows normal posterior tibial (*white arrowhead*), flexor digitorum longus (*white arrow*), and flexor hallucis longus (*black arrow*) tendons. **(B)** Axial proton density–weighted image with fat suppression in a patient with posterior tibial tendon rupture reveals the absence of the posterior tibial tendon and fluid-filled tendon sheath (*white arrowhead*). The flexor digitorum longus (*white arrow*) and flexor hallucis longus (*black arrow*) tendons are intact.

SUGGESTED READING

Garth WP. Flexor hallucis tendinitis in ballet dancers. *J Bone Joint Surg.* 1981;63A:1489.

Karasick D, Schweitzer ME. Tear of the posterior tibial tendon causing asymmetric flatfoot: radiographic findings. *AJR Am J Roentgenol.* 1993;161:1231–1240.

Schweitzer ME, Karasick D. MR imaging of disorders of the posterior tibialis tendon. *AJR Am J Roentgenol.* 2000;175:627–635.

Yao K, Yang TX, Yew WP. Posterior tibialis tendon dysfunction: overview of evaluation and management. *Orthopedics.* 2015;38(6):385–391.

■ SOFT TISSUE TRAUMA/OVERUSE SYNDROMES: ANTERIOR TENDON INJURIES

KEY FACTS

- The anterior tibial, extensor hallucis longus, and extensor digitorum longus tendons are enclosed in tendon sheaths.
- Tendon rupture is uncommon, but does occur in patients with previous fractures, patients with degenerative arthritis, and runners. Penetrating trauma may lacerate the tendons.
- Patients present with anterior ankle pain and swelling.
- The anterior tibial tendon accounts for 80% of dorsiflexion of the foot. It is this tendon that is most often injured. Injury is usually just below the superior retinaculum.
- Ultrasound or MRI is usually diagnostic.

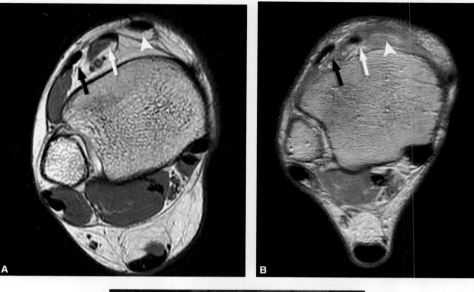

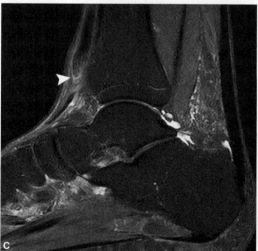

FIGURE 5-51. Magnetic resonance imaging (MRI) of anterior tibial tendon tear. **(A)** Axial proton density–weighted image shows normal anterior tibial (*white arrowhead*), extensor hallucis longus (*white arrow*), and extensor digitorum longus (*black arrow*) tendons. **(B)** Axial proton density–weighted image in a patient with anterior tibial tendon rupture reveals the absence of the anterior tibial tendon and fluid-filled tendon sheath (*white arrowhead*). The extensor hallucis longus (*white arrow*) and extensor digitorum longus (*black arrow*) tendons are intact. **(C)** Sagittal T2-weighted MR image with fat suppression demonstrates an abnormally thickened, retracted anterior tibial tendon at site of rupture (*arrowhead*).

SUGGESTED READING

Gallo RA, Kolman BH, Daffner RH, et al. MRI of tibialis anterior tendon rupture. *Skel Radiol.* 2004;33:102–106.

Khoury NJ, El-Khoury GY, Saltzman CL, et al. Rupture of the anterior tibial tendon: diagnosis with MR imaging. *AJR Am J Roentgenol.* 1996;167:351–354.

Ng JM, Rosenberg ZS, Bencardino JT, et al. US and MR imaging of the extensor compartment of the ankle. *Radiographics.* 2013;33(7):2047–2064.

■ SOFT TISSUE TRAUMA/OVERUSE SYNDROMES: PLANTAR FASCIITIS

KEY FACTS

- The plantar fascia is composed of medial, lateral, and central components that extend distally from the posteromedial calcaneal tuberosity. The central component is the strongest and 2 to 4 mm thick.
- Plantar fasciitis is a chronic and often disabling painful condition that may be related to exercise, standing, or walking. Pain is exaggerated by dorsiflexion of the great toe.
- Plantar fasciitis accounts for 7% to 9% of all running injuries.
- Plantar enthesophytes are evident in 25% to 37% of cases, but many asymptomatic patients demonstrate this finding.
- Differential diagnoses include calcaneal stress fracture, fascial rupture, and flexor hallucis longus tendinitis.
- Treatment includes rest, ice, heel pads, or orthotics.

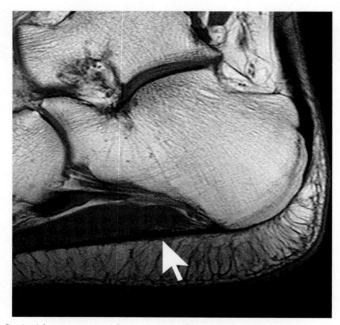

FIGURE 5-52. Sagittal fat-suppressed fast spin-echo T2-weighted image of the normal plantar fascia. There is uniform thickness with low signal intensity (*arrow*).

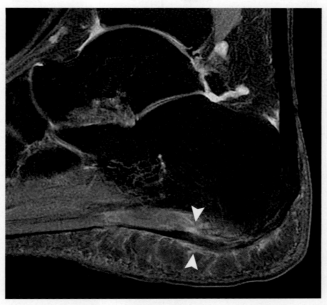

FIGURE 5-53. Active plantar fasciitis. Sagittal proton density–weighted image with fat suppression shows thickening of the plantar fascia with increased signal intensity above and below the fascia (*arrowheads*), as well as reactive edema at its calcaneal attachment.

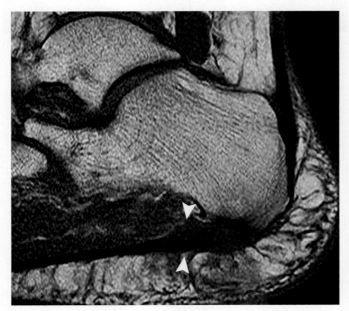

FIGURE 5-54. Chronic plantar fasciitis. Sagittal T1-weighted image shows thickening of the fascia (*arrowheads*) near the calcaneal attachment.

(continued)

■ SOFT TISSUE TRAUMA/OVERUSE SYNDROMES: PLANTAR FASCIITIS   *(Continued)*

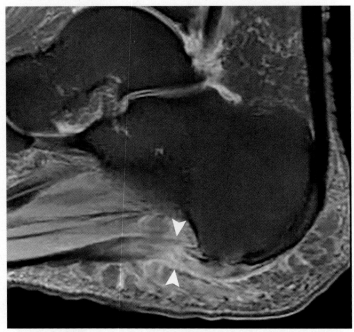

FIGURE 5-55. Ruptured plantar fascia. Sagittal proton density–weighted image with fat suppression demonstrates a complete tear (*arrowheads*) in the plantar fascia.

SUGGESTED READING

Berkowitz JF, Kier R, Radicel S. Plantar fasciitis: MR imaging. *Radiology.* 1991;179:665–667.

Lawrence DA, Rolen MF, Morshed KA, et al. MRI of heel pain. *AJR Am J Roentgenol.* 2013;200(4): 845–855.

Theodorou DJ, Theodorou SJ, Farooki S, et al. Disorders of the plantar fascia: review of MR imaging appearances. *AJR Am J Roentgenol.* 2001;176:97–104.

Theodorou DJ, Theodorou SJ, Kakitsubata Y, et al. Plantar fasciitis and fascial rupture: MR imaging findings in 26 patients supplemented with anatomic data in cadavers. *Radiographics.* 2000;20: S181–S197.

■ SOFT TISSUE TRAUMA/OVERUSE SYNDROMES: BURSITIS

KEY FACTS

- The heel has two bursae: one between the Achilles and calcaneus, and the other superficial to the Achilles tendon.
- Enlarged superficial bursae (Haglund disease) are common in younger women because of their footwear.
- Inflammation of the retrocalcaneal bursa is seen in patients with inflammatory arthropathies (reactive arthritis, gout, and rheumatoid arthritis) and heel varus deformities.
- Inflamed distended bursa may be evident on radiographs. However, MRI and ultrasound are more definitive.

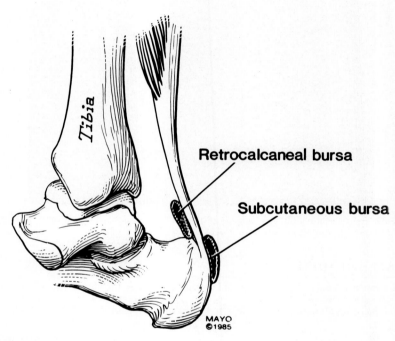

FIGURE 5-56. Bursae of the heel.

(continued)

■ SOFT TISSUE TRAUMA/OVERUSE SYNDROMES: BURSITIS *(Continued)*

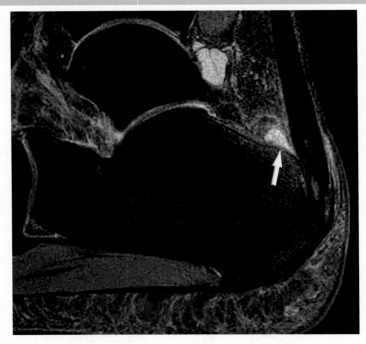

FIGURE 5-57. Retrocalcaneal bursitis. Sagittal proton density–weighted image with fat suppression shows fluid distending the retrocalcaneal bursa (*arrow*).

SUGGESTED READING

Bottger BA, Schweitzer ME, El-Nousam KI, et al. MR imaging of normal and abnormal retrocalcaneal bursae. *AJR Am J Roentgenol.* 1998;170:1239–1240.
Lawrence DA, Rolen MF, Morshed KA, et al. MRI of heel pain. *AJR Am J Roentgenol.* 2013;200(4):845–855.

■ SOFT TISSUE TRAUMA/OVERUSE SYNDROMES: OS TRIGONUM SYNDROME

KEY FACTS

- ■ The os trigonum is connected to the talus by a cartilaginous synchondrosis. Ossification of the process occurs from 7 to 13 years of age.
- ■ A separate ossicle remains in 7% to 14% of patients, and it is often bilateral.
- ■ Os trigonum syndrome may be the result of acute trauma or repetitive microtrauma. Process fracture, flexor hallucis tendinitis, and posterior impingement may all be evident.
- ■ Patients present with posterior ankle pain exaggerated by plantar flexion of the foot and soft tissue swelling.
- ■ Imaging is possible with several approaches.
    1. Routine radiographs with stress views to exaggerate symptoms, and there is edema in the pre-Achilles fat.
    2. Radionuclide scans are positive in the posterior talus. A negative scan excludes the diagnosis.
    3. MRI examinations show edema and flexor hallucis tendinitis.
    4. Diagnostic injection with anesthetic relieves symptoms.
- ■ Treatment is usually conservative with cast immobilization. If this fails, resection may be indicated.

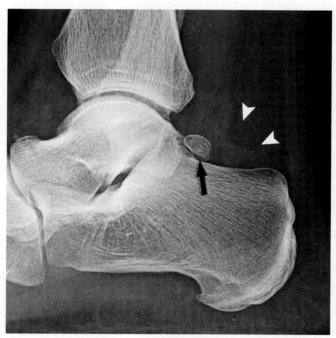

FIGURE 5-58. Lateral radiograph of the ankle shows an os trigonum (*black arrow*) with edema in the pre-Achilles fat (*arrowheads*) caused by os trigonum syndrome.

(continued)

■ SOFT TISSUE TRAUMA/OVERUSE SYNDROMES: OS TRIGONUM SYNDROME *(Continued)*

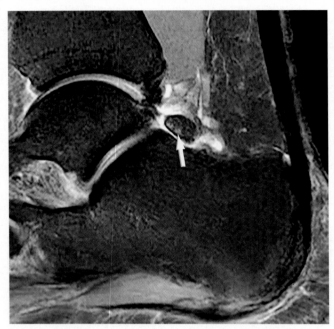

FIGURE 5-59. Magnetic resonance imaging (MRI) of os trigonum syndrome. Sagittal proton density–weighted image with fat suppression shows edema-like signal within an os trigonum (*arrow*) with surrounding fluid.

SUGGESTED READING

Cerezal L, Abascal F, Canga A, et al. MR imaging of ankle impingement syndromes. *AJR Am J Roentgenol*. 2003;181(2): 551–559.

Wakely CJ, Johnson DP, Watt I. The value of MR imaging in diagnosis of an os trigonum syndrome. *Skel Radiol*. 1996;25:133–136.

■ SOFT TISSUE TRAUMA/OVERUSE SYNDROMES: TARSAL TUNNEL SYNDROME

KEY FACTS

■ The tarsal tunnel is located in the posteromedial ankle and extends from just above the medial malleolus to the abductor hallucis muscle of the foot (Fig. 5-48). It is bounded medially by the flexor retinaculum and laterally by the talus and calcaneus. Contents of the tarsal tunnel include the posterior tibial, flexor digitorum longus, and flexor hallucis longus tendons and the posterior tibial nerve and vascular complex.

■ Tarsal tunnel syndrome is caused by posterior tibia neuropathy in the tarsal tunnel. The causes are summarized in Table 5-3.

■ Patients typically present with paresthesias, burning in the foot, or plantar anesthesia.

■ Imaging can be accomplished with ultrasound, CT, or MRI.

■ Treatment is usually surgical decompression. Best results (79% to 95%) are obtained when a definite mass or other cause (Table 5-3) can be defined.

Table 5-3   TARSAL TUNNEL SYNDROME CAUSES

Trauma

Fractures

Posttraumatic fibrosis

Talocalcaneal coalitions

Soft tissue masses

Ganglion cysts

Lipomas

Varicosities

Synovial hypertrophy

Hypertrophy of abductor hallucis muscle

Muscle anomalies

(continued)

■ SOFT TISSUE TRAUMA/OVERUSE SYNDROMES: TARSAL TUNNEL SYNDROME *(Continued)*

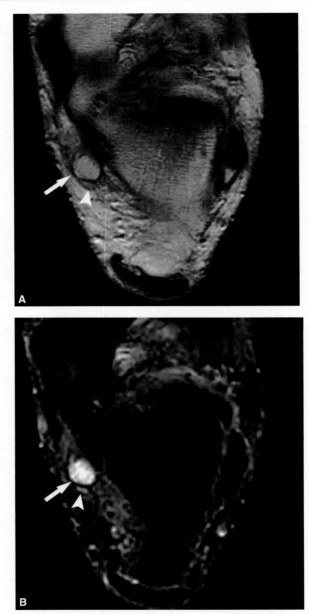

FIGURE 5-60. Ganglion cyst causing tarsal tunnel syndrome. Axial proton-density **(A)** and axial fat-suppressed T2-weighted **(B)** images show a ganglion cyst in the tarsal tunnel (*arrow*) abutting the posterior tibial nerve (*arrowhead*).

SUGGESTED READING

Erickson SJ, Quinn SF, Kneeland JB, et al. MR imaging of the tarsal tunnel and related spaces: normal and abnormal findings with anatomic correlation. *AJR Am J Roentgenol.* 1990;155(2): 323–328.

Pfeiffer WH, Cracchiolo A. Clinical results after tarsal tunnel decompression. *J Bone Joint Surg.* 1994;76A:1222–1230.

■ SOFT TISSUE TRAUMA/OVERUSE SYNDROMES: SINUS TARSI SYNDROME

KEY FACTS

- ■ The tarsal canal and sinus is bordered by the synovial capsules of the subtalar facets. It contains fat, neurovascular structures, and the five ligaments of the tarsal canal.
- ■ Patients with sinus tarsi syndrome present with lateral ankle or hindfoot pain and tenderness over the sinus tarsi to palpation. Most patients present with a history of ankle sprain or inversion injury (70%).
- ■ The cause may be related to calcaneofibular ligament tears, capsular hypertrophy, and space-occupying lesions.
- ■ Imaging of the tarsal canal and sinus can be accomplished with ultrasound, CT, or MRI. MRI is preferred in our experience.

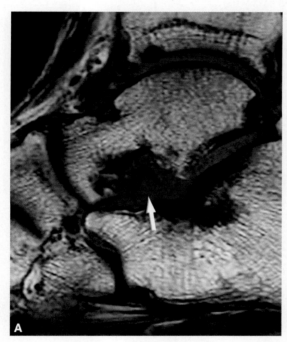

FIGURE 5-61. Sinus tarsi syndrome. Sagittal T1-weighted **(A)** and sagittal fat-suppressed proton density–weighted **(B)** images show abnormal signal intensity in the tarsal sinus (*arrows*).

(continued)

■ SOFT TISSUE TRAUMA/OVERUSE SYNDROMES: SINUS TARSI SYNDROME *(Continued)*

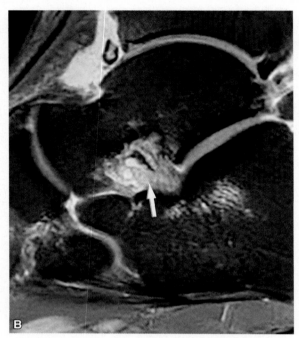

FIGURE 5-61. *(continued)*

SUGGESTED READING

Klein MA, Spreitzor AM. MR imaging of the tarsal canal and sinus: normal anatomy, pathologic findings, and features of sinus tarsi syndrome. *Radiology*. 1993;186:233–240.

Lee KB, Bai LB, Park JG, et al. Efficacy of MRI versus arthroscopy for evaluation of sinus tarsi syndrome. *Foot Ankle Int*. 2008;29(11):1111–1116.

Lektrakul N, Chung CB, Lai Y, et al. Tarsal sinus: arthrography, MR imaging, and pathologic findings in cadavers and retrospective study data in patients with sinus tarsi syndrome. *Radiology*. 2001;219:802–812.

■ SOFT TISSUE TRAUMA/OVERUSE SYNDROMES: IMPINGEMENT SYNDROMES

KEY FACTS

■ Impingement syndromes in the ankle may be related to bone or soft tissue abnormalities. There are five commonly described syndromes: anterior, anteromedial, anterolateral, posterior, and posteromedial.

- Anterior impingement syndrome: Common in athletes using repetitive dorsiflexion. Osseous beaklike changes in the anterior tibia and adjacent talus. Synovial scarring and hypertrophy.
- Anterolateral impingement syndrome: Usually related to prior inversion or plantar flexion injury. Associated tears in the capsule or ligaments. Chronic microtrauma with thickening of the ligaments and capsule is also implicated.
- Anteromedial impingement syndrome: Eversion injuries with partial ligament tears are implicated. Capsular thickening and osteophyte formation; 55% have associated talar dome defects.
- Posteromedial impingement syndrome: Uncommon, but seen with severe ankle injuries with crushing of the deep deltoid fibers.
- Posterior impingement syndrome: Acute and chronic trauma. Posterior talar process fractures, flexor hallucis longus tendinitis, and posterior tibiotalar impingement. Analogous to os trigonum syndrome.

■ Imaging can be accomplished with stress views, CT, or MRI. MRI is most useful to confirm diagnosis and exclude other causes of ankle pain.

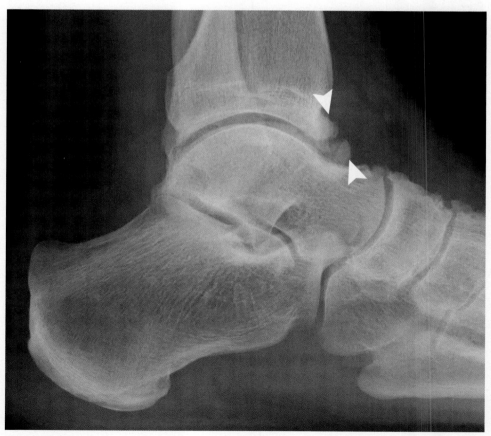

FIGURE 5-62. Anterior impingement syndrome. Lateral radiograph of the ankle shows beaklike osteophytes (*arrowheads*) along the anterior tibia and adjacent talus with associated anterior soft tissue edema.

(continued)

■ SOFT TISSUE TRAUMA/OVERUSE SYNDROMES: IMPINGEMENT SYNDROMES *(Continued)*

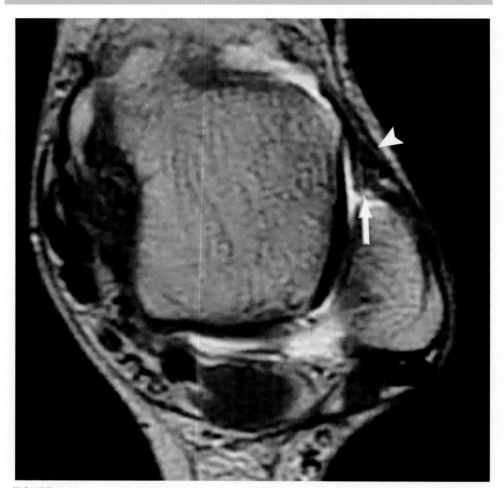

FIGURE 5-63. Anterolateral impingement syndrome. Axial T2-weighted image demonstrates low signal intensity meniscoid-shaped mass (*arrow*) extending from thickened anterior talofibular ligament (*arrowhead*) into the lateral gutter.

SUGGESTED READING

Dimmick S, Linklater J. Ankle impingement syndromes. *Radiol Clin North Am*. 2013;51:479–510.

Robinson P, White LM. Soft tissue and osseous impingement syndromes of the ankle: role of imaging in diagnosis and management. *Radiographics*. 2002;22:1457–1471.

Rubin DA, Tishkaff NW, Britton CA, et al. Anterolateral soft tissue impingement of the ankle: diagnosis using MR imaging. *AJR Am J Roentgenol*. 1997;169:829–835.

■ SOFT TISSUE TRAUMA/OVERUSE SYNDROMES: MIDFOOT AND FOREFOOT SYNDROMES

KEY FACTS

- ■ Overuse syndromes in the midfoot and forefoot are not uncommon.
- ■ Many conditions are clinically diagnosed and do not require imaging.
- ■ Table 5-4 summarizes conditions in which imaging studies may be required.

Table 5-4   FOREFOOT PAIN SYNDROMES

Condition	Imaging Approaches
Metatarsalgia	Clinical diagnosis and radiographs
Sesamoiditis	Sesamoid views, radionuclide scans, and MRI
Osteochondritis	Radiographs
Synovitis	Contrast-enhanced MRI
Hallux rigidus	Radiographs
Turf toe	Radiographs and MRI
Neuromas	Ultrasound and MRI
Stress fractures	Radiographs, MRI, and CT for midfoot

CT, computed tomography; MRI, magnetic resonance imaging.

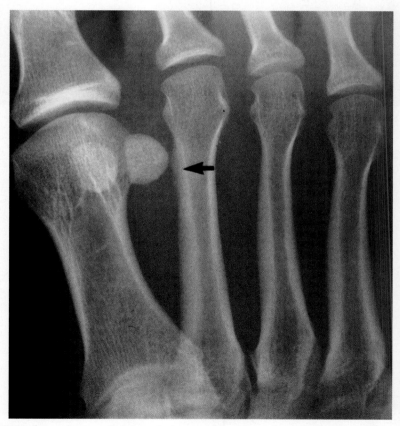

FIGURE 5-64. Stress fracture. Subtle periosteal new bone (*arrow*) in the distal second metatarsal as the result of a healing stress fracture.

(continued)

■ SOFT TISSUE TRAUMA/OVERUSE SYNDROMES: MIDFOOT AND FOREFOOT SYNDROMES *(Continued)*

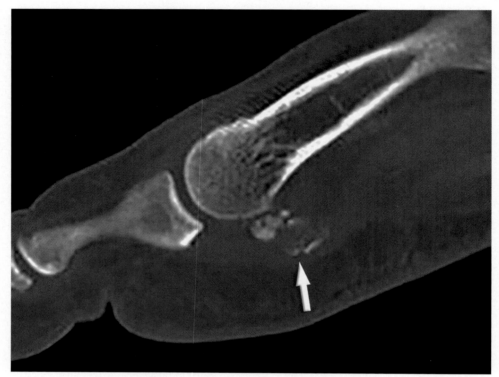

FIGURE 5-65. Sesamoid fracture. Sagittal computed tomography (CT) image through the forefoot demonstrates a comminuted fracture of the lateral (fibular) sesamoid (*arrow*).

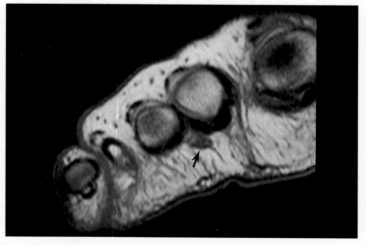

FIGURE 5-66. Axial T1-weighted image demonstrates a Morton neuroma (*arrow*).

SUGGESTED READING

Berquist TH. *Radiology of the Foot and Ankle*, 2nd ed. Philadelphia: Lippincott Williams & Wilkins; 2000:105–170.
Umans HR. Imaging sports medicine injuries of the foot and toes. *Clin Sports Med.* 2006;25(4):763–780.

■ NEOPLASMS/TUMORLIKE CONDITIONS: SKELETAL LESIONS—BENIGN

KEY FACTS

- ■ Skeletal neoplasms of the foot and ankle account for only 1% to 2% of primary skeletal neoplasms.
- ■ Benign lesions outnumber malignant lesions in the ratio 4:1.
- ■ Giant cell tumors and osteoid osteomas are most common in some series. Enchondroma is also frequently seen in the foot.
- ■ Malignant skeletal lesions in the foot and ankle are uncommon. Metastases are rare (0.007% to 0.3% of skeletal metastases). Myeloma involves the foot and ankle in 0.2% of patients.
- ■ Benign and malignant tumors and tumorlike conditions in the foot and ankle are as follows:

Benign Lesion	Malignant Neoplasm
Giant cell tumor	Osteosarcoma
Osteoid osteoma	Ewing sarcoma
Osteochondroma	Chondrosarcoma
Nonossifying fibroma	Hemangioendothelial sarcoma
Subungual exostosis	Fibrosarcoma
Aneurysmal bone cyst	Lymphoma
Enchondroma	Adamantinoma
Chondromyxoid fibroma	
Chondroblastoma	
Fibrous dysplasia	
Osteoblastoma	

- ■ Imaging of the skeletal lesions begins with routine radiographs. Features on radiographs are most useful for characterizing lesions.
- ■ CT and MRI are most useful for evaluating the extent of lesions and for staging.

(continued)

■ NEOPLASMS/TUMORLIKE CONDITIONS: SKELETAL LESIONS—BENIGN *(Continued)*

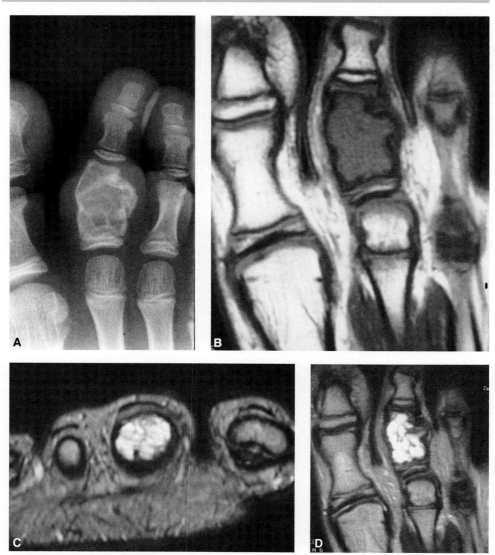

FIGURE 5-67. Aneurysmal bone cyst. **(A)** Radiograph shows an expanding lesion of the second proximal phalanx. Coronal T1-weighted **(B)**, axial **(C)**, and coronal **(D)** T2-weighted images show a septated lesion with fluid–fluid levels on the axial image **(C)**.

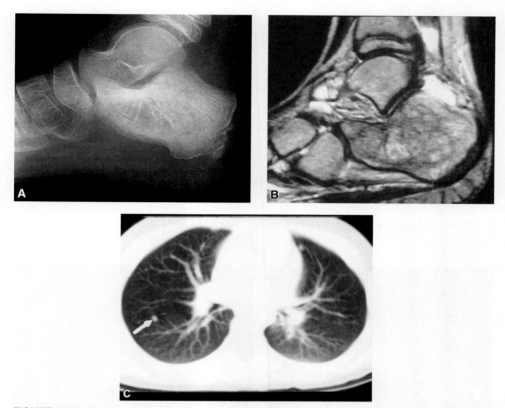

FIGURE 5-68. Ewing sarcoma of calcaneus. **(A)** Routine lateral radiograph shows bone sclerosis. **(B)** Sagittal T2-weighted image shows irregular signal intensity with joint fluid. **(C)** Computed tomography (CT) of chest shows a metastatic nodule (*arrow*).

SUGGESTED READING

Johnston MR. Epidemiology of soft-tissue and bone tumors of the foot. *Clin Podiatr Med Surg*. 1993;10:581–607.

Rhee JH, Lewis RB, Murphey MD. Primary osseous tumors of the foot and ankle. *Magn Reson Imaging Clin N Am*. 2008;16(1):71–91.

Unni KK. *Dahlin's Bone Tumors: General Aspects and Data on 11,087 Cases*. Philadelphia: Lippincott-Raven; 1996.

■ NEOPLASMS/TUMORLIKE CONDITIONS: SOFT TISSUE LESIONS—BENIGN

KEY FACTS

■ Soft tissue masses are more common than skeletal neoplasms in the foot and ankle.

■ Benign soft tissue lesions are much more common than malignant lesions (87% benign and 13% malignant).

■ Common benign lesions in the foot and ankle include lipomas, hemangiomas, fibromatosis, ganglion cysts, neuromas, and giant cell tumors of the tendon sheath.

■ Soft tissue malignancies in the foot and ankle are uncommon.

■ Malignant soft tissue tumors in the foot and ankle include synovial sarcoma, clear cell sarcoma, liposarcoma, angiosarcoma, and hemangiopericytoma.

■ Radiographs have limited value for characterizing soft tissue lesions. MRI and ultrasound (cystic vs. solid) are most useful. MRI is superior for characterizing the nature of the lesion. Malignant lesions typically have inhomogeneous signal intensity, irregular margins, and can encase neurovascular structures and bone.

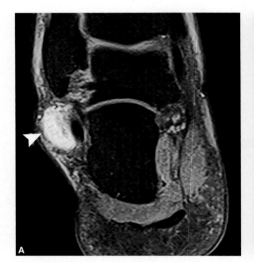 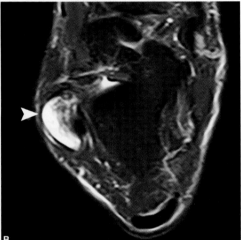

FIGURE 5-69. Peroneal tendon ganglion cyst. Coronal proton density–weighted image with fat suppression **(A)** and axial T2-weighted image with fat suppression **(B)** show a high signal intensity ganglion cyst (*arrowheads*) intimately associated with the peroneal tendons.

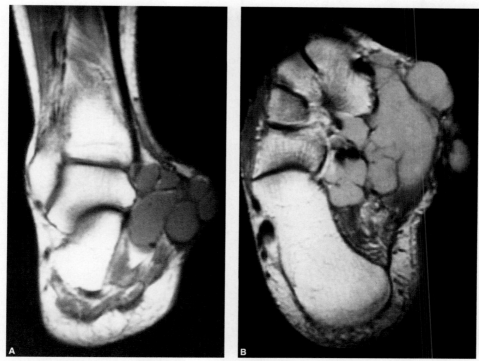

FIGURE 5-70. Synovial sarcoma. Coronal T1-weighted **(A)** and axial proton density **(B)** images show a multicystic loculated lesion that could be confused with a benign process.

SUGGESTED READING

Bancroft LW, Peterson JJ, Kransdorf MJ. Imaging of soft tissue lesions of the foot and ankle. *Radiol Clin North Am.* 2008;46(6):1093–1103.

Kirby SJ, Shereff MJ, Lewis MM. *Soft* tissue tumors and tumor-like conditions of the foot. Analysis of 83 cases. *J Bone Joint Surg.* 1989;71A:621–626.

Weiss SW, Goldblum JR. *Enzinger and Weiss's Soft Tissue Tumors.* 4th ed. St. Louis: Mosby; 2001.

■ ARTHRITIS: OSTEOARTHRITIS (DEGENERATIVE JOINT DISEASE)

KEY FACTS

- Radiographic features of osteoarthritis include increased bone density, osteophyte formation, subchondral sclerosis, asymmetric joint space narrowing, subchondral cysts, and loose bodies.
- The ankle, midfoot, and first MTP joints are affected most frequently.
- Calcaneal osteophytes at the Achilles insertion and plantar aponeurosis attachments are common. These are well defined compared with changes described in Reactive Arthritis.

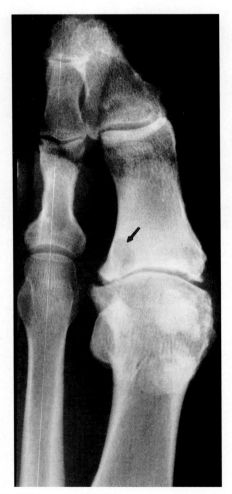

FIGURE 5-71. Anteroposterior (AP) view of the forefoot shows osteoarthritis of the first metatarsophalangeal (MTP) joint with asymmetric joint space narrowing, bone sclerosis, and a subchondral cyst (*arrow*).

SUGGESTED READING

Bancroft LW, McLeod RA. Arthritis. In: Berquist TH, ed. *Radiology of the Foot and Ankle*, 2nd ed. Philadelphia: Lippincott Williams & Wilkins; 2000:281–314.

Jacobson JA, Girish G, Jiang Y, et al. Radiographic evaluation of arthritis: degenerative joint disease and variations. *Radiology*. 2008;248:737–747.

■ ARTHRITIS: RHEUMATOID ARTHRITIS

KEY FACTS

- The foot is an early site of involvement in rheumatoid arthritis. The foot is involved in 90% of patients.
- The condition is symmetric and has characteristic joint distribution. The lateral aspect of the fifth MTP joint is frequently involved first. The interphalangeal joint of the great toe is commonly involved. The distal interphalangeal joints are spared.
- Proximal joints of the foot and ankle may also be affected with osteopenia joint space narrowing and, when present, ill-defined marginal erosions.
- Inflammatory changes in synovium, capsules, and ligaments may lead to subluxation.
- Subcutaneous rheumatoid nodules can occur, but only 1% involve the feet.

(continued)

■ ARTHRITIS: RHEUMATOID ARTHRITIS   (Continued)

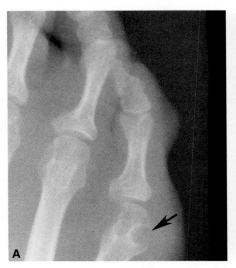 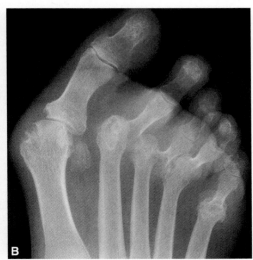

FIGURE 5-72. Rheumatoid arthritis limited to the fifth metatarsophalangeal (MTP) joint (*arrow*) **(A)** and involving all MTP joints with erosions and joint subluxation **(B)**.

SUGGESTED READING

Bancroft LW, McLeod RA. Arthritis. In: Berquist TH, ed. *Radiology of the Foot and Ankle*, 2nd ed. Philadelphia: Lippincott Williams & Wilkins; 2000:281–314.

Jacobson JA, Girish G, Jiang Y, et al. Radiographic evaluation of arthritis: inflammatory conditions. *Radiology*. 2008;248:378–389.

Sommer OJ, Kladosek A, Weiler V, et al. Rheumatoid arthritis: a practical guide to state-of-the-art imaging, image interpretation, and clinical implications. *RadioGraphics*. 2005;25:381–398.

■ ARTHRITIS: PSORIATIC ARTHRITIS

KEY FACTS

■ Psoriatic arthritis involves the hands and feet equally, is asymmetric, and involves the distal inter-phalangeal joints, with joint space widening, tuft erosion, and phalangeal ankylosis. Bone density is increased.

■ Three to five percent of patients with psoriasis develop arthropathy. In most, skin changes precede arthropathy.

■ Calcaneal changes may occur similar to reactive arthritis and ankylosing spondylitis.

■ In some patients, arthropathy resembles rheumatoid arthritis.

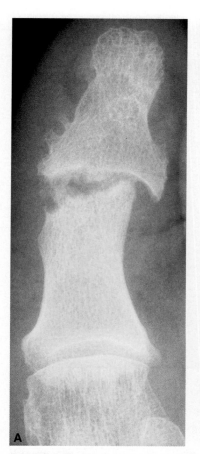 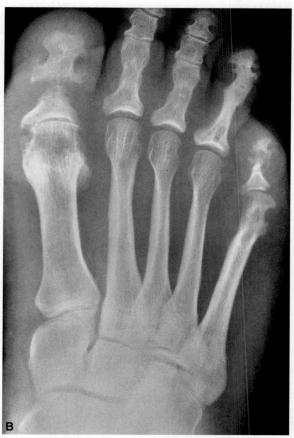

FIGURE 5-73. (A) Anteroposterior (AP) view of the great toe with asymmetric joint destruction and bone proliferation at the base of the distal phalanx characteristic of seronegative spondyloarthropathies. **(B)** Characteristic swelling and joint space changes in the great toe with ankylosis of the fourth toe caused by psoriatic arthritis.

SUGGESTED READING

Avila R, Pugh DG, Slocumb CH, et al. Psoriatic arthritis: a roentgenologic study. *Radiology*. 1960;75:691–701.

Jacobson JA, Girish G, Jiang Y, et al. Radiographic evaluation of arthritis: inflammatory conditions. *Radiology*. 2008;248:378–389.

■ ARTHRITIS: REACTIVE ARTHRITIS

KEY FACTS

- ■ Reactive arthritis involves the feet and, unlike psoriatic arthritis, typically spares the hands.
- ■ Key areas of involvement include the calcaneus, phalangeal joints, and sacroiliac joint.
- ■ Reactive arthritis is usually seen after a genitourinary infection. Arthropathy typically begins 2 to 4 weeks after infection.
- ■ Approximately one-third of patients present with the classic triad of urethritis, conjunctivitis, and arthritis. Forty percent of patients develop arthritis.
- ■ Erosions with bone proliferation differentiate reactive arthritis from rheumatoid arthritis.
- ■ Phalangeal involvement, especially the great toe, is common.
- ■ Calcaneal features are characteristic. Swelling, erosion, and osseous proliferation occur, usually at the plantar aspect.

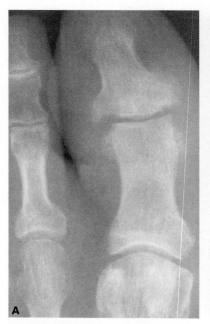 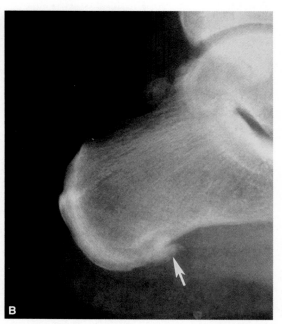

FIGURE 5-74. (A) Sausage digit with reactive arthritis. Characteristic diffuse swelling with erosions and proliferation of the distal joint. **(B)** Poorly defined spur (*arrow*) and swelling at the plantar aspect of the calcaneus caused by reactive arthritis.

SUGGESTED READING

Jacobson JA, Girish G, Jiang Y, et al. Radiographic evaluation of arthritis: inflammatory conditions. *Radiology.* 2008;248:378–389.

Peterson CC, Silbiger ML. Reiter's syndrome and psoriatic arthritis. Their roentgen spectra and some interesting similarities. *AJR Am J Roentgenol.* 1967;101:860–871.

■ ARTHRITIS: ANKYLOSING SPONDYLITIS

KEY FACTS

■ Ankylosing spondylitis involves both sacroiliac joints. There is asymmetric oligoarthropathy and calcaneal involvement.

■ Males 15 to 40 years of age are most commonly affected.

■ Peripheral joint involvement is most common in the hip and shoulder and is seen in 5% to 50% of patients.

■ In the foot, ankylosing spondylitis involves the MTP, first tarsometatarsal, and interphalangeal joints.

■ Calcaneal involvement is common when the foot is involved. Changes are similar to those in reactive arthritis.

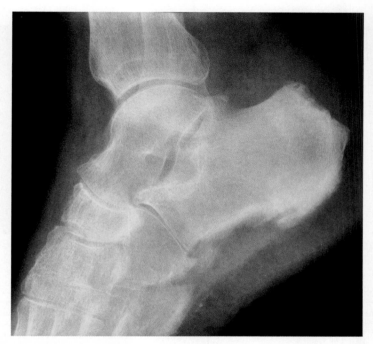

FIGURE 5-75. Poorly defined proliferative changes in the posterior and plantar aspects of the calcaneus caused by ankylosing spondylitis.

SUGGESTED READING

El-Khoury FV, Kathol MH, Brandser EA. Seronegative spondyloarthropathies. *Radiol Clin North Am.* 1996;34:343–357.
Jacobson JA, Girish G, Jiang Y, et al. Radiographic evaluation of arthritis: inflammatory conditions. *Radiology.* 2008;248:378–389.

■ ARTHRITIS: NEUROTROPHIC ARTHROPATHY

KEY FACTS

■ Neurotrophic arthropathy is caused by repetitive trauma secondary to sensory impairment.

■ Disorders may be the result of central (syphilis or meningomyelocele), peripheral (diabetes), or congenital insensitivity to pain.

■ The condition is most common in people with diabetes and involves the ankle (11%), hindfoot (24%), midfoot (30%), and forefoot (34%).

■ Neurotrophic arthropathy may be atrophic or hypertrophic. Bone sclerosis and degenerative changes predominate in the latter. The atrophic or osteopenic form is more common in the forefoot.

■ Atrophic or resorptive form is more difficult to differentiate from osteomyelitis.

■ Differentiation of neuropathic arthropathy from osteomyelitis may require combined radionuclide scans, positron emission tomography, or MRI with contrast enhancement.

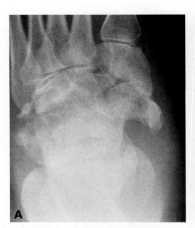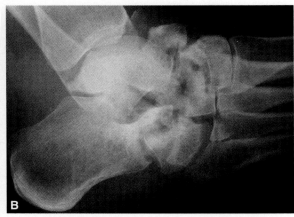

FIGURE 5-76. Anteroposterior (AP) **(A)** and lateral **(B)** radiographs show characteristic fragmentation in the midfoot as the result of neurotrophic arthritis.

SUGGESTED READING

Cofield RH, Morrison MJ, Beabout JW. Diabetic neuropathy in the foot: patient characteristics and patterns of radiographic change. *Foot Ankle*. 1983;4:15–22.

Jones EA, Manaster BJ, May DA, et al. Neuropathic osteoarthropathy: diagnostic dilemmas and differential diagnosis. *RadioGraphics*. 2000;20:S279–S293.

Moore TE, Yuh WTC, Kathol MH, et al. Abnormalities of the foot in patients with diabetes mellitus: findings on MR imaging. *AJR Am J Roentgenol*. 1991;157:813–816.

■ ARTHRITIS: GOUT

KEY FACTS

- ■ Gout is a common self-limited inflammatory arthropathy.
- ■ The arthropathy is most common in the lower extremities; 85% involve the foot.
- ■ Radiographic features include soft tissue swelling, tophi, and well-defined cortical erosions with overhanging margins.
- ■ Chronic gout results in deposition of monosodium urate crystals in synovial fluid, synovium, and periarticular tissues.
- ■ Involved digits demonstrate asymmetric swelling and joint involvement.
- ■ Dual Energy CT can be useful for detecting and characterizing urate deposition about the foot and ankle.

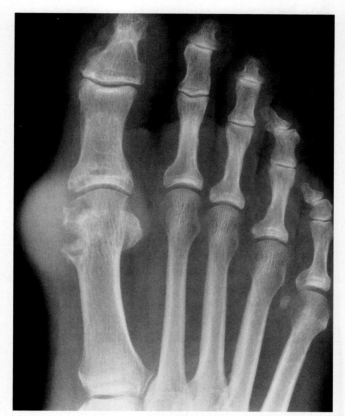

FIGURE 5-77. Gout. Extensive erosive changes in the first metatarsophalangeal (MTP) joint, primarily the metatarsal head. Note the tophaceous soft tissue mass medially.

SUGGESTED READING

Desai MA, Peterson JJ, Garner HW, Kransdorf MJ. Clinical utility of dual-energy CT for evaluation of tophaceous gout. *Radiographics*. 2011 Sep-Oct;31(5):1365–1375; discussion 1376–1377.
Girish G, Glazebrook KN, Jacobson JA. Advanced imaging in gout. *AJR Am J Roentgenol*. 2013;201:515–525.
Ya JS, Chung C, Recht M, et al. MR imaging of tophaceous gout. *AJR Am J Roentgenol*. 1997;168:523–527.

■ ARTHRITIS: CALCIUM PYROPHOSPHATE DEPOSITION DISEASE

KEY FACTS

- Calcium pyrophosphate deposition disease results in joint pain and calcification in fibrocartilage, hyaline cartilage, and periarticular soft tissues.
- Subchondral cystic changes are common and degenerative changes predominate.
- Calcium pyrophosphate deposition disease does not commonly involve the foot and ankle.
- Changes on radiographs or CT include degenerative change and subtle to gross calcifications.

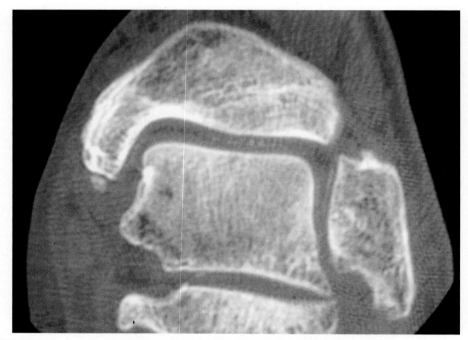

FIGURE 5-78. Computed tomography (CT) of ankle. Coronal CT image demonstrates cartilage calcification.

SUGGESTED READING

Magarelli N, Amelia R, Melillo N, et al. Imaging of chondrocalcinosis: calcium pyrophosphate dihydrate (CPPD) crystal deposition disease – imaging of common sites of involvement. *Clin Exp Rheumatol.* 2012;30:118–125.
Pascual E. The diagnosis of gout and CPPD arthropathy. *Br J Rheumatol.* 1996;35:306–308.

■ INFECTION: OSTEOMYELITIS

KEY FACTS

- Osteomyelitis is an infection involving the bone.
- Osteomyelitis may involve patients of any age. The route of infection may be hematogenous (children and older adults, calcaneus most commonly involved), direct extension from soft tissue infection or puncture wounds, or secondary to previous surgical procedures.
- Imaging of infections depends on suspected site (bone or soft tissue) and clinical condition.

Technique	Applications
CT	Subtle cortical destruction Cloacae Sequestra Gas in soft tissues
MRI	Early subtle changes in marrow, soft tissues, tendon sheaths, bursae, and fascia
Ultrasound	Joint fluid Fluid collections in soft tissues
Radionuclide scans	Early bone involvement (technetium-99m methylene diphosphate, gallium-67, indium-111 white blood cells, and Tc-99m white blood cells)

CT, computed tomography; MRI, magnetic resonance imaging; Tc-99m, technetium-99m.

- Confirmation of organism may require bone biopsy.
- *Staphylococcus aureus* is commonly isolated. Puncture wounds may result in organisms found in the soil (i.e., *Pseudomonas aeruginosa*).

(continued)

■ INFECTION: OSTEOMYELITIS *(Continued)*

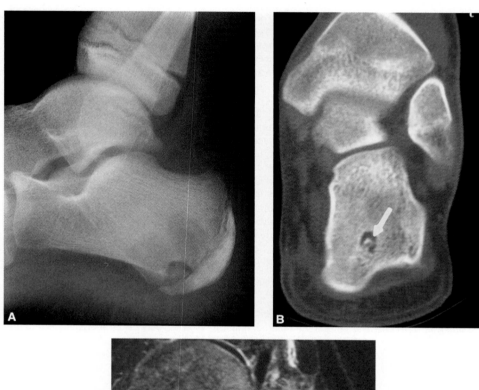

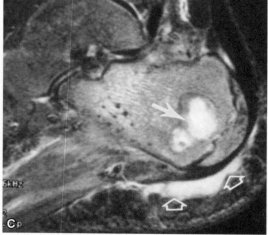

FIGURE 5-79. Osteomyelitis. **(A)** Lateral radiograph of the calcaneus shows lytic changes posteriorly. **(B)** Coronal computed tomography (CT) image demonstrates a sequestrum (*arrow*) in the area of infection. **(C)** Sagittal T2-weighted magnetic resonance (MR) image shows areas of bone infection (*arrow*) and fluid in the soft tissues (*open arrows*).

SUGGESTED READING

Kothari NA, Pelchovitz DJ, Meyer JS. Imaging of musculoskeletal infections. *Radiol Clin North Am.* 2001;39:653–671.

Ledermann HP, Morrison WB, Schweitzer ME. MR image analysis of pedal osteomyelitis: distribution, patterns of spread, and frequency of associated ulceration and septic arthritis. *Radiology.* 2002;223:747–755.

Stalcup ST, Pathria MN, Hughes TH. Musculoskeletal infections of the extremities: a tour from superficial to deep. *Appl Radiol.* 2011;40:12–22.

INFECTION: SOFT TISSUE INFECTION

KEY FACTS

- Soft tissue infection may involve distinct regions, such as tendon sheaths, bursae, or fascia. Infections may extend to involve bone.
- Soft tissue infections of the foot and ankle are particularly common in children with bare feet and adults with ischemic disease or diabetes mellitus.
- Necrotizing fasciitis is an uncommon, but serious, soft tissue infection. Older patients with preexisting conditions are most commonly affected. Seventy-five percent have mixed staphylococcal and streptococcal infections.
- Imaging of soft tissue infections can be accomplished with CT, contrast-enhanced MRI, or ultrasound. CT can be useful for detecting fascial changes and gas in the soft tissues in necrotizing fasciitis.

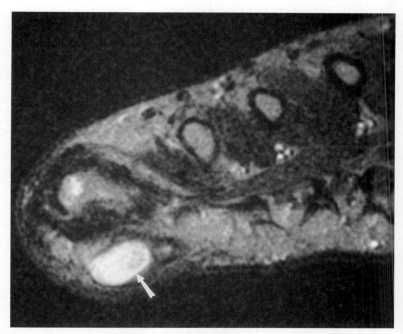

FIGURE 5-80. Axial T2-weighted magnetic resonance (MR) image demonstrates an abscess (*arrow*) after puncture wound to the foot.

SUGGESTED READING

Kothari NA, Pelchovitz DJ, Meyer JS. Imaging of musculoskeletal infections. *Radiol Clin North Am.* 2001;39:653–671.

Laughlin JT, Armstrong DG, Corporusso J, et al. Soft tissue and bone infection after puncture wounds in children. *West J Med.* 1997;166:126–128.

Ledermann HP, Morrison WB, Schweitzer ME. Is soft tissue inflammation in pedal infections contained by fascial planes? Analysis of compartmental involvement in 115 feet. *AJR Am J Roentgenol.* 2002;178:605–612.

Stalcup ST, Pathria MN, Hughes TH. Musculoskeletal infections of the extremities: a tour from superficial to deep. *Appl Radiol.* 2011;40:12–22.

■ INFECTION: JOINT SPACE INFECTION

KEY FACTS

- Joint space infections are most often caused by *S. aureus.*
- Infections are most common in children. Patients taking steroids or those with debilitating illnesses also have an increased incidence of joint space infection.
- Infections may be hematogenous, occur by puncture wound or direct extension from bone, or result from previous surgery.
- The earliest image findings are swelling and joint effusion. Early bone changes are most easily appreciated with radionuclide scans or MRI.
- Joint aspiration or synovial biopsy may be required to define the organism. Aspiration/biopsy can be accomplished with ultrasound or fluoroscopic guidance.

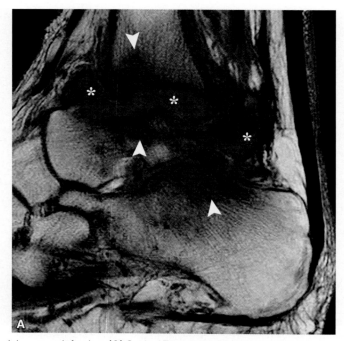

FIGURE 5-81. Joint space infection. **(A)** Sagittal T1-weighted image shows an ankle joint effusion (*asterisks*) with areas of bone involvement (*arrowheads*). **(B)** Coronal T1-weighted image shows extensive periarticular marrow signal abnormality and erosions at the ankle. **(C)** Corresponding coronal T1-weighted postcontrast image with fat suppression demonstrates abnormal enhancement of bone marrow and surrounding soft tissues.

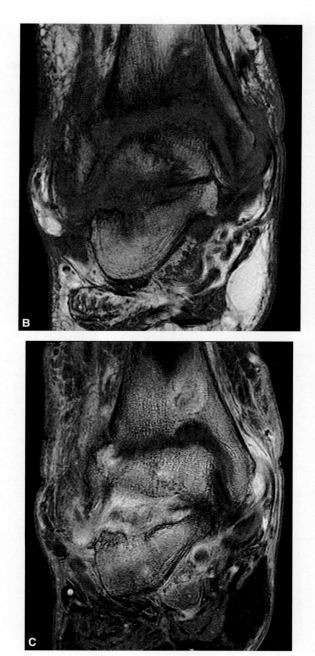

FIGURE 5-81. *(continued)*

SUGGESTED READING

Brower AC. Septic arthritis. *Radiol Clin North Am*. 1996;34:293–310.

Karchevsky M, Schweitzer ME, Morrison WB, et al. MRI findings of septic arthritis and associated osteomyelitis in adults. *AJR Am J Roentgenol*. 2004;182:119–122.

■ INFECTION: DIABETIC FOOT

KEY FACTS

- Diabetic foot disorders result in more hospitalizations than other diabetic complications.
- Up to 6% of diabetic persons undergo amputation because of infection and/or ischemic disease.
- Ulcerations tend to occur over pressure points (heel, metatarsal heads, and tips of toes) on the foot. More than 90% of cases of osteomyelitis in the diabetic foot result from contiguous spread from infected ulcers.
- Infection may be difficult to differentiate from neurotrophic arthropathy, especially the atrophic or osteopenic type.
- Table 5-5 presents imaging approaches to infection in the diabetic foot.

Table 5-5 DIABETIC FOOT INFECTIONS: IMAGING APPROACHES

A: Soft Tissue Swelling and/or Erythema with No Ulceration		
Radiograph	**Clinical Features**	**Next Steps**
Positive	Suspicious for infection	Biopsy and treat
Negative	Low index of suspicion	Three-phase bone scan
		If negative, stop
		If positive, MRI
Negative	High index of suspicion	MRI
		If positive, treat
		If negative, follow

B: Soft Tissue Ulceration		
Radiograph	**Clinical Features**	**Next Steps**
Positive	Suspicious for infection	Biopsy and treat
Negative	Low index of suspicion	Debride and treat ulcer (no drainage or obvious infection)
Negative	High index of suspicion	MRI or radionuclide WBC or granulocyte scans
		Positive, biopsy and treat
		Negative, treat ulcer

C: Neuropathic Arthropathy with or without Ulcer		
Radiograph	**Clinical Features**	**Next Steps**
Positive	Suspicious for infection	Biopsy and treat
Hypertrophic arthropathy	Suspicious for infection	Contrast-enhanced MRI or radionuclide WBC or granulocyte scans
		Positive, biopsy and treat
		Negative, follow

MRI, magnetic resonance imaging; WBC, white blood cell.

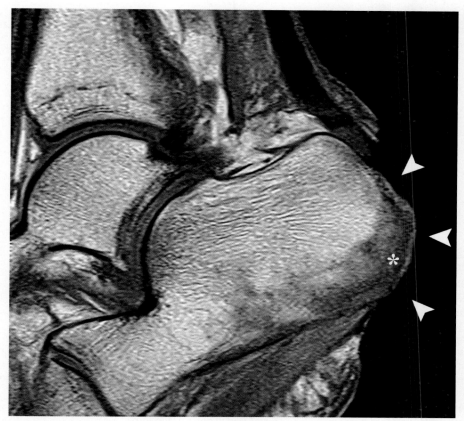

FIGURE 5-82. Sagittal T1-weighted image shows large diabetic heel ulcer (*arrowheads*) and abnormal signal intensity in the calcaneus (*asterisk*) caused by osteomyelitis.

SUGGESTED READING

Donovan A, Schweitzer ME. Use of MR imaging in diagnosing diabetes-related pedal osteomyelitis. *Radiographics.* 2010;30:723–736.

Lipsky BA, Pecasaro RE, Wheat LJ. The diabetic foot: soft tissue and bone infection. *Infect Dis Clin North Am.* 1990;4:409–432.

Morrison WB, Schweitzer ME, Wapner KL, et al. Osteomyelitis in feet of diabetics: clinical accuracy, surgical utility, and cost effectiveness of MR imaging. *Radiology.* 1995;196:557–564.

■ PEDIATRIC DISORDERS: TERMINOLOGY

KEY FACTS

- AP talocalcaneal angle
  - Newborn 40 degrees (range 25–55 degrees)
- Lateral talocalcaneal angle
  - 40 degrees (range 25–55 degrees)
- Talo–first metatarsal angle
  - Newborn 20 degrees (range 9–31 degrees)
- Tibiocalcaneal angle
  - Newborn 75 degrees
  - 6 years 65 degrees
- Lateral longitudinal arch
  - 150 to 175 degrees
  - Pes cavus ≤150 degrees
  - Pes planus >175 degrees

Term	Definition
Talipes	Congenital deformity of the foot
Pes	Acquired deformity of the foot
Valgus	Orientation of bones distal to a joint *away* from the midline
Varus	Orientation of bones distal to a joint *toward* the midline
Adduction	Displacement of bones or anatomic part in transverse plane toward the axis of the body
Abduction	Displacement of bones or anatomic part in a transverse plane away from the axis of the body
Equinus	Fixed plantar flexion of the foot
Calcaneus	Fixed dorsiflexion of the foot
Cavus	Raised longitudinal arch
Planus	Flattened longitudinal arch

■ PEDIATRIC DISORDERS: NORMAL ANGLES OF THE FOOT AND ANKLE

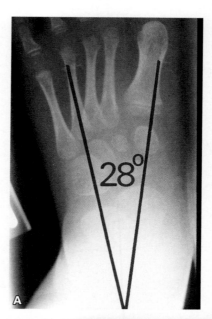

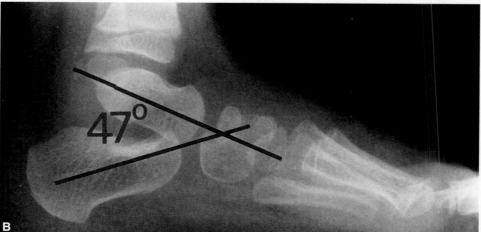

FIGURE 5-83. Normal simulated weight-bearing views of the pediatric foot. Normal anteroposterior (AP) **(A)** and lateral **(B)** talocalcaneal angles are 28 degrees (range 25–55 degrees) and 47 degrees (range 25–55 degrees), respectively.

(continued)

■ PEDIATRIC DISORDERS: NORMAL ANGLES
OF THE FOOT AND ANKLE   *(Continued)*

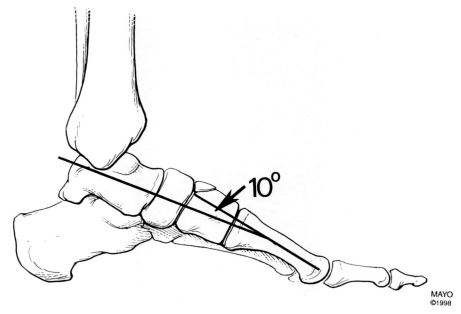

FIGURE 5-84. Lateral talo–first metatarsal angle is 10 degrees (range 9–31 degrees). Measured by lines along talar and first metatarsal axes.

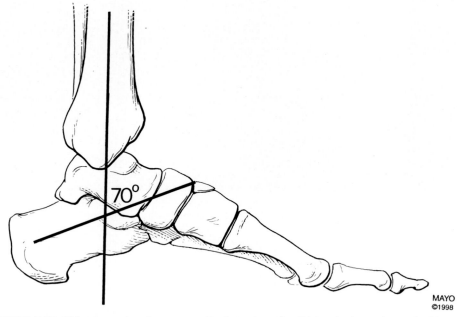

FIGURE 5-85. Tibiocalcaneal angle measured by lines along the tibial and calcaneal axes. In this case, 70 degrees; newborn, 75 degrees; 6 years, 65 degrees.

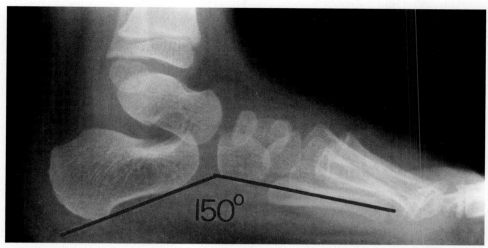

FIGURE 5-86. Longitudinal plantar arch angle measured by lines at the calcaneus and fifth metatarsal. Normal 150 to 170 degrees.

SUGGESTED READING

Harty MP. Imaging of pediatric foot disorders. *Radiol Clin North Am.* 2001;39:733–748.

Thapa MM, Pruthi S, Chew FS. Radiographic assessment of pediatric foot alignment: review. *AJR Am J Roentgenol.* 2010;194: S51–S58.

Vander Wilde R, Staheli LT, Chew DE, et al. Measurements on radiographs of the foot in normal infants and children. *J Bone Joint Surg.* 1998;70A:407–415.

■ PEDIATRIC DISORDERS: HINDFOOT ABNORMALITIES

KEY FACTS

■ Hindfoot valgus includes a group of disorders where the calcaneus is abducted and the distal bones move laterally. The talocalcaneal angle is increased on AP and lateral radiographs. Causes include congenital vertical talus, talipes calcaneovalgus, and neuromuscular disorders.

■ Hindfoot varus includes talipes equinovarus (clubfoot) and various neuromuscular disorders. The talocalcaneal angle is decreased on AP and lateral radiographs. When ossified, the navicular lies medial to the long axis of the talus.

■ Hindfoot equinus shows plantar flexion of the foot or declination of the calcaneus. The tibiocalcaneal angle is greater than 90 degrees. This disorder is seen with clubfoot, congenital vertical talus, and neuromuscular disorders.

■ Hindfoot calcaneus is a group of disorders resulting in increased calcaneal inclination or dorsiflexion. The anterior tibiocalcaneal angle is less than 65 degrees. Pes cavus is commonly associated with hindfoot calcaneus.

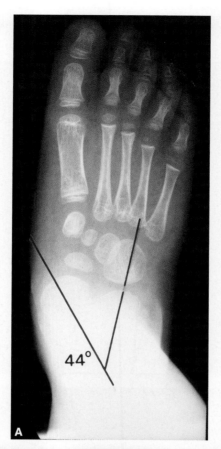

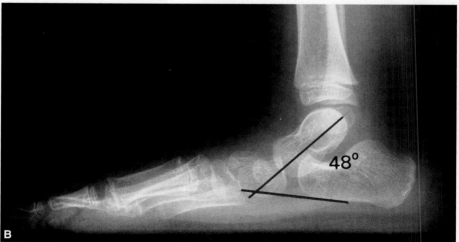

FIGURE 5-87. Hindfoot valgus. **(A)** Anteroposterior (AP) radiograph shows an increased talocalcaneal angle with the long axis of the talus directed medial to the navicular and first metatarsal. **(B)** Lateral view shows an increased angle with midfoot incongruency.

(continued)

■ PEDIATRIC DISORDERS: HINDFOOT ABNORMALITIES   *(Continued)*

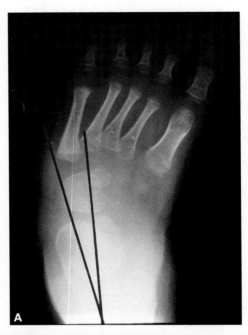

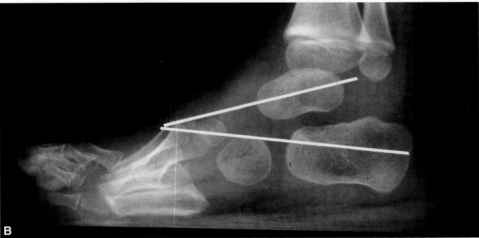

FIGURE 5-88. Hindfoot varus. **(A)** Anteroposterior (AP) radiograph shows a decreased talocalcaneal angle with metatarsus adductus. **(B)** Lateral radiograph shows a decreased talocalcaneal angle.

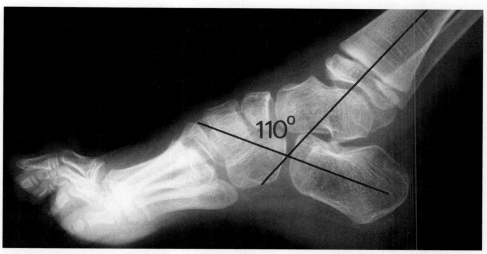

FIGURE 5-89. Hindfoot equinus. The foot is plantar flexed with tibiocalcaneal angle greater than 90 degrees (in this case, 110 degrees).

SUGGESTED READING

Ozonoff MB. *Pediatric Orthopedic Radiology.* Philadelphia: WB Saunders; 1992:397–460.

Thapa MM, Pruthi S, Chew FS. Radiographic assessment of pediatric foot alignment: review. *AJR Am J Roentgenol.* 2010;194: S51–S58.

Wainwright AM, Auld T, Benson MK, et al. The classification of congenital talipes equinovarus. *J Bone Joint Surg Br.* 2002;84:1020–1024.

■ PEDIATRIC DISORDERS: PLANTAR ARCH ABNORMALITIES

KEY FACTS

■ Pes planus (flatfoot) results with decreased calcaneal inclination. The normal arch is lost with a calcaneal–fifth metatarsal angle exceeding 175 degrees. Flatfoot may be flexible or rigid (often associated with tarsal coalition). "Rocker bottom" deformity occurs when the calcaneal–fifth metatarsal angle exceeds 180 degrees.

■ Pes cavus is an increased longitudinal arch with increased calcaneal inclination. Pes cavus is associated with neuromuscular disorders and peroneal muscle atrophy. Pes cavus can be associated with forefoot adduction and hindfoot varus (pes cavo varus).

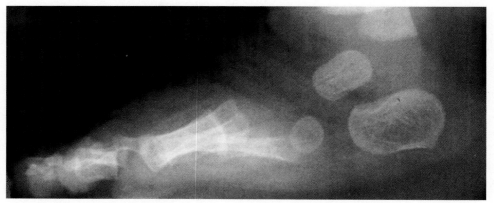

FIGURE 5-90. Lateral radiograph demonstrates pes planus with calcaneal–fifth metatarsal angle greater than 175 degrees.

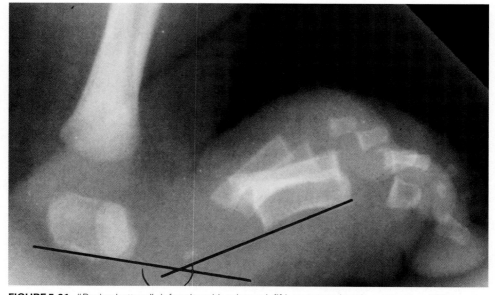

FIGURE 5-91. "Rocker bottom" deformity with calcaneal–fifth metatarsal angle greater than 180 degrees.

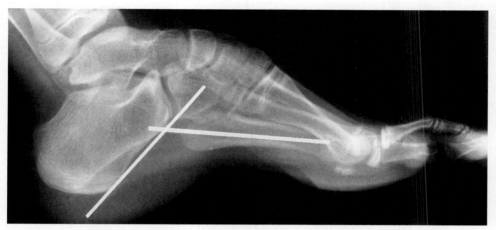

FIGURE 5-92. Pes cavus with increased calcaneal dorsiflexion and plantar flexion of the metatarsals. Calcaneal–fifth metatarsal angle is less than 150 degrees.

SUGGESTED READING

Harris EJ, Vanore JV, Thomas JL, et al. Diagnosis and treatment of pediatric flatfoot. *J Foot Ankle Surg*. 2004;43:341–373.
Vander Wilde R, Staheli LT, Chew DE, et al. Measurements on radiographs of the foot in normal infants and children. *J Bone Joint Surg*. 1988;70A:407–415.

■ PEDIATRIC DISORDERS: FOREFOOT ABNORMALITIES

KEY FACTS

- Metatarsus adductus (medial deviation of the forefoot) is the most common childhood foot deformity. The condition may be associated with midfoot and hindfoot disorders. There is no sex predilection; 50% are unilateral. The condition may be asymptomatic and resolve spontaneously.
- Skewfoot (hooked foot or "Z" foot) presents with forefoot adduction and associated deformities, such as hindfoot valgus, forefoot varus, or pes cavus.

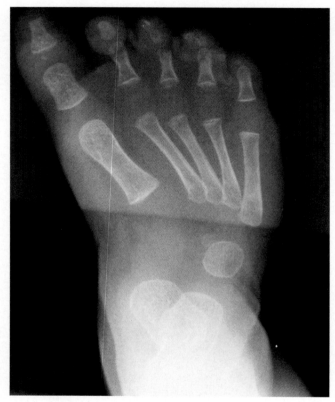

FIGURE 5-93. Anteroposterior (AP) radiograph demonstrates metatarsus adductus with hindfoot valgus.

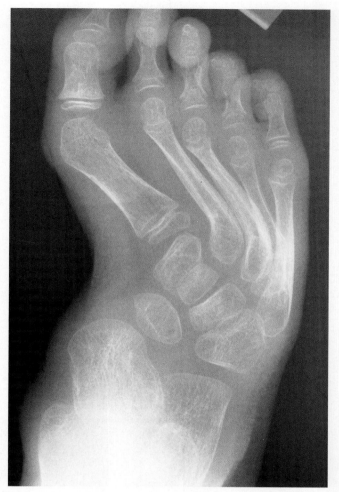

FIGURE 5-94. Anteroposterior (AP) radiograph of a patient with skewfoot (hooked or "Z" foot).

SUGGESTED READING

Hubbard AM, Davidson RS, Meyer JS, et al. Magnetic resonance imaging of skewfoot. *J Bone Joint Surg.* 1996;78A:389–397.
Napiontek M. Skewfoot. *J Pediatr Orthop.* 2002;22:130–133.

■ PEDIATRIC DISORDERS: TALIPES EQUINOVARUS

KEY FACTS

- Talipes equinovarus (clubfoot) consists of hindfoot equinus, hindfoot varus, and forefoot adductus. The incidence is 1 to 1.5 per 1,000 births. Males outnumber females in the ratio 2:1.
- The condition may be congenital or acquired.

Congenital	Acquired
Idiopathic	Polio
Meningocele	Cerebral palsy
Myelomeningocele	Sciatic nerve injury
Diastematomyelia	Vascular compromise
Abnormal muscle insertions	
Tarsal anomalies	

- Talipes equinovarus is seen in 30% of children with spina bifida and in 12% to 56% of children with constriction bands.
- Routine radiographs usually demonstrate the abnormalities. MRI is useful for unossified structures and muscle anomalies.
- Conservative therapy with manipulation and casting in newborns is attempted initially. Surgical release is considered when this fails.

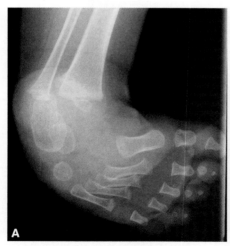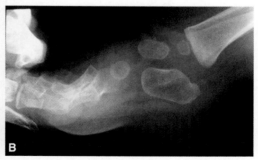

FIGURE 5-95. Anteroposterior (AP) **(A)** and lateral **(B)** radiographs show hindfoot equinus, hindfoot varus, and forefoot adductus.

SUGGESTED READING

Hersh A. The role of surgery in treatment of clubfoot. *Foot Ankle Int.* 1995;16:672–681.
Wainwright AM, Auld T, Benson MK, et al. The classification of congenital talipes equinovarus. *J Bone Joint Surg Br.* 2002;84:1020–1024.

■ PEDIATRIC DISORDERS: CONGENITAL VERTICAL TALUS

KEY FACTS

■ Congenital vertical talus consists of dorsal and lateral articulation with the navicular with a vertically oriented talus and flatfoot deformity.

■ The condition is not reducible and may be unilateral or bilateral.

■ The condition is often seen with arthrogryposis or myelomeningocele.

■ Radiographs demonstrate hindfoot valgus on the AP view and plantar flexion of the calcaneus and talus on the lateral view.

■ Surgical release and K-wire fixation is generally required for treatment.

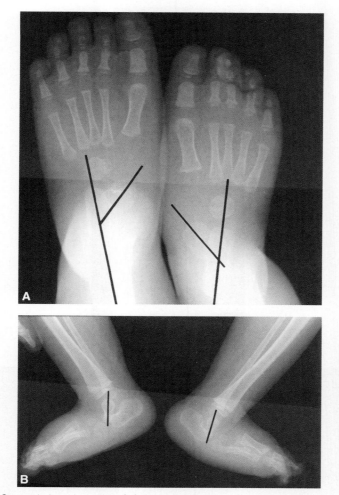

FIGURE 5-96. Congenital vertical talus. **(A)** Anteroposterior (AP) radiographs show hindfoot valgus (*lines*) greater on the right. **(B)** Lateral radiographs show vertically oriented tali (*lines*) and calcaneal plantar flexion with flatfoot deformities.

SUGGESTED READING

Mckie J, Radomisli T. Congenital vertical talus: a review. *Clin Podiatr Med Surg.* 2010;27:145–156.

Naptiontek M. Congenital vertical talus: a critical review of 32 feet operated by peritalar reduction. *J Pediatr Orthop.* 1995;4:179–185.

■ PEDIATRIC DISORDERS: PES PLANOVALGUS

KEY FACTS

- Pes planovalgus (flexible flatfoot deformity) presents with an increased talocalcaneal angle, hindfoot valgus, and forefoot abduction.
- The longitudinal and transverse arches flatten, so the metatarsals appear parallel on AP radiographs.
- The condition is flexible, painless, and the result of ligament laxity.
- The disorder is familial and often bilateral.
- Surgery is reserved for patients who become symptomatic or when orthotics fail.

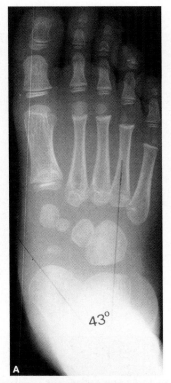

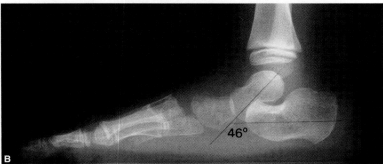

FIGURE 5-97. Pes planovalgus (flexible flatfoot). **(A)** Anteroposterior (AP) radiograph shows an increased talocalcaneal angle with lateral subluxation of the navicular. The forefoot is abducted and metatarsals parallel. **(B)** Lateral radiograph shows arch collapse with increased talocalcaneal angle.

SUGGESTED READING

Ozonoff MB. *Pediatric Orthopedic Radiology.* Philadelphia: WB Saunders; 1992:397–460.

Thapa MM, Pruthi S, Chew FS. Radiographic assessment of pediatric foot alignment: review. *AJR Am J Roentgenol.* 2010;194: S51–S58.

■ PEDIATRIC DISORDERS: TARSAL COALITIONS

KEY FACTS

- ■ Tarsal coalitions are abnormal fibrous, cartilaginous, or bony bars between the tarsal bones.
- ■ The condition may be congenital or acquired (infection, trauma, surgery).
- ■ Calcaneonavicular coalitions are most common. The condition may be bilateral and asymptomatic or associated with rigid flatfoot. Talar beaking may be associated.
- ■ Talocalcaneal coalitions are more common in males and bilateral in 20% to 25%. The midsubtalar joint is difficult to see, and talar beaking may be present.
- ■ Calcaneocuboid coalitions are rare.
- ■ Imaging may be accomplished with routine radiographs (oblique view best for calcaneonavicular coalitions), CT, or MRI. CT is used to define the extent of the coalition. MRI can differentiate fibrous, cartilaginous, and osseous coalitions.

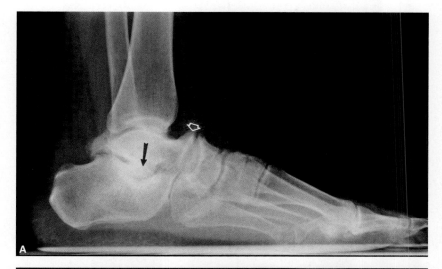

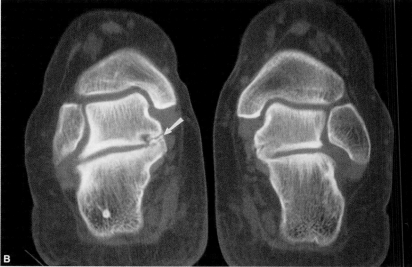

FIGURE 5-98. Talocalcaneal coalition. **(A)** Lateral radiograph shows flatfoot deformity with osseous density (*arrow*) in the midsubtalar joint and a prominent talar beak (*open arrow*). **(B)** Coronal computed tomography (CT) image confirms the coalition (*arrow*).

(continued)

■ PEDIATRIC DISORDERS: TARSAL COALITIONS   *(Continued)*

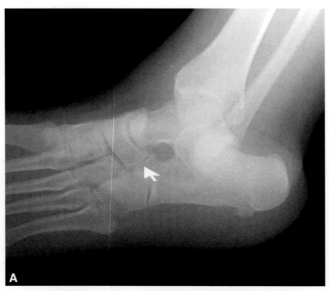

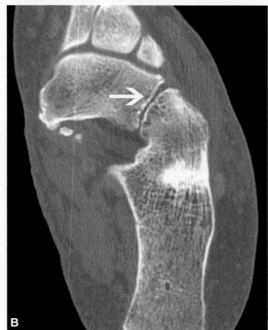

FIGURE 5-99. Calcaneonavicular fibrous coalition. Oblique radiograph **(A)** shows elongation of the anterior calcaneal process and abnormal articulation between the navicular and the calcaneus (*arrow*). Axial computed tomography (CT) image **(B)** depicting the fibrous or cartilaginous calcaneonavicular coalition to better advantage (*arrow*).

SUGGESTED READING

Crim J, Kjeldsberg K. Radiographic diagnosis of tarsal coalition. *AJR Am J Roentgenol.* 2004;18:323–328.
Newman SJ, Newberg AH. Congenital tarsal coalition: multimodality evaluation with emphasis on CT and MR imaging. *Radiographics.* 2000;20:321–332.

■ PEDIATRIC DISORDERS: OVERGROWTH/HYPOPLASIA/APLASIA

KEY FACTS

- ■ Macrodactyly: Overgrowth of soft tissues or osseous structures may be generalized or focal. In the foot, all structures in one or more digits may be affected. The condition may be idiopathic or associated with hemangiomas, arteriovenous malformations, or neurofibromatosis.
- ■ Bradydactyly: Abnormal shortening of the toes. Digits and phalanges affected are variable. Bradydactyly may be associated with trisomy 13 and 18, fetal alcohol syndrome, and certain mucopolysaccharidoses.
- ■ Syndactyly: Lack of differentiation between two or more digits. The condition may involve only soft tissues or soft tissue and bone. Males are affected more often than females. The condition may be isolated or associated with conditions such as Apert syndrome, Poland syndrome, and mesomelic dysplasia.
- ■ Polydactyly: Common, resulting in supernumerary digits or metatarsals. The condition is seen in 1.7 per 1,000 births and is bilateral in 25% to 50%. It is usually an isolated condition, but 15% are associated with other congenital anomalies.

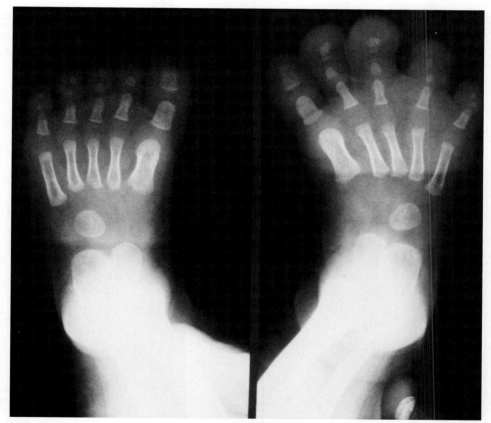

FIGURE 5-100. Macrodactyly. Anteroposterior (AP) radiographs show increased size of the right toes.

(continued)

■ PEDIATRIC DISORDERS: OVERGROWTH/HYPOPLASIA/ APLASIA   *(Continued)*

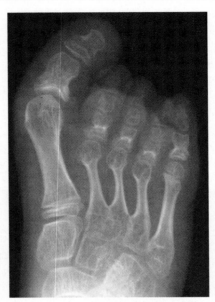

FIGURE 5-101. Bradydactyly. Anteroposterior (AP) radiograph shows generalized shortening of the second to fourth rays.

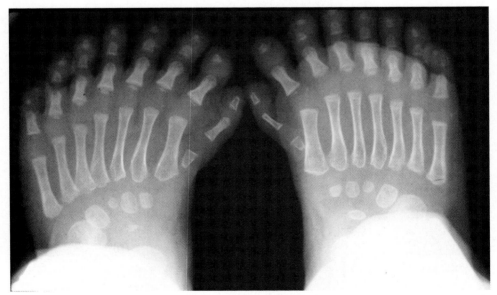

FIGURE 5-102. Polydactyly. Anteroposterior (AP) radiographs show bilateral supernumerary metatarsals and digits.

SUGGESTED READING

Taybi H, Lachman RS. *Radiology of Syndromes, Metabolic Disorders, and Skeletal Dysplasias.* St. Louis: CV Mosby-Yearbook; 1996.

■ PEDIATRIC DISORDERS: FREIBERG INFRACTION

KEY FACTS

■ Freiberg infraction is posttraumatic osteonecrosis of the metatarsal head. The condition is three to four times more common in females than in males.

■ Patients present in late childhood or adolescence. The condition is bilateral in 10%.

■ The second metatarsal is involved most often, followed by the third and fourth metatarsal heads.

■ Radiographs demonstrate flattening of the metatarsal head with sclerosis and fragmentation.

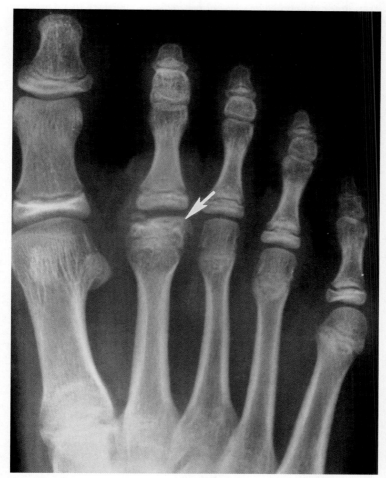

FIGURE 5-103. Freiberg infraction. Anteroposterior (AP) radiograph shows a flattened sclerotic second metatarsal head (*arrow*).

SUGGESTED READING

Cerrato RA. Freiberg's disease. *Foot Ankle Clin*. 2011;16:647–658.
Smillie IS. Freiberg's infraction (Köhler's second disease). *J Bone Joint Surg*. 1957;39B:580.

■ PEDIATRIC DISORDERS: KÖHLER DISEASE

KEY FACTS

- Köhler disease is an osteochondrosis of the navicular.
- Patients present at 5 years of age. Males outnumber females in the ratio 6:1.
- Patients have pain, swelling, and local tenderness.
- It may be difficult to differentiate this process from normal variants in appearance of the navicular.
- Radiographs demonstrate a flattened, sclerotic, fragmented navicular. Radionuclide scans may demonstrate a photopenic region.
- The navicular returns to normal or near-normal configuration over 3 to 4 months, regardless of treatment.

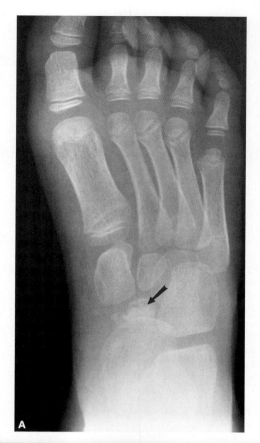

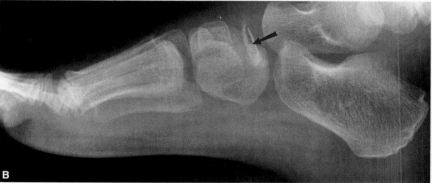

FIGURE 5-104. Köhler disease. Anteroposterior (AP) **(A)** and lateral **(B)** radiographs show a sclerotic flattened navicular (*arrow*).

SUGGESTED READING

Borges JL, Guille JT, Bowen JR. Köhler's bone disease of the tarsal navicular. *J Pediatr Orthop.* 1995;15:596–598.

6 Shoulder/Arm

Francesca D. Beaman, Jeffrey J. Peterson, and Thomas H. Berquist

■ FRACTURES/DISLOCATIONS: PROXIMAL HUMERAL FRACTURES

KEY FACTS

- Fractures of the proximal humerus usually occur in the elderly.
- Proximal humeral fractures account for 5% of all skeletal fractures.
- Fractures in the elderly are usually caused by a fall.
- Fractures tend to follow the physeal lines dividing the humerus into four parts: humeral head, greater tuberosity, lesser tuberosity, and humeral shaft.
- Fragments are considered displaced if separated by 1 cm or angulated 45 degrees or greater (Table 6-1).
- The majority of fractures (85%) are undisplaced.
- Undisplaced fractures are treated conservatively. Displaced, especially comminuted or four-part fractures, require surgery or arthroplasty.
- Complications:
  - Adhesive capsulitis
  - Neurovascular injury
  - Malunion, nonunion
  - Avascular necrosis

Table 6-1   NEER CLASSIFICATION

Fracture Type	Description
One-part (80% of cases)	No fragment displacement
	>1 cm or angulated
	>45 degrees
Two-part (13% of cases)	One fragment displaced
	>1 cm or angulated
	>45 degrees
Three-part (3% of cases)	Two fragments displaced or angulated as in "two part"
Four-part (4% of cases)	Three fragments displaced or angulated as above

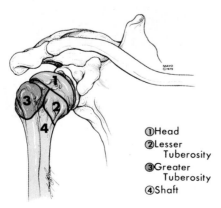

①Head
②Lesser
  Tuberosity
③Greater
  Tuberosity
④Shaft

FIGURE 6-1. The four parts of proximal humeral fractures.

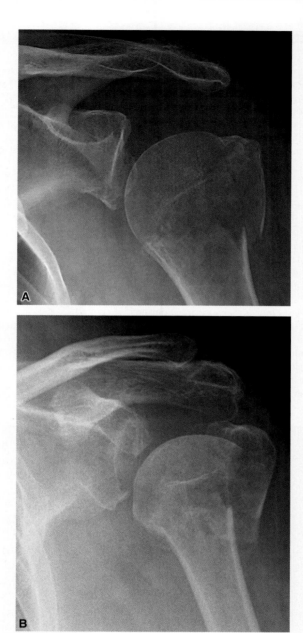

FIGURE 6-2. Proximal humeral fracture. Grashey views of a four-part proximal humeral fracture in two different patients with **(A)** minimal and **(B)** moderate displacement of the fragments.

SUGGESTED READING

Berquist TH. *MRI of the Musculoskeletal System.* 6th ed. Philadelphia: Lippincott Williams & Wilkins; 2012.

Lin DJ, Wong TT, Kazam JM. Shoulder arthroplasty, from indications to complications: what the radiologist needs to know. *Radiographics.* 2016;36(1):192–208.

Sandstrom CK, Kennedy SA, Gross JA. Acute shoulder trauma: what the surgeon wants to know. *Radiographics.* 2015;35(2):475–492.

■ FRACTURES/DISLOCATIONS: GLENOHUMERAL DISLOCATIONS

KEY FACTS

- Dislocations of the glenohumeral joint are the most common dislocation (50% of all dislocations).
- Dislocations may be anterior (96%), posterior (2% to 4%), or, less frequently, superior or inferior.
- Anterior dislocations are usually the result of falls with the arm abducted and externally rotated.
  - The humeral head is frequently impacted against the labrum, resulting in a posterolateral impaction fracture (67% to 76%) or Hill–Sachs lesion.
  - The anterior inferior labrum or glenoid may also be injured (50%), and such an injury is referred to as a Bankart lesion (may be cartilaginous or osseous).
  - Most anterior dislocations are obvious on routine radiographs.
- Posterior dislocations occur with seizures, shock therapy, or falls with the arm abducted and internally rotated. The patient's arm is internally rotated, and external rotation is blocked.
  - Radiographic features may be subtle.
    - ❖ Humeral head fixed in internal rotation (100%)
    - ❖ Joint may appear widened
    - ❖ Overlap of humeral head and glenoid absent or distorted
    - ❖ "Trough line" oriented vertically in the humeral head, caused by impaction fracture of the anteromedial humeral head resulting from contact with the posterior glenoid
    - ❖ Lesser tuberosity fracture (25%)
  - Scapular "Y" view makes diagnosis most obvious.
  - Treatment of dislocations is closed reduction unless there are significant associated fractures.
- Complications of dislocations:
  - Associated fractures: lesser tuberosity, coracoid, greater tuberosity, subscapularis avulsion
  - Recurrent dislocation
  - Degenerative arthritis
  - Neurovascular injury

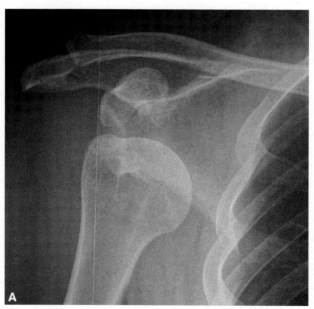

FIGURE 6-3. Anterior dislocation. Anteroposterior (AP) **(A)** and axillary **(B)** radiographs show an anterior dislocation of the humeral head. **(C)** AP radiograph in another patient shows an anterior dislocation with fracture fragments laterally. **(D)** Axial T2 fat-saturated magnetic resonance (MR) image shows a Hill–Sachs lesion (*arrow*) in the posterior humeral head.

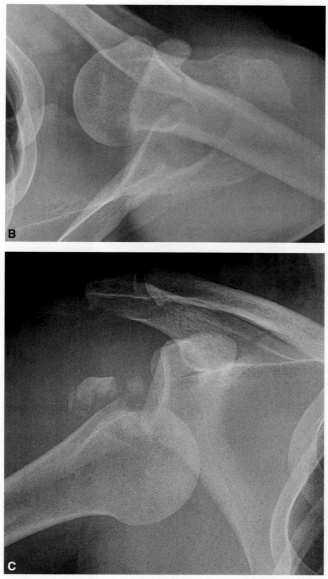

FIGURE 6-3. *(continued)*

(continued)

■ FRACTURES/DISLOCATIONS: GLENOHUMERAL DISLOCATIONS *(Continued)*

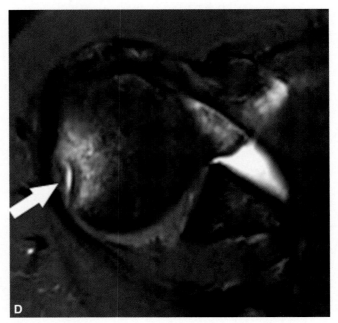

FIGURE 6-3. *(continued)*

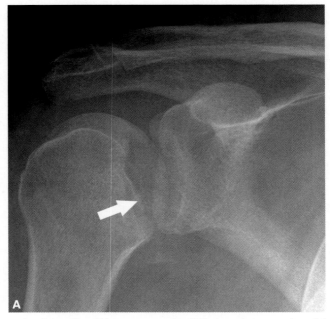

FIGURE 6-4. Posterior dislocation. **(A)** Anteroposterior (AP) view shows overlap of the glenoid and humeral head with an anteromedial impaction fracture *(arrow)*. **(B)** Axillary view shows the humeral head fracture impacted into the posterior glenoid locking the shoulder in internal rotation.

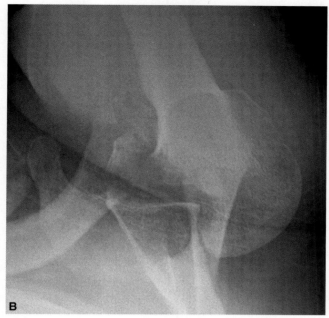

FIGURE 6-4. (*continued*)

SUGGESTED READING

Atef A, El-Tantawy A, Gad H, Hefeda M. Prevalence of associated injuries after anterior shoulder dislocation: a prospective study. *Int Orthop*. 2016;40(3):519–524.

Gyftopoulos S, Wang A, Babb J. Hill–Sachs lesion location: does it play a role in engagement? *Skeletal Radiol*. 2015;44(8):1129–1134.

Sebro R, Oliveira A, Palmer WE. MR arthrography of the shoulder: technical update and clinical applications. *Semin Musculoskelet Radiol*. 2014;18(4):352–364.

■ FRACTURES/DISLOCATIONS: ACROMIOCLAVICULAR DISLOCATION

KEY FACTS

- Dislocations of the acromioclavicular (AC) joint (12%) are less common than glenohumeral (85%) shoulder dislocations.
- Most commonly results from a fall striking the point (AC joint region) of the shoulder.
- Injuries may be partial or complete (Table 6-2).
- Routine clavicle radiographs may be normal with incomplete ligament injury. Weight-bearing views are useful to classify injuries (Types I and II).
- Closed reduction is usually used for Types I and II injuries. Internal fixation is frequently required for Types III to VI lesions.

Table 6-2 ACROMIOCLAVICULAR DISLOCATIONS

Classification	Radiographic Features
Type I, few fibers torn	Normal
Type II, rupture of the capsule and AC ligaments	Joint widened, clavicle may be slightly subluxed
Type III, same as Type II, but coracoclavicular ligaments also disrupted	Elevated clavicle, coracoclavicular space ↑
Types III and V, same as Type III	Same as Type III, but posterior clavicular displacement with Type IV and superior with Type V
Type VI, disruption of all ligaments with anterior entrapment	Clavicle trapped below coracoid

AC, acromioclavicular.

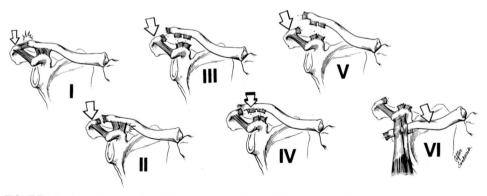

FIGURE 6-5. Acromioclavicular (AC) joint injuries. Type I: AC sprain, few fibers torn. Type II: disruption of the AC ligaments with coracoclavicular ligaments intact. Type III: disruption of the AC and coraco-clavicular ligaments. Type IV: disruption of both ligament complexes with posterior clavicular displacement. Type V: disruption of both ligament complexes with marked superior clavicular displacement. Type VI: disruption of both ligament complexes with anterior entrapment beneath the coracoid.

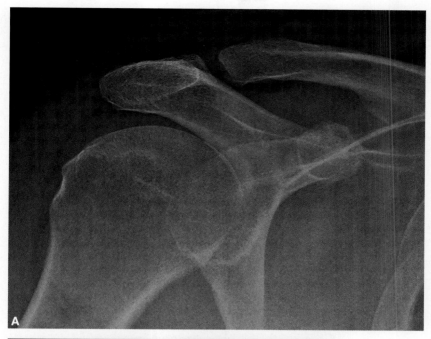

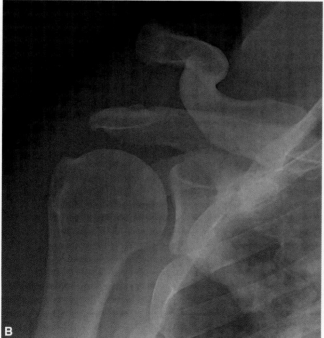

FIGURE 6-6. Acromioclavicular (AC) separation. **(A)** Anteroposterior (AP) radiograph shows a normal AC joint space. **(B)** Grashey and scapular-Y **(C)** views show marked superior displacement of the clavicle (Type V).

(continued)

■ FRACTURES/DISLOCATIONS: ACROMIOCLAVICULAR DISLOCATION *(Continued)*

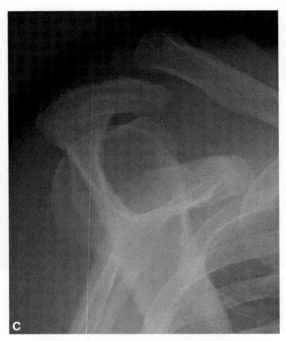

FIGURE 6-6. *(continued)*

SUGGESTED READING

Kim AC, Matcuk G, Patel D, et al. Acromioclavicular joint injuries and reconstructions: a review of expected imaging findings and potential complications. *Emerg Radiol.* 2012;19(5):399–413.

Loriaut P, Casabianca L, Alkhaili J, et al. Arthroscopic treatment of acute acromioclavicular dislocations using a double button device: clinical and MRI results. *Orthop Traumatol Surg Res.* 2015;101(8):895–901.

Nemec U, Oberleitner G, Nemec SF, et al. MRI versus radiography of acromioclavicular joint dislocation. *Am J Roentgenol.* 2011;197(4):968–973.

FRACTURES/DISLOCATIONS: STERNOCLAVICULAR DISLOCATIONS

KEY FACTS

- Dislocations of the sternoclavicular joint are uncommon (3% of shoulder dislocations).
- Usually occurs with indirect shoulder trauma. Anterior dislocation is the result of posterolateral forces transmitted medially. Posterior dislocation is the result of direct anterior trauma. A majority of dislocations are anterior (>90%).
- Radiographic evaluation is difficult with routine views because of bone overlap. Computed tomography (CT) is the technique of choice to evaluate the sternoclavicular joint.
- Treatment is usually conservative.
- Complications are most common with posterior dislocations: tracheal rupture, arch vessel laceration, and neural injury.

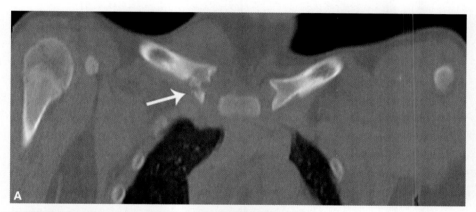

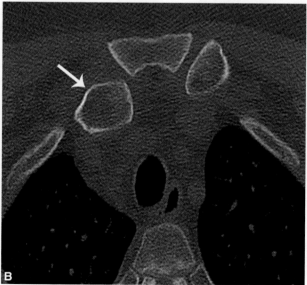

FIGURE 6-7. Sternoclavicular fracture dislocation. **(A)** Coronal reformatted computed tomography (CT) image shows a fracture (*arrow*) of the right clavicular head with disruption of the sternoclavicular joint. **(B)** Axial and sagittal-reformatted **(C)** CT images in another patient show posterior dislocation of the right clavicular head (*arrow*). Note normal alignment of the left sternoclavicular joint in **(B)**.

(continued)

■ FRACTURES/DISLOCATIONS: STERNOCLAVICULAR DISLOCATIONS *(Continued)*

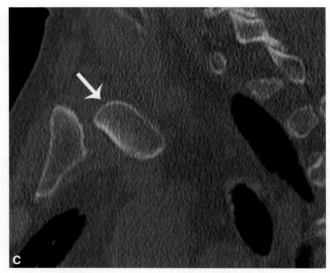

FIGURE 6-7. *(continued)*

SUGGESTED READING

Khorashadi L, Burns EM, Heaston DR, et al. Posterior dislocation of the sternoclavicular joint. *Radiol Case Rep.* 2015;6(3):439.

Morell DJ, Thyagarajan DS. Sternoclavicular joint dislocation and its management: a review of the literature. *World J Orthop.* 2016;7(4):244–250.

Restrepo CS, Martinez S, Lemos DF, et al. Imaging appearances of the sternum and sternoclavicular joints. *Radiographics.* 2009;29(3):839–859.

■ FRACTURES/DISLOCATIONS: CLAVICLE FRACTURES

KEY FACTS

- ■ Clavicle fractures are especially common in children.
- ■ Injury occurs after a fall on the outstretched hand.
- ■ Fractures most commonly involve the middle third (80%). The distal clavicle is involved in 15%, and medial clavicle in 5%.
- ■ Routine anteroposterior (AP) radiographs are usually adequate for diagnosis.
- ■ Most clavicle fractures can be treated with closed reduction. Distal fractures involving the AC joint and ligaments may require internal fixation.
- ■ Complications include malunion, nonunion (1% to 2%), and degenerative arthritis when there is joint involvement.

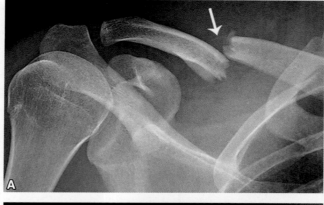

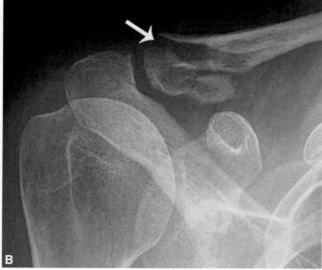

FIGURE 6-8. Clavicle fractures. Anteroposterior (AP) radiographs show mildly displaced mid **(A)** and distal **(B)** clavicular fractures (*arrow*) without widening of the acromioclavicular (AC) joint. **(C)** AP radiograph in another patient shows a midclavicular fracture with override of the fracture fragments, which was treated with hardware fixation **(D)**.

(continued)

▪ FRACTURES/DISLOCATIONS: CLAVICLE FRACTURES *(Continued)*

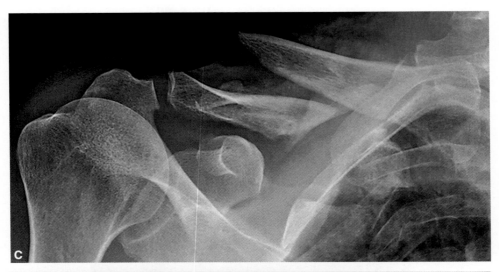

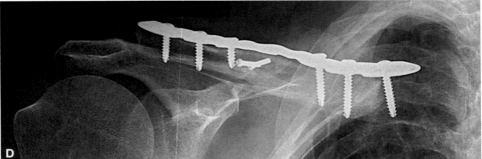

FIGURE 6-8. *(continued)*

SUGGESTED READING

Melenevsky Y, Yablon CM, Ramappa A, et al. Clavicle and acromioclavicular joint injuries: a review of imaging, treatment, and complications. *Skeletal Radiol*. 2011;40(7):831–842.

Suppan CA, Bae DS, Donohue KS, et al. Trends in the volume of operative treatment of midshaft clavicle fractures in children and adolescents: a retrospective, 12-year, single-institution analysis. *J Pediatr Orthop B*. 2016;25(4):305–309.

■ FRACTURES/DISLOCATIONS: POSTTRAUMATIC OSTEOLYSIS

KEY FACTS

- ■ Posttraumatic osteolysis occurs in the distal clavicle.
- ■ Patients present with pain and weakness.
- ■ Differential diagnosis includes rotator cuff tear and AC separation.
- ■ Routine radiographs may be normal early, but later erosive changes occur in the distal clavicle. Magnetic resonance imaging (MRI) shows edema (increased signal on T2-weighted images) in the distal clavicle and joint.
- ■ When conservative therapy fails, the distal clavicle can be resected.

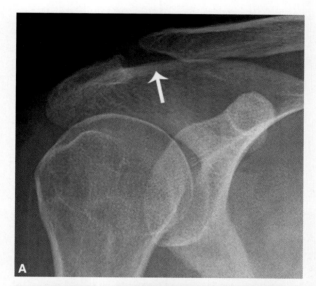

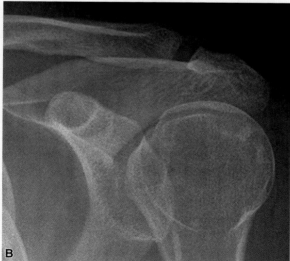

FIGURE 6-9. Posttraumatic osteolysis. Anteroposterior (AP) radiographs of the same patient show widening (arrow) of the right acromioclavicular (AC) joint **(A)** and a normal left **(B)** joint. **(C)** AP radiograph in another patient shows irregularity of the distal clavicle (*arrow*). Coronal T2 fat-saturated **(D)** and axial proton density fat-saturated **(E)** magnetic resonance (MR) images in the same patient as **(C)** show irregularity of the distal clavicle with joint inflammation (*arrow*). A = acromion.

(continued)

■ FRACTURES/DISLOCATIONS: POSTTRAUMATIC OSTEOLYSIS *(Continued)*

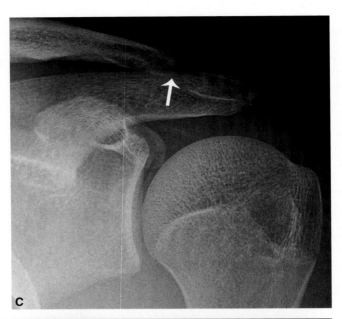

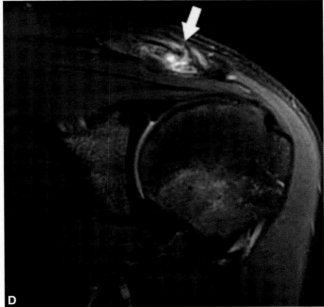

FIGURE 6-9. *(continued)*

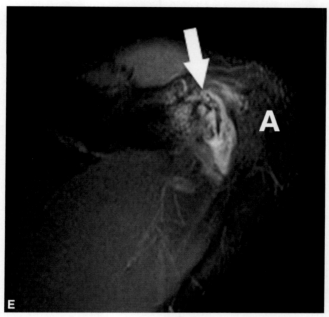

FIGURE 6-9. (*continued*)

SUGGESTED READING

Kassarjian A, Llopis E, Palmer WE. Distal clavicular osteolysis: MR evidence for subchondral fracture. *Skeletal Radiol.* 2007;36(1):17–22.

Rios CG, Mazzocca AD. Acromioclavicular joint problems in athletes and new methods of management. *Clin Sports Med.* 2008;27(4):763–788.

■ FRACTURES/DISLOCATIONS: SCAPULAR FRACTURES

KEY FACTS

- Fractures of the scapula are uncommon (1% of all skeletal fractures).
- Injury is the result of direct trauma.
- Scapular fractures can be overlooked on AP and lateral radiographs.
- Associated fractures of the clavicle and ribs occur in 88%.
- Articular involvement is best evaluated with CT.
- Conservative therapy is usually preferred unless there is significant articular deformity or displacement.

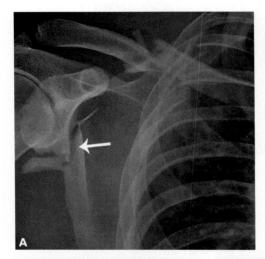

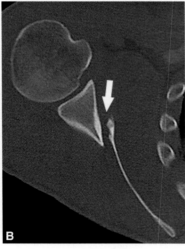
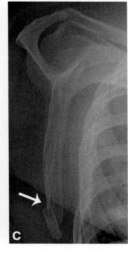

FIGURE 6-10. Scapular fracture. Anteroposterior (AP) radiograph **(A)** and axial computed tomography (CT) image **(B)** show a displaced fracture of the scapular neck (*arrow*). Note, a midclavicular fracture and rib fractures can also be seen on the radiograph. **(C)** Lateral radiograph in another patient shows a fracture (*arrow*) of the inferior scapular body.

SUGGESTED READING

Armitage BM, Wijdicks CA, Tarkin IS, et al. Mapping of scapular fractures with three-dimensional computed tomography. *J Bone Joint Surg Am.* 2009;91(9):2222–2228.

Lewis S, Argintar E, Jahn R, et al. Intra-articular scapular fractures: outcomes after internal fixation. *J Orthop.* 2013;10(4):188–192.

Ropp AM, Davis DL. Scapular fractures: what radiologists need to know. *Am J Roentgenol.* 2015;205(3):491–501.

■ FRACTURE/DISLOCATIONS: HUMERAL SHAFT FRACTURES

KEY FACTS

- ■ Humeral shaft fractures account for 1% of all fractures.
- ■ Location of the fracture in relation to muscle attachments affects the direction of displacement. Proximal third fractures displace medially because of pectoral muscle forces. Fractures distal to the deltoid insertion are abducted by the deltoid muscle.
- ■ 69% of fractures involve the midshaft.
- ■ Fractures at the mid/distal third junction are difficult to manage. Radial nerve and nutrient artery injury may occur.
- ■ Complication of humeral shaft fractures includes nonunion, malunion, infection, radial nerve injury (5% to 10%), and compartment syndrome.

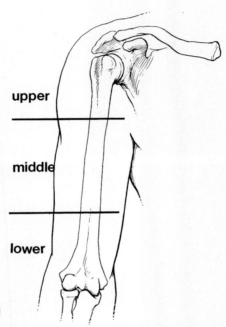

FIGURE 6-11. Fractures of the humerus are described by location as upper, middle, or lower third.

(continued)

■ FRACTURE/DISLOCATIONS: HUMERAL SHAFT FRACTURES *(Continued)*

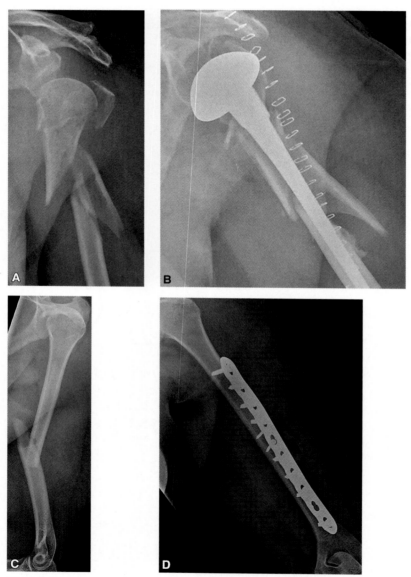

FIGURE 6-12. Anteroposterior (AP) radiographs show a four-part proximal humeral fracture extending into the proximal diaphysis **(A)** treated with shoulder prosthesis **(B)**. **C)** AP radiograph in another patient shows a midhumeral shaft fracture with separation and angulation of the fragments. This can result in soft tissue interposition and nonunion and was treated with open reduction and internal fixation using a compression plate **(D)**.

SUGGESTED READING

Ricci FP, Barbosa RI, Elui VM, et al. Radial nerve injury associated with humeral shaft fracture: a retrospective study. *Acta Ortop Bras.* 2015;23(1):19–21.

Walker M, Palumbo B, Badman B, et al. Humeral shaft fractures: a review. *J Shoulder Elbow Surg.* 2011;20(5):833–844.

■ ROTATOR CUFF DISEASE: BASIC CONCEPTS

KEY FACTS

- ■ The rotator cuff is composed of the supraspinatus, infraspinatus, teres minor, and subscapularis tendons.
- ■ The rotator cuff is responsible for up to 50% of muscle effort for abduction and 80% for external rotation.
- ■ Rotator cuff tear (Table 6-3) most commonly results from impingement of the cuff between the coracoacromial arch and the humeral head. Vascular insufficiency may play a role. Chronic sports trauma and occupational overuse may result in cuff tears. Acute trauma is an infrequent cause of isolated rotator cuff tears.
- ■ Imaging of rotator cuff disease can be accomplished with routine radiographs, ultrasound, CT arthrography, and conventional MRI or magnetic resonance (MR) arthrography. MRI is the technique of choice at most institutions.

Table 6-3   ETIOLOGY OF ROTATOR CUFF TEARS

Primary Impingement

Abnormal acromial configuration

Acromioclavicular osteophytes

Os Acromiale

Thickened coracoacromial ligament

Secondary extrinsic impingement

Ischemia

Trauma

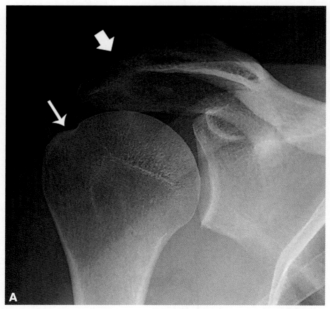

FIGURE 6-13. (A) Normal Grashey view of the shoulder shows a preserved humeroacromial distance, normal greater tuberosity (*thin arrow*), and no abnormality of the acromioclavicular (AC) joint (*thick arrow*). **(B)** Grashey view radiograph in a patient with chronic rotator cuff disease shows a narrowed humeroacromial distance, prominent subacromial osteophyte (*white arrow*) causing impingement, significant AC joint degenerative hypertrophy and bony irregularity of the greater tuberosity (*black arrow*).

(continued)

■ ROTATOR CUFF DISEASE: BASIC CONCEPTS *(Continued)*

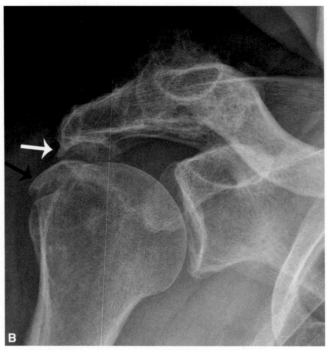

FIGURE 6-13. *(continued)*

SUGGESTED READING

Llopis E, Montesinos P, Guedez MT, et al. Normal shoulder MRI and MR arthrography: anatomy and technique. *Semin Musculoskelet Radiol.* 2015;19(3):212–230.

Tuite MJ. Magnetic resonance imaging of rotator cuff disease and external impingement. *Magn Reson Imaging Clin N Am.* 2012;20(2):187–200.

■ ROTATOR CUFF DISEASE: IMPINGEMENT

KEY FACTS

■ Ninety-five percent of rotator cuff tears are attributed to chronic impingement.
■ Impingement is the result of anomalies or abnormalities in the coracoacromial arch (clavicle, anterior acromion, coracoacromial ligaments, and coracoid).
■ Abnormalities may be osseous or soft tissue:
- Os acromiale
- Hooked acromion
- Subacromial osteophytes
- Soft tissue masses (ganglion cysts)
- Thickened coracoacromial ligament
■ Acromial shape has been classified as straight (Type 1), curved (Type 2), hooked (Type 3), convex inferior surface (Type 4), or downward sloping. The scapular Y view may be superior to MRI for classification of the acromial shape.
■ Features of impingement may be identified on routine radiographs, ultrasound, CT, and MRI.

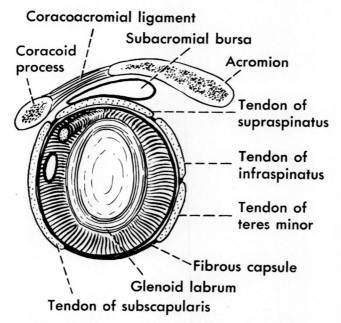

FIGURE 6-14. Sagittal illustration demonstrates the capsule, labrum, and coracoacromial arch (coracoid, coracoacromial ligament, and acromion).

(continued)

■ ROTATOR CUFF DISEASE: IMPINGEMENT *(Continued)*

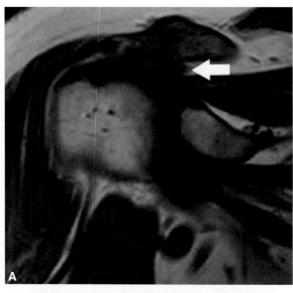

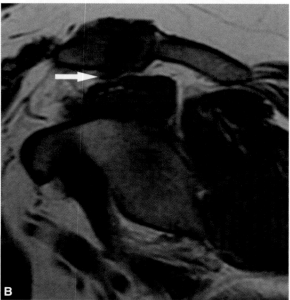

FIGURE 6-15. Impingement syndrome. **(A)** Coronal proton density and sagittal T1 **(B)** magnetic resonance (MR) images show hypertrophy of the acromioclavicular (AC) joint with inferior osteophytes (*arrow*) reducing the humeroacromial space causing impingement.

SUGGESTED READING

Beltran LS, Nikac V, Beltran J. Internal impingement syndromes. *Magn Reson Imaging Clin N Am.* 2012;20(2):201–211.
Dietrich TJ, Jonczy M, Buck FM, et al. Ultrasound of the coracoacromial ligament in asymptomatic volunteers and patients with shoulder impingement. *Acta Radiol.* 2016;57(8):971–977.
Harrison AK, Flatow EL. Subacromial impingement syndrome. *J Am Acad Orthop Surg.* 2011;19(11):701–708.

■ ROTATOR CUFF DISEASE: ROTATOR CUFF TEARS— FULL THICKNESS TEARS

KEY FACTS

- Patients with rotator cuff tears present with chronic pain. Pain is increased with forward flexion and abduction. Night pain that prevents sleep is common. Reduced strength and crepitation may be evident on physical examination.
- Imaging of complete rotator cuff tears can be accomplished with CT arthrography, MRI, or MR arthrography and ultrasound. It is important to document the size of the tear and tendon morphology (≤1 cm = small; 1–3 cm = moderate; 3–5 cm = large; >5 cm = massive). Contrast media extending through the torn segment into the subacromial subdeltoid bursa can be seen during an arthrogram.
- Ultrasound features:
  - Disruption (anechoic) separating tendon ends
  - Volume loss with flattening or concavity of echogenic subdeltoid fat
  - Subdeltoid bursa fluid
  - Irregularity of greater tuberosity
- MRI features:
  - Fluid signal intensity on T2-weighted images involving full thickness. Signal intensity increased from proton density to T2-weighted sequence.
  - Tendon retraction or muscle atrophy may be present.
  - Size measured on axial, sagittal, and coronal images.
  - Fluid (increased signal on T2-weighted sequence) is typically present in subacromial subdeltoid bursa.
- Treatment is most commonly surgical repair.

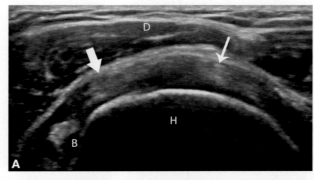

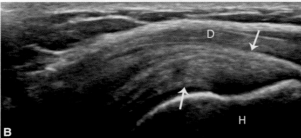

FIGURE 6-16. Ultrasound of the rotator cuff. **(A)** Transverse ultrasound image shows normal supraspinatus (*thick arrow*) and infraspinatus (*thin arrow*) tendons. **(B)** Longitudinal image shows a normal supraspinatus tendon and footprint (*arrows*). **(C)** Transverse image shows full thickness tearing of the supraspinatus (*thick arrow*) and infraspinatus (*thin arrow*) tendons with the absence of tendon adjacent to the humeral head. **(D)** Longitudinal image shows tearing of the supraspinatus tendon from the footprint (*thin arrow*) with tendon retraction (*thick arrow*). A, anterior; B, biceps tendon; D, deltoid muscle; H, humeral head; P, posterior.

(continued)

■ ROTATOR CUFF DISEASE: ROTATOR CUFF TEARS— FULL THICKNESS TEARS *(Continued)*

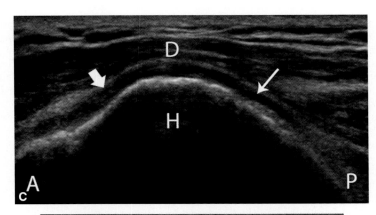

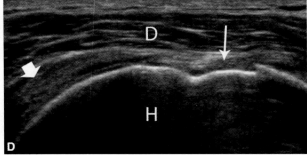

FIGURE 6-16. *(continued)*

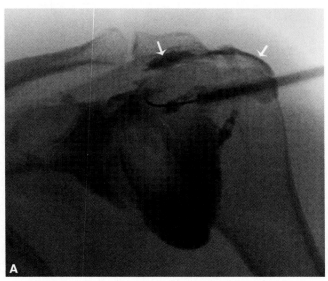

FIGURE 6-17. Computed tomography (CT) arthrogram. **(A)** Anteroposterior (AP) arthrogram shows contrast in the subacromial subdeltoid bursa *(arrows)*. **(B)** CT performed following the arthrogram shows a full thickness supraspinatus tear *(arrow)*. Note the anchors present in the humeral head from prior rotator cuff repair.

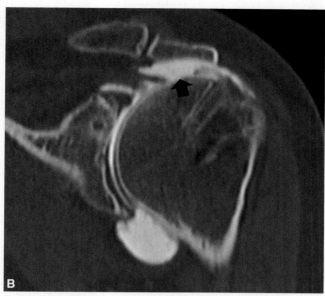

FIGURE 6-17. (*continued*)

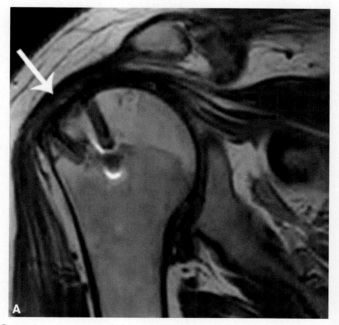

FIGURE 6-18. Coronal proton density **(A)** and T2 fat-saturated **(B)** magnetic resonance (MR) images show full thickness tearing of the supraspinatus tendon (*arrow*) with an absent tendon at the footprint adjacent to the humeral head anchors from prior tendon repair.

(*continued*)

■ ROTATOR CUFF DISEASE: ROTATOR CUFF TEARS— FULL THICKNESS TEARS *(Continued)*

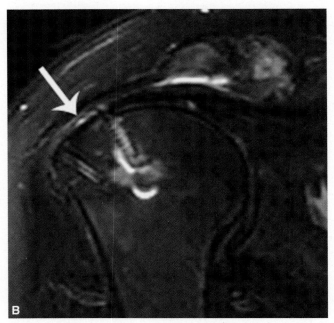

FIGURE 6-18. *(continued)*

SUGGESTED READING

Chung CB, Steinbach LS. *MRI of the Upper Extremity: Shoulder, Elbow, Wrist and Hand.* Philadelphia: Lippincott Williams & Wilkins; 2009.

Keener JD, Wei AS, Kim HM, et al. Proximal humeral migration in shoulders with symptomatic and asymptomatic rotator cuff tears. *J Bone Joint Surg Am.* 2009;91(6):1405–1413.

Morrison WB, Sanders TG. *Problem Solving in Musculoskeletal Imaging.* Philadelphia: Mosby; 2008.

■ ROTATOR CUFF DISEASE: PARTIAL THICKNESS TEARS

KEY FACTS

- Partial tears of the rotator cuff may involve the superior (bursal) (28%), inferior (articular) surface (33%), both surfaces (39%), or intrasubstance. Tears involve only a portion of the tendon thickness. Arthroscopic classification for partial tears is Grade 1 if less than 25% of the fibers are involved, Grade 2 if less than 50% of the fibers are involved, and Grade 3 if more than 50% of fibers are involved.
- It is not unusual for partial tears to be asymptomatic in patients more than 60 years of age.
- Partial tears can be evaluated with ultrasound, conventional MRI, or MR arthrography.
- MR arthrography is most accurate for evaluating partial tears and associated abnormalities, such as impingement.
- Conventional MRI is 94% specific and 89% accurate for full-thickness tears, but only 69% specific and 84% accurate for partial tears.

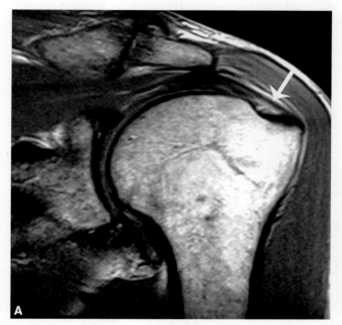

FIGURE 6-19. Partial thickness tear. Coronal proton density **(A)** and T2 fat-saturated **(B)** magnetic resonance (MR) images show a partial thickness tear of the supraspinatus tendon footprint (*arrow*).

(continued)

■ ROTATOR CUFF DISEASE: PARTIAL THICKNESS TEARS *(Continued)*

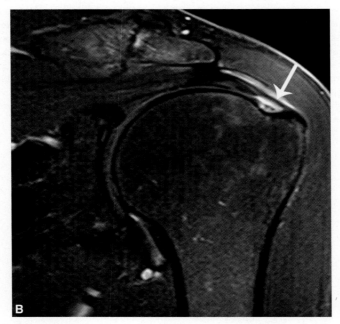

FIGURE 6-19. *(continued)*

SUGGESTED READING

Bauer S, Wang A, Butler R, et al. Reliability of a 3 T MRI protocol for objective grading of supraspinatus tendonosis and partial thickness tears. *J Orthop Surg Res.* 2014;9:128.

Choo HJ, Lee SJ, Kim JH, et al. Delaminated tears of the rotator cuff: prevalence, characteristics, and diagnostic accuracy using indirect MR arthrography. *Am J Roentgenol.* 2015;204(2):360–366.

■ ROTATOR CUFF DISEASE: TENDINOSIS

KEY FACTS

- ■ Tendinosis is common with aging and related to mucoid degeneration in the tendons.
- ■ Tendon degeneration shows thickening with heterogeneous echotexture on ultrasound. There is increased signal intensity on proton density MR images, but not on T2-weighted images.
- ■ Tendon inflammation may be difficult to differentiate from tendinosis on MR images.

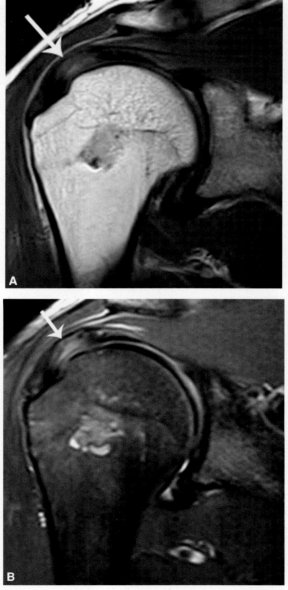

FIGURE 6-20. Tendinosis. Coronal proton density **(A)** and T2 fat-saturated **(B)** magnetic resonance (MR) images show heterogeneity of the supraspinatus tendon consistent with tendinopathy arrow. **(C)** Longitudinal ultrasound image shows thickening and heterogeneity of the subscapularis tendon consistent with tendinopathy. *D*, deltoid muscle; H, humeral head.

(continued)

■ ROTATOR CUFF DISEASE: TENDINOSIS *(Continued)*

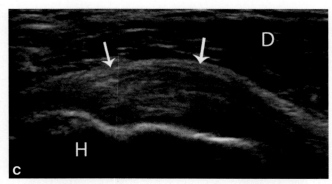

FIGURE 6-20. *(continued)*

SUGGESTED READING

Sein ML, Walton J, Linklater J, et al. Reliability of MRI assessment of supraspinatus tendinopathy. *Br J Sports Med.* 2007;41(8):e9.

Yablon CM, Jacobson JA. Rotator cuff and subacromial pathology. *Semin Musculoskelet Radiol.* 2015;19(3):231–242.

■ ROTATOR CUFF DISEASE: POSTOPERATIVE CHANGES

KEY FACTS

- Rotator cuff repairs may be accomplished with open techniques or arthroscopy.
- Resection of the distal clavicle and a portion of the acromion may be required to relieve impingement.
- Up to 26% of patients have recurrent symptoms after repair.
- Complications seen after cuff repair include
  - Recurrent rotator cuff tear
  - Impingement
  - Bursitis
  - Tendinitis
  - Suprascapular nerve palsy
  - Adhesive capsulitis
  - Deltoid muscle dehiscence
  - Scarring
  - Biceps tendon subluxation
- Postoperative imaging can be difficult because small leaks can be defined arthrographically that mimic tears.
- Ultrasound or MRI is best suited to evaluate postoperative complications.

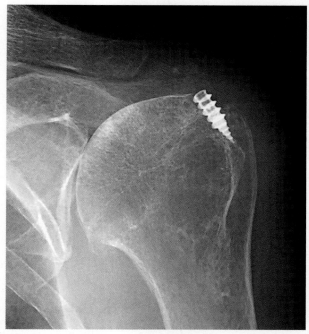

FIGURE 6-21. Postoperative change. Grashey view radiograph shows a soft tissue anchor in the humeral head from prior rotator cuff repair. Note the loss of the humeroacromial space consistent with a cuff tear and advanced degenerative changes of the glenohumeral joint.

(continued)

■ **ROTATOR CUFF DISEASE: TENDINOSIS** *(Continued)*

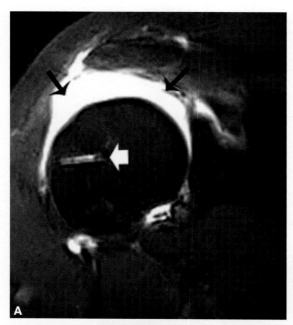

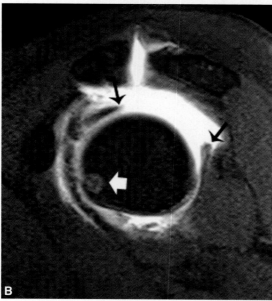

FIGURE 6-22. **(A)** Coronal and sagittal T1 fat-saturated **(B)** magnetic resonance (MR) arthrogram images show a large recurrent tear (*black arrows*) and artifact (*white arrow*) from the soft tissue anchor.

SUGGESTED READING

Collin P, Yoshida M, Delarue A, et al. Evaluating postoperative rotator cuff healing: prospective comparison of MRI and ultrasound. *Orthop Traumatol Surg Res*. 2015;101(suppl 6):S265–S268.

Mellado JM, Calmet J, Olona M, et al. MR assessment of the repaired rotator cuff: prevalence, size, location, and clinical relevance of tendon rerupture. *Eur Radiol*. 2006;16(10):2186–2196.

■ INSTABILITY: BASIC CONCEPTS

KEY FACTS

- Shoulder stability depends on an intact capsule, labrum, pericapsular soft tissues, and glenohumeral osseous structures.
- Instability may be anterior (>90%), posterior (5%), or multidirectional.
- Anterior stability depends on the capsule, three glenohumeral ligaments (superior, middle, and inferior), anterior labrum, and subscapularis.
- Posterior stability is maintained by the capsule, posterior labrum, and rotator cuff muscles.
- Instability can be categorized into four types:

Type I	Involuntary unidirectional (usually anterior) instability caused by trauma
Type II	Overuse or repetitive trauma in throwing athletes and swimmers
Type III	Multidirectional instability caused by generalized ligament laxity
Type IV	Voluntary instability

SUGGESTED READING

Field LD, Ryu RK, Abrams JS, et al. Arthroscopic management of anterior, posterior, and multidirectional shoulder instabilities. *Instr Course Lect.* 2016;65:411–435.

Pavic R, Margetic P, Bensic M, et al. Diagnostic value of US, MR and MR arthrography in shoulder instability. *Injury.* 2013;44(suppl 3):S26–S32.

■ INSTABILITY: RECURRENT SUBLUXATION/DISLOCATIONS—CAPSULAR ABNORMALITIES

KEY FACTS

- Recurrent anterior dislocation is reported in 50% to 90% of patients after anterior dislocation.
- Hill–Sachs lesions, Bankart lesions, and associated labral, capsular, and rotator cuff abnormalities are common.
- The shoulder capsule is categorized into three types:

Type I	Capsules attach at the labral margin
Type II	Capsules attach just medial to the labral margin
Type III	Capsules attach more than 1 cm medial to the labrum. These patients are more susceptible to anterior subluxation.

- Imaging of capsular abnormalities can be accomplished with MRI or MR arthrography. MR arthrography is preferred to better demarcate the capsule size and attachments.

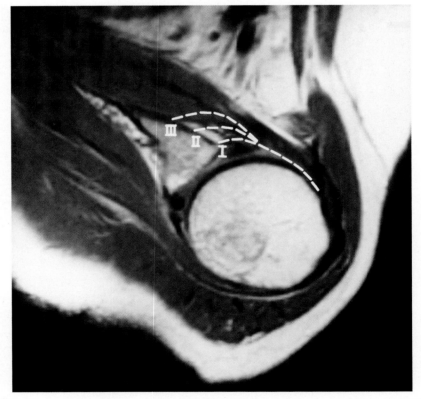

FIGURE 6-23. Axial magnetic resonance (MR) image demonstrates the types of capsular attachment (*broken lines*): Type I at glenoid margin, Type II just medial to margin, and Type III more than 1 cm beyond the glenoid margin.

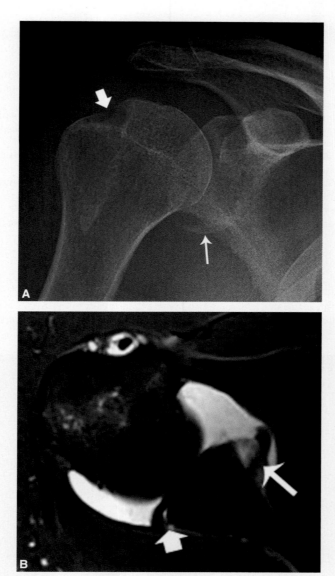

FIGURE 6-24. Anterior dislocation. **(A)** Anteroposterior (AP) radiograph shows a Hill–Sachs lesion in the humeral head (*thick arrow*) and a displaced glenoid fracture (bony Bankart lesion) (*thin arrow*). **(B)** Axial T1 fat-saturated magnetic resonance (MR) arthrogram image shows sequela of recurrent anterior dislocation with stripping of the anterior capsule and displacement of the anterior labrum (*thin arrow*). Note there is also a posterior labral tear (*thick arrow*).

SUGGESTED READING

Davis DE, Abboud JA. Operative management options for traumatic anterior shoulder instability in patients younger than 30 years. *Orthopedics*. 2015;38(9):570–576.

Roy EA, Cheyne I, Andrews GT, et al. Beyond the cuff: MR imaging of labroligamentous injuries in the athletic shoulder. *Radiology*. 2016;278(2):316–332.

■ INSTABILITY: LABRAL TEARS

KEY FACTS

■ The anterior labrum is triangular, and the posterior labrum is slightly rounded in most patients.

■ Labral tears may involve the anterior inferior labrum (anterior instability) or extend over a larger area, resulting in multidirectional instability.

■ Bankart lesions may be labral or osteochondral in nature. There are also several variants.

   ● Perthes lesion: periosteum of the scapula is stripped but remains in place. The labrum may be detached or remain in normal position.

   ● Anterior labroligamentous periosteal sleeve avulsion: periosteum is stripped, resulting in rotation of labroligamentous structures.

■ Superior labral lesions may also involve the biceps tendon. Superior labral lesions are often referred to as superior labrum anterior posterior (SLAP) lesions because of the extension into the anterior and posterior labrum.

■ SLAP lesions are divided into 10 types, but the 4 types initially described are still most commonly used:

Type I	Localized tears or fraying at junction of biceps tendon
Type II	Tear extends anteriorly and posteriorly
Type III	Tear with a bucket-handle configuration
Type IV	Tear extends into biceps tendon

■ SLAP lesions are associated with rotator cuff tears and instability in 15% to 25% of patients.

■ Imaging of labral injuries and the capsule is best accomplished with MRI or MR arthrography.

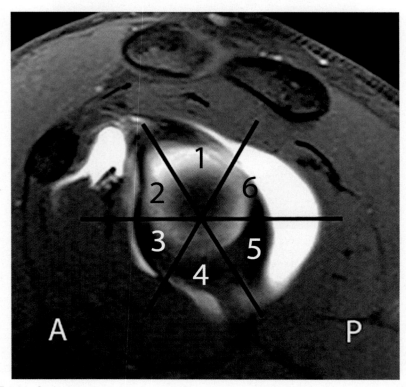

FIGURE 6-25. Sagittal magnetic resonance (MR) arthrogram demonstrates the six labral quadrants: *1*, superior; *2*, anterior superior; *3*, anterior inferior; *4*, inferior; *5*, posterior inferior; *6*, posterior superior. Most unstable injuries occur in segment 3. The lesions may also be described like the face of a clock. *A*, anterior; *P*, posterior.

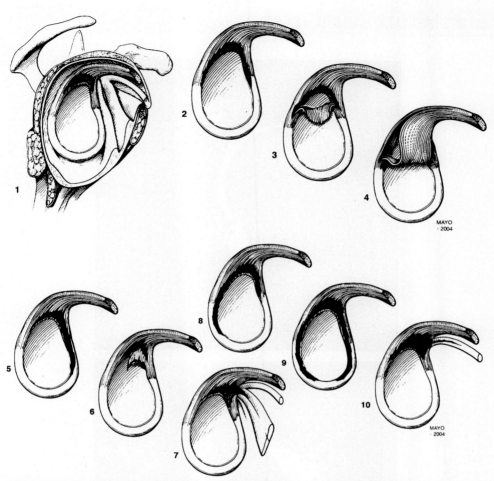

FIGURE 6-26. Categories of superior labrum anterior posterior (SLAP) lesions: *1*, fraying of the superior labrum; *2*, stripping of the superior labrum and biceps tendon from the glenoid; *3*, bucket-handle tear of the labrum and intact biceps tendon; *4*, bucket-handle tear extending into the biceps tendon; *5*, Bankart with superior extension to include the superior labrum and biceps tendon; *6*, anterior and posterior flap tear with superior biceps involvement; *7*, biceps labral complex tear with extension into the middle glenohumeral ligament; *8*, superior labral tear with posterior extension; *9*, nearly complete labral detachment; *10*, SLAP with extension of the tear to the rotator interval and involved structures.

(continued)

■ INSTABILITY: LABRAL TEARS *(Continued)*

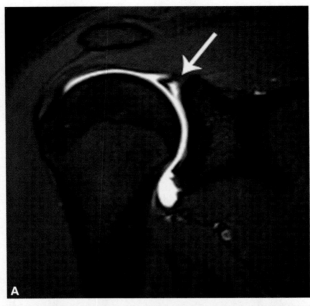

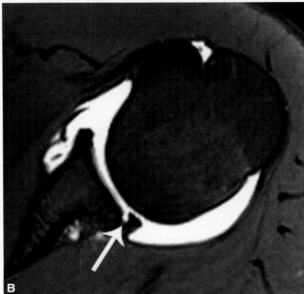

FIGURE 6-27. Labral tears. **(A)** Coronal T1 fat-saturated magnetic resonance (MR) arthrogram image shows a superior labral tear (*arrow*); **(B)** axial T1 fat-saturated MR arthrogram image shows a posterior tear (*arrow*).

SUGGESTED READING

Clavert P. Glenoid labrum pathology. *Orthop Traumatol Surg Res.* 2015;101(suppl 1):S19–S24.

Magee T. How often do surgeons intervene on shoulder labral lesions detected at MR examination? A retrospective review of MR examinations correlated with arthroscopy. *Br J Radiol.* 2014;87(1038):20130736.

Rowbotham EL, Grainger AJ. Superior labrum anterior to posterior lesions and the superior labrum. *Semin Musculoskelet Radiol.* 2015;19(3):269–276.

■ INSTABILITY: HUMERAL OSTEOCHONDRAL OR LIGAMENT AVULSIONS

KEY FACTS

- Avulsion of the glenohumeral ligament may involve soft tissue (humeral avulsion of glenohumeral ligament) or bony (bony humeral avulsion of glenohumeral ligament) avulsion.
- Lesions are seen in 7.5% to 9.4% of patients with anterior instability.
- Prior anterior dislocations are evident in 67% of patients.
- Rotator cuff tears and fractures may be associated.
- MR images may show thickening, irregularity, or disruption of the glenohumeral ligament.
- MR arthrograms demonstrate extravasation at the humeral attachment and capsular stripping.

(continued)

■ INSTABILITY: HUMERAL OSTEOCHONDRAL OR LIGAMENT AVULSIONS *(Continued)*

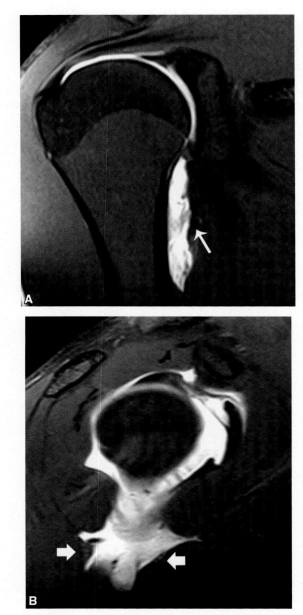

FIGURE 6-28. Coronal **(A)** and sagittal T1 **(B)** fat-saturated magnetic resonance (MR) arthrogram images show humeral avulsion of the glenohumeral ligament (*thin arrow*) with contrast extravasation inferiorly (*thick arrows*).

SUGGESTED READING

Magee T. Prevalence of HAGL lesions and associated abnormalities on shoulder MR examination. *Skeletal Radiol.* 2014;43(3):307–313.

Pouliart N, Boulet C, Maeseneer MD, et al. Advanced imaging of the glenohumeral ligaments. *Semin Musculoskelet Radiol.* 2014;18(4):374–397.

■ INSTABILITY: POSTERIOR INSTABILITY

KEY FACTS

- ■ Posterior dislocations account for 2% to 4% of dislocations.
- ■ Recurrent subluxation is common in throwing athletes and in patients with repetitive microtrauma.
- ■ Posterior labrocapsular sleeve avulsion has also been described as a cause of posterior instability.
- ■ Bennett lesion–posterior labral injury with calcification/ossification at the posterior–inferior glenoid margin. This is most frequently seen in baseball pitchers.
- ■ MR arthrography is the technique of choice for evaluating posterior instability. Bennett lesions may be more easily identified with CT.

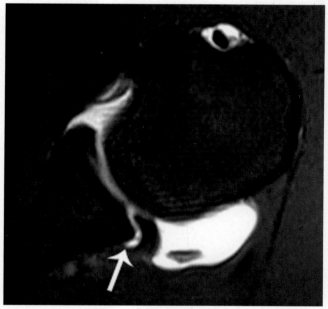

FIGURE 6-29. Posterior instability. Axial T1 fat-saturated magnetic resonance (MR) arthrogram image shows a large posterior capsule and a posterior labral tear with periosteal stripping (*arrow*). Note that there is also a loose body posteriorly in the joint.

SUGGESTED READING

Gottschalk MB, Ghasem A, Todd D, et al. Posterior shoulder instability: does glenoid retroversion predict recurrence and contralateral instability? *Arthroscopy*. 2015;31(3):488–493.

Rebolledo BJ, Nwachukwu BU, Konin GP, et al. Posterior humeral avulsion of the glenohumeral ligament and associated injuries: assessment using magnetic resonance imaging. *Am J Sports Med.* 2015;43(12):2913–2917.

Saupe N, White LM, Bleakney R, et al. Acute traumatic posterior shoulder dislocation: MR findings. *Radiology.* 2008;248(1):185–193.

■ INSTABILITY: MULTIDIRECTIONAL INSTABILITY

KEY FACTS

- Multidirectional instability is typically atraumatic and accounts for 2% of cases of instability.
- Instability may be anterior and posterior or inferior and superior.
- Multidirectional instability occurs with labrocapsular laxity in segments 3 to 5.
- SLAP lesions may also be evident.

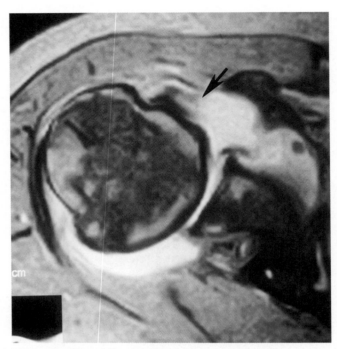

FIGURE 6-30. Multidirectional instability. Axial magnetic resonance (MR) arthrogram image demonstrates anterior and posterior capsular enlargement with posterior humeral subluxation. There is a subscapularis tendon tear (*arrow*).

SUGGESTED READING

Merolla G, Cerciello S, Chillemi C, et al. Multidirectional instability of the shoulder: biomechanics, clinical presentation, and treatment strategies. *Eur J Orthop Surg Traumatol.* 2015;25(6):975–985.

Walz DM, Burge AJ, Steinbach L. Imaging of shoulder instability. *Semin Musculoskelet Radiol.* 2015;19(3):254–268.

■ INSTABILITY: LABRAL VARIANTS

KEY FACTS

- ■ The normal labrum is triangular. However, the posterior labrum may appear more rounded.
- ■ The anterior superior labrum may be absent with associated thickening of the middle glenohumeral ligament. This anatomic variant is called a Buford complex.
- ■ A sublabral foramen (focal detachment anterosuperiorly) is present in 8% to 12% of patients. The middle glenohumeral ligament is not thickened in this case.

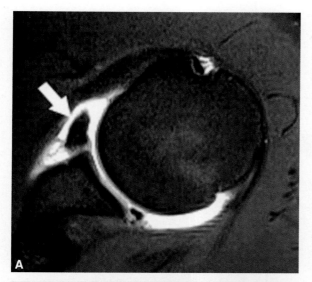

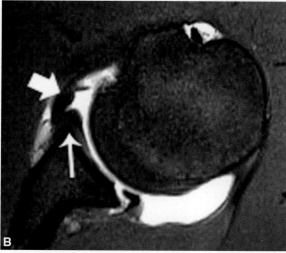

FIGURE 6-31. (A) Axial T1 fat-saturated magnetic resonance (MR) image shows a Buford complex with an absent anterosuperior labrum and thickening of the middle glenohumeral ligament (*arrow*). **(B)** Axial MR image more inferiorly shows the middle glenohumeral ligament (*thick arrow*) separating from the anterior labrum (*thin arrow*). Note that there is also a posterior labral tear in this case.

SUGGESTED READING

Gustas CN, Tuite MJ. Imaging update on the glenoid labrum: variants versus tears. *Semin Musculoskelet Radiol.* 2014;18(4):365–373.

Tuite MJ, Currie JW, Orwin JF, et al. Sublabral clefts and recesses in the anterior, inferior, and posterior glenoid labrum at MR arthrography. *Skeletal Radiol.* 2013;42(3):353–362.

■ BICEPS TENDON

KEY FACTS

■ The biceps muscle has two bellies. The tendon of the short head attaches to the coracoid. The tendon of the long head extends over the humeral head and passes through the bicipital groove hooded by the transverse ligament.

■ Biceps tendon abnormalities include
  ● Tendinopathy
  ● Tenosynovitis
  ● Subluxation/dislocation
  ● Tendon rupture
  ● Stenosing tenosynovitis

■ Tendinopathy may be the result of impingement, subluxation, or attrition. The latter is caused by inflammation in the groove leading to stenosis, osteophyte formation, or tendon thinning.

■ Tendon rupture most commonly occurs proximally (96%).

■ Imaging of the osseous groove and tendon can be accomplished with CT, MRI, or ultrasound. Images in the axial plane are most useful for evaluating the bicipital groove and tendon.

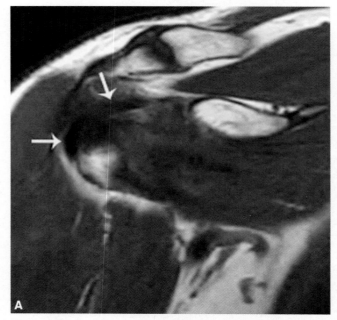

FIGURE 6-32. Biceps tendon. Coronal proton density **(A)** and sagittal T1 **(B)** magnetic resonance (MR) images show the normal course and low signal intensity of the long head of the biceps tendon (*arrows*). Ultrasound images show a normal biceps tendon (*arrows*) in long **(C)** and short **(D)** axes.

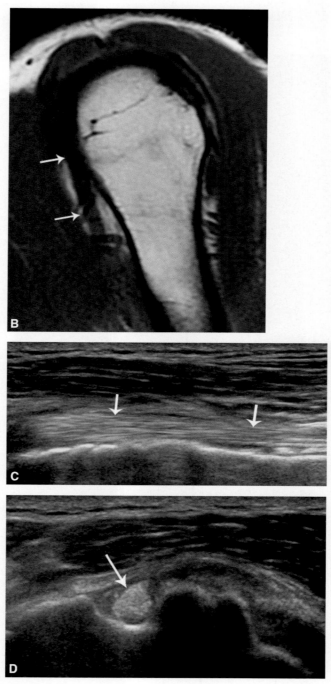

FIGURE 6-32. (*continued*)

(*continued*)

■ BICEPS TENDON *(Continued)*

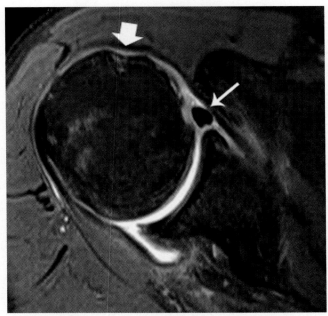

FIGURE 6-33. Axial proton density fat-saturated magnetic resonance (MR) image shows dislocation of the biceps tendon (*thin arrow*) with an empty bicipital groove (*thick arrow*) caused by a full thickness subscapularis tendon tear.

SUGGESTED READING

Malavolta EA, Assunção JH, Guglielmetti CL, et al. Accuracy of preoperative MRI in the diagnosis of disorders of the long head of the biceps tendon. *Eur J Radiol*. 2015;84(11):2250–2254.
Schaeffeler C, Waldt S, Holzapfel K, et al. Lesions of the biceps pulley: diagnostic accuracy of MR arthrography of the shoulder and evaluation of previously described and new diagnostic signs. *Radiology*. 2012;264(2):504–513.

■ ADHESIVE CAPSULITIS

KEY FACTS

- Adhesive capsulitis (frozen shoulder) may develop after trauma, or present as an idiopathic condition.
- Idiopathic adhesive capsulitis is most common in the nondominant shoulder of middle-aged or older females.
- The condition is bilateral in 34%.
- Patients present with pain and reduced motion.
- Imaging of capsulitis requires evaluation of capsular volume (normal >10 mL); therefore, contrast should be injected, and the volume injected should be documented. This can be done with conventional or CT arthrography or MR arthrography. Conventional MRI is not as useful compared with these techniques.
- Findings at arthrography may include decreased joint volume, no or limited distension of the axillary pouch, and no or limited contrast in the biceps tendon sheath.
- Findings on MR may include soft tissue thickening of the axillary capsule, capsular or rotator interval edema/enhancement, and thickening of the coracohumeral ligament.
- Distension arthrography (gradual increased pressure and volume injected) is useful in mild to moderately severe cases.

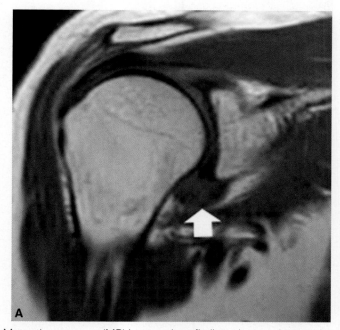

FIGURE 6-34. Magnetic resonance (MR) images show findings that may be seen in adhesive capsulitis. Coronal proton density **(A)** and T2 fat-saturated **(B)** images show thickening and inflammation of the axillary soft tissues (*arrow*), and sagittal T2 fat-saturated **(C)** image shows edema in the rotator interval (*arrow*).

(continued)

■ ADHESIVE CAPSULITIS *(Continued)*

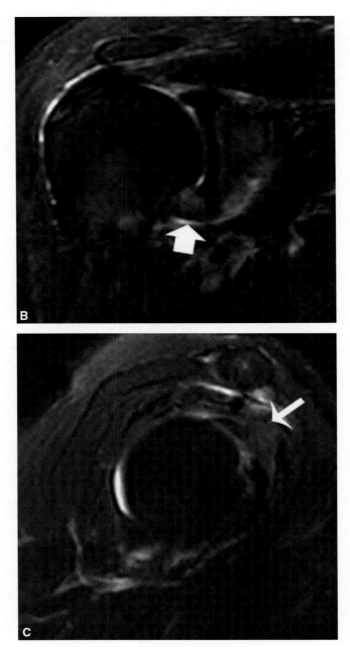

FIGURE 6-34. *(continued)*

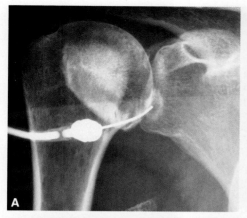
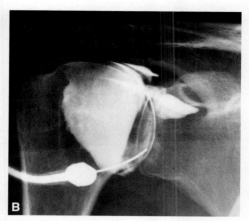
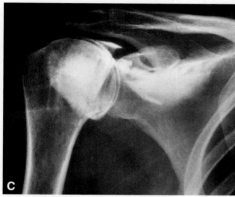

FIGURE 6-35. Female with adhesive capsulitis treated with distension arthrography. **(A)** Initial arthrogram shows a small tight capsule (4 mL injected). **(B)** and **(C)** Increased volumes of contrast mixed with anesthetic show volume increase **(B)** and eventual capsular rupture **(C)**, which is the end point of the procedure.

SUGGESTED READING

Gondim Teixeira PA, Balaj C, Chanson A, et al. Adhesive capsulitis of the shoulder: value of inferior glenohumeral ligament signal changes on T2-weighted fat-saturated images. *Am J Roentgenol*. 2012;198(6):W589–W596.

Lee SY, Park J, Song SW. Correlation of MR arthrographic findings and range of shoulder motions in patients with frozen shoulder. *Am J Roentgenol*. 2012;198(1):173–179.

Ueda Y, Sugaya H, Takahashi N, et al. Rotator cuff lesions in patients with stiff shoulders: a prospective analysis of 379 shoulders. *J Bone Joint Surg Am*. 2015;97(15):1233–1237.

■ NERVE ENTRAPMENT SYNDROMES

KEY FACTS

- Neural injury may occur with fractures and dislocations.
- Nerve compression syndromes may involve the axillary nerve, or branches, as it passes between the teres minor and major (quadrilateral space syndrome), or the suprascapular nerve in the supraspinous notch, or in its course to supply the supraspinatus and infraspinatus muscles.
- Quadrilateral space syndrome: The axillary nerve and posterior humeral circumflex artery and vein pass between the teres minor and teres major in the quadrilateral space. Nerve compression in this region results in pain, paresthesias, and muscle atrophy in the teres muscles. Clinical diagnosis is difficult.
- Suprascapular nerve compression: The suprascapular nerve has motor and sensory fibers. The nerve enters the supraspinous fossa through the suprascapular notch and passes beneath the superior transverse scapular ligament. The nerve supplies the supraspinatus and infraspinatus. Anterior compression (lesion in the suprascapular notch) affects both muscles, and posterior compression (lesion in the spinoglenoid notch) affects the infraspinatus. Compression may be secondary to trauma, soft tissue masses, or dilated veins. Patients present with pain, which may mimic rotator cuff disease, and muscle atrophy.
- MRI is the technique of choice for evaluating the neuromuscular structures of the shoulder and excluding other causes of shoulder pain.

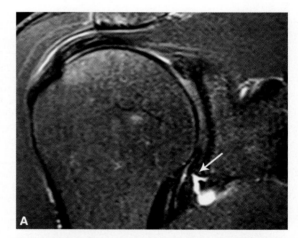

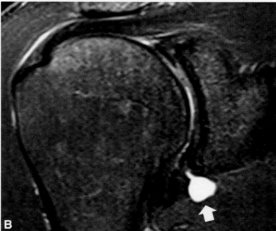

FIGURE 6-36. Coronal T2 fat-saturated magnetic resonance (MR) images show a paralabral cyst extending through a tear in the inferior labrum (*arrow* in **A**) into the quadrilateral space (*arrow* in **B**).

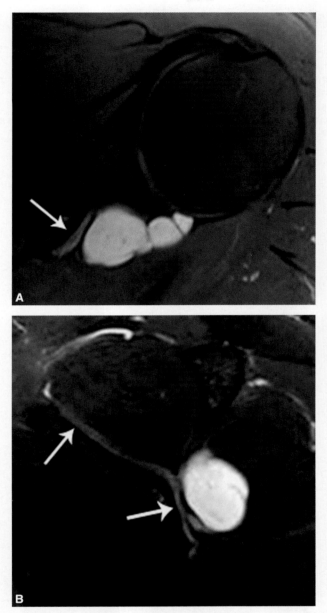

FIGURE 6-37. Axial proton density fat-saturated **(A)** and sagittal T2 fat-saturated **(B)** magnetic resonance (MR) images show a large paralabral cyst in the spinoglenoid notch compressing the infraspinatus nerve (*arrows* on nerve).

SUGGESTED READING

Budzik JF, Wavreille G, Pansini V, et al. Entrapment neuropathies of the shoulder. *Magn Reson Imaging Clin N Am.* 2012;20(2):373–391.

Friend J, Francis S, McCulloch J, et al. Teres minor innervation in the context of isolated muscle atrophy. *Surg Radiol Anat.* 2010;32(3):243–249.

■ INFLAMMATORY ARTHROPATHIES

KEY FACTS

- The shoulder is frequently involved with degenerative and other arthropathies.
- Early changes may be difficult to detect on conventional radiographs. MRI or MR arthrography may detect early synovial and bone changes more clearly.
- Bursal inflammatory changes may also result in shoulder pain.
- Bursal abnormalities may be detected with ultrasound or MRI. Routine radiographs may demonstrate calcification in bursae, tendons, or peritendinous soft tissues.

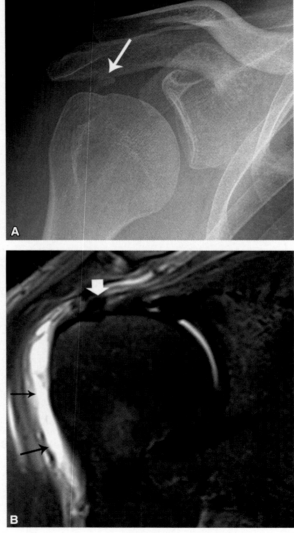

FIGURE 6-38. **(A)** Grashey view radiograph shows hydroxyapatite crystal deposition (*arrow*) in the supraspinatus tendon. Coronal T2 fat-saturated **(B)** and sagittal T2 fat-saturated **(C)** magnetic resonance (MR) images show the hypointense crystal deposition (*thick arrow*) within the supraspinatus tendon with associated inflammation (edema) (*thin arrows*) throughout the subdeltoid space.

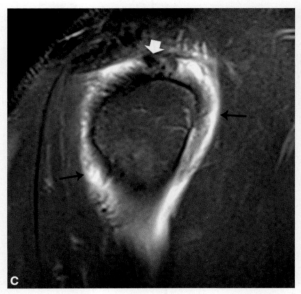

FIGURE 6-38. (*continued*)

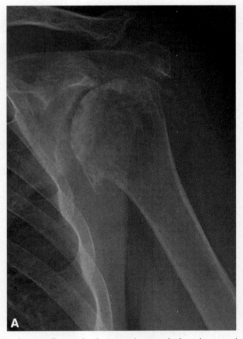

FIGURE 6-39. **(A)** Grashey view radiograph shows advanced glenohumeral degenerative arthritis. Axial proton density fat-saturated **(B)** and sagittal T2 fat-saturated **(C)** magnetic resonance (MR) images in the same patient show the glenohumeral degenerative arthritis with extensive synovitis (*arrows*). This patient was treated with a reverse shoulder arthroplasty **(D)**.

(continued)

■ INFLAMMATORY ARTHROPATHIES *(Continued)*

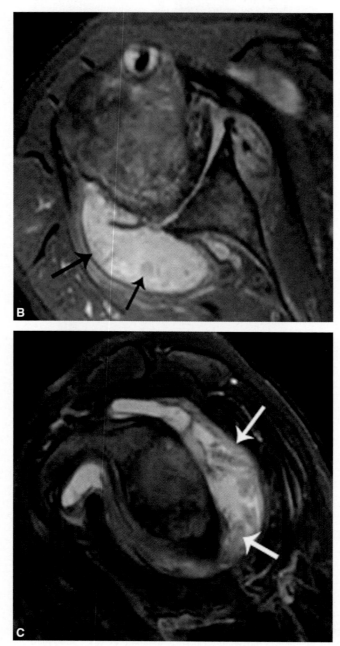

FIGURE 6-39. *(continued)*

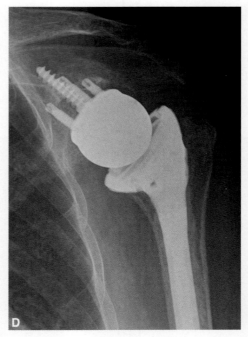

FIGURE 6-39. (*continued*)

SUGGESTED READING

Bazzocchi A, Pelotti P, Serraino S, et al. Ultrasound imaging-guided percutaneous treatment of rotator cuff calcific tendinitis: success in short-term outcome. *Br J Radiol*. 2016;89(1057):20150407.

Brower AC, Flemming DJ. *Arthritis in Black and White*. 3rd ed. Philadelphia: WB Saunders; 2012.

Nörenberg D, Ebersberger HU, Walter T, et al. Diagnosis of calcific tendonitis of the rotator cuff by using susceptibility-weighted MR imaging. *Radiology*. 2016;278(2):475–484.

■ OSTEONECROSIS

KEY FACTS

- Detection of early osteonecrosis can be difficult with routine radiographs (see Chapter 3 for a more complete discussion).
- MRI is the technique of choice for detection and classification of early avascular necrosis.
- MR images in the axial and coronal planes using T1- and T2-weighted or short T1 inversion recovery sequences are sufficient for diagnosis.

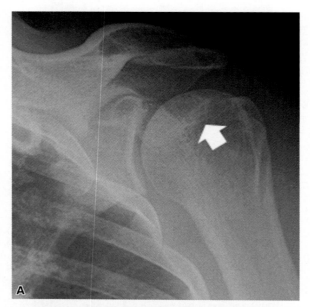

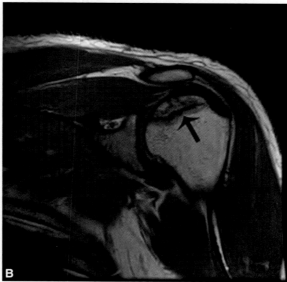

FIGURE 6-40. Osteonecrosis. **(A)** Grashey view radiograph shows increased density in the superior medial humeral head (*arrow*) consistent with avascular necrosis (AVN). Coronal T1 **(B)** and coronal T2 **(C)** fat-saturated magnetic resonance (MR) images show the crescent-shaped region (*arrow*) of abnormal signal in the humeral head caused by AVN.

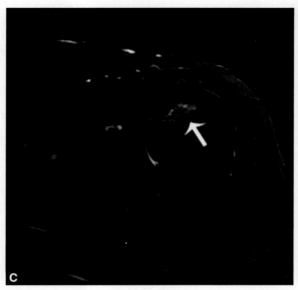

FIGURE 6-40. (*continued*)

SUGGESTED READING

Murphey MD, Foreman KL, Klassen-Fischer MK, et al. From the radiologic pathology archives imaging of osteonecrosis: radiologic-pathologic correlation. *Radiographics*. 2014;34(4):1003–1028.

Poignard A, Flouzat-Lachaniette CH, Amzallag J, et al. The natural progression of symptomatic humeral head osteonecrosis in adults with sickle cell disease. *J Bone Joint Surg Am*. 2012;94(2):156–162.

■ NEOPLASMS

KEY FACTS

- ■ Routine radiographs are essential for evaluating skeletal neoplasms and may show abnormalities (calcification, fat, mass) when soft tissue neoplasms are present.
- ■ Soft tissue neoplasms in the shoulder include lipoma, hemangioma, nodular fasciitis, nerve sheath tumors, and soft tissue sarcomas.
- ■ MRI is the technique of choice for evaluating soft tissue masses. T1- and T2-weighted images are essential. Intravenous gadolinium is used routinely in our practice.
- ■ MRI, CT, or nuclear medicine examinations may be used for staging skeletal neoplasms.
- ■ Common skeletal lesions are as follows:

Neoplasm	No. in Upper Arm (Humerus, Scapula, Clavicle)/ Total/% in Upper Arm
Benign	
Chondroblastoma	35/147/24
Osteochondroma	194/884/22
Chondroma	83/426/19
Giant cell tumor	36/682/5
Osteoid osteoma	40/397/10
Hemangioma	8/149/5
Malignant	
Primary chondrosarcoma	194/1,072/18
Ewing sarcoma	94/614/15
Lymphoma	136/905/15
Osteosarcoma	235/1,984/12
Fibrosarcoma	31/286/11
Myeloma	150/1,057/14

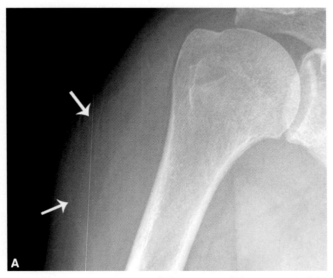

FIGURE 6-41. Lipoma. Grashey view radiograph **(A)**, sagittal T1 **(B)**, and axial T2 **(C)** fat-saturated magnetic resonance (MR) images show a fat lesion (*arrows*) within the lateral deltoid muscle, which was a lipoma.

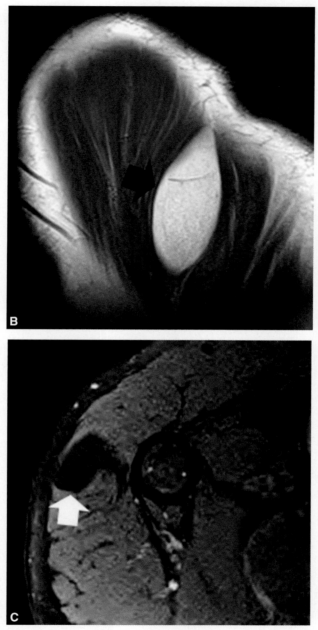

FIGURE 6-41. (*continued*)

(*continued*)

■ NEOPLASMS *(Continued)*

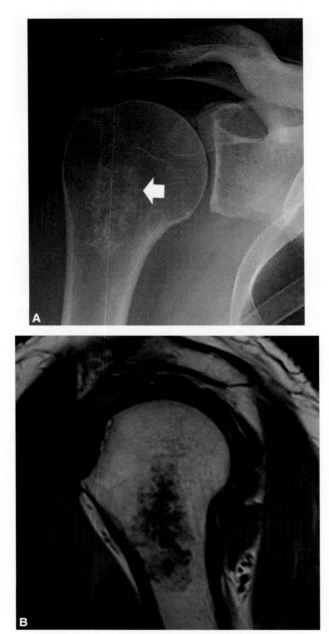

FIGURE 6-42. Enchondroma. Grashey view radiograph **(A)**, sagittal T1 **(B)**, and axial T2 **(C)** fat-saturated magnetic resonance (MR) images show a chondroid lesion (*arrow* in **A**) in the proximal humerus, which was isointense to skeletal muscle on T1 and hyperintense on T2 consistent with an enchondroma.

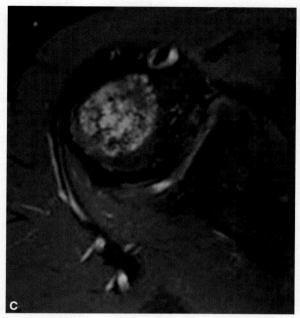

FIGURE 6-42. (*continued*)

SUGGESTED READING

Unni KK and Inwards CY. *Dahlin's Bone Tumors: General Aspects and Data on 10,165 Cases.* 6th ed. Philadelphia: Lippincott Williams & Wilkins; 2009
Vanhoenacker FM, Verstraete KL. Soft tissue tumors about the shoulder. *Semin Musculoskelet Radiol.* 2015;19(3):284–299.

■ BRACHIAL PLEXUS

KEY FACTS

- The brachial plexus arises from the anterior rami of the fifth to eighth cervical and first thoracic nerves. The nerve roots form trunks (upper, middle, and lower) in the brachial plexus. Each trunk has anterior and posterior divisions.
- The brachial plexus is a difficult area to image using CT or other conventional techniques. MR is the optimal imaging method.
- The lower neck through the shoulder needs to be imaged to evaluate the neural structures of the brachial plexus. This can be accomplished with T1-weighted sagittal and T2-weighted axial images. Sagittal T1-weighted images are also very helpful.
- MRI is useful for evaluating primary or metastatic lesions, trauma, and inflammatory changes involving the brachial plexus.

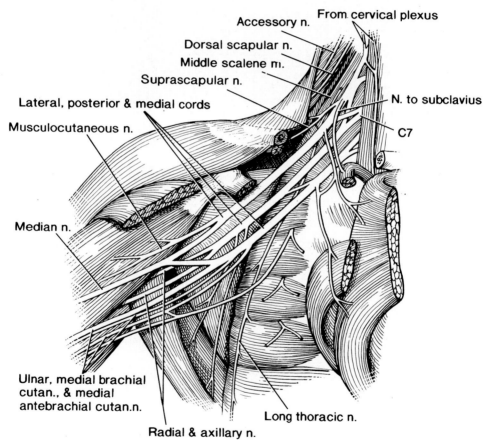

FIGURE 6-43. Anatomic illustration of the brachial plexus.

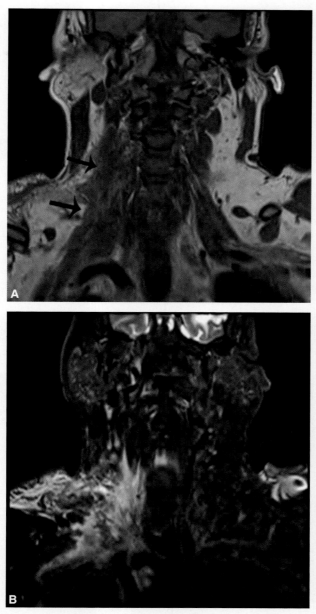

FIGURE 6-44. Brachial plexus. Coronal T1 **(A)** and coronal T2 **(B)** fat-saturated magnetic resonance (MR) images show extensive edema (*arrows* in **A**) throughout the right-side brachial plexus secondary to trauma with poor definition of individual nerves.

SUGGESTED READING

Martinoli C, Gandolfo N, Perez MM, et al. Brachial plexus and nerves about the shoulder. *Semin Musculoskelet Radiol.* 2010;14(5):523–546.

Vargas MI, Gariani J, Delattre BA, et al. Three-dimensional MR imaging of the brachial plexus. *Semin Musculoskelet Radiol.* 2015;19(2):137–148.

Elbow/Forearm

Jeffrey J. Peterson, Thomas H. Berquist, and Laura W. Bancroft

■ FRACTURES/DISLOCATIONS: DISTAL HUMERAL FRACTURES

KEY FACTS

- Eighty percent of distal humeral fractures occur in children.
- Fifteen percent of physeal fractures in children involve the distal humerus.
- The mechanism of injury is a fall on the outstretched hand.
- Fractures may be flexion or extension injuries. Extension injuries are 10 times more common than flexion injuries.
  - Extension fracture: oblique fracture with posterior displacement of the distal fragment
  - Flexion fracture: older age group; transverse fracture line; distal fragment anterior
- Fractures are usually obvious on anteroposterior (AP) and lateral radiographs. Computed tomography (CT) with coronal and sagittal reformatting is helpful for evaluating subtle injuries. Magnetic resonance imaging (MRI) is useful for physeal fractures in young children.
- Treatment: closed reduction.
- Complications: neurovascular injury, premature physeal closure, arthrosis, malunion, nonunion.

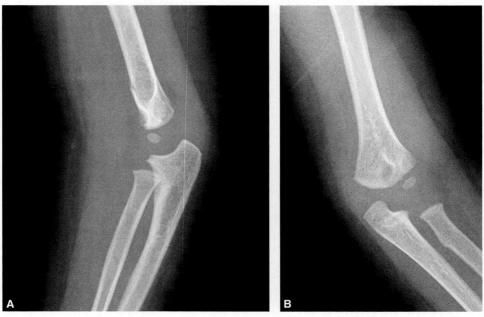

FIGURE 7-1. Distal humeral fracture. Lateral **(A)** and anteroposterior (AP) **(B)** radiographs show a non-displaced supracondylar fracture.

■ FRACTURES/DISLOCATIONS: DISTAL HUMERAL FRACTURES (Continued)

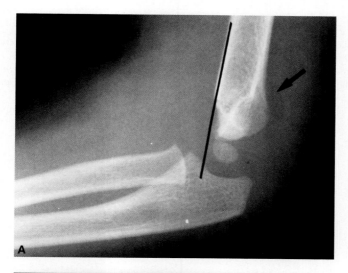

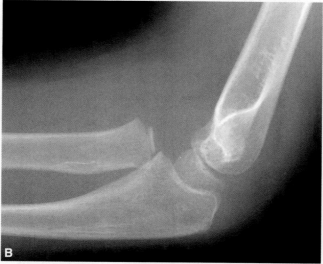

FIGURE 7-2. Supracondylar fracture. Lateral radiograph **(A)** does not depict a supracondylar fracture line, but the capitulum lies posterior to the anterior humeral line (*black line*), indicating a supracondylar fracture. The anterior humeral line should intersect the midcapitellum. There is also a positive posterior fat pad sign (*arrow*). Lateral radiograph **(B)** in another patient depicts a joint effusion with subtle supracondylar fracture associated with dislocation of the radial head.

SUGGESTED READING

Anderson SE, Otsuka NY, Steinbach LS. MR imaging of pediatric elbow trauma. *Semin Musculoskel Radiol.* 1998;2:185–198.

Kinik H, Atalar H, Mergen E. Management of distal humeral fractures in adults. *Arch Orthop Trauma Surg.* 1999;119:467–469.

Murphy BJ. MR imaging of the elbow. *Radiology.* 1992;184:525–529.

Neviaser RJ, Resch H, Neviaser AS, Crosby LA. Proximal humeral fractures: pin, plate, or replace. *Instr Course Lect.* 2015;64:203–214.

■ FRACTURES/DISLOCATIONS: EPICONDYLAR FRACTURES

KEY FACTS

- ■ Avulsion fractures of the epicondyle are common in children.
- ■ The injury is common in throwing athletes, specifically pitchers.
- ■ The medial epicondyle is particularly vulnerable between ages 9 and 14 years.
- ■ Mechanism of injury is varus and valgus forces. Medial epicondylar fractures are common; lateral epicondylar fractures are rare.
- ■ Displaced medial epicondylar fragments may be trapped in the joint.
- ■ Routine radiographs are usually adequate for diagnosis. MRI is useful for subtle undisplaced fractures and associated soft tissue injuries.
- ■ Treatment: closed reduction for undisplaced fractures; pinning of displaced (>3 mm) fractures.
- ■ Complications: fragment entrapped in joint, instability.

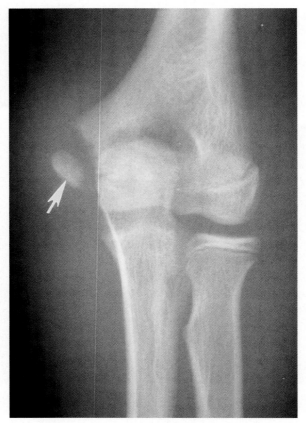

FIGURE 7-3. Anteroposterior (AP) radiograph of the elbow in a young pitcher with an avulsed medial epicondyle (*arrow*).

SUGGESTED READING

Larson RL. Epiphyseal fractures in the adolescent athlete. *Orthop Clin North Am.* 1973;4:839–851.
Stevens MA, El-Khoury GY, Kathol MH et-al. Imaging features of avulsion injuries. *Radiographics.* 1999;19(3):655–672.

■ FRACTURES/DISLOCATIONS: ADULT DISTAL HUMERAL FRACTURES

KEY FACTS

■ The distal humerus consists of medial and lateral columns with the trochlea between the two columns.

■ The mechanism of injury is trochlear impaction into the humeral articular surface with flexor and extensor muscles causing displacement of the epicondyles.

■ Fractures may be nonarticular, involve one condyle, or have a "T" or "Y" configuration with varying degrees of comminution.

■ Treatment: internal fixation commonly required.

■ Routine radiographs are usually diagnostic. CT with coronal and sagittal reformatting is important for operative planning.

■ Complications: poor reduction, exuberant callus, reduced range of motion, arthrosis, nonunion (2% to 10%), nerve compression (15%), and postoperative infection.

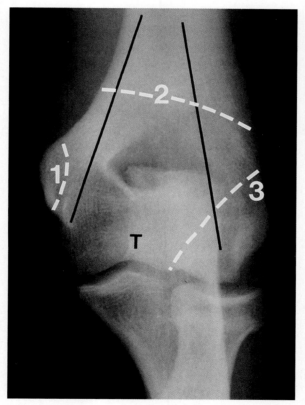

FIGURE 7-4. Anteroposterior (AP) radiograph demonstrates the medial and lateral columns (*black lines*) with the trochlea (*T*) between the columns. Fractures may be extra-articular (*1*), across both columns (*2*), or intra-articular (*3*), involving one or both columns.

(continued)

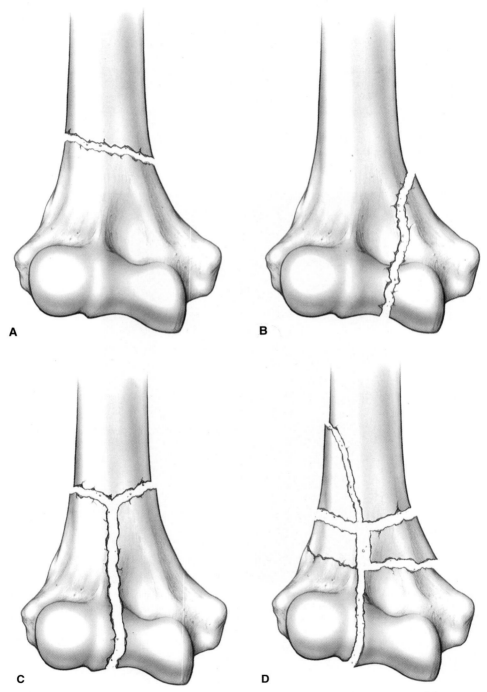

FIGURE 7-5. Adult distal humeral fracture patterns. **(A)** Extra-articular. **(B)** One condyle. **(C)** Both condyles. **(D)** and **(E)** Both condyles with comminution.

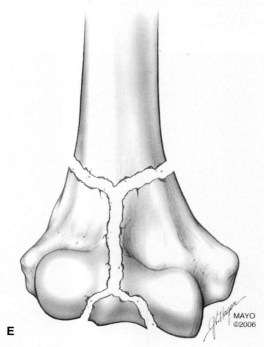

E

FIGURE 7-5. (*continued*)

(*continued*)

■ FRACTURES/DISLOCATIONS: ADULT DISTAL HUMERAL FRACTURES   *(Continued)*

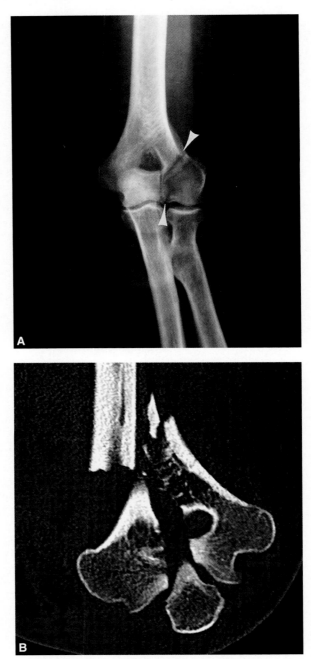

FIGURE 7-6. (A) Anteroposterior (AP) radiograph of a lateral column fracture entering the margin of the trochlea (*arrowheads*). **(B)** Coronal reformatted computed tomography (CT) of an intra-articular "T" fracture.

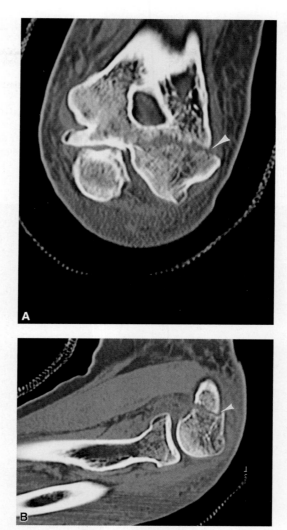

FIGURE 7-7. Computed tomography (CT) images of a lateral column fracture reformatted in the coronal **(A)** and **(B)** sagittal planes.

SUGGESTED READING

Helfet DL, Kloen P, Anand N, et al. Open reduction and internal fixation of delayed unions and nonunions of fractures of the distal part of the humerus. *J Bone Joint Surg.* 2003;85A:33–44.

Ring D, Jupiter JB. Complex fractures of the distal humerus and their complications. *J Shoulder Elbow Surg.* 1999;8:85–97.

■ FRACTURES/DISLOCATIONS: CAPITELLAR FRACTURES

KEY FACTS

- ■ Capitellar fractures account for 1% of elbow injuries.
- ■ Fractures may involve the entire capitellum or the articular surface, or be comminuted and involve the radial head.
- ■ Mechanism of injury: direct blow or fall on the outstretched hand with force transmitted from the radius to the capitellum.
- ■ Subtle fractures may present with a positive fat pad sign and may require CT or MRI for detection.
- ■ Treatment: Loose fragments may require removal. K-wire fixation of large fragments may be necessary in certain cases.

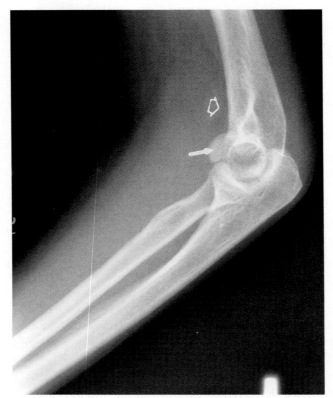

FIGURE 7-8. Lateral view of the elbow demonstrates a capitellar fracture (*arrow*) and displaced fat pad (*open arrow*).

SUGGESTED READING

Fowles JV, Dassab MT. Fractures of the capitellum humeria. *J Bone Joint Surg.* 1975;56A:794–798.

■ FRACTURES/DISLOCATIONS: FRACTURES OF THE PROXIMAL RADIUS

KEY FACTS

■ Fractures of the radial head and neck are common, accounting for one-third of elbow fractures. Fractures are categorized as three types on the basis of displacement or comminution of the radial head or neck. Type I, undisplaced (<2 mm) head or neck fracture; Type II, displaced head or neck fracture; Type III, comminuted head or neck fracture.

■ Mechanism of injury: fall on the outstretched hand with the elbow partially flexed and pronated.

■ Associated elbow, forearm, and wrist injuries may be present.

■ Routine radiographs may be normal, except for a positive fat pad sign. Follow-up in 10 to 14 days may demonstrate the fracture. MRI or CT may be required for detection of subtle fractures and for operative planning with complex fractures.

■ Treatment: Undisplaced fractures are treated with closed reduction. Displaced or comminuted fractures may require internal fixation, resection, or arthroplasty.

■ Complications include associated ulnar fracture, heterotopic ossification, instability, and arthrosis.

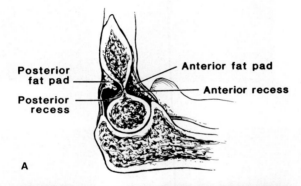

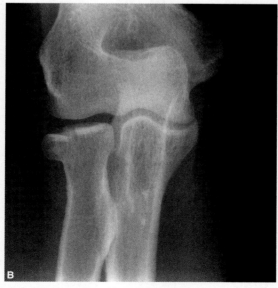

FIGURE 7-9. Fat pad sign. **(A)** Normal position of the fat pads. Anteroposterior (AP) **(B)** and lateral **(C)** radiographs of a radial head fracture with displaced fat pads on the lateral view (*arrows*).

(continued)

■ FRACTURES/DISLOCATIONS: FRACTURES OF THE PROXIMAL RADIUS *(Continued)*

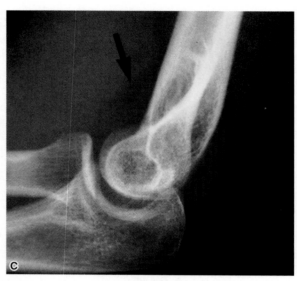

FIGURE 7-9. *(continued)*

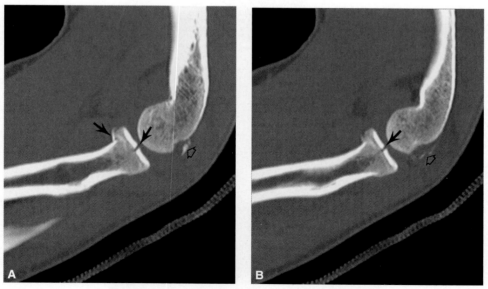

FIGURE 7-10. Computed tomography (CT) images in the sagittal plane **(A, B)** demonstrate a minimally displaced comminuted radial head fracture *(arrows)* with associated capitellar fragments *(open arrow)*.

SUGGESTED READING

Corbett RH. Displaced fat pads in elbow trauma. *Injury.* 1978;9:297–298.
Geel CW, Palmer AK. Radial head fractures and their effect on the radioulnar joint: a rationale for treatment. *Clin Orthop.* 1992;275:79–84.

■ FRACTURES/DISLOCATIONS: ULNAR FRACTURES

KEY FACTS

- ■ The ulna is susceptible to trauma because of its superficial location.
- ■ Mechanism of injury: direct blow after fall on the flexed elbow.
- ■ Most fractures are intra-articular.
- ■ Triceps fascia disruption leads to significant displacement and articular deformity.
- ■ Routine radiographs are usually diagnostic. The lateral view is most useful.
- ■ Treatment: Joint congruity must be restored, which usually requires internal fixation for displaced fractures.
- ■ Complications: Instability, decreased range of motion (3% to 50%), articular deformity and arthrosis, ulnar neuropathy (10%), and nonunion (5%).

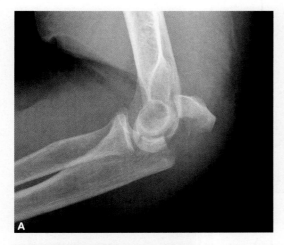

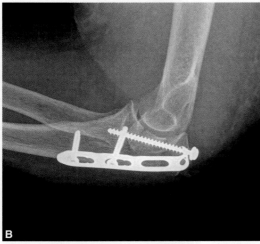

FIGURE 7-11. (A) Lateral view of the elbow shows a displaced olecranon fracture. **(B)** Fractures were internally fixed using plate and screw fixation.

SUGGESTED READING

Rettig AC, Waugh TR, Evanski PM. Fracture of the olecranon: a problem of management. *J Trauma.* 1979;19:23–28.

▪ FRACTURES/DISLOCATIONS: CORONOID FRACTURES

KEY FACTS

- ▪ Isolated coronoid fractures are uncommon. There are three categories of fracture. Type I: small avulsion of the coronoid tip. Type II: fracture involves 50% of the coronoid, but does not extend to the base. Type III: fracture of the coronoid base.
- ▪ Coronoid fractures are seen most commonly with posterior dislocations.
- ▪ Recurrent dislocation is common after coronoid fracture/dislocation.
- ▪ Displaced fractures can be detected on radiographs. The lateral view is most useful. CT may be required for detection of undisplaced fractures.
- ▪ Treatment: Closed reduction is adequate in most cases.
- ▪ Complications: instability, arthrosis, and recurrent dislocation.

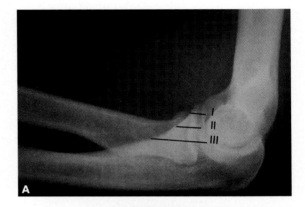

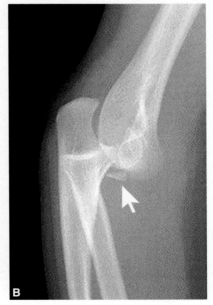

FIGURE 7-12. Lateral radiograph demonstrates the locations of Types I to III coronoid fractures **(A)**. Lateral radiograph of the elbow **(B)** depicts a posterior dislocation of the elbow with a small avulsion fracture of the coronoid process (*arrow*) (Type II).

SUGGESTED READING

Doornberg JN, Ring D. Coronoid fracture patterns. *J Hand Surg Am.* 2006;31(1):45–52.
Regan W, Morrey BF. Fractures of the coronoid process of the ulna. *J Bone Joint Surg.* 1989;71A:1348–1354.

■ FRACTURE/DISLOCATIONS: ELBOW DISLOCATIONS

KEY FACTS

- ■ Dislocation classifications refer to the position of the dislocation.
- ■ Most elbow dislocations are posterior and involve both the radius and the ulna.
- ■ The mechanism of injury is a fall with the elbow extended.
- ■ Anterior, medial, and lateral dislocations are uncommon.
- ■ Associated injuries include coronoid, radial head, epicondylar fractures, and neurovascular injuries.
- ■ Postreduction CT imaging is important to fully assess the joint space and associated fractures.
- ■ Complications include arthrosis, instability, decreased range of motion, neurovascular injury, and extensive heterotopic ossification.

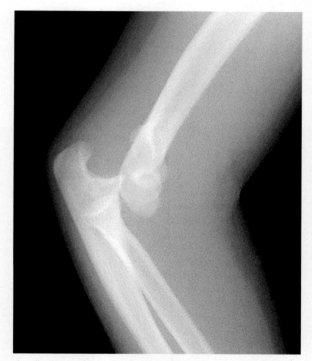

FIGURE 7-13. Lateral radiograph of the elbow depicting a posterior dislocation.

SUGGESTED READING

Koyle SG. Posterior dislocations of the elbow. *Clin Orthop.* 1991;269:201.

O'Driscoll SW, Morrey BF, Korinek S, et al. Elbow subluxations and dislocations: a spectrum of instability. *Clin Orthop.* 1992;280:186–197.

Pugh DMW, Wild LM, Schemitsch EH, et al. Standard surgical protocols for treatment of elbow dislocations with radial head and coronoid fractures. *J Bone Joint Surg.* 2004;86A:1122–1130.

■ FRACTURES/DISLOCATIONS: MONTEGGIA FRACTURES

KEY FACTS

■ Monteggia fracture or lesion is a dislocation of the radial head with an associated proximal ulnar fracture.

■ This injury accounts for only 7% of ulnar fractures and 0.7% of elbow injuries.

■ Four injury patterns are commonly described:

Type I	Fracture of the ulna with anterior dislocation of the radial head (50% to 75% of cases)
Type II	Fracture of the ulna with posterior or posterolateral radial head dislocation (10% to 15% of cases)
Type III	Fracture of the ulna with lateral or anterolateral radial head dislocation (6% to 20%); more common in children
Type IV	Anterior dislocation with radial and ulnar fractures (5% of cases)

■ Mechanism of injury: direct blow to posterior ulna, fall on the outstretched hand with elbow flexed, or hyperextension.

■ Routine radiographs are diagnostic. Keep in mind, the dislocation may reduce during radiographic positioning (20% of cases).

■ Treatment: closed reduction in children; open reduction usually required in adults.

■ Complications: recurrent dislocation, arthrosis, nonunion, and neurovascular injury.

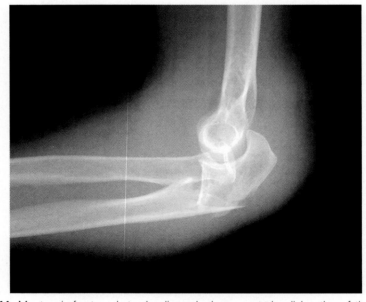

FIGURE 7-14. Monteggia fracture. Lateral radiograph shows posterior dislocation of the radial head with a proximal ulnar fracture.

SUGGESTED READING

Bado J. The Monteggia lesion. *Clin Orthop.* 1967;50:71–86.

Iyer RS, Thapa MM, Khanna PC, et al. Pediatric bone imaging: imaging elbow trauma in children—a review of acute and chronic injuries. *Am J Roentgenol.* 2012;198(5):1053–1068.

■ FRACTURES/DISLOCATIONS: FOREARM FRACTURES

KEY FACTS

- Forearm fractures typically involve both the radius and the ulna (75%), or one osseous structure with dislocation at the wrist or elbow.
- Mechanism of injury: direct blow or fall on the outstretched arm.
- Fractures may be undisplaced, but muscle forces tend to cause angulation and rotation of fragments.
- AP and lateral radiographs are diagnostic. The elbow and wrist should be included to avoid overlooking associated subluxation or dislocation.
- Treatment: Internal fixation is commonly required to prevent displacement.
- Complications: reduced pronation and supination, nonunion, cross union, and neurovascular injuries.

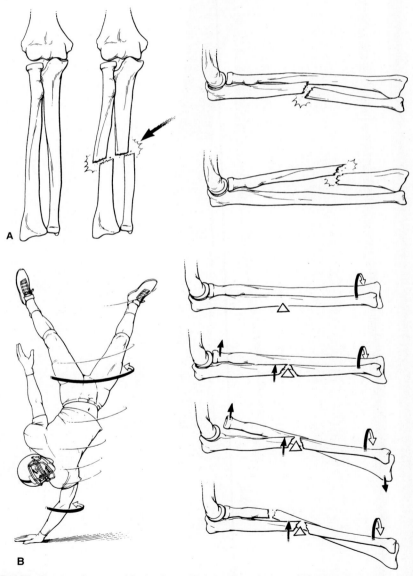

FIGURE 7-15. Forearm fracture. Mechanism of injury: direct blow in **(A)** and fall on the outstretched arm **(B)** with forces that tend to displace the fracture.

(continued)

■ FRACTURES/DISLOCATIONS: FOREARM FRACTURES *(Continued)*

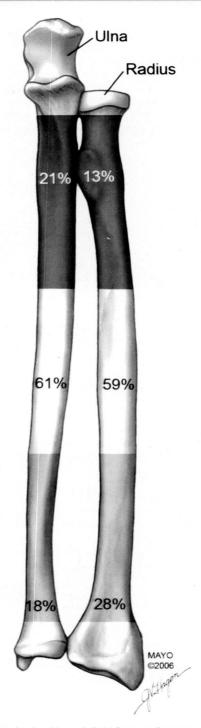

FIGURE 7-16. Incidence of proximal, mid-, and distal forearm fractures.

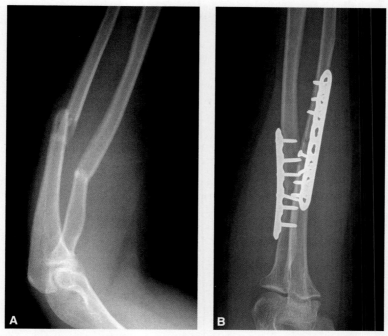

FIGURE 7-17. Anteroposterior (AP) radiograph **(A)** of a mildly displaced and angulated mid-diaphyseal ulnar and proximal diaphyseal radial fractures. Radiograph **(B)** following open reduction and internal fixation shows significantly improved alignment.

SUGGESTED READING

Chapman MW, Gordon JE, Zissimos AG. Compression plate fixation of acute forearm fractures of the diaphysis of the radius and ulna. *J Bone Joint Surg.* 1989;71A:159–169.

■ OSTEOCHONDRITIS DISSECANS

KEY FACTS

■ Osteochondritis dissecans is common in adolescents, especially throwing athletes; 10% to 20% are bilateral.

■ Patients present with dull, aching pain in the involved elbow. Swelling and reduced motion are common.

■ The capitellum is most often involved.

■ Staging is important for treatment planning:

Stage I	Intact cartilage with no displacement
Stage II	Fissure in articular cartilage with slight displacement
Stage III	Displaced

■ Routine radiographs may not detect the lesion, and staging is difficult. MRI or magnetic resonance (MR) arthrography is preferred for detection and staging.

■ Treatment: conservative treatment for Type I; arthroscopic repair for Types II and III.

■ Complications: early arthrosis.

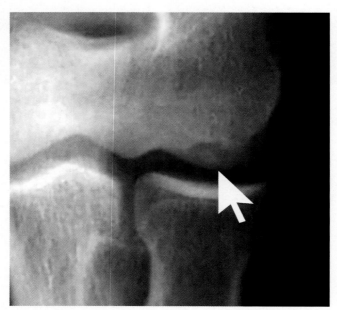

FIGURE 7-18. Axial T1 demonstrates an undisplaced osteochondritis dissecans of the capitellum (*arrow*).

SUGGESTED READING

Herzog RJ. Magnetic resonance imaging of the elbow. *Magn Reson Q.* 1993;9:188–210.
Kijowski R, De Smet AA. Radiography of the elbow of patients with osteochondritis dissecans of the capitellum. *Skel Radiol.* 2005;34:266–271.

■ SOFT TISSUE TRAUMA: BICEPS TENDON

KEY FACTS

- The biceps tendon is the most commonly injured tendon of the elbow. Injuries are more common in men aged more than 40 years.
- Injuries are most common at the radial tuberosity after catching a heavy weight with the elbow flexed and supinated.
- Patients present with acute pain, fullness, and ecchymosis in the antecubital fossa.
- Chronic microtrauma may result in degeneration, partial tears, bursitis, or ganglion formation. Bicipitoradial bursitis (55%) and micro bone avulsion (50%) are common with partial tears.
- Imaging of biceps tendon pathology may be accomplished with routine radiographs, ultrasound, or MRI.
- Radiographs: irregularity of the radial tuberosity.
- Ultrasound: abnormal echo texture or cyst in case of ganglion.
- MRI: T2-weighted images show increased signal in tendon or disruption. Ganglion cysts are well-defined, high-intensity masses.
- Treatment: Operative intervention is often required for complete tears or partial tears with 30% to 40% function loss.

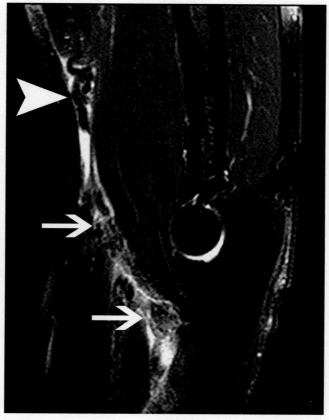

FIGURE 7-19. Sagittal fluid-sensitive magnetic resonance (MR) image depicts a complete tear of the distal biceps tendon with proximal retraction of the torn tendon fibers (*arrowhead*) and hemorrhage along the previous tract of the distal biceps tendon (*arrows*).

(continued)

■ SOFT TISSUE TRAUMA: BICEPS TENDON *(Continued)*

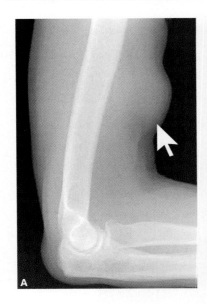

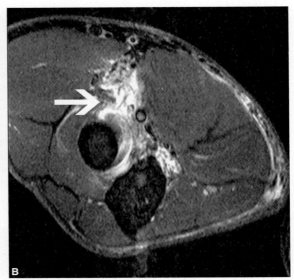

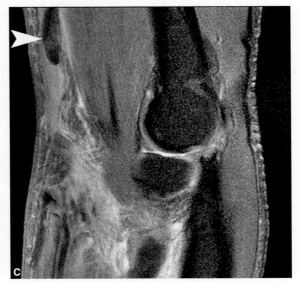

FIGURE 7-20. Biceps tendon tear. Lateral radiograph **(A)** shows the "Popeye Sign" *(arrow)* with retraction of the torn distal biceps muscle and tendon into the mid-upper arm. Axial **(B)** T2-weighted image shows fluid and hemorrhage in the expected location of the distal biceps tendon *(arrow)*. Sagittal **(C)** T2-weighted image depicts complete rupture of the distal biceps tendon with proximal retraction *(arrowhead)*.

SUGGESTED READING

Chew ML, Giuffre BM. Disorders of the distal biceps brachii tendon. *Radiographics.* 2005;25:1227–1237.

Fitzgerald SW, Curry DR, Erickson SJ, et al. Distal biceps tendon injury: MR imaging diagnosis. *Radiology.* 1994;191:203–206.

■ SOFT TISSUE TRAUMA: TRICEPS TENDON INJURIES

KEY FACTS

- ■ Inflammation of the triceps tendon is common, but tendon ruptures are rare.
- ■ Triceps ruptures occur with deceleration forces while the triceps is contracted.
- ■ Triceps tears are more common in patients with systemic diseases or patients on steroid therapy.
- ■ Imaging of triceps injuries can be accomplished using radiographs, ultrasound, or MRI.
- ■ Radiographs: Up to 80% of triceps injuries have an avulsed olecranon fragment visible on the lateral view.
- ■ Ultrasound: abnormal echo texture or loss of tendon substance with complete disruption.
- ■ MRI: T2-weighted or short-TI inversion recovery (STIR) sequences show increased signal intensity in tendon (varies with extent of tear). Axial and sagittal image planes are most useful.
- ■ Treatment of inflammatory and partial tears may be conservative. Complete tears are corrected surgically.

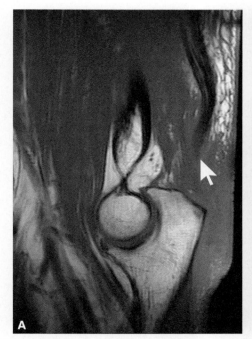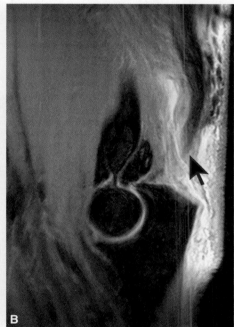

FIGURE 7-21. Sagittal T1-weighted **(A)** and T2-weighted **(B)** magnetic resonance (MR) images show a complete tear of the distal triceps tendon with minimal proximal retraction (*arrow*).

SUGGESTED READING

Rajasekhar C, Kakarlapudi TK, Bhamra MS. Avulsion of the triceps tendon. *Emerg Med J.* 2002;19(3):271–272.

Tiger E, Mayer DP, Glazer R. Complete avulsion of the triceps tendon: MRI diagnosis. *Comput Med Imaging Graphics.* 1993;17:51–54.

■ SOFT TISSUE TRAUMA: FLEXOR/EXTENSOR TENDON INJURIES

KEY FACTS

- Tendinopathy or tears of the flexor or extensor tendons are common.
- Injury to the common extensor tendon (lateral epicondylitis and tennis elbow) is common with repetitive microtrauma. Injury most commonly involves the origin of the extensor carpi radialis brevis. Lateral epicondylitis affects 50% of throwing athletes, and 50% of tennis players older than 30 years will develop symptoms.
- Injury to the common flexor tendon (medial epicondylitis) occurs less frequently. The injury usually involves the flexors and pronator teres. The syndrome occurs in 1% to 3% of adults, especially golfers and throwing athletes.
- Four stages of epicondylitis have been described by Kraushaar and Nirschl.
  - Stage 1: inflammatory, resolves
  - Stage 2: tendinosis and angiofibroblastic degeneration
  - Stage 3: tendinosis with rupture
  - Stage 4: a combination of 2 and 3 plus scarring and calcification
- Ultrasound or MRI is most useful when imaging studies are performed. Axial and coronal T2-weighted or STIR images are most useful.
- Treatment of most tendinopathies is conservative. Partial or complete tears in athletes may require surgical repair.

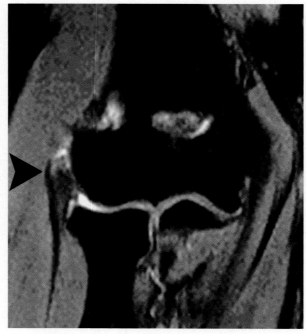

FIGURE 7-22. Extensor tendinopathy. Coronal T2-weighted magnetic resonance (MR) image in a patient with a clinical history of lateral epicondylitis shows thickening and abnormal signal intensity involving the common extensor tendon (*arrowhead*) compatible with low-grade partial tear of the tendon.

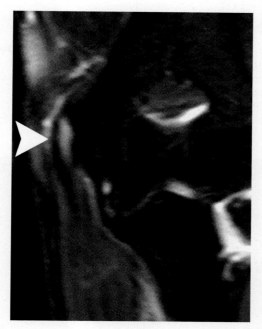

FIGURE 7-23. Flexor tendinopathy. Coronal T2-weighted magnetic resonance (MR) image in a patient with a clinical history of medial epicondylitis shows thickening and increased signal intensity involving the common flexor origin (*arrowhead*) compatible with tendinopathy.

SUGGESTED READING

Kijowski R, DeSmet AA. Magnetic resonance imaging findings in patients with medial epicondylitis. *Skeletal Radiol.* 2005;34:196–202.

Kraushaar BS, Nirschl RL. Tendinosis of the elbow (tennis elbow). *J Bone Joint Surg.* 1999;81A:259–278.

Struijs PAA, Spruyt M, Assendelft WJJ, et al. The predictive value of diagnostic sonography for effectiveness of conservative treatment of tennis elbow. *Am J Roentgenol.* 2005;185:1113–1118.

■ SOFT TISSUE TRAUMA: MUSCLE INJURIES

KEY FACTS

- Muscle injuries to the upper extremity are infrequent compared with injuries to the lower extremity.
- Muscle strains are usually stretch injuries resulting from eccentric overload.
- MRI is most useful for detection and staging (partial and complete) of muscle injuries. Axial and coronal or sagittal T2-weighted or STIR sequences show increased signal intensity in the involved muscle.
- Treatment is conservative for partial tears. Surgery may be required for complete tears.

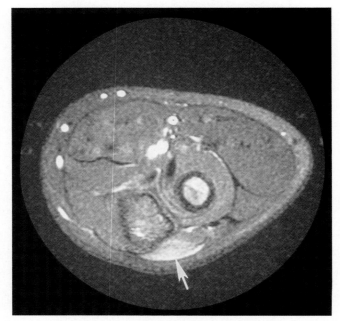

FIGURE 7-24. Anconeus strain. Axial T2-weighted image of the elbow shows increased signal intensity (*arrow*) resulting from repetitive microtrauma.

SUGGESTED READING

El-Khoury GY, Brandser EA, Kathol MH, et al. Imaging of muscle injuries. *Skeletal Radiol.* 1996;25(1):3–11.
Herzog RJ. Magnetic resonance imaging of the elbow. *Magn Reson Q.* 1993;9:188–210.

■ SOFT TISSUE TRAUMA: LIGAMENT INJURIES

KEY FACTS

- ■ The radial and ulnar collateral ligaments provide important support for elbow stability.
- ■ The ulnar collateral ligament complex is most important for stability. Injuries usually occur when valgus force is applied to the elbow. Such injuries are commonly seen in athletes involved in throwing sports or javelin throwing. Causes of medial elbow pain in throwing athletes include:
  - ● Medial tendon overuse
  - ● Flexor/pronator muscle tears
  - ● Ulnar collateral ligament tears
  - ● Avulsion of the coronoid tubercle
  - ● Posteromedial impingement
  - ● Ulnar neuropathy
  - ● Ulnar nerve subluxation
  - ● Medial antebrachial cutaneous nerve injury
- ■ Radial collateral ligament injuries occur less frequently. Injuries are the result of varus stress.
- ■ Imaging can be accomplished with conventional arthrography, ultrasound, MRI, or MR arthrography. The anterior band of the ulnar collateral ligament is optimally imaged in the coronal plane. The transverse band is less clinically significant and sometimes absent. This may be difficult to identify on MR images.
- ■ Treatment: Partial tears may be treated conservatively. Complete tears may require surgical intervention.

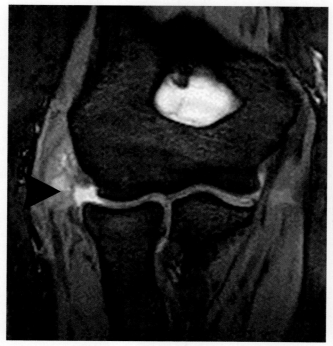

FIGURE 7-25. Radial collateral ligament tear. Coronal T2-weighted magnetic resonance (MR) image depicts a complete tear of the radial collateral ligament (*arrowhead*) in a tennis player who sustained a severe varus injury of the elbow.

(continued)

■ SOFT TISSUE TRAUMA: LIGAMENT INJURIES *(Continued)*

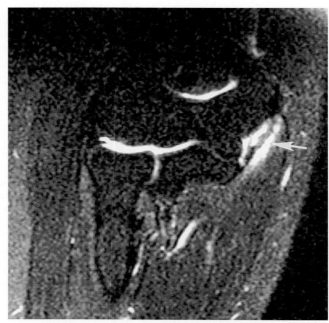

FIGURE 7-26. Partial tear of the anterior band of the ulnar collateral ligament. Coronal T2-weighted image shows increased signal intensity about and in the ligament (*arrow*) resulting from a partial tear.

SUGGESTED READING

Carrino JA, Morrison WB, Zon KH, et al. MR imaging and MR arthrography of the ulnar collateral ligament of the elbow: prospective evaluation of 2-dimensional pulse sequences for detection of complete tears. *Skeletal Radiol.* 2001;30:625–632.

Cotton A, Jacobson J, Brossmann J, et al. Collateral ligaments of the elbow: conventional MR imaging and MR arthrography with oblique coronal plane and elbow flexion. *Radiology.* 1997;204:806–812.

Ward SI, Teefey SA, Paletta GA, et al. Sonography of the medial collateral ligament of the elbow: a study of cadavers and healthy male volunteers. *Am J Roentgenol.* 2002;180:389–394.

■ NEOPLASMS: BONE TUMORS

KEY FACTS

- ■ Osseous neoplasms of the elbow are rare.
- ■ Characterization of lesions is accomplished most easily with routine radiographs.
- ■ CT or MRI is most useful for staging of lesions.
- ■ Table 7-1 summarizes malignant and benign osseous neoplasms in the elbow and forearm.

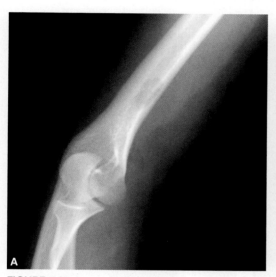 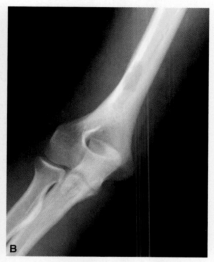

FIGURE 7-27. Langerhans cell histiocytosis. Anteroposterior (AP) and lateral radiographs **(A, B)** show an intramedullary well-circumscribed lytic lesion in the distal humeral metadiaphysis compatible with Langerhans cell histiocytosis.

Table 7-1   SKELETAL NEOPLASMS OF THE ELBOW AND FOREARM

	No. in Elbow and Forearm/Total/%
Benign	
Osteoid osteoma	23/331/7
Chondromyxoid fibroma	2/45/4.4
Giant cell tumor	12/568/2
Osteochondroma	12/872/1.4
Chondroma	2/290/0.6
Malignant	
Ewing sarcoma	22/512/4
Lymphoma	28/694/4
Myeloma	15/814/2
Osteosarcoma	19/1,649/1
Chondrosarcoma	9/895/1
Fibrosarcoma	3/255/1

SUGGESTED READING

Unni KK. *Dahlin's Bone Tumors: General Aspects and Data on 11,087 Cases.* 5th ed. Philadelphia: Lippincott-Raven; 1996.

■ NEOPLASMS: SOFT TISSUE TUMORS

KEY FACTS

- ■ Soft tissue tumors are most effectively identified and categorized with MRI.
- ■ As a general rule, benign lesions are well defined, with homogeneous signal intensity.
- ■ Malignant tumors are inhomogeneous, especially on T2-weighted sequences, have irregular margins, and may encase neurovascular structures and bone.
- ■ Intravenous gadolinium is useful to define cysts (do not enhance) and areas of necrosis. We routinely use contrast-enhanced fat-suppressed T1-weighted images in patients with neoplasms.

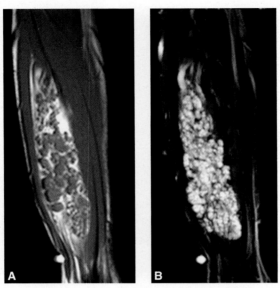

FIGURE 7-28. Hemangioma. Axial T1-weighted **(A)** and T2-weighted **(B)** magnetic resonance (MR) images show a multilobulated mass with numerous nodular foci of bright signal on T2-weighted images and extensive adipose tissue throughout the lesion on T1-weighted images.

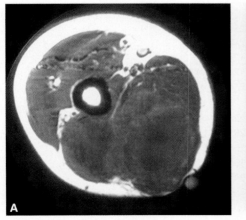
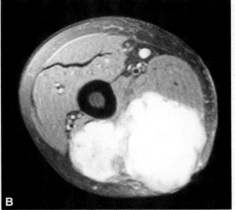

FIGURE 7-29. Malignant fibrous histiocytoma. Axial T1- **(A)** and T2-weighted **(B)** images of this malignant lesion. Signal inhomogeneity is most easily appreciated on the T2-weighted image **(B)**.

SUGGESTED READING

Berquist TH. Magnetic resonance imaging of musculoskeletal neoplasms. *Clin Orthop.* 1989;244:101–118.

■ INFECTION

KEY FACTS

- ■ Musculoskeletal infections may present as an acute or insidious process.
- ■ Skeletal infections typically present in medullary bone with hyperemia and edema.
- ■ Soft tissue infections may be diffuse or result in more localized abscess formation.
- ■ Joint space infections may present with soft tissue changes, joint effusion, or joint and bone involvement.
- ■ Routine radiographs are usually normal early, except for soft tissue swelling. MRI is most useful for early detection and evaluation of bone and soft tissue involvement.

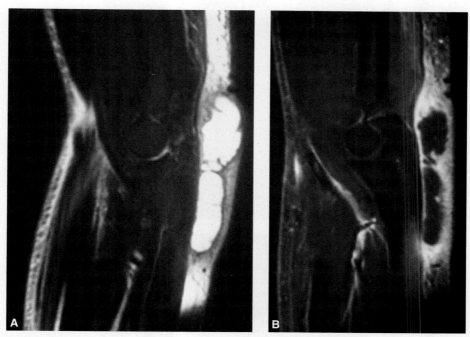

FIGURE 7-30. Soft tissue abscess. Sagittal T2-weighted **(A)** and post–gadolinium-enhanced fat-suppressed **(B)** images show a large nonenhancing fluid collection.

(continued)

■ **INFECTION** *(Continued)*

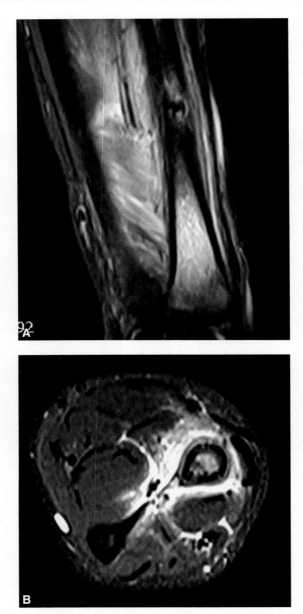

FIGURE 7-31. Osteomyelitis. Coronal proton density **(A)** and axial T2-weighted **(B)** magnetic resonance (MR) images in a navy patient with a history of a forearm puncture wound demonstrate focal abnormal signal within the distal radial diaphysis with surrounding periosteal reaction and sclerosis. There is diffuse surrounding soft tissue edema.

SUGGESTED READING

Berquist TH, Broderick DF. Musculoskeletal infection. In: Berquist TH, ed. *MRI of the Musculoskeletal System.* 5th ed. Philadelphia: Lippincott Williams & Wilkins; 2006:916–947.

■ ARTHROPATHIES

KEY FACTS

- Arthropathies involving the elbow include degenerative arthritis secondary to trauma and systemic arthropathies, such as rheumatoid arthritis, hemophiliac arthropathy, gout, and arthropathy secondary to dialysis.
- Routine radiographs remain the primary screening technique for detection and characterization of arthropathies.
- Radionuclide scans and MRI detect changes earlier than radiographs. Intravenous gadolinium studies show changes in articular cartilage and synovial pathology more readily.

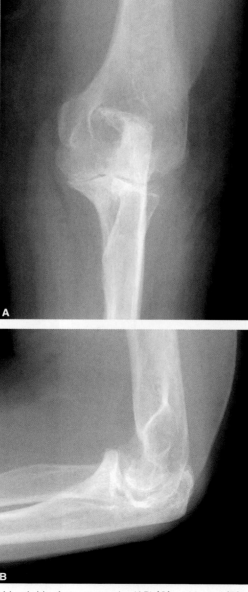

FIGURE 7-32. Rheumatoid arthritis. Anteroposterior (AP) **(A)** and lateral **(B)** radiographs show diffuse osteopenia with joint space narrowing and erosive changes.

(continued)

■ ARTHROPATHIES *(Continued)*

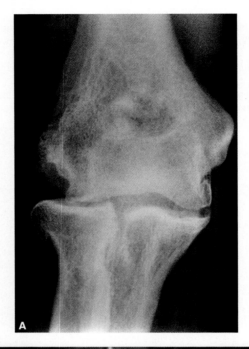

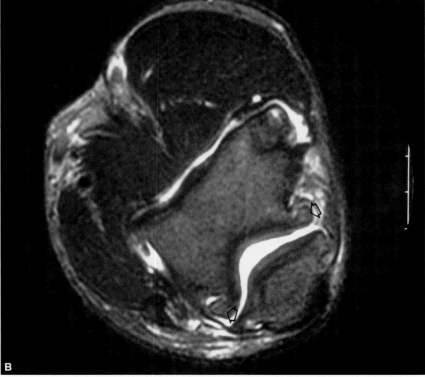

FIGURE 7-33. Osteoarthritis. **(A)** Anteroposterior (AP) radiograph shows bone sclerosis and osteophytes typical of osteoarthritis. **(B)** Axial T2-weighted magnetic resonance (MR) image shows a joint effusion with osteophytes (*open arrows*).

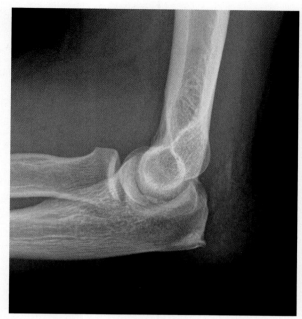

FIGURE 7-34. Gout. Lateral radiograph demonstrates prominent nodular swelling posterior to the olecranon with internal high attenuation and subtle calcification compatible with gouty tophi and olecranon bursitis.

SUGGESTED READING

Brower AC. *Arthritis in Black and White.* 2nd Ed. Philadelphia: WB Saunders; 1997:325–342.

■ NERVE ENTRAPMENT SYNDROMES

KEY FACTS

- Nerve compression or entrapment syndromes fall into four categories:
  - First degree (neurapraxic): conduction defects with no structural abnormalities evident. Cause may be blunt trauma or ischemia.
  - Second degree (axonometric): disruption of nerve fibers with connective tissue intact. Regeneration can occur.
  - Third/fourth degree: complete motor and sensory loss.
- Cause of nerve compression syndromes about the elbow varies to some degree depending on the nerve involved (ulnar, median, or radial).
  - Ulnar Nerve:
    - ❖ The nerve passes from anterior to posterior through the arcade of Struthers (Fig. 7-35). At the elbow the nerve lies posterior to the medial epicondyle before entering the cubital tunnel (Fig. 7-36). Causes of ulnar nerve compression include:
      - ◆ Fibrous adhesions
      - ◆ Muscle anomalies (anconeus epitrochlearis)
      - ◆ Absent cubical retinaculum (10%)
      - ◆ Thickened cubical retinaculum

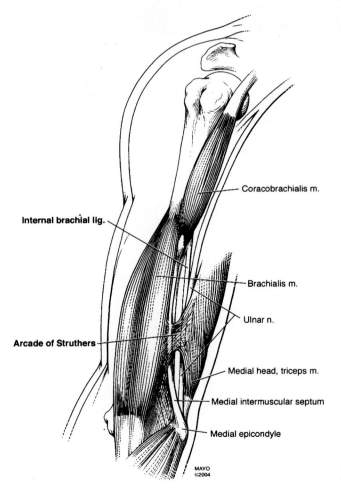

Coracobrachialis m.

Internal brachial lig.

Brachialis m.

Ulnar n.

Arcade of Struthers

Medial head, triceps m.

Medial intermuscular septum

Medial epicondyle

MAYO
©2004

FIGURE 7-35. Ulnar nerve in the arm and the arcade of Struthers.

(continued)

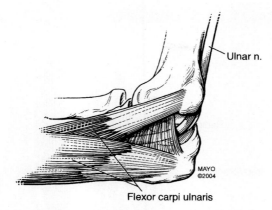

FIGURE 7-36. Ulnar nerve in the cubital tunnel.

- ◆ Thickened ulnar collateral ligament
- ◆ Vascular anomalies
- ◆ Bursitis
- ◆ Myotendinous inflammation
- ◆ Ganglion cysts
- ◆ Inflammatory arthropathies
- ◆ Neoplasms
- ◆ Prior fractures
- ◆ Loose bodies
- ● Median Nerve:
    - ❖ The median nerve lies beneath the brachialis muscle accompanied by the brachial artery and vein and biceps tendon.
    - ❖ Median nerve compression occurs at the supracondylar process and ligament of Struthers. Fractures of the humerus and elbow commonly injure the median nerve.
    - ❖ The median nerve may also be compressed between the two heads of the pronator muscle (pronator syndrome). Patients present with anterior elbow pain and tingling in the median nerve distribution.
    - ❖ The anterior interosseous nerve is a motor branch of the median nerve and innervates the flexor pollicis longus, the radial flexor digitorum profundus, and the pronator quadratus. Denervation leads to weakness of flexion of the index and middle fingers and patient present with weakness inability to pinch the thumb and index finger together. This can be tested by having the patient make the "OK" sign.
- ● Radial Nerve:
    - ❖ The radial nerve takes an anterior course 10 cm above the lateral epicondyle (Fig. 7-37) dividing into superficial and posterior interosseous branches. The radial nerve is vulnerable to compression from the lateral head of the triceps to the distal forearm. More proximally, radial nerve injury is associated with humeral fractures. Causes of radial nerve compression include:
        - ◆ Humeral shaft fractures
        - ◆ Fracture/dislocations of the radius
        - ◆ Cast immobilization
        - ◆ Thickening of the arcade of Frohse
        - ◆ Radiocapitellar pannus
        - ◆ Vascular anomalies
        - ◆ Muscle anomalies
        - ◆ Bursitis
        - ◆ Soft tissue masses
        - ◆ Synovial chondromatosis

(continued)

■ NERVE ENTRAPMENT SYNDROMES *(Continued)*

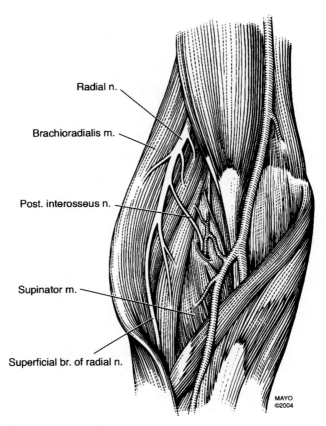

FIGURE 7-37. Radial and posterior interosseous nerves.

- 2 common syndromes about the elbow:
  ❖ Radial Tunnel Syndrome/Radial Nerve Sensory Syndrome
  ❖ Sensory neuropathy with no motor deficits. Patient present with burning sensation in the lateral elbow and forearm
  ❖ Difficult clinical diagnosis—mimics lateral epicondylitis
  ❖ Typically no imaging findingsMuscle anomalies
  ❖ Posterior Interosseous Nerve Syndrome/Radial Nerve Motor Syndrome
  ❖ AKA Supinator Syndrome
  ❖ Motor neuropathy—deficits of Supinator, Extensor digitorum communis (EDC), extensor pollucis longus (EPL), extensor indicis proprius (EIP), extensor digitorum digiti quinti proprius (EDQP)
  ❖ Wrist drop and loss of extension of the MCP joints

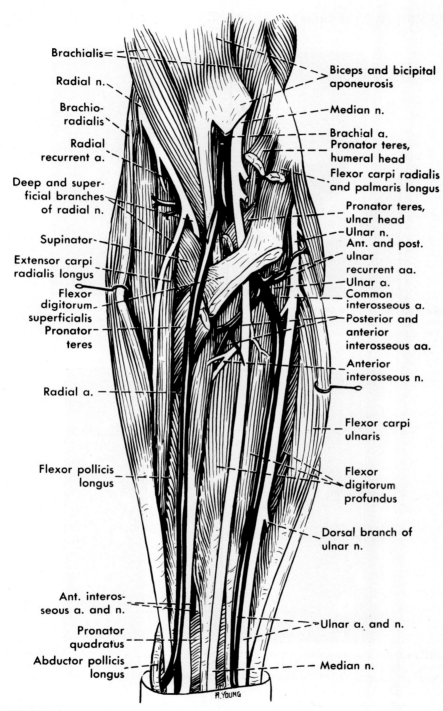

Brachialis

Radial n.

Brachio-
radialis

Radial
recurrent a.

Deep and super-
ficial branches
of radial n.

Supinator

Extensor carpi
radialis longus

Flexor
digitorum
superficialis

Pronator
teres

Radial a.

Flexor pollicis
longus

Ant. interos-
seous a. and n.

Pronator
quadratus

Abductor pollicis
longus

Biceps and bicipital
aponeurosis

Median n.

Brachial a.
Pronator teres,
humeral head

Flexor carpi radialis
and palmaris longus

Pronator teres,
ulnar head

Ulnar n.
Ant. and post.
ulnar
recurrent aa.

Ulnar a.
Common
interosseous a.

Posterior and
anterior
interosseous aa.

Anterior
interosseous n.

Flexor carpi
ulnaris

Flexor
digitorum
profundus

Dorsal branch of
ulnar n.

Ulnar a. and n.

Median n.

R. YOUNG

FIGURE 7-38. Neurovascular anatomy of the elbow and forearm.

(continued)

■ NERVE ENTRAPMENT SYNDROMES *(Continued)*

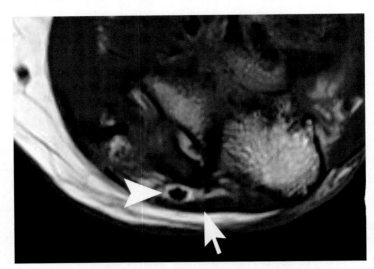

FIGURE 7-39. Ulnar nerve compression. Axial T1-weighted images show an accessory anconeus epi-trochlearis muscle (*arrow*) overlying the ulnar nerve (*arrowhead*), resulting in occasional symptoms of ulnar nerve compression.

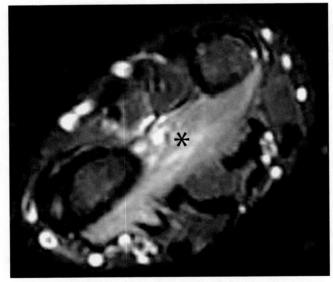

FIGURE 7-40. Anterior intraosseous nerve syndrome. Axial T2-weighted magnetic resonance (MR) im-age through the distal forearm shows denervation edema through the pronator quadratus musculature resulting from compression of the anterior intraosseous nerve proximally in the forearm.

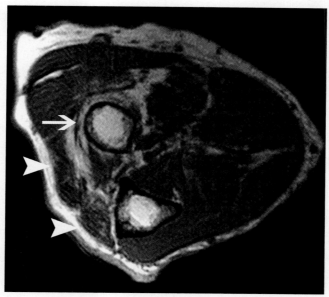

FIGURE 7-41. Posterior intraosseous nerve syndrome. Axial T1-weighted magnetic resonance (MR) image of the proximal forearm shows marked atrophy of supinator muscle as well as the extensor musculature of the forearm compatible with chronic compression of the posterior intraosseous nerve in the proximal forearm.

SUGGESTED READING

Beltran J, Rosenberg ZS. Diagnosis of compression and entrapment neuropathies of the upper extremity: value of MR imaging. *Am J Roentgenol.* 1994;163:525–531.

Major N. Magnetic resonance imaging of the elbow. *Curr Probl Diagn Radiol.* 2000;1:27–40.

Miller TT, Reinus WR. Nerve entrapment syndromes of the elbow, forearm, and wrist. *Am J Roentgenol.* 2010;195(3):585–594.

O'Driscoll SW, Horii E, Carmichael S, et al. The cubital tunnel and ulnar neuropathy. *J Bone Joint Surg.* 1991;73A:613–617.

8 Hand and Wrist

Jeffrey J. Peterson and Thomas H. Berquist

■ FRACTURES/DISLOCATIONS: DISTAL RADIUS/ULNAR FRACTURES—COLLES FRACTURE

KEY FACTS

- Fractures of the distal radius are common. In elderly patients, osteopenia results in fracture from minor trauma. In children, incomplete or physeal fractures are common. Fractures of the ulna or ulnar styloid commonly occur with distal radial fractures.
- Distal radial fractures have multiple eponyms, such as Colles, Smith, Barton, and Chauffeur's fractures. Today, most are categorized by the extent of articular involvement. Type A fractures are extra-articular, Type B fractures are partial articular, and Type C fractures involve both the radiocarpal joints and distal radioulnar joint (DRUJ).
- Colles fracture is a term applied to fractures to distal radial, with or without articular involvement, and dorsal displacement of the distal fragment.
- Mechanism of injury: fall on the outstretched hand.
- Anteroposterior (AP) and lateral radiographs are diagnostic. However, computed tomography (CT) is often performed to completely evaluate articular involvement.
- Treatment: traction to reduce and reachieve radial length and palmar tilt. Closed reduction is usually successful.
- Complications: occur in up to 33% of patients and include
  - Compressive neuropathy
  - Arthrosis
  - Malunion
  - Tendon rupture
  - Ligament injuries
  - Ischemic contractures

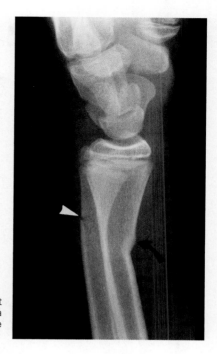

FIGURE 8-1. Lateral radiograph of the wrist demonstrates incomplete fractures of the ulna (*arrowhead*) and a torus (buckle) fracture of the radius (*curved arrow*).

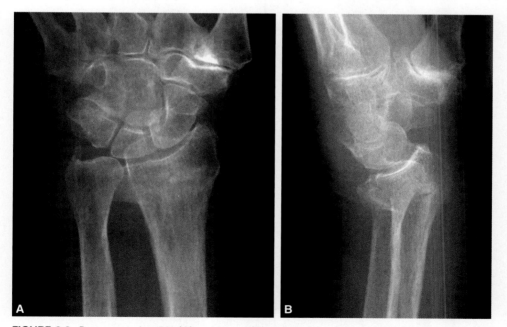

FIGURE 8-2. Posteroanterior (PA) **(A)** and lateral **(B)** radiographs of the wrist show a typical Colles fracture with dorsal impaction of the radius and an ulnar styloid fracture. The fracture extends into the distal radioulnar joint (DRUJ) (Type B).

(continued)

■ FRACTURES/DISLOCATIONS: DISTAL RADIUS/ULNAR FRACTURES—COLLES FRACTURE *(Continued)*

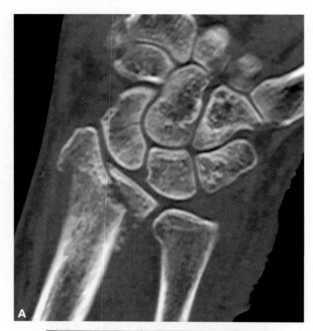

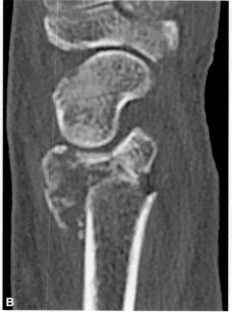

FIGURE 8-3. Coronal **(A)** and sagittal **(B)** computed tomography (CT) images clearly demonstrate the fracture fragments and the extent of articular separation.

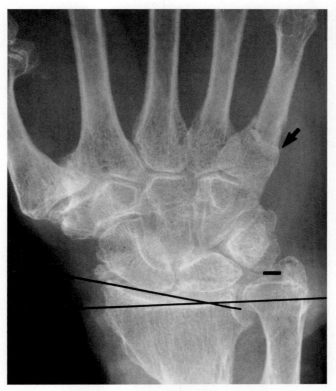

FIGURE 8-4. Posteroanterior (PA) radiograph of an old Colles fracture with shortening of the radius and decreased radial inclination (*lines*). There is degenerative arthritis and an associated fifth metacarpal fracture (*arrow*).

SUGGESTED READING

Cooney WP, Dobyns JH, Linscheid RL. Complications of Colles' fractures. *J Bone Joint Surg.* 1980;62A:613–619.
Orthopedic Trauma Association Committee for Coding and Classification. Fracture and dislocation compendium. *J Orthop Trauma.* 1996;10:26–30.

■ FRACTURES/DISLOCATIONS: DISTAL RADIUS/ULNAR FRACTURES—SMITH FRACTURE

KEY FACTS

■ Smith fracture is a "reverse Colles fracture" with palmar displacement of the distal radial fragment.

■ Mechanism of injury: fall on a palmar flexed wrist.

■ Treatment: closed reduction; restore radial length. Internal fixation may be required with significant displacement or articular involvement.

■ Complications: identical to Colles fracture complications.

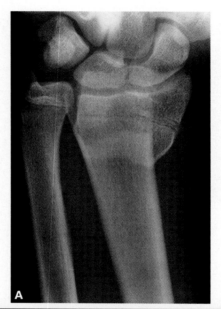

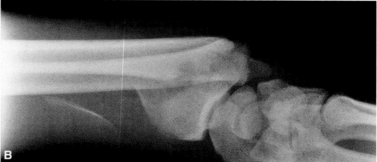

FIGURE 8-5. Anteroposterior (AP) **(A)** and lateral **(B)** radiographs of a Smith fracture with palmar displacement of the distal radius.

SUGGESTED READING

Thomas FB. Reduction of Smith's fracture. *J Bone Joint Surg.* 1957;37B:463–470.

■ FRACTURES/DISLOCATIONS: DISTAL RADIUS/ULNAR FRACTURES—BARTON FRACTURE

KEY FACTS

■ A Barton fracture is an intra-articular fracture of the radius involving the dorsal or volar lip of the radial styloid.

■ Radial styloid fractures are divided into three zones. Zone I fractures may be stable without associated ligament injuries. Zone II fractures commonly have associated ligament injury. Zone III fractures are likely to have ligament injury and joint incongruency (Fig. 8-6).

■ Mechanism of injury: Palmar fractures occur similar to Smith fractures. Dorsal fractures result from a fall on the outstretched hand with the forearm pronated.

■ Treatment: closed reduction unless the articular surface cannot be restored. In the latter setting, internal fixation may be required.

■ Complications: similar to Colles fracture, except subluxation and arthrosis are more common.

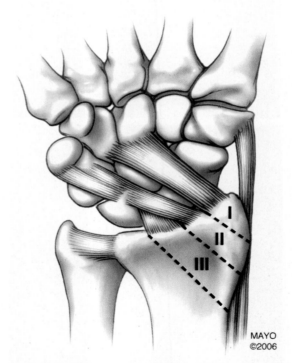

FIGURE 8-6. Zones of radial styloid (Barton fracture). Zone I: styloid tip, may be stable with no ligament injury. Zone II: possible ligament injury, may have articular deformity. Zone III: likely to have ligament injury and joint deformity.

(continued)

■ FRACTURES/DISLOCATIONS: DISTAL RADIUS/ULNAR FRACTURES—BARTON FRACTURE *(Continued)*

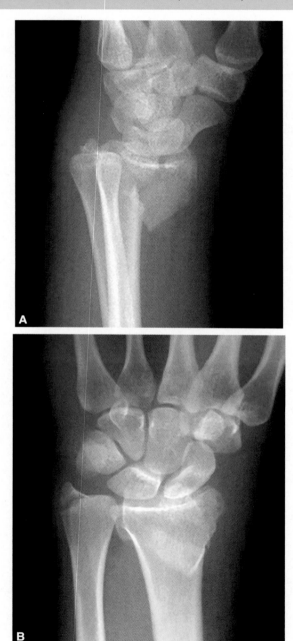

FIGURE 8-7. Volar Barton fracture. Anteroposterior (AP) **(A)** and lateral **(B)** radiographs of an intra-articular fracture of the lateral aspect of the radius.

SUGGESTED READING

DeOliveira JC. Barton's fracture. *J Bone Joint Surg.* 1973;55A:586–594.

Putnam MD. Radial styloid fractures. In: Blair WF, ed. *Techniques in Hand Surgery.* Baltimore: Williams and Wilkins; 1996:322–329.

■ FRACTURES/DISLOCATIONS: DISTAL RADIUS/ULNAR FRACTURES—CHAUFFEUR'S FRACTURE

KEY FACTS

- A Chauffeur's fracture is an intra-articular fracture of the distal radius that predominately involves the radial styloid.
- The fracture line typically enters the joint at the junction of the scaphoid and lunate fossae.
- Mechanism of injury: axial compression transmitted through the scaphoid. Decades ago, the injury was associated with backfires resulting in the automobile starting crank striking the wrist.
- AP and lateral radiographs are adequate for diagnosis.
- Treatment: cast immobilization if minimally displaced. Percutaneous K-wires may be required to maintain reduction.

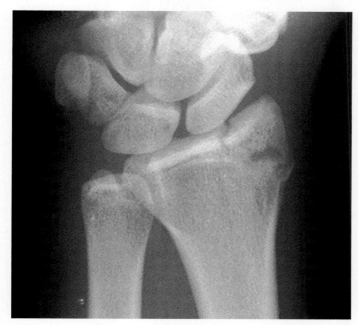

FIGURE 8-8. Posteroanterior (PA) radiograph of a Chauffeur's fracture during reduction with an external fixation.

SUGGESTED READING

Wood MB, Berquist TH. The hand and wrist. In: Berquist TH, ed. *Imaging of Orthopedic Trauma,* 2nd ed. New York: Raven Press; 1992:749–870.

■ FRACTURES/DISLOCATIONS: GALEAZZI FRACTURES

KEY FACTS

- ■ The Galeazzi fracture is a fracture of the distal radius, usually diaphysis, with associated subluxation or dislocation of the DRUJ.
- ■ Mechanism of injury: fall on the outstretched hand with hyperpronation of the forearm.
- ■ Treatment: reduction and internal fixation.
- ■ Routine radiographs are diagnostic.
- ■ Complications: malunion of the fracture and residual subluxation of the DRUJ.

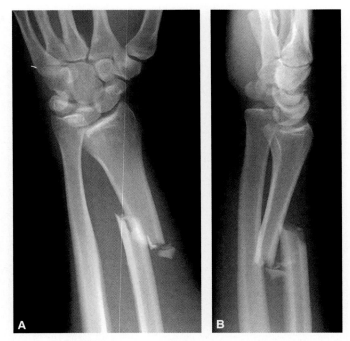

FIGURE 8-9. Posteroanterior (PA) **(A)** and lateral **(B)** radiographs show a distal radial fracture with dislocation of the distal radioulnar joint (DRUJ).

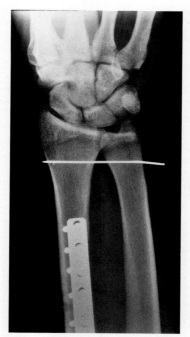

FIGURE 8-10. Posteroanterior (PA) radiograph in a patient with a prior Galeazzi fracture after plate and screw fixation of the radial fracture and K-wire fixation of the joint.

SUGGESTED READING

Wood MB, Berquist TH. The hand and wrist. In: Berquist TH, ed. *Imaging of Orthopedic Trauma*. 2nd ed. New York: Raven Press; 1992:749–870.

▪ FRACTURES/DISLOCATIONS: DISTAL RADIOULNAR JOINT SUBLUXATION/DISLOCATIONS

KEY FACTS

▪ Subluxation or dislocation of the DRUJ may be dorsal (most common) or volar.
▪ Mechanism of injury:
  ● Dorsal—hyperpronation injury
  ● Volar—hypersupination injury to the forearm
▪ Routine radiographic findings may be subtle. Axial CT or magnetic resonance imaging (MRI) with the wrist in pronation, neutral, and supinated positions is most useful to confirm the diagnosis.
▪ Treatment: Closed reduction and cast immobilization may be successful. Open repair may be best for long-term results and optimal stability.

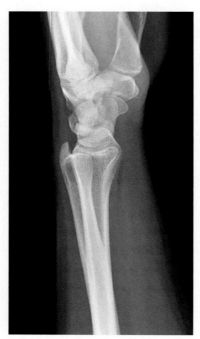

FIGURE 8-11. Lateral radiograph shows distal radioulnar joint subluxation with dorsal subluxation of the distal ulna in relation to the distal radius.

SUGGESTED READING

Hamlin C. Traumatic disruption of the distal radioulnar joint. *Am J Sports Med.* 1977;5:93–96.
Nakamura R, Horie E, Imaeda T, et al. Criteria for diagnosing distal radioulnar joint subluxation by computed tomography. *Skeletal Radiol.* 1996;25:649–653.

■ FRACTURES/DISLOCATIONS: SCAPHOID FRACTURES

KEY FACTS

- The scaphoid is the most commonly fractured carpal bone in adults, accounting for 70% of all carpal injuries. Scaphoid fractures in children account for only 2.9% of hand and wrist fractures.
- Mechanism of injury: fall on the outstretched hand.
- Scaphoid fractures may be difficult to detect and treat. Nonunion and avascular necrosis (AVN) are common complications.
- Scaphoid fractures are classified by fracture location and orientation of the fracture line. Fractures may involve the (1) tubercle, (2) distal articular surface, (3) fracture of the distal third, (4) waist fracture, or (5) proximal pole fracture (Fig. 8-12).
- Imaging of scaphoid fractures requires AP, lateral, and scaphoid views. Displacement or obliteration of the navicular fat stripe is a useful sign for subtle fractures. Radionuclide scans, MRI, or CT may be useful for detecting subtle fractures and evaluating complications.
- Treatment: cast immobilization for undisplaced fractures. Displaced fractures (>1 mm step-off or angulation) are treated with internal fixation.
- Complications: delayed union (failure to unite in 3 months), nonunion, malunion, AVN (most common with proximal pole fractures), radioscaphoid impingement, and arthrosis.

(continued)

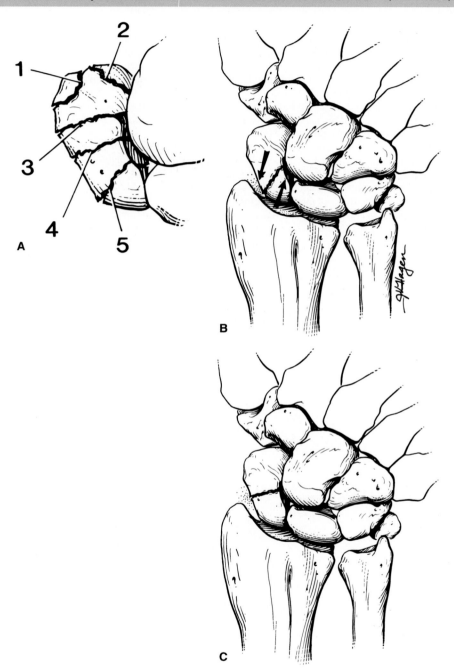

FIGURE 8-12. (A) Locations of scaphoid fractures: 1, tubercle; 2, distal articular surface; 3, distal third; 4, waist; 5, proximal pole. **(B)** Oblique fracture. Shearing forces (*arrows*) lead to instability and displacement. **(C)** Transverse waist fracture is more stable.

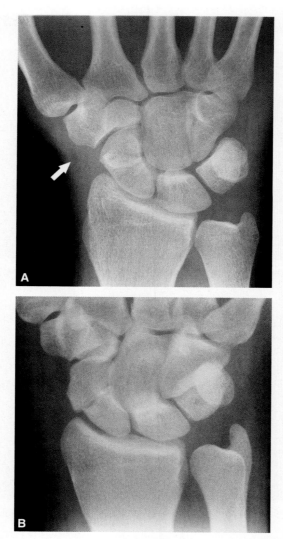

FIGURE 8-13. (A) Subtle scaphoid fracture with absent navicular fat stripe (*arrow*). **(B)** Displaced scaphoid waist fracture.

(continued)

■ FRACTURES/DISLOCATIONS: SCAPHOID FRACTURES *(Continued)*

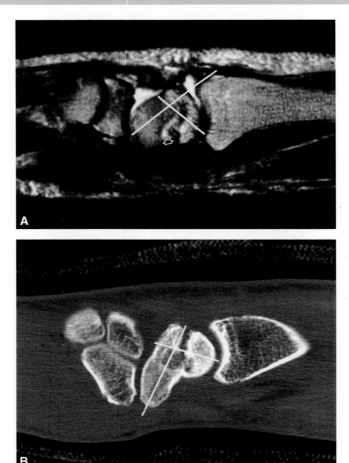

FIGURE 8-14. Humpback deformity. **(A)** Sagittal proton density–weighted magnetic resonance (MR) image demonstrates fluid (*open arrow*) in the fracture line and deformity (*white lines*) caused by dorsal separation of the fracture's fragments. **(B)** Sagittal reformatted computed tomography (CT) image demonstrates a similar humpback deformity (*lines*) with sclerosis of the proximal fragment caused by avascular necrosis (AVN).

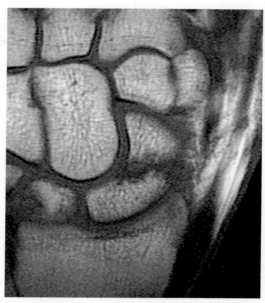

FIGURE 8-15. Coronal T1-weighted magnetic resonance (MR) image shows nondisplaced scaphoid fracture, which was radiographically occult.

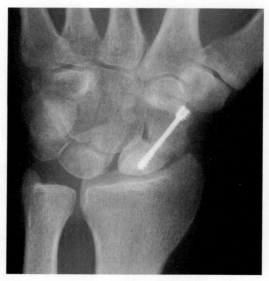

FIGURE 8-16. Posteroanterior (PA) view of a displaced scaphoid fracture with Herbert screw fixation. The proximal pole is sclerotic because of avascular necrosis (AVN).

SUGGESTED READING

Cooney WP III. Isolated carpal fractures. In: Cooney WP III, Linscheid RL, Dobyns JH, eds. *The Wrist: Diagnosis and Operative Treatment*. St. Louis: Mosby; 1998:474–487.

Fisk GR. An overview of injuries of the wrist. *Clin Orthop*. 1980;149:137–144.

■ FRACTURES/DISLOCATIONS: OTHER CARPAL FRACTURES

KEY FACTS

- Other carpal fractures occur less frequently than scaphoid fractures.
- The triquetrum is the second most common carpal bone fractured followed by the capitate and lunate.
- Mechanism of injury: fall on the outstretched hand; compressive or shearing forces.
- Treatment: closed reduction and cast immobilization.
- Imaging usually can be accomplished with radiographs. The lateral view is most useful for triquetral avulsion fractures. Subtle injuries may require CT or MRI.
- Complications: nonunion, arthrosis, and carpal tunnel syndrome.

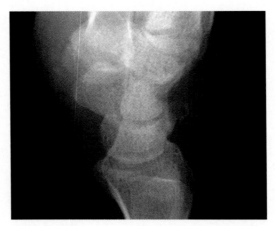

FIGURE 8-17. Lateral radiograph shows a triquetral fracture (*arrow*) seen only on the lateral radiograph.

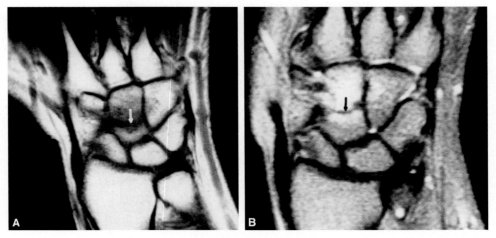

FIGURE 8-18. Coronal T1-weighted **(A)** and T2-weighted **(B)** images of a capitate fracture (*arrow*) with surrounding edema. Radiographs were normal.

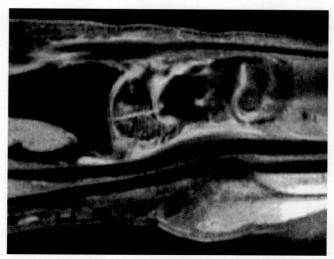

FIGURE 8-19. Sagittal T2-weighted fast spin-echo image with fat suppression demonstrates an undisplaced lunate fracture (*arrow*).

SUGGESTED READING

Berquist TH. *Imaging of Orthopedic Trauma,* 2nd ed. New York: Raven Press; 1992:749–870.

■ FRACTURES/DISLOCATIONS: CARPAL AND CARPOMETACARPAL DISLOCATIONS

KEY FACTS

- Dislocations of the carpus are most often associated with perilunate injury.
- The transscaphoid perilunate dislocation is most common. The proximal scaphoid maintains its lunate relationship, and the distal scaphoid and remainder of the carpal bones displace dorsally.
- Carpometacarpal dislocations are most often associated with distal carpal or metacarpal base fractures.
- Mechanism of injury: fall on the outstretched hand.
- Imaging may be accomplished with posteroanterior (PA) and lateral radiographs. CT is best for subtle cases, evaluation of osteochondral fractures, treatment planning, and postreduction evaluation.
- Treatment: closed reduction if alignment can be restored; otherwise internal fixation.
- Complications: arthrosis, AVN, and instability.

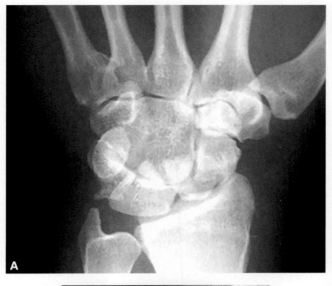

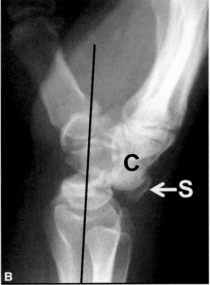

FIGURE 8-20. Transscaphoid perilunate dislocation seen on posteroanterior (PA) **(A)** and lateral **(B)** radiographs. The PA view shows a fracture of the scaphoid with the lunate and proximal scaphoid in nearly normal position **(A)**. The lateral view shows preservation of radiolunate alignment (*line*) but dorsal dislocation of the capitate and second carpal row (*C*). The distal scaphoid fracture fragment **(S)** remains attached to the capitate and is also displaced dorsally **(B)**.

(continued)

■ FRACTURES/DISLOCATIONS: CARPAL AND CARPOMETACARPAL DISLOCATIONS   *(Continued)*

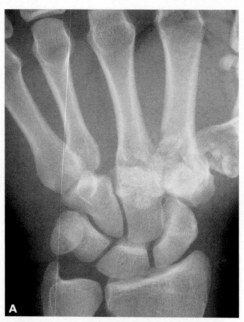

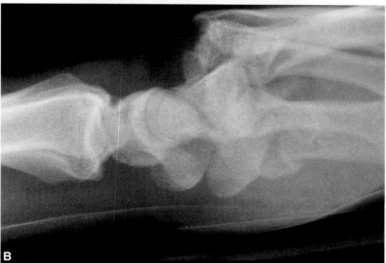

FIGURE 8-21. Posteroanterior (PA) **(A)** and lateral **(B)** radiographs of a carpometacarpal fracture/dislocation.

SUGGESTED READING

Gregor DP, O'Brien ET. Classification and management of carpal dislocations. *Clin Orthop.* 1980;149:55–72.

■ FRACTURES/DISLOCATIONS: METACARPAL FRACTURES

KEY FACTS

- Metacarpal fractures are common. The fourth and fifth metacarpals are most often injured.
- Fractures are generally categorized as thumb, mobile rays (fourth and fifth), and stable rays (second and third).
- Thumb fractures are described by location. In order of decreasing frequency, fractures occur as follows:
  - Intra-articular basilar fractures
  - Proximal metaphyseal fractures
  - Transverse or spiral diaphyseal fractures
  - First metacarpal neck fractures
- Second and third (stable rays) metacarpal fractures
  - Considered stable because of lack of motion at the carpometacarpal joints.
  - Neck fractures are most common.
  - Spiral fractures are less common.
- Fourth and fifth (mobile rays) metacarpal fractures
  - Considered mobile because of motion at carpometacarpal joints.
  - Fractures of the neck and metacarpal bases occur more frequently.
  - Fracture of the fifth metacarpal neck (boxer's fracture) is most common.
- Mechanism of injury: direct trauma and axial loading.
- Imaging with routine radiographs generally is diagnostic. CT may be required to more completely evaluate articular fractures.
- Treatment: closed reduction of nonangulated or nonarticular fractures. Angulated or articular fractures require internal fixation.
- Complications: shortening, rotation (especially spiral fractures), decreased function, malunion, and arthrosis.

(continued)

■ FRACTURES/DISLOCATIONS: METACARPAL FRACTURES *(Continued)*

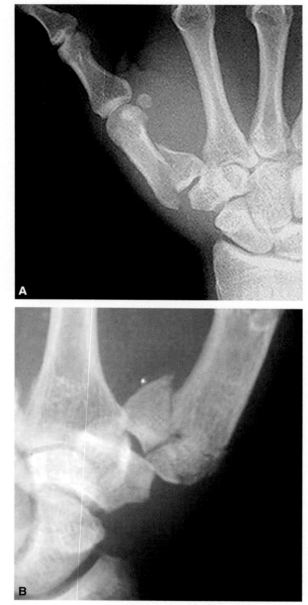

FIGURE 8-22. Radiograph of the thumb **(A)** demonstrates a Bennett fracture with a two-part intra-articular fracture/dislocation at base of first metacarpal with a small fragment remaining articulated with the trapezium and lateral retraction of first metacarpal by abductor pollicis longus. Radiograph in another patient **(B)** depicts a Rolando fracture with a Y-shaped three-fragment fracture of the first metacarpal, which extends to the articular surface of the first carpometacarpal (CMC) articulation.

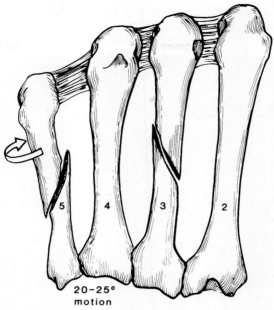

FIGURE 8-23. The second to fifth metacarpals. There is laxity in the transverse metacarpal ligament between the fourth and fifth metacarpals, which leads to shortening and rotation with oblique or spiral factures. There is more motion allowed at the fourth and fifth metacarpal bases.

FIGURE 8-24. Posteroanterior (PA) view of a fifth metacarpal neck fracture (boxer's fracture). Note the apex dorsal angulation at the fracture site (*lines*) with volar displacement of the fifth metacarpal head (*arrow*).

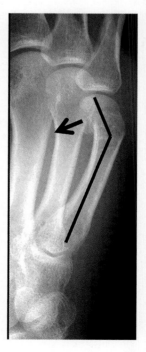

(continued)

■ FRACTURES/DISLOCATIONS: METACARPAL FRACTURES *(Continued)*

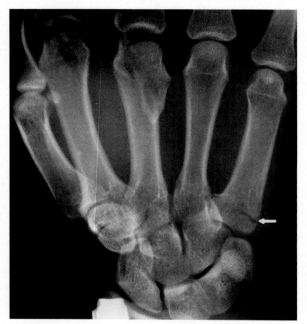

FIGURE 8-25. Posteroanterior (PA) radiograph shows intra-articular fractures of the second and third metacarpals and an undisplaced fracture of the fifth metacarpal base (*arrow*).

SUGGESTED READING

Berquist TH. *Imaging of Orthopedic Trauma.* 2nd ed. New York: Raven Press; 1992:749–870.

■ FRACTURES/DISLOCATIONS: PHALANGEAL FRACTURES/ DISLOCATIONS

KEY FACTS

- Phalangeal fractures are the most common fractures in the hand. Fractures of the proximal phalanx are most common.
- Dislocations of the phalangeal and metacarpophalangeal (MCP) joints are usually dorsal.
- Mechanism of injury: direct blows, falls, and athletic injuries.
- Imaging with PA and lateral radiographs is usually adequate. CT may be required after reduction for osteochondral evaluation.
- Treatment: closed reduction unless there is shortening, angulation, or significant articular involvement.
- Complications: shortening, rotation, arthrosis, and decreased joint function.

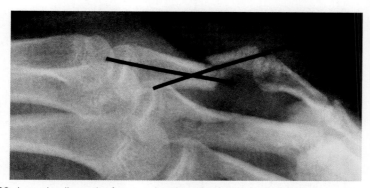

FIGURE 8-26. Lateral radiograph of an angulated proximal phalangeal fracture.

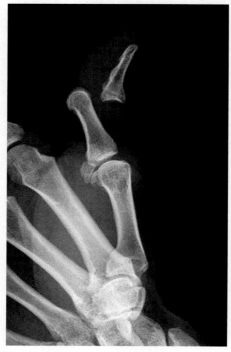

FIGURE 8-27. Lateral view of a dorsal phalangeal dislocation.

(continued)

▪ FRACTURES/DISLOCATIONS: PHALANGEAL FRACTURES/ DISLOCATIONS   *(Continued)*

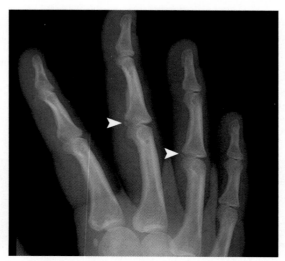

FIGURE 8-28. Oblique radiograph of the hand depicts volar plate injuries involving the third and fourth middle phalanges (*arrowheads*) related to a hyperextension injury.

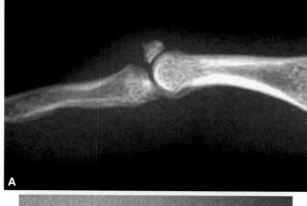

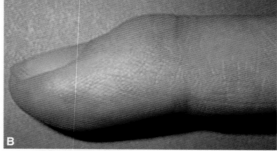

FIGURE 8-29. Lateral view **(A)** of a hyperflexion Mallet fracture of the distal phalanx. A photograph of the finger **(B)** depicts the residual flexion deformity at the distal interphalangeal (DIP) joint due to disruption of the extensor mechanism of the finger at the level of the DIP joint.

SUGGESTED READING

Ruby LK. Common hand injuries in athletes. *Orthop Clin North Am.* 1980;11:819–839.

■ CARPAL INSTABILITY

KEY FACTS

■ Carpal instability can be seen after fractures and ligament injuries, or in association with inflammatory arthropathies.

■ Dorsal intercalated segment instability (DISI) is most common. On the lateral radiographs, the scapholunate angle is increased (>60 degrees), and the lunate–capitate angle is increased (>30 degrees). The abnormal lunate–capitate angle is apex dorsal and the lunate faces dorsally.

■ Volar intercalated segment instability is seen less frequently. The scapholunate angle is decreased (<30 degrees), and the lunate–capitate angle is increased (>30 degrees). The abnormal lunate–capitate angle is apex volar and the lunate faces volarly.

■ Scapholunate advanced collapse (SLAC) results from chronic scapholunate dissociation and results in radioscapoid arthropathy with sparing of the radiolunate space. The captitate migrates proximally into the widened scapholunate space resulting from the chronic scapholunate ligament tear.

■ Scaphoid nonunion advanced collapse (SNAC) results from chronic scaphoid fracture nonunion and results in similar instability pattern as SLAC, except the capitate migrates proximally into the space created by the collapsed proximal pole of the scaphoid.

■ Diagnosis can be accomplished on PA and lateral radiographs.

■ Treatment options include proximal row carpectomy, wrist fusion, or limited carpal (four corner) fusion.

(continued)

■ CARPAL INSTABILITY   *(Continued)*

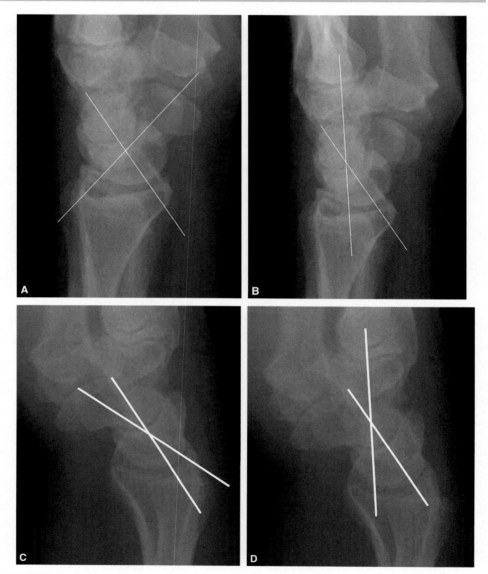

FIGURE 8-30. Lateral radiographs of the wrist demonstrate dorsal intercalated segmental instability (DISI) with dorsal tilt of the lunate and an abnormally increased scapholunate angle measuring greater than 60 degrees **(A)**, and an abnormally increased lunate–capitate angle measuring greater than 30 degrees with apex dorsal angulation **(B)**. Lateral radiographs in another patient demonstrate volar intercalated segmental instability (VISI) with volar tilt of the lunate and an abnormally decreased scapholunate angle measuring less than 30 degrees **(C)**, and an abnormally decreased lunate–capitate angle measuring less than 30 degrees with apex volar angulation **(D)**.

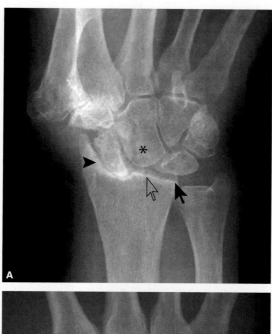

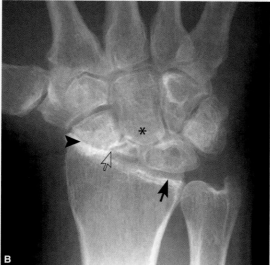

FIGURE 8-31. Scapholunate advanced collapse (SLAC) **(A)** and scaphoid nonunion advanced collapse (SNAC) **(B)**. Posteroanterior (PA) radiograph of the wrist in a patient with SLAC **(A)** demonstrates marked widening of the scapholunate space (*open arrow*) compatible with disruption of the scapholunate ligament. There is proximal migration of the capitate (*asterisk*) with narrowing of the radioscaphoid articulation (*arrowhead*), but relative sparing of the radiolunate articulation (*arrow*). PA radiographs in another patient with SNAC **(B)** demonstrate marked chronic nonunion of a scaphoid fracture (*open arrow*). There is narrowing of the radioscaphoid articulation (*arrowhead*) with relative sparing of the radiolunate articulation (*arrow*). There is associated proximal migration of the capitate (*asterisk*) into the defect created by the collapse of the proximal pole of the scaphoid.

SUGGESTED READING

Cohen MS. Degenerative arthritis of the wrist: proximal row carpectomy versus scaphoid excision and four corner arthrodesis. *J Hand Surg.* 2001;26A:94–104.

Linscheid RL, Dobyns JH, Beabout JW, et al. Traumatic instability of the wrist: diagnosis, classification, and pathomechanics. *J Bone Joint Surg.* 1972;54A:1612–1632.

■ SOFT TISSUE TRAUMA/MISCELLANEOUS CONDITIONS: LIGAMENT INJURIES

KEY FACTS

- ■ Ligament injuries of the hand and wrist may occur as isolated injuries or in association with fractures.
- ■ Ligament anatomy of the wrist is complex, including dorsal and volar capsular ligaments and interosseous ligaments.
- ■ Ligamentous support of the MCP and phalangeal joints is similar with collateral ligaments, accessory collateral ligaments, and the volar plate.
- ■ Common ligament injuries of the hand and wrist are as follows:
  - ● Scapholunate ligament tear
  - ● Lunotriquetral ligament tear
  - ● Triangular fibrocartilage complex tears
  - ● "Gamekeeper's thumb"—tear of the ulnar collateral ligament of the first MCP joint
- ■ Imaging of ligament injuries may be accomplished with several approaches.
  - ● Stress views—varus and valgus of the involved joint (MCP and interphalangeal).
  - ● Motion series of the wrist—PA radial and ulnar deviation, flexion and extension lateral, and clenched-fist PA.
  - ● Arthrography—involved wrist of the hand or wrist is injected with iodinated contrast. Extravasation is seen with capsule and ligament tears. Anesthetic can be injected to confirm source of pain.
  - ● MRI, magnetic resonance (MR) arthrography, or CT arthrography—fluid (T2-weighted image) or contrast passes through ligament and capsular defects.

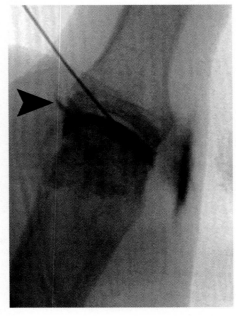

FIGURE 8-32. Arthrogram of the first metacarpophalangeal (MCP) joint shows extravasation (*arrowhead*) resulting from gamekeeper's thumb with an ulnar collateral ligament tear.

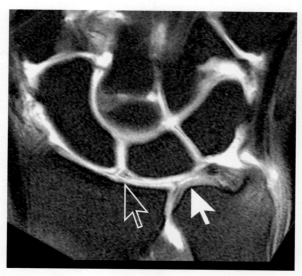

FIGURE 8-33. Coronal image from a magnetic resonance (MR) arthrogram of the wrist shows a tear of the scapholunate ligament allowing contrast to spill from the radiocarpal joint into the midcarpal articulation (*open arrow*). There is also a central perforation of the triangular fibrocartilage allowing contrast to spill from the radiocarpal joint into the distal radioulnar joint (*arrow*).

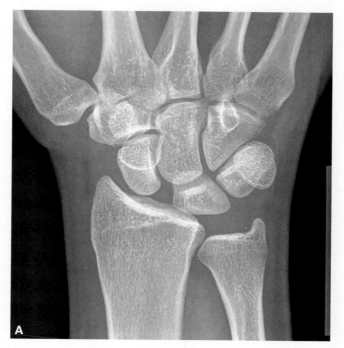

FIGURE 8-34. Scapholunate tear. **(A)** Posteroanterior (PA) radiograph of the wrist shows widening of the scapholunate space. **(B)** Coronal reformatted image from a computed tomography (CT) arthrogram in another patient depicts a tear of the scapholunate ligament allowing contrast to spill from the radiocarpal articulation into the midcarpal joint (*arrow*).

(continued)

■ SOFT TISSUE TRAUMA/MISCELLANEOUS CONDITIONS: LIGAMENT INJURIES   *(Continued)*

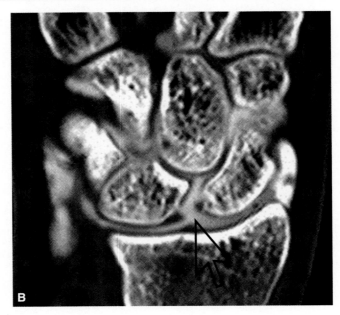

FIGURE 8-34. *(continued)*

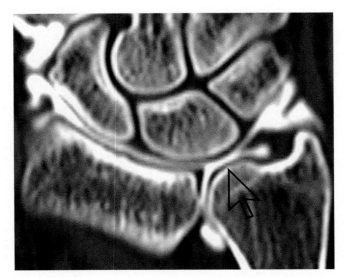

FIGURE 8-35. Triangular fibrocartilage tear. Coronal reformatted image from a computed tomography (CT) arthrogram of the wrist shows a central perforation of the triangular fibrocartilage. Following injection of the radiocarpal joint, contrast passes through a triangular fibrocartilage tear (*arrow*) into the distal radioulnar joint.

SUGGESTED READING

Girgis W, Epstein RE. Magnetic resonance imaging of the hand and wrist. *Semin Roentgenol.* 2000;35:286–296.
Schweitzer ME, Brahine SK, Holder J, et al. Chronic wrist pain: spin-echo and short TI inversion recovery MR imaging and conventional and MR arthrography. *Radiology.* 1992;182:205–211.

■ SOFT TISSUE TRAUMA/MISCELLANEOUS CONDITIONS: TENDON INJURIES

KEY FACTS

- Tendon injuries include partial and complete tears, subluxation or dislocation, and tendinitis. The last is most common.
- Tendinitis may be the result of infection, previous fracture, or overuse.
- Imaging of tendon injuries can be performed with tenography, ultrasound, or MRI. The latter is noninvasive and preferred in most cases. T2-weighted sequences in the axial and coronal or sagittal planes can detect inflammation and tears. With tears, both ends of the tendon must be demonstrated for operative planning.
- Tears in the pulley systems of the flexor tendons may also occur. Patients should be studied in the sagittal plane with the finger in flexion and extension. The "bowstring sign" may be seen with widening of the space between the flexor tendon and the phalanges on flexion images.

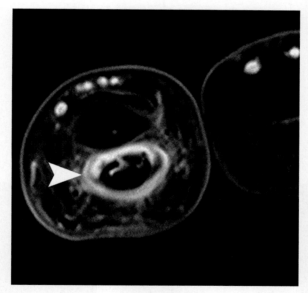

FIGURE 8-36. Flexor tenosynovitis. Axial postcontrast T1-weighted image with fat saturation depicts enhancement and synovitis surrounding the flexor tendon sheath of the index finger (*arrowhead*) compatible with flexor tenosynovitis.

(continued)

■ SOFT TISSUE TRAUMA/MISCELLANEOUS CONDITIONS: TENDON INJURIES *(Continued)*

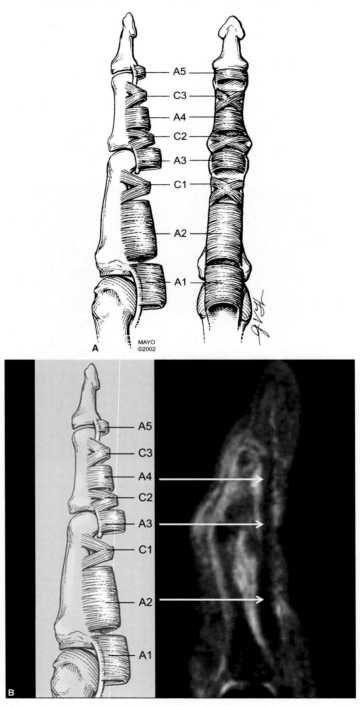

FIGURE 8-37. Flexor tendon and pulley injuries. **(A)** The pulley system maintains position of the flexor tendons. There are five annular and three cruciform pulleys. **(B)** Sagittal fat-suppressed fast spin-echo T2-weighted image demonstrates a tear of the A2, A3, and A4 flexor tendon pulleys with separation of the flexor tendon from the phalanges (*arrows*).

SUGGESTED READING

Clavero JA, Alomar X, Moukill JM, et al. MR imaging of ligament and tendon injuries of the fingers. *Radiographics.* 2002;22:237–257.

Klauser A, Frauscher F, Bodner G, et al. Finger pulley injuries in extreme rock climbers: depiction with dynamic US. *Radiology.* 2002; 222:755–761.

Paradella JA, Balkisoon ARA, Hayes CW, et al. Bowstring injury of the flexor tendon pulley system: MR imaging. *Am J Roentgenol.* 1996;167:347–349.

■ SOFT TISSUE/MISCELLANEOUS CONDITIONS: DE QUERVAIN TENOSYNOVITIS AND INTERSECTION SYNDROME

KEY FACTS

- De Quervain tenosynovitis involves the first dorsal extensor compartment.
- Patients present with pain and restriction of the extensor pollicis brevis and abductor pollicis longus.
- The condition is most common in women 30 to 50 years of age involved in overuse of motions such as grasp and radial and ulnar deviation of the wrist.
- Clinical symptoms may mimic a scaphoid fracture, flexor carpi radialis tendinitis, or intersection syndrome (squeaker's wrist).
- Intersection syndrome occurs related to friction between the first and second extensor compartment tendons, where they cross several centimeters proximal to the wrist joint (Fig. 8-38). This typically results in tendinopathy and tenosynovitis of the second extensor compartment tendons, the extensor carpi radialis longus and brevis. A bursa may form between the extensor carpi radialis longus and brevis and the abductor pollicis longus and extensor pollicis brevis.
- Patients with intersection syndrome are frequently involved in racket sports, and present with pain, weak grip, and crepitation (squeaker's wrist).
- MRI or ultrasound may be used to confirm the diagnosis. The region of the radial styloid may have abnormal signal intensity as the result of chronic tendon thickening. A fluid-filled bursa is typical in intersection syndrome.

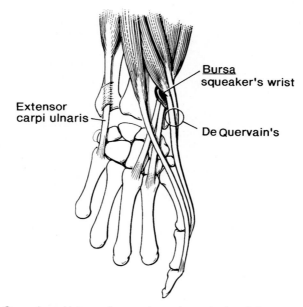

FIGURE 8-38. De Quervain and intersection syndrome (squeaker's wrist).

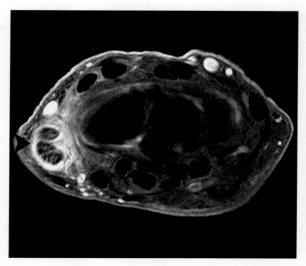

FIGURE 8-39. De Quervain tenosynovitis. Axial fast spin-echo fat-suppressed T2-weighted image demonstrates fluid and synovitis surrounding the abductor pollicis longus and extensor pollicis brevis tendons (*arrowhead*).

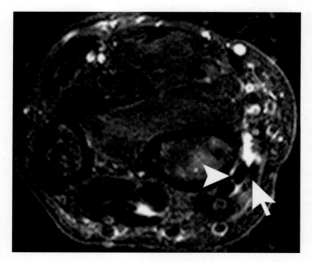

FIGURE 8-40. Intersection syndrome. Axial fat-suppressed T2-weighted image demonstrates inflammatory changes about the first (*arrow*) and second (*arrowhead*) extensor tendon compartments where they cross in the distal forearm.

SUGGESTED READING

Costa CR, Morrison WB, Carrino JA. MRI features of intersection syndrome of the forearm. *Am J Roentgenol.* 2003;181:1245–1249.

Glajchen N, Schweitzer ME. MRI features in de Quervain's tenosynovitis of the wrist. *Skeletal Radiol.* 1996;25:63–65.

■ NEOPLASMS: BONE TUMORS

KEY FACTS

- Bone tumors are uncommon in the hand and wrist compared with the axial skeleton and lower extremity.
- Benign tumors are more common than malignant tumors.
- Table 8-1 lists common tumor and tumorlike conditions in the hand and wrist.
- Routine radiographs remain the main screening technique for patients with suspected bone neoplasms. CT or MRI is useful for treatment planning.

Table 8-1 BONE TUMOR AND TUMORLIKE CONDITIONS IN THE HAND AND WRIST

	No. in Hand and Wrist/Total/%
Benign	
Enchondroma	130/290/45
Giant cell tumor	84/568/15
Aneurysmal bone cyst	34/289/12
Osteoid osteoma	29/331/9
Chondromyxoid fibroma	3/45/7
Osteochondroma	30/872/3
Osteoblastoma	3/87/3
Chondroblastoma	1/119/0.8
Benign vascular tumors	0/108/0
Fibrous defects	0/125/0
Malignant	
Hemangioendothelioma	6/80/7.5
Malignant fibrous histiocytoma	2/83/2
Chondrosarcoma	18/895/2
Fibrosarcoma	5/255/2
Osteosarcoma	17/1,649/1
Ewing sarcoma	6/512/1
Lymphoma	6/694/0.8
Metastasis	2/3,000/0.06
Myeloma	0/814/0

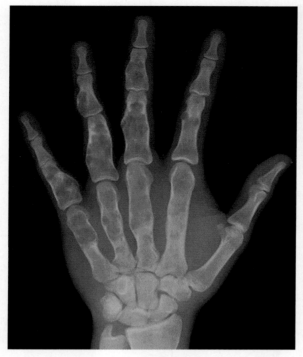

FIGURE 8-41. Ollier disease. Posteroanterior (PA) radiograph of the hand demonstrates multiple lytic expansile lesions throughout the hand compatible with multiple enchondromas.

SUGGESTED READING

Peterson JJ, Bancroft LW, Kransdorf MJ. Principles of bone and soft tissue imaging. *Hand Clin.* 2004;(20):147–166.
Pozanski AK. *The Hand in Radiologic Diagnosis.* Philadelphia: WB Saunders; 1984.
Unni KK. *Dahlin's Bone Tumors: General Aspects and Data on 11,087 Cases.* 5th ed. Philadelphia: Lippincott-Raven; 1996.

■ NEOPLASMS: SOFT TISSUE MASSES

KEY FACTS

- Most soft tissue masses of the hand and wrist are benign.
- Imaging of soft tissue masses is difficult with radiographs. Ultrasound is useful, but MRI is preferred for detection and classification of these lesions.
- Common soft tissue masses of the hand and wrist include
  - Ganglion cysts (commonly associated with internal derangements of the wrist)
  - Epidermoid cysts (distal finger)
  - Glomus tumors (subungual or palmar aspect of finger)
  - Giant cell tumor of the tendon sheath
  - Mucoid cysts (distal joints of hand)
  - Lipomas
  - Hemangiomas
  - Neuromas

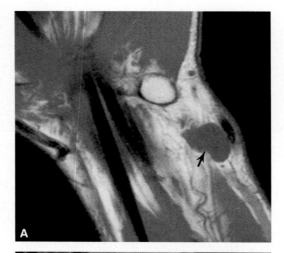

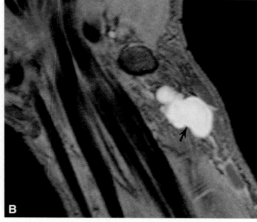

FIGURE 8-42. Coronal T1-weighted **(A)** and fat-suppressed fast spin-echo T2-weighted **(B)** images of the wrist demonstrate a lobulated ganglion cyst (*arrow*).

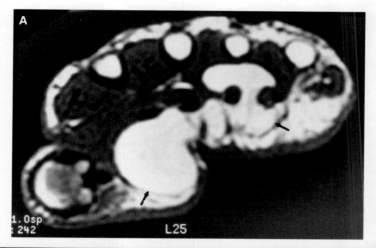

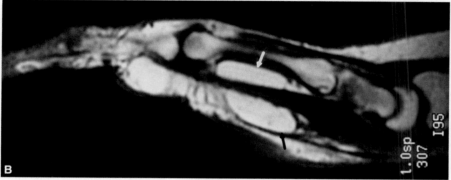

FIGURE 8-43. Lipoma. Axial **(A)** and sagittal **(B)** T1-weighted images of a lobulated fatty lesion (*arrows*) characteristic of a lipoma.

SUGGESTED READING

Butler ED, Hamell JP, Seipel RS, et al. Tumors of the hand. A 10-year survey and report of 437 cases. *Am J Surg.* 1960;100:293–302.

Peterson JJ, Bancroft LW, Kransdorf MJ. Principles of bone and soft tissue imaging. *Hand Clin.* 2004;(20):147–166.

■ ARTHROPATHIES

KEY FACTS

- Numerous arthropathies affect the hand and wrist (Table 8-2).
- Routine radiographs of the hands provide the best screening tool for patients with arthritis. Dynamic contrast-enhanced MRI can detect synovial changes early and monitor disease activity.
- Image features and distribution of involvement are useful in determining the type of arthritis.
- Swelling: uniform, periarticular, fusiform (sausage digit—psoriasis), and lumpy (rheumatoid nodules and sarcoid)
- Subluxation: common with rheumatoid arthritis and systemic lupus erythematosus
- Mineralization: usually normal except infection or rheumatoid arthritis
- Calcification: seen in gouty tophi, scleroderma, mixed connective tissue disease, tumoral calcinosis, and chondrocalcinosis
- Distal joints: osteoarthritis and psoriasis
- Proximal joints: rheumatoid arthritis

Table 8-2 ARTHROPATHIES OF THE HAND AND WRIST

Image Features	Rheumatoid	Psoriasis	Osteoarthritis	CPPD	Gout
Soft tissues	Symmetric wrist, MCP, PIP	Fusiform, Sausage digit	DIP and PIP joints	Mild swelling	Nodular
Subluxation	MCP late	Distal if present	DIP and PIP joints	No	uncommon
Bone density	Decreased	Normal to ↑	Normal to ↑	Normal	Normal
Erosions	Poorly defined	Large, pencil in cup	Central in erosive OA	No	Well defined, overhanging edge
Joint space	Uniformly narrowed	Widened	Narrowed	Narrowed	Narrowed
Calcifications	No	No	No	Yes	Tophi
New bone formation	No	Yes	Osteophytes	Osteophytes	±
Distribution	PIP, MCP, wrist	Distal	DIP, PIP, MCP, wrist, variable	MCP, wrist	Random

CPPD, calcium pyrophosphate dihydrate deposition; DIP, distal interphalangeal; MCP, metacarpophalangeal; PIP, proximal interphalangeal; OA, osteoarthritis.

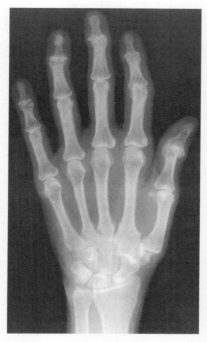

FIGURE 8-44. Posteroanterior (PA) view of the hand and wrist with changes of osteoarthritis in the distal phalangeal joints and wrist. There are changes of erosive osteoarthritis in the second through fourth distal phalangeal joints.

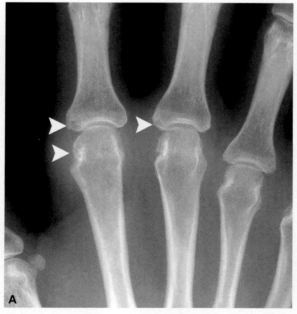

FIGURE 8-45. Rheumatoid arthritis. **(A)** Early changes in the hand with soft tissue swelling and erosions (*arrowheads*). **(B)** Advanced rheumatoid arthritis with subluxation and extensive erosions about the hand and wrist.

(continued)

■ ARTHROPATHIES *(Continued)*

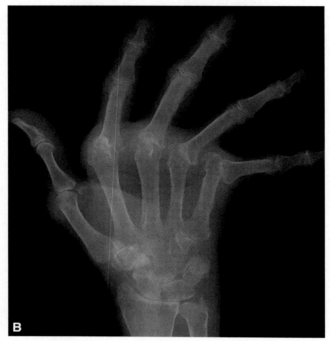

FIGURE 8-45. (*continued*)

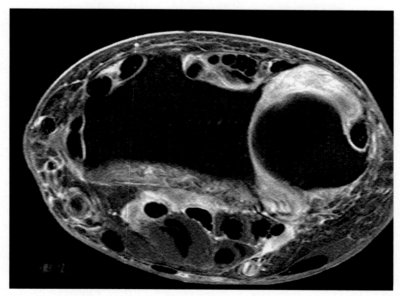

FIGURE 8-46. Rheumatoid arthritis. Axial T1-weighted image with fat saturation following gadolinium administration demonstrates erosion and synovitis involving the distal radioulnar joint. Tenosynitis is also present in several flexor and extensor tendon compartments.

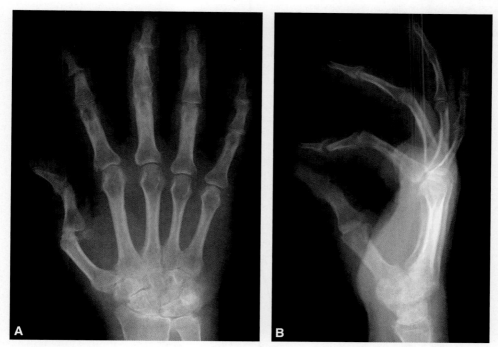

FIGURE 8-47. Psoriatic arthritis. Posteroanterior (PA) **(A)** and lateral **(B)** radiographs demonstrate fusiform swelling of the index finger with erosive changes in the distal interphalangeal joint of the index and long fingers resulting in pencil in cup deformities. There is ankylosis of the first and forth distal interphalangeal joints.

SUGGESTED READING

Brower AC. *Arthritis in Black and White.* Philadelphia: WB Saunders; 1997:33–67.

■ AVASCULAR NECROSIS

KEY FACTS

■ AVN can involve any osseous structure in the hand and wrist. AVN commonly involves the lunate (Kienböck disease), the proximal scaphoid after fracture (Preiser disease), and, to a lesser extent, the capitate and metacarpal heads.

■ Kienböck disease is considered traumatic. Patients present with vague wrist pain. AVN of the lunate is associated with ulnar minus variance (ulna shorter than radius).

■ Routine radiographs are often normal in early stages of AVN. Later, bone sclerosis and fragmentation occur. Early detection can be accomplished with radionuclide scans, but MRI is the technique of choice for early detection and after the healing process.

■ MRI of AVN can be performed using T1- and T2-weighted sequences. The coronal plane is most useful for the lunate, proximal scaphoid, and other carpal bones. Intravenous gadolinium is useful for evaluating flow and subtle changes.

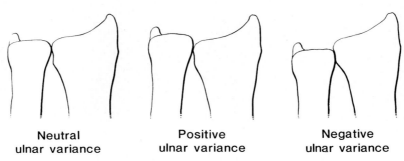

Neutral ulnar variance   **Positive ulnar variance**   **Negative ulnar variance**

FIGURE 8-48. Normal (neutral), ulnar positive, and ulnar negative variance. Ulnar negative variance is associated with avascular necrosis (AVN) of the lunate. Ulnar positive variance is associated with ulnar lunate abutment syndrome.

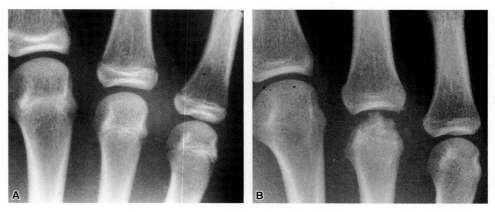

FIGURE 8-49. Baseball player with hand pain after trauma. **(A)** Initial radiograph is normal. **(B)** Repeat radiograph one year later, there is fragmentation of the fourth metacarpal head as the result of avascular necrosis (AVN).

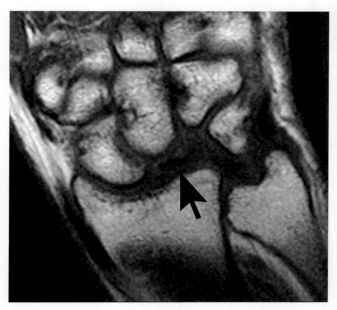

FIGURE 8-50. Avascular necrosis (AVN) of the lunate. T1-weighted magnetic resonance (MR) image shows collapse and sclerosis (*arrow*) in the lunate related to AVN.

SUGGESTED READING

Barnes NA, Howes AJ, Jeffers H, et al. Avascular necrosis of the third metacarpal head. *Eur Radiol.* 2000;3:115–117.
Reinus WR, Conway WF, Totty WG, et al. Carpal avascular necrosis: MR imaging. *Radiology.* 1986;160:689–693.

■ NERVE COMPRESSION SYNDROMES: CARPAL TUNNEL SYNDROME

KEY FACTS

■ Patients with carpal tunnel syndrome present with chronic discomfort and tingling in the distribution of the median nerve. Nocturnal symptoms are common. Muscle atrophy may be present on physical examination.

■ Most patients are 30 to 60 years of age. Females outnumber males in the ratio 5:1. The condition is bilateral in 50% of the cases.

■ Cause may be related to tenosynovitis, soft tissue masses, ganglion cysts, fracture deformity, anomalous muscles, or ischemia.

■ Diagnosis is based on physical examination and nerve conduction studies. Imaging, when necessary, can be accomplished with ultrasound or MRI.

■ Treatment: decompression of carpal tunnel.

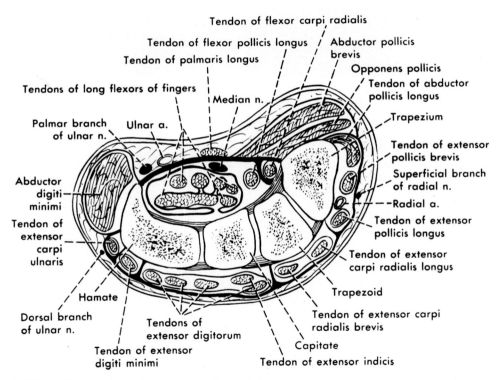

FIGURE 8-51. The relationships of the median and ulnar nerves in the wrist.

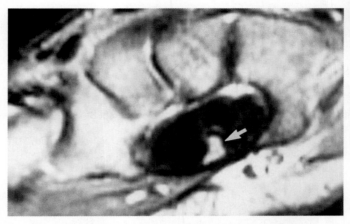

FIGURE 8-52. Axial T2-weighted magnetic resonance (MR) image shows deformity and increased signal intensity in the median nerve (*arrow*) causing carpal tunnel syndrome.

SUGGESTED READING

Campagna R, Pessis E, Feydy A, et al. MRI assessment of recurrent carpal tunnel syndrome after open surgical release of the median nerve. *Am J Roentgenol.* 2009;193(3):644–650.

Ikeda K, Haughton VM, Hu KC, et al. Correlative MR anatomic study of the median nerve. *Am J Roentgenol.* 1996;167:1233–1236.

Mauer J, Bleochkowski A, Tempka A, et al. High-resolution MR imaging of the carpal tunnel and wrist. *Acta Radiol.* 2000;41:78–83.

■ NERVE COMPRESSION SYNDROMES: ULNAR NERVE COMPRESSION

KEY FACTS

- Ulnar nerve compression causes pain and tingling in the distribution of the nerve.
- Compression most commonly occurs in Guyon canal (Fig. 8-53).
- Cause is similar to carpal tunnel syndrome. Primary neural pathology or compression form and adjacent mass are most common.
- Imaging of Guyon canal and the ulnar nerve is most easily accomplished with MRI.
- T2-weighted axial and coronal or sagittal images are most useful.

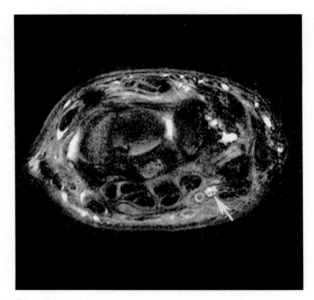

FIGURE 8-53. Axial T2-weighted image demonstrates increased signal intensity and enlargement of the ulnar nerve (*arrow*) resulting from trauma. Findings correlated with electromyography.

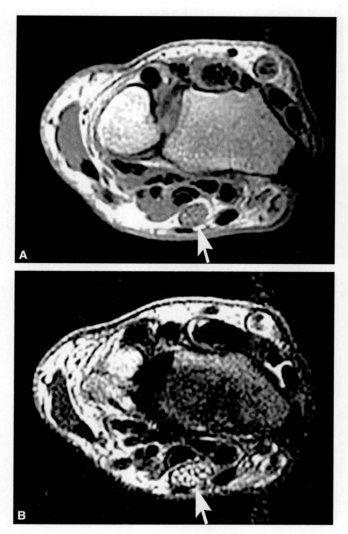

FIGURE 8-54. Lipomatosis of the median nerve. Axial T1-weighted **(A)** and T2-weighted **(B)** images demonstrate an enlarged median nerve with associated fatty tissue interdigitating with the individual fibers of the nerve (*arrow*).

SUGGESTED READING

Andreisek G, Crook DW, Burg, D, et al. Peripheral neuropathies of the median, radial, and ulnar nerves: MR imaging features. *Radiographics.* 2006;26:1267–1287.

Berquist TH. *MRI of the Musculoskeletal System,* 5th ed. Philadelphia: Lippincott Williams & Wilkins; 2006:789–797.

■ ULNAR LUNATE ABUTMENT SYNDROME

KEY FACTS

- Ulnar lunate abutment syndrome is associated with ulnar positive variance (Fig. 8-55).
- Patients present with ulnar wrist pain that is often exaggerated by ulnar deviation of the wrist.
- Radiographs show ulnar positive variance and sclerosis or cystic change in the lunate and triquetrum. Features are more easily demonstrated with MRI for early bone, cartilage, and triangular fibrocartilage abnormalities.
- Treatment: ulnar shortening when conservative treatment fails.

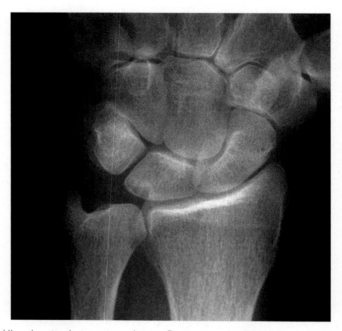

FIGURE 8-55. Ulnar lunate abutment syndrome. Posteroanterior (PA) radiograph demonstrates ulnar positive variance, prominent ulnar styloid, and sclerotic changes in the lunate and triquetrum caused by cartilage loss.

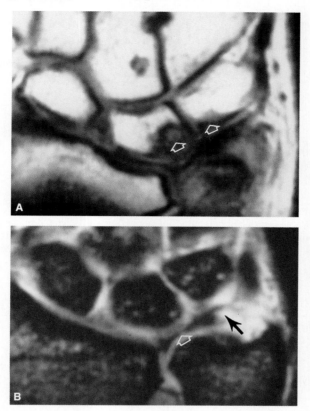

FIGURE 8-56. Magnetic resonance (MR) images in patients with ulnar lunate abutment syndrome. **(A)** T1-weighted image shows low signal intensity in the lunate and adjacent triquetrum. **(B)** Gradient echo coronal shows displacement of the radial aspect of the triangular fibrocartilage (*open arrow*) and a peripheral tear (*black arrow*).

SUGGESTED READING

Cerezal L, del Pinal F, Abascal F, et al. Imaging findings in the ulnar-sided wrist impaction syndromes. *Radiographics.* 2002;22:105–121.

Palmer AK, Werner FW. Triangular fibrocartilage complex of the wrist—anatomy and function. *J Hand Surg.* 1981;16:153–162.

Musculoskeletal Neoplasms

Hillary W. Garner, Jeffrey J. Peterson, Thomas H. Berquist, and Mark J. Kransdorf

■ BONE TUMORS/TUMORLIKE CONDITIONS: IMAGING APPROACHES

KEY FACTS

- Imaging studies are essential for detecting, characterizing, and staging bone lesions.
- Radiographs, computed tomography (CT), magnetic resonance imaging (MRI), and radionuclide scans all play a role. Angiography is useful for evaluating tumor vascularity and for preoperative embolization.
- Effectiveness of imaging studies for evaluating features of bone tumors is as follows:

Radiographs	CT	MRI	Nuclear Medicine
Lesion morphology	Thin cortical bone	Lesion extent	Early detection in marrow and soft tissues
Site (cortical, marrow, diaphysis, metaphysis, epiphysis)	Bone destruction or production	Joint space involvement	Skip lesions
Bone production or destruction	Periosteal response	Marrow edema patterns	Metastasis
Periosteal response	Calcifications/ matrix	Cortical destruction	
Soft tissue calcification or ossifications	Trabecular destruction		

CT, computed tomography; MRI, magnetic resonance imaging.

SUGGESTED READING

Fitzgerald JJ, Roberts CC, Daffner RH, et al. *Follow-Up of Malignant or Aggressive Musculoskeletal Tumors*. Reston: American College of Radiology; 2011.

Garner HW, Kransdorf MJ. Musculoskeletal sarcoma: update on imaging of the post-treatment patient. *Can Assoc Radiol J*. 2016;67(1):12–20.

Hwang S, Panicek DM. The evolution of musculoskeletal tumor imaging. *Radiol Clin North Am*. 2009;47(3):435–453.

Kransdorf MJ, Bridges MD. Current developments and recent advances in musculoskeletal tumor imaging. *Semin Musculoskelet Radiol*. 2013;17(2):145–155.

Mintz DN, Hwang S. Bone tumor imaging, then and now. *HSS J*. 2014;10(3):230–239.

Morrison WB, Weissman BN, Kransdorf MJ, et al. ACR appropriateness criteria—primary bone tumors. Reston: American College of Radiology; 2013.

■ BONE TUMORS/TUMORLIKE CONDITIONS: RADIOGRAPHIC FEATURES

KEY FACTS

■ Patient's age and lesion location are the two most helpful pieces of information when evaluating a bone lesion. Routine radiographs provide additional important information to further narrow the diagnostic possibilities. Key discriminatory radiographic features are as follows:
- Patterns of bone destruction:
  ❖ Geographic: least aggressive. Margins may be sclerotic, well defined without sclerosis, or ill defined.
  ❖ Moth-eaten: more aggressive, less well defined. Wider zone of transition. Seen with malignant lesions and osteomyelitis.
  ❖ Permeative: most aggressive with more rapid destruction. Margins not defined. Seen with aggressive malignancies and infections.
- Bone formation
  ❖ Matrix—calcification or ossification
  ❖ Trabeculation—seen with giant cell tumors, chondromyxoid fibroma, aneurysmal bone cyst, hemangioma, nonossifying fibroma
  ❖ Cortical breach/penetration
  ❖ Periosteal response
  ❖ Soft tissue mass
- Distribution:
  ❖ Central, eccentric, cortical, and juxtacortical
  ❖ Diaphyseal, metaphyseal, and epiphyseal
  ❖ Skeletal location (e.g., tibia and calcaneus)

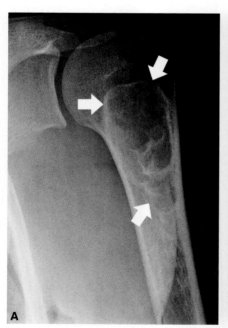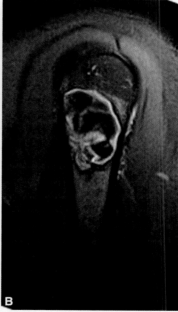

FIGURE 9-1. Patterns of bone destruction—geographic. Anteroposterior (AP) radiograph of the left shoulder **(A)** shows a well-defined geographic lucent lesion with sclerotic septations and a sclerotic margin (*arrows*) in the proximal humeral metaphysis. Corresponding sagittal fat-saturated T2-weighted magnetic resonance (MR) image **(B)** more clearly shows the geographic nature of this nonossifying fibroma.

(continued)

■ BONE TUMORS/TUMORLIKE CONDITIONS: RADIOGRAPHIC FEATURES *(Continued)*

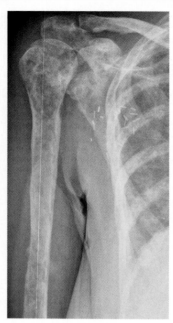

FIGURE 9-2. Patterns of bone destruction—moth-eaten. Anteroposterior (AP) radiograph of the right humerus shows a moth-eaten appearance of the proximal humerus with poorly defined margins as the result of breast cancer metastasis.

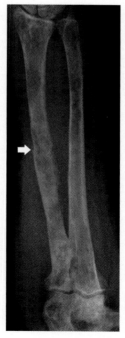

FIGURE 9-3. Patterns of bone destruction—permeative. Anteroposterior (AP) radiograph of the left forearm shows poorly defined lytic lesions in the radius and ulna with permeative cortical changes corresponding to breast cancer metastases. There is a pathologic minimally displaced transverse fracture of the radial shaft (*arrow*).

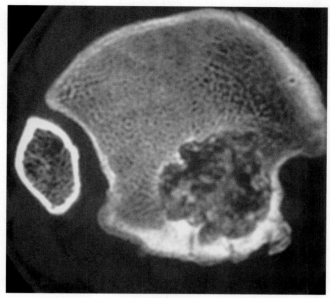

FIGURE 9-4. Matrix calcifications. Axial computed tomography (CT) image of the distal tibial epiphysis shows a well-defined geographic lesion with calcifications. Appearance and location are characteristic of chondroblastoma.

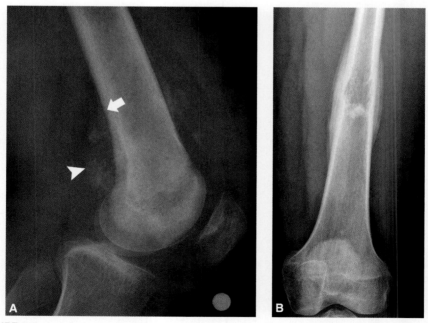

FIGURE 9-5. Aggressive periosteal response. Lateral view of the left knee **(A)** shows an osteogenic sarcoma with osteoid matrix, soft tissue extension, triangular elevation (Codman triangles) (*arrow*), and sunburst periosteal reaction (*arrowhead*). Anteroposterior (AP) view of the left femur **(B)** shows an osteogenic sarcoma with onion-skin periosteal reaction. Codman triangles, sunburst periosteal reaction, and onion-skin periosteal reaction are associated with aggressive lesions.

(continued)

■ BONE TUMORS/TUMORLIKE CONDITIONS: RADIOGRAPHIC FEATURES *(Continued)*

SUGGESTED READING

Caracciolo JT, Temple HT, Letson GD, et al. A modified Lodwick–Madewell grading system for the evaluation of lytic bone lesions. *Am J Roentgenol.* 2016;207(1):150–156.

Miller TT. Bone tumors and tumorlike conditions: analysis with conventional radiography. *Radiology.* 2008;246(3):662–674.

Morrison WB, Weissman BN, Kransdorf MJ, et al. *ACR Appropriateness Criteria—Primary Bone Tumors.* Reston: American College of Radiology; 2013.

Sundaram M, McLeod RA. MR imaging of tumors and tumorlike lesions of bone and soft tissue. *Am J Roentgenol.* 1990;155(4):817–824.

■ BONE TUMORS/TUMORLIKE CONDITIONS: MAGNETIC RESONANCE IMAGING PROTOCOLS

KEY FACTS

■ MRI of bone tumors often requires individualized customization of the imaging protocol compared with other indications for MRI.

■ The coil and the field of view should be selected to best center the lesion of concern for optimal characterization. However, at least one sequence of the MRI examination should be obtained with a large field of view of the entire bone in question to evaluate for skip lesions and possible joint involvement.

■ Image planes should be selected to demonstrate the entire bone of interest on one image, particularly for long bones. This often requires doing oblique rather than "straight" coronal and/or sagittal imaging.

■ Coil selection should account for the anatomic area of interest.

■ Contrast enhancement is used routinely.

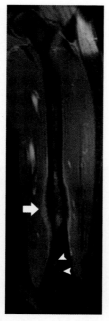

FIGURE 9-6. Optimal imaging protocol. Patients with a diaphyseal femoral sarcoma (*arrow*) and distal metaphyseal femoral skip lesions (*arrowheads*) confirmed after femoral resection. The skip lesions may be missed unless at least one sequence of the magnetic resonance (MR) examination is obtained with a large field of view of the entire bone in question.

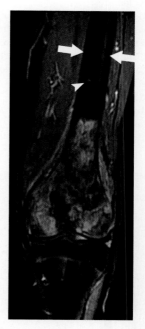

FIGURE 9-7. Optimal imaging planes. Optimal coronal magnetic resonance (MR) image of distal femoral sarcoma with proximal skip lesion (*arrowhead*) shows the entire area of interest on one image with the level of excision marked for limb salvage (*arrows*). At least 3 cm of normal marrow is usually included in the resection.

SUGGESTED READING

Garner HW, Kransdorf MJ. Musculoskeletal sarcoma: update on imaging of the post-treatment patient. *Can Assoc Radiol J.* 2016;67(1):12–20.

Kransdorf MJ, Bridges MD. Current developments and recent advances in musculoskeletal tumor imaging. *Semin Musculoskelet Radiol.* 2013;17(2):145–155.

Morrison WB, Weissman BN, Kransdorf MJ, et al. *ACR Appropriateness Criteria—Primary Bone Tumors.* Reston: American College of Radiology; 2013.

■ BONE TUMORS/TUMORLIKE CONDITIONS: OSTEOID OSTEOMA

KEY FACTS

- ■ Clinical:
  - ● Osteoid osteoma is a relatively common lesion accounting for 10% of benign bone tumors. Patients present with pain, worse at night, often relieved by anti-inflammatory medications (75%).
- ■ Age: 5 to 35 years, peak second decade
- ■ Sex: Males outnumber females in the ratio 3:1.
- ■ Common locations: majority in lower extremity; proximal femur, femoral neck
- ■ Three types of osteoid osteoma:
  - ● Cortical: fusiform cortical thickening with a lucent nidus arising from the cortex
  - ● Cancellous: intramedullary in location. Often involve the femoral neck and small bones of the hand, foot, and posterior elements of the spine.
  - ● Subperiosteal: arise on the surface of bone. Often associated with surrounding solid continuous periosteal reaction.
- ■ Imaging features:
  - ● Radiographic features: small round lucent area with surrounding sclerosis and periosteal reaction. May have central calcification or ossification.
  - ● CT: technique of choice for detection and characterization
  - ● MRI: small focal lesion with surrounding reactive edema on fluid-sensitive sequences. Subtle lesions enhance with dynamic contrast studies.
- ■ Differential diagnosis:
  - ● Brodie abscess
  - ● Osteoblastoma
  - ● Stress fracture
- ■ Treatment: complete resection of nidus; percutaneous radiofrequency ablation

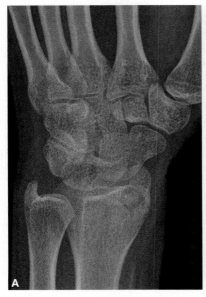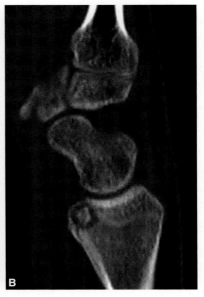

FIGURE 9-8. Osteoid osteoma. Oblique radiograph **(A)** and sagittal computed tomography (CT) **(B)** of the distal forearm demonstrate a lucent nidus with central mineralization in the radial volar aspect of the distal radial epiphysis. Sagittal T1-weighted magnetic resonance (MR) image **(C)** shows mild T1 hyperintensity relative to muscle of the nidus rim (*arrowhead*) with central T1 signal loss (*arrow*) corresponding to the mineralization seen on radiograph and CT. Axial T2-weighted image **(D)** shows edema-like signal in the marrow surrounding the lesion and the volar soft tissues adjacent to the lesion, but the lesion itself (*arrow*) is not well defined.

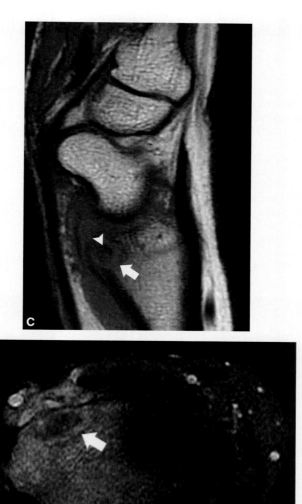

FIGURE 9-8. (*continued*)

SUGGESTED READING

Hakim DN, Pelly T, Kulendran M, Caris JA. Benign tumours of the bone: a review. *J Bone Oncol.* 2015;4(2):37–41.
Jordan RW, Koç T, Chapman AW, et al. Osteoid osteoma of the foot and ankle—a systematic review. *Foot Ankle Surg.* 2015;21(4):228–234.
Liu PT, Chivers FS, Roberts CC, et al. Imaging of osteoid osteoma by dynamic gadolinium-enhanced imaging. *Radiology.* 2003;277:691–700.

▪ BONE TUMORS/TUMORLIKE CONDITIONS: OSTEOBLASTOMA

KEY FACTS

- ▪ Clinical:
  - ● Osteoblastomas account for 3.5% of benign bone tumors. Patients present with chronic local pain.
- ▪ Age: any age, most common second decade
- ▪ Sex: Males outnumber females in the ratio 3:1.
- ▪ Common locations: vertebrae (42.5%), posterior elements most commonly involved
- ▪ Imaging features:
  - ● Radiographic features: may be similar to osteoid osteoma, but larger (>1.5 cm). May have malignant appearance. Bone expanded; 55% have an ossified matrix.
  - ● CT: cortical expansion, ossified matrix
  - ● MRI: variable, not well defined
- ▪ Differential diagnosis:
  - ● Osteoid osteoma
  - ● Aneurysmal bone cyst
  - ● Osteosarcoma
- ▪ Treatment: en bloc resection, bone grafting

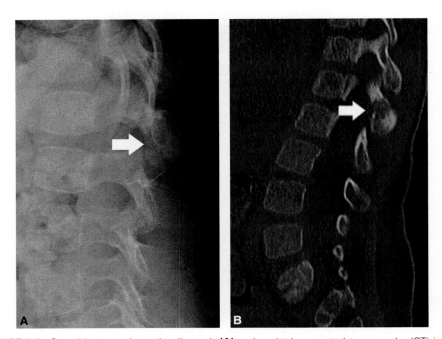

FIGURE 9-9. Osteoblastoma. Lateral radiograph **(A)** and sagittal computed tomography (CT) image **(B)** of the lumbar spine demonstrate a rounded lucent lesion (*arrow*) in the left lamina of the L1 vertebral body. There is subtle internal mineralization and a thin cortical rim seen on the CT. Sagittal T1-weighted magnetic resonance (MR) image **(C)** shows a rounded lesion (*arrow*) with mild T1 hyperintensity relative to the paraspinal musculature (not shown). Sagittal postcontrast T1-weighted MR image **(D)** shows marked reactive enhancement in the soft tissues surrounding the lesion and only mild intralesional enhancement (*arrow*).

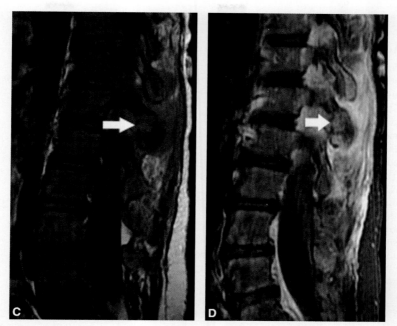

FIGURE 9-9. (*continued*)

SUGGESTED READING

Hakim DN, Pelly T, Kulendran M, Caris JA. Benign tumours of the bone: a review. *J Bone Oncol.* 2015;4(2):37–41.

McLeod RA, Dahlin DC, Beabout JW. The spectrum of osteoblastoma. *Am J Roentgenol.* 1976;126:321–335.

Unni KK. *Dahlin's Bone Tumors: General Aspects and Data on 11,087 Cases.* Philadelphia: Lippincott-Raven; 1996:131–142.

■ BONE TUMORS/TUMORLIKE CONDITIONS: OSTEOCHONDROMA

KEY FACTS

- Clinical:
  - Osteochondromas are the most common, accounting for 35% of benign skeletal neoplasms. Patients present with a palpable mass that may be painful.
- Age: 5 to 50 years, peak second decade
- Sex: Males outnumber females in the ratio 2:1.
- Common locations: distal femur, proximal tibia, proximal humerus
- Imaging features:
  - Radiographic features: bony projection with contiguous marrow and cortex from bone of origin
  - CT: similar to radiograph. Cartilaginous cap more easily appreciated (normal cap thickness <1.5 to 2 cm).
  - MRI: cartilage cap low intensity on T1-weighted and high intensity on T2-weighted sequences. Other features similar to radiographs.
- Differential diagnosis:
  - Usually characteristic
- Treatment: Observe unless symptoms or cosmetic deformity, then resect.

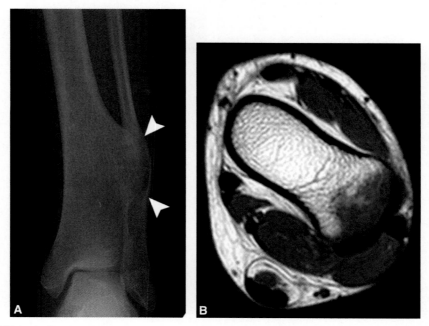

FIGURE 9-10. Osteochondroma. Anteroposterior (AP) radiograph **(A)** and axial T1-weighted **(B)** and axial fluid-sensitive **(C)** magnetic resonance (MR) images of the left lower leg show a distal tibial sessile lesion with corticomedullary continuity typical of osteochondroma. Note the chronic remodeling of the adjacent fibula on the radiograph (*arrowheads*). A thin hyperintense cartilage cap (*arrow*) is best seen on the fluid-sensitive MR image just deep to the chronically remodeled hypointense fibula (*arrowheads*).

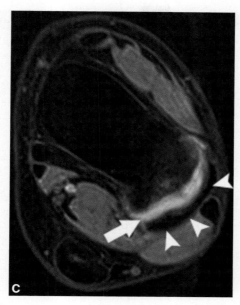

FIGURE 9-10. (*continued*)

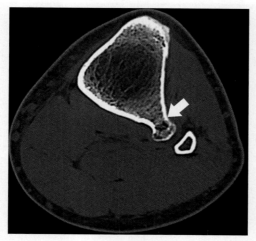

FIGURE 9-11. Osteochondroma. Axial computed tomography (CT) image of a proximal left tibial osteo-chondroma in a different patient again demonstrates the typical corticomedullary continuity (*arrow*).

SUGGESTED READING

Bernard SA, Murphey MD, Flemming DJ, et al. Improved differentiation of benign osteochondromas from second-ary chondrosarcomas with standardized measurement of cartilage cap at CT and MR imaging. *Radiology.* 2010;255(3):857–865.

Douis H, Saifuddin A. The imaging of cartilaginous bone tumours. I. Benign lesions. *Skeletal Radiol.* 2012;41(10):1195–1212.

Unni KK. *Dahlin's Bone Tumors: General Aspects and Data on 11,087 Cases.* 5th ed. Philadelphia: Lippincott-Raven; 1996:11–24, 121–130, 355–432.

■ BONE TUMORS/TUMORLIKE CONDITIONS: ENCHONDROMA

KEY FACTS

- Clinical:
  - Enchondromas account for 13.4% of benign bone tumors. Most are asymptomatic. If painful, low-grade chondrosarcoma should be excluded. Chondrosarcomas have more intense uptake on radionuclide scans and typically erode two-thirds of the cortical thickness. There may also be periosteal reaction and a soft tissue mass.
- Age: all age groups, 55% in the second through fourth decades
- Sex: no sex predilection
- Common locations: small bones of hand and feet (50%) with 87% in the hand, proximal femur, and humerus
- Imaging features:
  - Radiographic features: medullary with sharp margins. Calcification common. May be multiple.
  - CT: well-defined lesion with central calcified matrix. Cortical erosion easily measured.
  - MRI: lobulated low intensity on T1-weighted and high intensity on T2-weighted images. Useful for differentiating enchondroma from chondrosarcoma. Mineralized areas show decreased signal intensity on all pulse sequences.
- Differential diagnosis:
  - Bone infarct
  - Chondrosarcoma
- Treatment: observe. Curettage and bone graft if symptomatic.

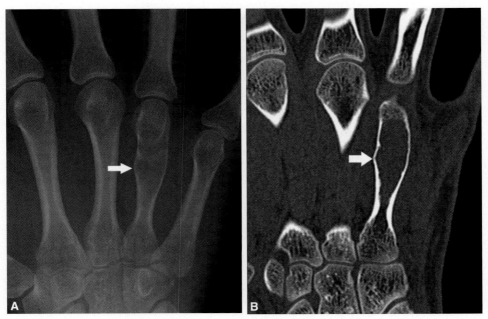

FIGURE 9-12. Enchondroma. Anteroposterior (AP) radiograph **(A)** of the right hand demonstrates a lucent expansile lesion in the fourth metacarpal with endosteal scalloping (*arrow*), better delineated on the corresponding coronal computed tomography (CT) image **(B)**. There is no associated intralesional matrix demonstrated on the radiograph or CT. The lesion is isointense to muscle on the coronal T1-weighted magnetic resonance (MR) image **(C)** and markedly hyperintense on fat-saturated T2-weighted MR image **(D)**. The lesion demonstrates heterogeneous globular enhancement on the coronal postcontrast fat-saturated T1-weighted MR image **(E)**. These radiographic, CT, and MR imaging features are typical of enchondroma in the small bones of the hands and feet.

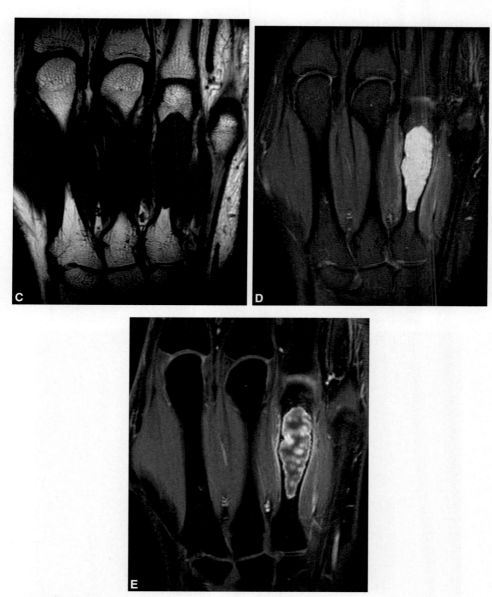

FIGURE 9-12. *(continued)*

(continued)

■ BONE TUMORS/TUMORLIKE CONDITIONS: ENCHONDROMA *(Continued)*

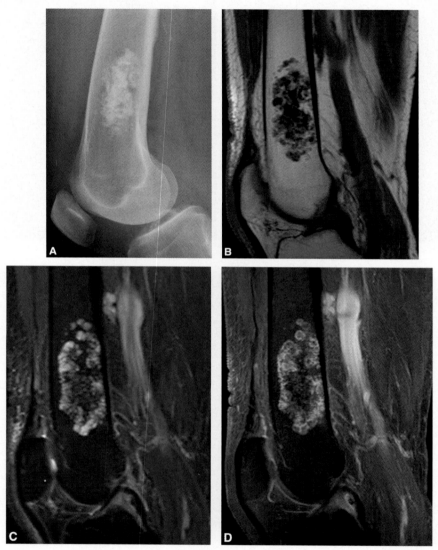

FIGURE 9-13. Enchondroma. Lateral radiograph **(A)** of the right knee demonstrates a geographic lesion in the distal femur with chondroid matrix and no endosteal scalloping. Sagittal T1-weighted **(B)**, fat-saturated T2-weighted **(C)**, and postcontrast fat-saturated T1-weighted **(D)** magnetic resonance (MR) images show the characteristic arc-and-ring morphology of enchondroma, with the peripheral areas of nonmineralized cartilage demonstrating typical iso- to slight hyperintensity on T1, hyperintensity on T2, and rim-like enhancement of the individual cartilage floccules. The central areas of mineralized cartilage demonstrate expected hypointensity on both T1 and T2 without enhancement. There is no marrow edema, cortical destruction, or soft tissue mass.

SUGGESTED READING

Douis H, Saifuddin A. The imaging of cartilaginous bone tumours. I. Benign lesions. *Skeletal Radiol.* 2012;41(10):1195–1212.

Murphy MD, Flemming DJ, Boyea SR, et al. Enchondroma vs. chondrosarcoma in the appendicular skeleton: differentiating features. *Radiographics.* 1998;18:1213–1237.

Stomp W, Reijnierse M, Kloppenburg M, et al. Prevalence of cartilaginous tumours as an incidental finding on MRI of the knee. *Eur Radiol.* 2015;25(12):3480–3487.

■ BONE TUMORS/TUMORLIKE CONDITIONS: CHONDROBLASTOMA

KEY FACTS

- ■ Clinical:
  - ● Patients present with chronic local pain.
- ■ Age: 90% occur from 5 to 25 years of age, approximately 70% in second decade
- ■ Sex: Males outnumber females in the ratio 2 to 3:1.
- ■ Common locations: epiphyseal with 40% in the knee and 16% in the proximal humerus
- ■ Imaging features:
  - ● Radiographic features: epiphyseal location. Sharp margins with sclerotic rim. Calcification in approximately 50% to 60%.
  - ● CT: well-defined lesion with sclerotic margins and, frequently, central calcification
  - ● MRI: well-defined low-intensity lesion on T1-weighted and variably high signal intensity on T2-weighted sequences, with extensive surrounding edema in the majority of cases
- ■ Differential diagnosis:
  - ● Giant cell tumor
  - ● Avascular necrosis
  - ● Clear cell chondrosarcoma
- ■ Treatment: curettage and bone grafting

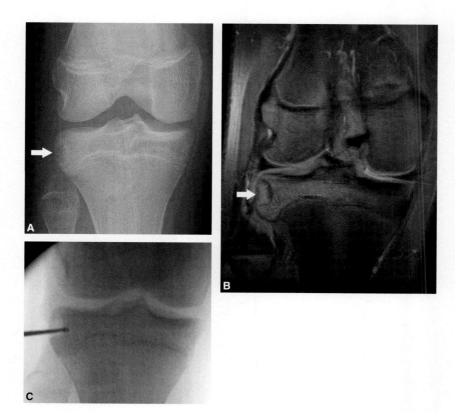

FIGURE 9-14. Chondroblastoma. Anteroposterior (AP) radiograph **(A)** demonstrates a subtle lucent lesion (*arrow*) in the lateral aspect of the right proximal tibial epiphysis with a sclerotic margin and faint intralesional calcifications. Coronal proton density fat-saturated magnetic resonance (MR) image **(B)** demonstrates a well-defined hyperintense lesion (*arrow*) with prominent edema-like signal in the surrounding marrow and adjacent soft tissues. Intraoperative radiograph **(C)** obtained during the later stage of curettage demonstrates a curette within the lesion cavity.

(continued)

■ BONE TUMORS/TUMORLIKE CONDITIONS: CHONDROBLASTOMA *(Continued)*

SUGGESTED READING

Douis H, Saifuddin A. The imaging of cartilaginous bone tumours. I. Benign lesions. *Skeletal Radiol.* 2012;41(10):1195–1212.

Suneja R, Grimer RJ, Belthur M, et al. Chondroblastoma of bone: long-term results and functional outcome after intralesional curettage. *J Bone Joint Surg Br.* 2005;87:974–978.

Unni KK. *Dahlin's Bone Tumors: General Aspects and Data on 11,087 Cases.* Philadelphia: Lippincott-Raven; 1996:47–57.

Weatherall PT, Moole GE, Mendelsohn DB, et al. Chondroblastoma: classic and confusing appearance at MR. *Radiology.* 1994;190:467–474.

Xu H, Nugent D, Monforte HL, et al. Chondroblastoma of bone in the extremities: a multicenter retrospective study. *J Bone Joint Surg Am.* 2015;97(11):925–931.

■ BONE TUMORS/TUMORLIKE CONDITIONS: CHONDROMYXOID FIBROMA

KEY FACTS

- ■ Clinical:
  - ● Patients present with local pain and swelling.
- ■ Age: 5 to 50 years, most common (55%) in the second and third decades
- ■ Sex: slightly more common in males
- ■ Common locations: metaphysis of the knee and distal tibia
- ■ Imaging features:
  - ● Radiographic features: eccentric metaphyseal lesion with well-defined sclerotic margins. Calcifications seen in 12%, more common in those aged more than 40 years.
  - ● CT: eccentric metaphyseal lesion with well-defined sclerotic margins. Calcifications easily appreciated.
  - ● MRI: well-defined lesion with uniform low intensity on T1-weighted and high or intermediate intensity on T2-weighted sequences
- ■ Differential diagnosis:
  - ● Fibrous defect
  - ● Fibrous dysplasia
  - ● Chondroblastoma
  - ● Aneurysmal bone cyst
- ■ Treatment: curettage and bone grafting

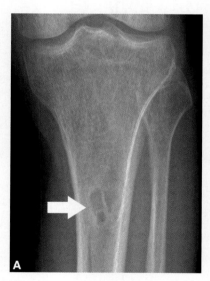

FIGURE 9-15. Chondromyxoid fibroma. Anteroposterior (AP) radiograph of the left lower leg **(A)** shows a lucent lesion (*arrow*) in the proximal tibial diaphysis with sclerotic septations. Axial computed tomography (CT) image **(B)** shows a soft tissue density mass replacing the normal marrow fat density with no matrix calcifications and causing endosteal scalloping (*arrow*). The vertical sclerotic septation seen on radiograph is at the anterior aspect of the mass (*arrowhead*). Axial T1-weighted **(C)**, fat-saturated T2-weighted **(D)**, and postcontrast fat-saturated T1-weighted **(E)** images show a central area of nonenhancing cystic change. The peripheral tissue demonstrates T1 isointensity to muscle, heterogeneous T2 hyperintensity, and enhancement.

(continued)

■ BONE TUMORS/TUMORLIKE CONDITIONS: CHONDROMYXOID FIBROMA *(Continued)*

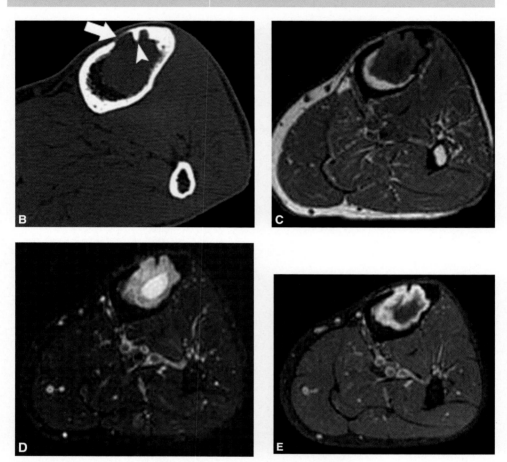

FIGURE 9-15. *(continued)*

SUGGESTED READING

Cappelle S, Pans S, Sciot R. Imaging features of chondromyxoid fibroma: report of 15 cases and literature review. *Br J Radiol.* 2016;20160088. [Epub ahead of print]

Douis H, Saifuddin A. The imaging of cartilaginous bone tumours. I. Benign lesions. *Skeletal Radiol.* 2012;41(10):1195–1212.

Rahimi A, Beabout JW, Ivens JC, et al. Chondromyxoid fibroma: a clinicopathological study of 76 cases. *Cancer.* 1972;30:726–736.

Yamaguchi T, Dorfman HD. Radiographic and histologic patterns of calcification in chondromyxoid fibroma. *Skeletal Radiol.* 1998;27:559–564.

■ BONE TUMORS/TUMORLIKE CONDITIONS: NONOSSIFYING FIBROMA

KEY FACTS

■ Clinical:
- Nonossifying fibroma, fibrous cortical defect, and fibroxanthoma describe similar metaphyseal or metadiaphyseal lesions. Lesions are common and typically discovered incidentally.
■ Age: 5 to 35 years, peak second decade
■ Sex: no sex predilection
■ Common locations: distal femur, distal tibia
■ Imaging features:
- Radiographic features: well-defined eccentric lytic defect with scalloped sclerotic margins in the metaphysis or metadiaphysis of a long bone
- CT: well-defined eccentric lytic defect with scalloped sclerotic margins in the metaphysis or metadiaphysis of a long bone
- MRI: well-defined cortical lesion with low to intermediate intensity on T1-weighted and low to intermediate signal intensity on T2-weighted sequences
■ Differential diagnosis:
- Fibrous dysplasia
- Chondromyxoid fibroma
- Eosinophilic granuloma
■ Treatment: none unless potential for pathologic fracture

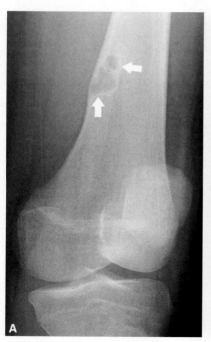
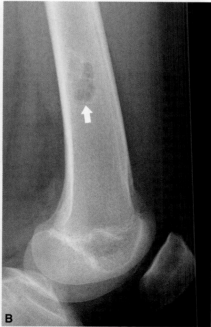

FIGURE 9-16. Nonossifying fibroma. Anteroposterior (AP) **(A)** and lateral **(B)** radiographs show an eccentric, geographic, mildly expansile lucent lesion in the distal femoral diaphysis with sclerotic septation and well-defined sclerotic margins (*arrows*). The lesion is largely hypointense on both coronal T1-weighted **(C)** and fat-saturated T2-weighted **(D)** magnetic resonance (MR) images, but has a thin T1- and T2-hyperintense rim (*arrows*) of tissue immediately subjacent to the T1- and T2-hypointense margin (*arrowheads*).

(continued)

■ BONE TUMORS/TUMORLIKE CONDITIONS: NONOSSIFYING FIBROMA *(Continued)*

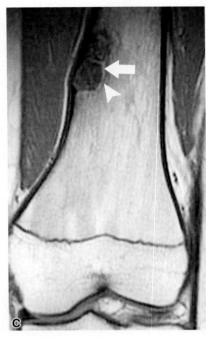 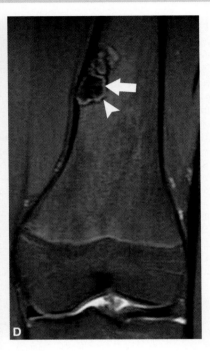

FIGURE 9-16. *(continued)*

SUGGESTED READING

Jee W, Choe B, Kang H, et al. Nonossifying fibroma: characteristics at MR imaging with pathologic correlation. *Radiology.* 1998;209:197–202.

Wootton-Gorges SL. MR imaging of primary bone tumors and tumor-like conditions in children. *Magn Reson Imaging Clin N Am.* 2009;17(3):469–487.

■ BONE TUMORS/TUMORLIKE CONDITIONS: SOLITARY BONE CYST

KEY FACTS

- Also known as a simple bone cyst or unicameral bone cyst
- Clinical:
  - Patients are asymptomatic unless pathologic fracture occurs.
- Age: first two decades
- Sex: Males outnumber females in the ratio 3:1.
- Common locations: proximal humerus, femur, or tibia (90% in humerus or femur)
- Imaging features:
  - Radiographic features: well-defined lytic lesion frequently near the physis. May have internal septations. If fracture has occurred, the "fallen fragment sign" (bone fragment in the dependent portion of the cyst) is virtually pathognomonic.
  - CT: fluid density, well-defined lesion with or without bony septations
  - MRI: uniformly iso- to low intensity on T1-weighted and high intensity on T2-weighted sequences. Internal septations may be seen. Fluid–fluid level or "fallen fragment" after fracture.
- Differential diagnosis:
  - Aneurysmal bone cyst
  - Fibrous dysplasia
- Treatment: aspiration and steroid injection. If in a weight-bearing region, consider curettage and bone grafting.

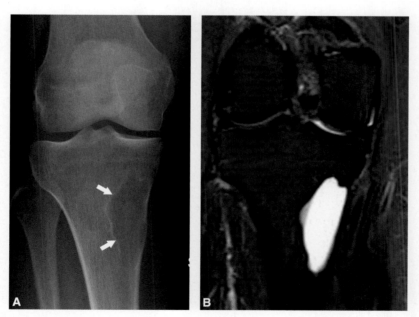

FIGURE 9-17. Unicameral bone cyst. Anteroposterior (AP) radiograph **(A)** of the right knee shows an eccentric, geographic, mildly expansile lucent lesion in the proximal tibial metaphysis with a thin sclerotic margin (*arrows*). Coronal short-TI inversion recovery (STIR) **(B)** magnetic resonance (MR) image demonstrates homogeneous hyperintensity compatible with a fluid-filled cyst. Axial postcontrast fat-saturated T1-weighted image **(C)** demonstrates a thin rim of peripheral enhancement (*arrow*).

(continued)

■ BONE TUMORS/TUMORLIKE CONDITIONS: SOLITARY BONE CYST (Continued)

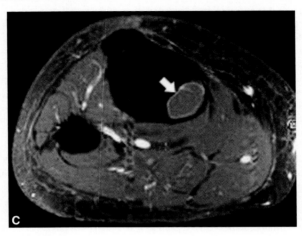

FIGURE 9-17. (continued)

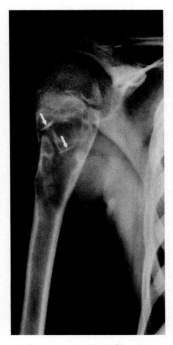

FIGURE 9-18. Unicameral bone cyst. Anteroposterior (AP) radiograph of the humerus demonstrates a bone cyst with pathologic fracture and the associated "fallen fragment sign" (arrows).

SUGGESTED READING

Conway WF, Hayes CW. Miscellaneous lesions of the bone. *Radiol Clin North Am.* 1993;31:299–323.

Kileen K. The fallen fragment sign. *Radiology.* 1998;207:261–262.

Mascard E, Gomez-Brouchet A, Lambot K. Bone cysts: unicameral and aneurysmal bone cyst. *Orthop Traumatol Surg Res.* 2015;101(1 suppl):S119–S127.

Wootton-Gorges SL. MR imaging of primary bone tumors and tumor-like conditions in children. *Magn Reson Imaging Clin N Am.* 2009;17(3):469–487.

■ BONE TUMORS/TUMORLIKE CONDITIONS: ANEURYSMAL BONE CYST

KEY FACTS

- Clinical:
  - Patients present with pain.
- Age: 5 to 35 years, 80% in the first two decades
- Sex: Females slightly outnumber males.
- Common locations: more than 50% in the long bones; 12% to 30% in the spine
- Imaging features:
  - Radiographic features: eccentric lytic lesion with expanded or "ballooned" bony contour. Sclerotic rim and periosteal response are common.
  - CT: same features as radiographs but with fluid–fluid levels of varying fluid density reflective of varying blood product age
  - MRI: well-defined expansile lesion with fluid–fluid levels of varying T1 and T2 intensity reflective of varying blood product age
- Differential diagnosis:
  - Bone cyst
  - Giant cell tumor
  - Osteoblastoma (vertebral location)
- Treatment: curettage and bone grafting

(continued)

■ BONE TUMORS/TUMORLIKE CONDITIONS:
ANEURYSMAL BONE CYST *(Continued)*

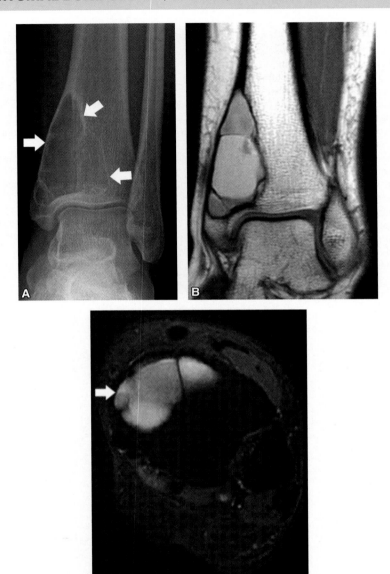

FIGURE 9-19. Aneurysmal bone cyst. Anteroposterior (AP) radiograph **(A)** shows an eccentric expansile lucent lesion (*arrows*) in the distal tibia with thin septations. The lesion demonstrates several discrete areas of variable T1 hyperintensity on the coronal T1-weighted magnetic resonance (MR) image **(B)**, which reflects blood products of varying age. Axial fat-saturated T2-weighted MR image **(C)** demonstrates a septated cystic lesion with a fluid–fluid level (*arrow*).

SUGGESTED READING

Mascard E, Gomez-Brouchet A, Lambot K. Bone cysts: unicameral and aneurysmal bone cyst. *Orthop Traumatol Surg Res.* 2015;101(1 suppl):S119–S127.

Munk PL, Helms CA, Holt RG, et al. MR imaging of aneurysmal bone cysts. *Am J Roentgenol.* 1989;153:99–101.

Wootton-Gorges SL. MR imaging of primary bone tumors and tumor-like conditions in children. *Magn Reson Imaging Clin N Am.* 2009;17(3):469–487.

■ BONE TUMORS/TUMORLIKE CONDITIONS: FIBROUS DYSPLASIA

KEY FACTS

- ■ Clinical:
  - ● Typically asymptomatic. Abnormal bone growth may cause deformity. Lesions may be single (monostotic) in which case the femur, tibia, ribs, and skull base are most commonly involved. Multiple lesions (polyostotic) involve one side of the skeleton in 90% of patients. These lesions are more often symptomatic and may enlarge until skeletal maturity.
- ■ Associated syndromes:
  - ● Mazabraud syndrome: fibrous dysplasia and multiple intramuscular myxomas
  - ● Albright–McCune: females with polyostotic dysplasia, skin lesions, and precocious puberty
- ■ Age: most often second or third decade
- ■ Sex: slightly more common in females
- ■ Common locations: skull, mandible, ribs, femoral neck, tibia
- ■ Imaging features:
  - ● Radiographic features: metaphyseal or diaphyseal lytic or "ground glass" density with sharp margins and bone expansion. May affect multiple bones in approximately 15% of patients. "Long lesion in long bone."
  - ● CT: well-defined lesion with sclerotic margins
  - ● MRI: well-defined lesion with low-intensity margins. Low signal intensity on T1-weighted and intermediate signal intensity on T2-weighted sequences.
- ■ Differential diagnosis:
  - ● Nonossifying fibroma
  - ● Bone cyst
  - ● Aneurysmal bone cyst
  - ● Chondromyxoid fibroma
- ■ Treatment: observation

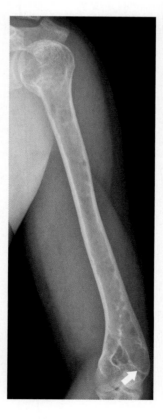

FIGURE 9-20. Fibrous dysplasia. Anteroposterior (AP) radiograph of the left humerus demonstrates a long mildly expansile lucent lesion with "ground-glass" density involving nearly the entire length of the bone. There is a well-defined thin sclerotic margin distally (*arrow*).

(continued)

■ BONE TUMORS/TUMORLIKE CONDITIONS: FIBROUS DYSPLASIA *(Continued)*

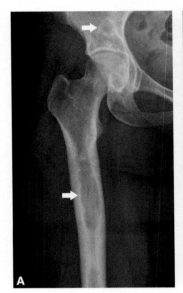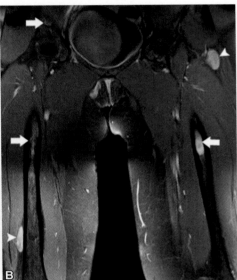

FIGURE 9-21. Mazabraud syndrome. Anteroposterior (AP) radiograph **(A)** of the right hip and femur demonstrates fibrous dysplasia in the right ilium and proximal femoral diaphysis (*arrows*). Coronal short-TI inversion recovery magnetic resonance (STIR MR) image **(B)** of both thighs demonstrates the right-sided lesions seen on radiograph as well as one in the contralateral left femur (*arrows*). There are also homogeneous T2-hyperintense soft tissue masses compatible with myxomas in the right thigh and left lateral hip region (*arrowheads*).

SUGGESTED READING

Bousson V, Rey-Jouvin C, Laredo JD, et al. Fibrous dysplasia and McCune-Albright syndrome: imaging for positive and differential diagnoses, prognosis, and follow-up guidelines. *Eur J Radiol.* 2014;83(10):1828–1842.

Campanacci M, Laus M. Osteofibrous dysplasia of the tibia and fibula. *J Bone Joint Surg.* 1981;63A:367–375.

Gober GA, Nicholas RW. Case report 800: skeletal fibrous dysplasia associated with intramuscular myxomas (Mazabraud's syndrome). *Skeletal Radiol.* 1993;22:452–455.

Greenspan A, Remagen W. *Differential Diagnosis of Tumors and Tumor-like Lesions in Bone and Joints.* Philadelphia: Lippincott-Raven; 1998:215–223.

Wootton-Gorges SL. MR imaging of primary bone tumors and tumor-like conditions in children. *Magn Reson Imaging Clin N Am.* 2009;17(3):469–487.

■ BONE TUMORS/TUMORLIKE CONDITIONS: GIANT CELL TUMOR

KEY FACTS

- ■ Clinical:
  - ● Giant cell tumors account for 22.7% of benign bone tumors. Patients present with pain and swelling in the involved site. A tender palpable mass commonly present.
- ■ Age: 20 to 40 years
- ■ Sex: females affected slightly more frequently than males
- ■ Common locations: Most involve the distal femur or proximal tibia (46%) followed by the distal radius and sacrum. Arise in the metaphysis. Eventually extend into the epiphysis and to the subchondral cortex of the adjacent articular surface.
- ■ Imaging features:
  - ● Radiographic features: lytic lesion with nonsclerotic margins originating in the metaphysis but extending to subchondral bone. Cortical breakthrough in 33% to 50% of cases.
  - ● CT: similar to radiographs. No tumor matrix.
  - ● MRI: iso- to slightly higher signal intensity relative to muscle on T1-weighted and intermediate signal on T2-weighted sequences. T2 sequences may show decreased signal because of hemosiderin deposition. In some cases, signal intensity increased on T2-weighted images. May have secondary aneurysmal bone cyst formation with fluid–fluid levels. Enhances with postcontrast images.
- ■ Differential diagnosis:
  - ● Chondroblastoma
  - ● Osteosarcoma
  - ● Fibrosarcoma
  - ● Malignant fibrous histiocytoma
- ■ Treatment: resection with grafting or, in some cases, joint prosthesis

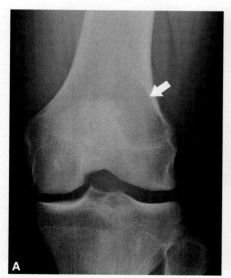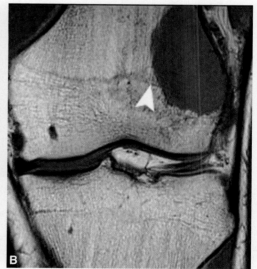

FIGURE 9-22. Giant cell tumor. Anteroposterior (AP) radiograph **(A)** of the left knee demonstrates a geographic lucent lesion with a nonsclerotic margin (*arrow*) involving the distal femoral metaphysis. The coronal T1-weighted magnetic resonance (MR) image **(B)** better demonstrates the distal aspect of the lesion crossing the physeal scar (*arrowhead*) and involving the epiphysis.

(continued)

■ BONE TUMORS/TUMORLIKE CONDITIONS: GIANT CELL TUMOR *(Continued)*

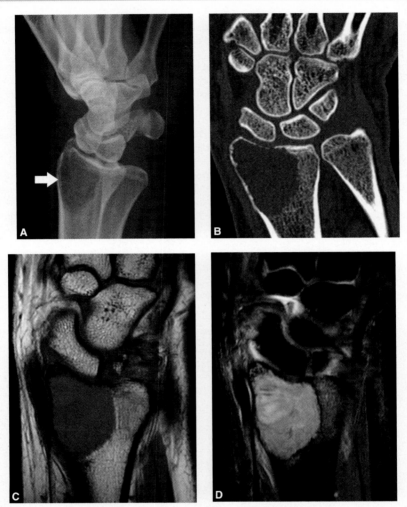

FIGURE 9-23. Giant cell tumor. Oblique radiograph **(A)** of the left wrist demonstrates a geographic lucent lesion (*arrow*) with a nonsclerotic margin involving the distal radial metaphysis and epiphysis. Coronal computed tomography (CT) image **(B)** better delineates the homogeneous soft tissue density lesion and the associated cortical thinning. The lesion shows homogeneous mild hyperintensity relative to muscle on the coronal T1-weighted magnetic resonance (MR) image **(C)** and heterogeneous T2 hyperintensity on the coronal fat-saturated T2-weighted MR image **(D)**. There is edema-like signal in the surrounding marrow and adjacent soft tissues.

SUGGESTED READING

Aoki J, Tanikawa H, Ishü K, et al. MR findings indicative of hemosiderin in giant-cell tumor of bone: frequency, cause, and diagnostic significance. *Am J Roentgenol.* 1996;166:145–148.

Chakarun JC, Forrester DM, Gottsegen CJ, et al. Giant cell tumor of bone: review, mimics, and new developments in treatment. *Radiographics.* 2013;33:197–211.

Murphey MD, Nomikos GC, Flemming DJ, et al. From the archives of AFIP. Imaging of giant cell tumor and giant cell reparative granuloma of bone: radiologic-pathologic correlation. *Radiographics.* 2001;21(5):1283–1309.

Wootton-Gorges SL. MR imaging of primary bone tumors and tumor-like conditions in children. *Magn Reson Imaging Clin N Am.* 2009;17(3):469–487.

■ BONE TUMORS/TUMORLIKE CONDITIONS: EOSINOPHILIC GRANULOMA/LANGERHANS CELL HISTIOCYTOSIS

KEY FACTS

- ■ Clinical:
  - ● Patients present with pain. Multisystem disease is associated with Hand–Schüller–Christian or Letterer–Siwe variants.
- ■ Age: 1 to 20 years
- ■ Sex: Males outnumber females in the ratio 2:1.
- ■ Common locations: skull most common; any bone may be involved
- ■ Imaging features:
  - ● Radiographic features: variable, but lesions usually lytic with variable margins. May be multiple (one-third). Medullary expansion, periosteal response, and sclerosis in long bones. Epiphysis usually involved. Lesions may have double contour margins.
  - ● CT: similar to radiographic features. Cortical and periosteal changes more easily appreciated.
  - ● MRI: well-defined lesions with intermediate or high signal intensity on T1- and T2-weighted images (increased signal on T1 because of xanthomatous histiocytes)
- ■ Differential diagnosis:
  - ● Osteomyelitis
  - ● Malignancy
  - ● Metastasis
- ■ Treatment: resection and bone grafting for solitary lesion. Patients with multiple lesions observed as lesions may regress.

(continued)

■ BONE TUMORS/TUMORLIKE CONDITIONS: EOSINOPHILIC GRANULOMA/LANGERHANS CELL HISTIOCYTOSIS *(Continued)*

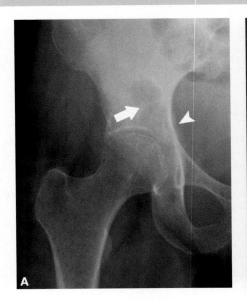
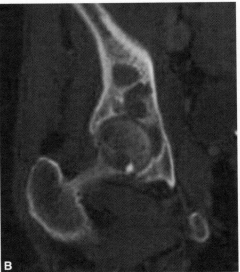

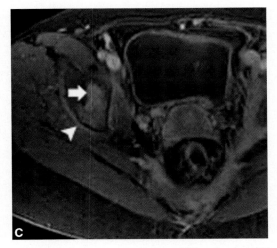

FIGURE 9-24. Eosinophilic granuloma. Anteroposterior (AP) radiograph **(A)** of the right hip shows a lucent lesion with a sclerotic septation (*arrow*) and sclerotic margins in the right acetabulum. There is subtle periosteal new bone along the iliopubic line (*arrowhead*). The lesion is better delineated on the coronal computed tomography (CT) **(B)**. The lesion (*arrow*) is mildly hyperintense on the axial T2-weighted magnetic resonance (MR) image **(C)**. There is edema-like signal in the adjacent marrow, periosteum (*arrowhead*), and soft tissues.

SUGGESTED READING

Azouz EM, Saigal G, Rodriguez MM, Podda A. Langerhans' cell histiocytosis: pathology, imaging and treatment of skeletal involvement. *Pediatr Radiol.* 2005;35(2):103–115.

DeSchepper AMA, Ramon F, Van Marck E. MR imaging of eosinophilic granuloma in bone: report of 11 cases. *Skeletal Radiol.* 1993;22:163–166.

Haupt R, Minkov M, Astigarraga I, et al. Langerhans cell histiocytosis (LCH): guidelines for diagnosis, clinical work-up, and treatment for patients till the age of 18 years. *Pediatr Blood Cancer.* 2013;60(2):175–184. doi:10.1002/pbc.24367.

■ BONE TUMORS/TUMORLIKE CONDITIONS: OSTEOSARCOMA

KEY FACTS

- ■ Clinical:
  - ● Osteosarcomas account for 19% of sarcomas and, with the exception of myeloma, are the most common primary bone malignancy. Patients present with pain and swelling in the affected region.
- ■ Age: Second decade is the peak incidence.
- ■ Sex: Males slightly outnumber females.
- ■ Common locations: distal femur or proximal tibia (48%), pelvis and proximal femur (14%), shoulder and proximal humerus (10%)
- ■ Imaging features:
  - ● Radiographic features: metaphyseal lytic, blastic, or mixed appearance. Lesions poorly defined with aggressive periosteal response (spiculations or Codman triangles). Soft tissue extension common.
  - ● CT: similar to radiographic features
  - ● MRI: Imaging features are nonspecific. Signal intensity varies with matrix (decreased with blastic, increased with lytic on T2-weighted sequence). Staging of marrow and soft tissue involvement is the primary indication for MRI.
- ■ Differential diagnosis:
  - ● Ewing sarcoma
  - ● Fibrosarcoma
  - ● Chondrosarcoma
  - ● Giant cell tumor
  - ● Osteomyelitis
- ■ Treatment: limb salvage or amputation. Radiation and chemotherapy as adjuvant therapy or for nonoperable lesions.

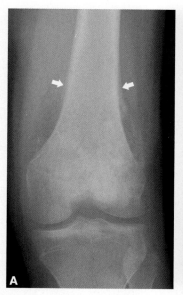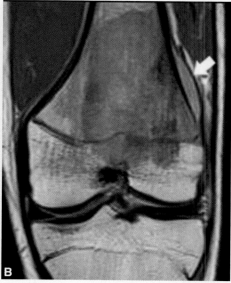

FIGURE 9-25. Osteosarcoma. Anteroposterior (AP) radiograph **(A)** of the left knee shows a poorly defined sclerotic lesion with osteoid matrix involving the distal femoral metaphysis, open physis, and epiphysis in this skeletally immature (16-year-old) patient. There is associated aggressive periosteal reaction both medially and laterally (*arrows*). Coronal proton density magnetic resonance (MR) image **(B)** better delineates the mass, its invasion across the physis into the epiphysis, and the associated periosteal elevation (*arrow*).

(continued)

■ BONE TUMORS/TUMORLIKE CONDITIONS: OSTEOSARCOMA *(Continued)*

SUGGESTED READING

Azouz ME, Esseltine DW, Chevalier L. Radiographic evaluation of osteosarcoma. *J Can Assoc Radiol*. 1982;33:167–171.

Kaste SC. Imaging pediatric bone sarcomas. *Radiol Clin North Am*. 2011;49(4):749–765.

Suresh S, Saifuddin A. Radiological appearances of appendicular osteosarcoma: a comprehensive pictorial review. *Clin Radiol*. 2007;62(4):314–323.

Unni KK. *Dahlin's Bone Tumors: General Aspects and Data on 1,087 Cases*. Philadelphia: Lippincott-Raven; 1996:143–183.

■ BONE TUMORS/TUMORLIKE CONDITIONS: PAROSTEAL OSTEOSARCOMA

KEY FACTS

- ■ Clinical:
  - ● Patients typically present with a painless mass in the distal posterior thigh.
- ■ Age: third decade (older than conventional osteosarcoma)
- ■ Sex: Females outnumber males in the ratio 2:1.
- ■ Common locations: majority in distal posterior femur (67%), proximal tibia or fibula (12%), proximal humerus (10%)
- ■ Imaging features:
  - ● Radiographic features: large ossified mass on the surface of a long bone. Cortex thick and deformed. Larger masses may surround bone.
  - ● CT: similar to radiographs. Lucent zone (periosteum) separates the tumor from the cortex (string sign).
  - ● MRI: often not required because of characteristic CT features and lack of improved specificity for MRI
- ■ Differential diagnosis:
  - ● Myositis ossificans
  - ● Periosteal osteosarcoma
  - ● Osteosarcoma
  - ● Periosteal chondrosarcoma
- ■ Treatment: limb salvage resection

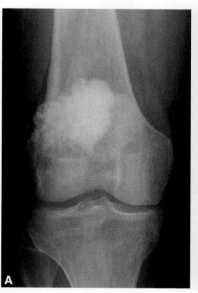 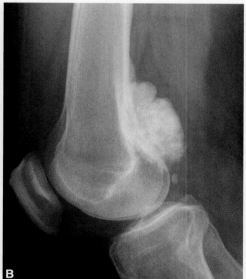

FIGURE 9-26. Parosteal osteosarcoma. Anteroposterior (AP) **(A)** and lateral **(B)** radiographs of the right knee show a cortically based dense osseous mass with lobular margins involving the posterior aspect of the distal femur. Axial computed tomography (CT) image **(C)** and axial T1-weighted **(D)** and fat-saturated T2-weighted **(E)** magnetic resonance (MR) images better delineate the relationship of the densely ossified tumor with the cortex. There is a focal area where the cortex and the mass are indistinguishable (*arrow*), whereas the remainder of the mass is discrete from the cortex. Of note, the subjacent marrow demonstrates normal signal.

(continued)

■ BONE TUMORS/TUMORLIKE CONDITIONS: PAROSTEAL OSTEOSARCOMA *(Continued)*

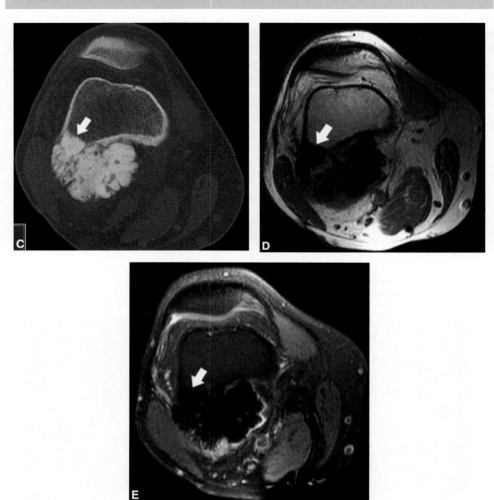

FIGURE 9-26. *(continued)*

SUGGESTED READING

Greenfield GB, Arrington JA. *Imaging of Bone Tumors: A Multimodality Approach*. Philadelphia: JB Lippincott; 1995:43–166.
Yarmish G, Klein MJ, Landa J, et al. Imaging characteristics of primary osteosarcoma: nonconventional subtypes. *Radiographics*. 2010;30(6):1653–1672. doi:10.1148/rg.306105524.

■ BONE TUMORS/TUMORLIKE CONDITIONS: PERIOSTEAL OSTEOSARCOMA

KEY FACTS

- Clinical:
  - Periosteal osteosarcomas account for only 1.5% of osteosarcomas. Patients present with local pain over involved bone.
- Age: 15 to 30 years, peak in the second decade
- Sex: Females outnumber males in the ratio 1.6:1.
- Common locations: diaphysis of femur and tibia (73%)
- Imaging features:
  - Radiographic features: surface lesion on the diaphysis with partial calcification or ossification. Medullary bone not involved.
  - CT: similar to radiographic features. Confirms marrow sparing.
  - MRI: normal marrow with variable signal intensity in periosteum and soft tissues, depending on calcifications
- Differential diagnosis:
  - Myositis ossificans
  - Parosteal osteosarcoma
  - Periosteal chondrosarcoma
- Treatment: wide excision and bone graft (allograft)

(continued)

■ BONE TUMORS/TUMORLIKE CONDITIONS: PERIOSTEAL OSTEOSARCOMA *(Continued)*

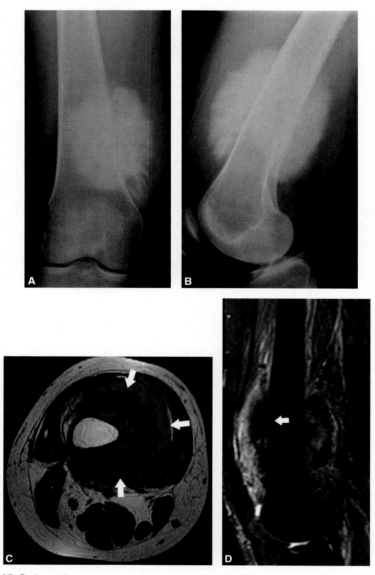

FIGURE 9-27. Periosteal osteosarcoma. Anteroposterior (AP) **(A)** and lateral **(B)** radiographs of the right knee show a large soft tissue mass with spiculated, sunburst-like mineralization partially encasing the distal right femur. The exact relationship of the mass with the bone is not well delineated, but there is no obvious cortical destruction. Corresponding axial T1-weighted magnetic resonance (MR) image **(C)** shows a large soft tissue mass (*arrows*) with heterogeneous T1 signal partially encasing the distal femur without cortical or marrow signal abnormalities. Sagittal short-TI inversion recovery (STIR) MR image **(D)** again shows the large soft tissue mass with heterogeneous T2 signal, with central low signal reflecting the areas of mineralization and peripheral high signal reflecting aggressive tumor. Note the subtle linear areas of edema-like signal in the subcortical marrow (*arrow*).

SUGGESTED READING

Murphey MD, Jelinek JS, Temple HT, et al. Imaging of periosteal osteosarcoma: radiologic-pathologic comparison. *Radiology.* 2004;233(1):129–138.

Unni KK, Dahlin DC, Beabout JW. Periosteal osteogenic sarcoma. *Cancer.* 1976;37:2476–2485.

Yarmish G, Klein MJ, Landa J, et al. Imaging characteristics of primary osteosarcoma: nonconventional subtypes. *Radiographics.* 2010;30(6):1653–1672. doi:10.1148/rg.306105524.

■ BONE TUMORS/TUMORLIKE CONDITIONS: TELANGIECTATIC OSTEOSARCOMA

KEY FACTS

■ Clinical:
  ● Telangiectatic osteosarcomas account for 3.5% of all osteosarcomas. Patients present with pain.
■ Age: 15 to 35 years, peak incidence in the second decade
■ Sex: Males outnumber females in the ratio 2:1.
■ Common locations: distal femur and proximal tibia (61%), humerus (14%)
■ Imaging features:
  ● Radiographic features: large lytic or permeative metaphyseal lesion. Cortical destruction with aggressive periosteal response and soft tissue mass.
  ● CT: similar to radiographic features
  ● MRI: high-intensity bone and soft tissue lesion on T2-weighted images; low intensity on T1-weighted images. Signal intensity may be mixed, especially on T1-weighted images because of clotted blood. Fluid–fluid levels.
■ Differential diagnosis:
  ● Osteosarcoma
  ● Fibrosarcoma
  ● Aneurysmal bone cyst
■ Treatment: limb salvage with wide excision

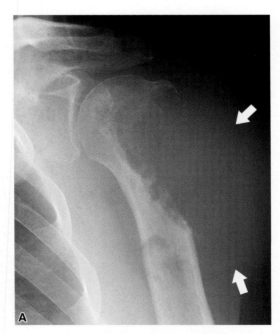

FIGURE 9-28. Telangiectatic osteosarcoma. Anteroposterior (AP) radiograph **(A)** of the left shoulder demonstrates a permeative lytic lesion in the proximal humerus with a large soft tissue mass (*arrows*). Axial T1-weighted **(B)** and fat-saturated T2-weighted **(C)** magnetic resonance (MR) images show tumor replacement of the lateral aspect of the proximal humerus with an associated large soft tissue mass and multiple fluid–fluid levels.

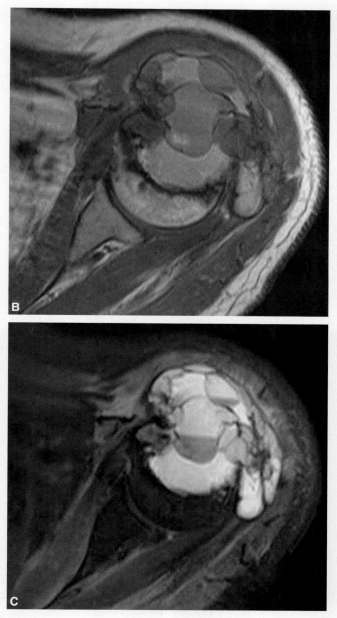

FIGURE 9-28. (*continued*)

SUGGESTED READING

Huvos AG, Rosen G, Bretsky SS, et al. Telangiectatic osteosarcoma: a clinicopathologic study of 124 cases. *Cancer.* 1982;49:1679–1689.

Murphey MD, wan Jaovisidha S, Temple HT, et al. Telangiectatic osteosarcoma: radiologic-pathologic comparison. *Radiology.* 2003;229(2):545–553.

Yarmish G, Klein MJ, Landa J, et al. Imaging characteristics of primary osteosarcoma: nonconventional subtypes. *Radiographics.* 2010;30(6):1653–1672. doi:10.1148/rg.306105524.

■ BONE TUMORS/TUMORLIKE CONDITIONS: EWING SARCOMA

KEY FACTS

- ■ Clinical:
  - ● Ewing sarcomas account for 9.1% of all primary malignant bone tumors. Patients present with local pain and swelling. Patients may also have fever and increased white counts suggesting infection.
- ■ Age: 5 to 30 years, 75% in the first two decades and 60% in the second decade
- ■ Sex: no sex predilection
- ■ Common locations: pelvis and sacrum (25%), femur and tibia (27%), humerus and forearm (12%), foot and ankle (8%)
- ■ Imaging features:
  - ● Radiographic features: long diaphyseal lesion with permeative pattern. May have sclerosis or mixed appearance. Aggressive periosteal (laminated characteristic of Ewing sarcoma) response and soft tissue mass common.
  - ● CT: similar to radiographic features; periosteum and soft tissue better defined
  - ● MRI: signal intensity variable in mixed or sclerotic lesions. High signal intensity on T2-weighted and low signal intensity on T1-weighted with lytic permeative lesions.
- ■ Differential diagnosis:
  - ● Lymphoma
  - ● Osteosarcoma
  - ● Osteomyelitis
- ■ Treatment: radiation or radiation plus chemotherapy. Surgical therapy is more often considered recently.

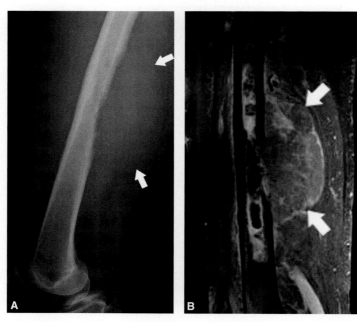

FIGURE 9-29. Ewing sarcoma. Lateral radiograph **(A)** of the right femur shows a permeative lesion in the mid diaphysis with periosteal reaction anteriorly and cortical destruction and a large soft tissue mass posteriorly (*arrows*). Both the osseous and soft tissue (*arrows*) components of the mass demonstrate heterogeneous enhancement on sagittal postcontrast fat-saturated T1-weighted magnetic resonance (MR) image **(B)**.

SUGGESTED READING

Fletcher BD. Responses of osteosarcoma and Ewing's sarcoma to chemotherapy: imaging evaluation. *Am J Roentgenol.* 1991;157:825–833.

Kaste SC. Imaging pediatric bone sarcomas. *Radiol Clin North Am.* 2011;49(4):749–765.

Murphey MD, Senchak LT, Mambalam PK, et al. From the radiologic pathology archives: Ewing sarcoma family of tumors: radiologic-pathologic correlation. *Radiographics.* 2013;33(3):803–831.

Unni KK. *Dahlin's Bone Tumors: General Aspects and Data on 11,087 Cases.* Philadelphia: Lippincott-Raven; 1996:249–261.

■ BONE TUMORS/TUMORLIKE CONDITIONS: CHONDROSARCOMA (PRIMARY, CENTRAL)

KEY FACTS

- Clinical:
  - Chondrosarcomas account for 9.2% of malignant bone tumors. Osteosarcomas are twice as common. Patients present with pain.
- Age: more common in adults 40 to 60 years old (62%)
- Sex: Males outnumber females in the ratio 1.5:1.
- Common locations: pelvic region most common (23%), proximal femur (13.5%), proximal humerus (12%), trunk (10.6%), proximal tibia and fibula (7%)
- Imaging features:
  - Radiographic features: Two-thirds are calcified. Cortical erosion or destruction usually is present. Typically, little periosteal response. Soft tissue extension common with large lesions.
  - CT: superior for evaluation of cortex and matrix calcification
  - MRI: intermediate to high intensity on T2-weighted sequences. Calcification seen as low intensity on T1- and T2-weighted sequences. Soft tissue extension more easily evaluated compared with CT.
- Differential diagnosis:
  - Osteosarcoma
  - Fibrosarcoma
  - Metastasis
- Treatment: wide excision with reconstruction

(continued)

■ BONE TUMORS/TUMORLIKE CONDITIONS: CHONDROSARCOMA (PRIMARY, CENTRAL) *(Continued)*

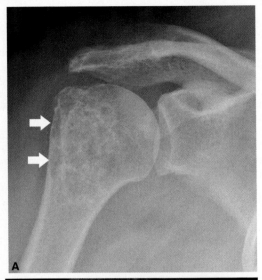

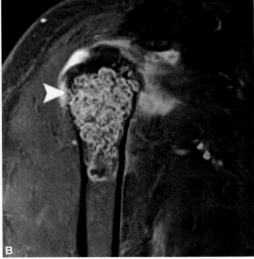

FIGURE 9-30. Low-grade chondrosarcoma. Anteroposterior (AP) radiograph **(A)** of the right shoulder shows a lesion with chondroid matrix and endosteal scalloping (*arrows*). Sagittal oblique postcontrast fat-saturated T1-weighted magnetic resonance (MR) image **(B)** shows focal cortical destruction (*arrowhead*) indicating a malignant lesion.

SUGGESTED READING

Collins MS, Koyama T, Swee RG, Inwards CY. Clear cell chondrosarcoma: radiographic, computed tomographic, and magnetic resonance findings in 34 patients with pathologic correlation. *Skeletal Radiol.* 2003;32(12):687–694.

Hudson TM, Manaster BJ, Springfield DS, et al. Radiology of medullary chondrosarcoma: preoperative treatment planning. *Skeletal Radiol.* 1983;10:69–78.

Littrell LA, Wenger DE, Wold LE, et al. Radiographic, CT, and MR imaging features of dedifferentiated chondrosarcomas: a retrospective review of 174 de novo cases. *Radiographics.* 2004;24(5):1397–1409.

Murphey MD, Flemming DJ, Boyea SR, et al. Enchondroma versus chondrosarcoma in the appendicular skeleton: differentiating features. *Radiographics.* 1998;18:1213–1237.

■ BONE TUMORS/TUMORLIKE CONDITIONS: CHONDROSARCOMA (SECONDARY)

KEY FACTS

- ■ Clinical:
  - ● Secondary chondrosarcomas originate from osteochondromas or enchondromas. Patients with enchondromas present with pain. Patients with osteochondromas present with enlarging masses and pain. Malignant changes are more common in patients with multiple osteochondromas.
- ■ Age: 30 to 50 years
- ■ Sex: Males outnumber females in the ratio 2:1.
- ■ Common locations: shoulder and proximal humerus (10.4%), pelvis and proximal femur (33%), spine (10.4%)
- ■ Imaging features:
  - ● Radiographic features: Irregular cartilage cap with streaky calcific densities and lucent areas in an osteochondroma suggest malignant transformation. With enchondromas, endosteal scalloping, disappearing calcifications, and increasing area of lucency suggest malignancy.
  - ● CT: similar to radiographs but more useful for evaluating matrix, cartilage cap, and cortical involvement
  - ● MRI: Lesions have increased intensity on T2-weighted and decreased intensity on T1-weighted sequences. Osteochondroma cartilage cap is easily defined (high signal intensity) and measured greater than 1.5 to 2 cm suggests malignancy. Gadolinium-enhanced T1-weighted images show ring and arc septal pattern of chondrosarcoma.
- ■ Treatment: surgical resection with wide margins

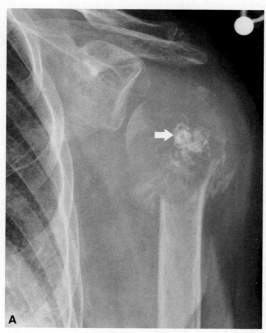

A

FIGURE 9-31. Secondary chondrosarcoma. Anteroposterior (AP) radiograph **(A)** of the left shoulder shows a large expansile lytic lesion of the humeral head and neck with cortical destruction. There is a small central area of chondroid matrix (*arrow*) compatible with underlying enchondroma. Sagittal short-TI inversion recovery magnetic resonance (STIR MR) image **(B)** shows the large soft tissue component with heterogeneous mild T2 hyperintensity. The hypointense chondroid matrix (*arrow*) of the underlying enchondroma is well visualized.

(continued)

■ BONE TUMORS/TUMORLIKE CONDITIONS: CHONDROSARCOMA (SECONDARY) *(Continued)*

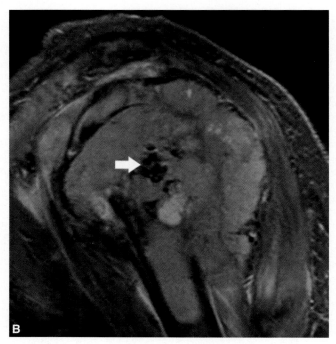

FIGURE 9-31. *(continued)*

SUGGESTED READING

Aoki JA, Sone S, Fujioka F, et al. MR of enchondroma and chondrosarcoma: rings and arcs of Gd-DTPA enhancement. *J Comput Assist Tomogr.* 1991;15:1011–1016.

Ferrer-Santacreu EM, Ortiz-Cruz EJ, Díaz-Almirón M, et al. Enchondroma versus chondrosarcoma in long bones of appendicular skeleton: clinical and radiological criteria—a follow-up. *J Oncol.* 2016;2016:8262079. doi: 10.1155/2016/8262079.

Lin PP, Moussallem CD, Deavers MT. Secondary chondrosarcoma. *J Am Acad Orthop Surg.* 2010;18(10):608–615.

Murphey MD, Flemming DJ, Boyea SR, et al. Enchondroma versus chondrosarcoma in the appendicular skeleton: differentiating features. *Radiographics.* 1998;18(5):1213–1237.

Staals EL, Bacchini P, Mercuri M, et al. Dedifferentiated chondrosarcomas arising in preexisting osteochondromas. *J Bone Joint Surg Am.* 2007;89(5):987–993.

Unni KK. *Dahlin's Bone Tumors: General Aspects and Data on 11,087 Cases.* Philadelphia: Lippincott-Raven; 1996:71–108.

■ BONE TUMORS/TUMORLIKE CONDITIONS: FIBROSARCOMA AND MALIGNANT FIBROUS HISTIOCYTOMA OF BONE

KEY FACTS

- ■ Clinical:
  - ● These are uncommon malignancies of bone (1% of malignant bone tumors). Up to 30% arise from lesions such as radiation, bone infarcts, Paget disease, or chronic osteomyelitis. Patients present with pain and swelling.
- ■ Age: peaks in those aged in their 40s and 60s
- ■ Sex: no sex predilection
- ■ Common locations: distal femur and proximal tibia (35%), pelvis and proximal femur (27%), shoulder and humerus (10%)
- ■ Imaging features:
  - ● Radiographic features: large, eccentrically located lytic lesion with poorly defined margins. Cortical disruption and soft tissue mass common.
  - ● CT: similar to radiographic features
  - ● MRI: high signal intensity on T2-weighted and typically low on T1-weighted sequences. Areas of hemorrhage may be high intensity on T1-weighted sequences. Marrow extent and soft tissue extension optimally imaged.
- ■ Differential diagnosis:
  - ● Osteosarcoma
  - ● Giant cell tumor
  - ● Metastasis
- ■ Treatment: limb salvage with joint reconstruction

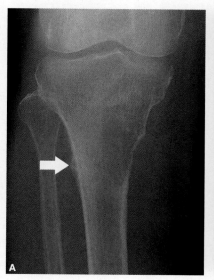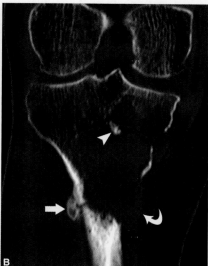

FIGURE 9-32. Malignant fibrous histiocytoma of bone. Anteroposterior (AP) radiograph **(A)** of the right lower leg shows an ill-defined lytic lesion with a healing pathologic fracture (*arrow*) in the proximal tibia. Coronal computed tomography (CT) image **(B)** shows a soft tissue density mass with osseous sequestra (*arrowhead*), cortical destruction, pathologic fracture with callus formation (*arrow*), and soft tissue mass (*curved arrow*).

SUGGESTED READING

Smith SE, Kransdorf MJ. Primary musculoskeletal tumors of fibrous origin. *Semin Musculoskelet Radiol.* 2000;4(1):73–88.

Taconia WK, Mulder JD. Fibrosarcoma and malignant fibrous histiocytoma of long bones: radiographic features and grading. *Skeletal Radiol.* 1984;11:237–245.

Unni KK. *Dahlin's Bone Tumors: General Aspects and Data on 11,087 Cases.* Philadelphia: Lippincott-Raven; 1996:217–224.

■ BONE TUMORS/TUMORLIKE CONDITIONS: ADAMANTINOMA

KEY FACTS

- Clinical:
  - Adamantinomas account for less than 1% of all malignant bone tumors. Patients present with local pain.
- Age: 74% in the second and third decades
- Sex: no sex predilection
- Common locations: tibial diaphysis (90%)
- Imaging features:
  - Radiographic features: eccentric lytic areas with sclerosis. Bone expanded. Typically dominant central lesion. May be multiple. Both the tibia and fibula may be involved.
  - CT: defines cortical and soft tissue involvement
  - MRI: features variable and not well documented
- Differential diagnosis:
  - Fibrous dysplasia
  - Fibroma
- Treatment: excision with wide margins

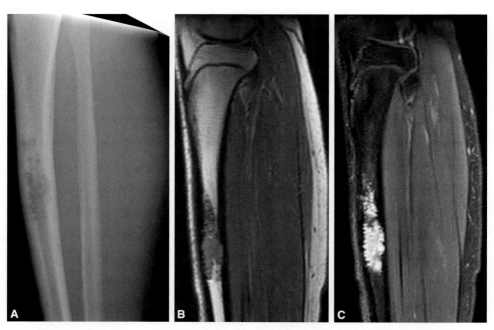

FIGURE 9-33. Adamantinoma. Lateral radiograph **(A)** of the right lower leg shows a moth-eaten lytic, mildly expansile lesion with cortical involvement in the tibial shaft. The lesion demonstrates mild hyperintensity relative to muscle on the sagittal T1-weighted magnetic resonance (MR) image **(B)** and prominent T2 hyperintensity on the fat-saturated T2-weighted MR image **(C)**.

SUGGESTED READING

Levine SM, Lambiase RE, Petchprapa CN. Cortical lesions of the tibia: characteristic appearances on radiography. *Radiographics.* 2003;23:157–177.

Most MJ, Sim FH, Inwards CY. Osteofibrous dysplasia and adamantinoma. *J Am Acad Orthop Surg.* 2010;18(6):358–366.

Weiss SW, Dorfman HD. Adamantinoma of long bones: an analysis of nine cases with emphasis on metastasizing lesions and fibrous dysplasia-like changes. *Hum Pathol.* 1977;8:141–153.

■ BONE TUMORS/TUMORLIKE CONDITIONS: PAGET SARCOMA

KEY FACTS

- ■ Clinical:
  - ● Malignant degeneration occurs in 1% to 6% of patients with Paget disease. Most (50%) are osteosarcomas, followed by fibrosarcoma, chondrosarcoma, and other histologic types. Patients present with increasing or new pain in the region of Paget involvement.
- ■ Age: elderly
- ■ Sex: Males outnumber females in the ratio 2:1.
- ■ Common locations: pelvis, proximal humerus
- ■ Imaging features:
  - ● Radiographic features: Most lesions are lytic, but mixed lytic and sclerotic occur. Soft tissue involvement common. Originate in bone affected by Paget disease.
  - ● CT: cortical destruction and soft tissue involvement more clearly defined
  - ● MRI: variable signal intensity. Soft tissue extension easily identified. Low signal intensity on T1-weighted images in areas of lucency on the radiograph suggests malignant degeneration.
- ■ Treatment: wide excision or amputation. Radiation for nonsurgical cases.

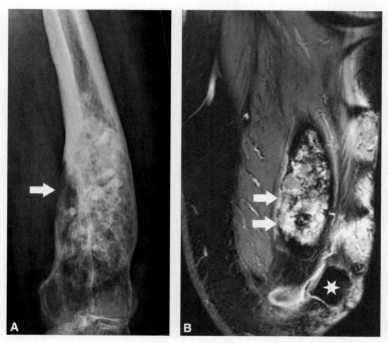

FIGURE 9-34. Paget sarcoma. Anteroposterior (AP) radiograph **(A)** of the left femur shows changes of Paget disease with a lytic area and cortical destruction medially (*arrow*). Coronal postcontrast fat-saturated T1-weighted magnetic resonance (MR) image **(B)** shows the areas of cortical breakthrough (*arrows*). The left patella is indicated by the *star*.

SUGGESTED READING

Hall FM. Incidence of bone sarcoma in Paget's disease. *Radiology.* 1983;148:865.

López C, Thomas DV, Davies AM. Neoplastic transformation and tumour-like lesions in Paget's disease of bone: a pictorial review. *Eur Radiol.* 2003;13(4 suppl):L151–L163.

Sundarum M, Khanna G, El-Khoury GY. T1-weighted MR imaging for distinguishing large osteolysis of Paget disease from sarcomatous degeneration. *Skeletal Radiol.* 2001;30:378–383.

■ BONE TUMORS/TUMORLIKE CONDITIONS: METASTASIS

KEY FACTS

- Clinical:
  - Pain is the most frequent presenting symptom.
- Age: adults
- Sex: no sex predilection
- Common locations: axial skeleton, proximal long bones
- Imaging features:
  - Radiographic features: solitary or multiple lesions. Lesions may be lytic, sclerotic, or mixed, depending on primary tumor.
  - Radionuclide scans: best screening technique for most metastatic lesions. Seen as areas of increased scintigraphic activity.
  - CT: useful for treatment planning of focal lesions
  - MRI: signal intensity varies:
    - ❖ Sclerotic, decreased signal on T1- and T2-weighted images
    - ❖ Lytic, decreased T1- and increased signal on T2-weighted images
    - ❖ Enhancement variable for lytic and sclerotic. Diffusion or chemical shift imaging may assist in differentiating between benign and malignant compression fractures in the spine.
- Differential diagnosis:
  - Multiple myeloma
  - Lymphoma
  - Brown tumors

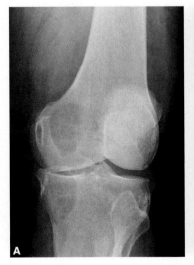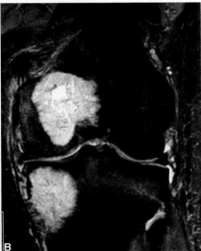

FIGURE 9-35. Metastases from a primary lung cancer. Anteroposterior (AP) radiograph **(A)** of the left knee shows lytic lesions in the medial aspects of the distal femur and proximal tibia. Both lesions demonstrate similar irregular margins and heterogeneous hyperintensity on the coronal fat-saturated T2-weighted magnetic resonance (MR) image **(B)**.

SUGGESTED READING

Roberts CC, Daffner RH, Weissman BN, et al. ACR appropriateness criteria on metastatic bone disease. *J Am Coll Radiol.* 2010;7(6):400–409.

Simon MA, Karluk MB. Skeletal metastasis of unknown origin: diagnostic strategy for orthopedic surgeons. *Clin Orthop.* 1983;166:96–103.

Yang HL, Liu T, Wang XM, et al. Diagnosis of bone metastases: a meta-analysis comparing [18]FDG PET, CT, MRI and bone scintigraphy. *Eur Radiol.* 2011;21(12):2604–2617.

Zajick DC, Morrison WB, Schweitzer ME. Benign and malignant processes: normal values and differentiation with chemical shift MR imaging in vertebral marrow. *Radiology.* 2005;237:590–596.

■ BONE TUMORS/TUMORLIKE CONDITIONS: MYELOMA

KEY FACTS

- ■ Clinical:
  - Myeloma is the most common primary bone malignancy. Patients present with local pain and often associated weakness and weight loss.
- ■ Age: usually more than 60 years; rare in those aged less than 40 years
- ■ Sex: Males outnumber females in the ratio 2:1.
- ■ Common locations: skull, axial skeleton, ribs
- ■ Imaging features:
  - Radiographic features: typically multiple small lytic foci. May be a solitary lesion. Bone expansion and soft tissue mass common, especially in the ribs.
  - CT: generally not performed unless focal lesion
  - MRI: lesions low intensity on T1-weighted and high intensity on T2-weighted sequences, although variable
- ■ Differential diagnosis:
  - Metastasis
  - Lymphoma
- ■ Treatment: chemotherapy. Surgical intervention for pending pathologic fractures.

(continued)

■ BONE TUMORS/TUMORLIKE CONDITIONS: MYELOMA *(Continued)*

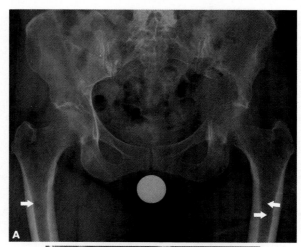

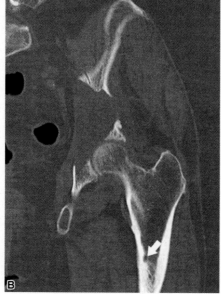

FIGURE 9-36. Multiple myeloma. Anteroposterior (AP) radiograph **(A)** of the pelvis demonstrates several small lytic lesions (*arrows*) in the proximal femora and a large permeative mass compatible with plasmacytoma in the left acetabulum and ilium with broad cortical loss along the iliopubic line. Coronal computed tomography (CT) image **(B)** of the left hip shows cortical loss and soft tissue density replacement of the normal left acetabular and ilial marrow from the plasmacytoma, as well as the small focal myelomatous lesion in the proximal left femur (*arrow*).

SUGGESTED READING

Ferraro R, Agarwal A, Martin-Macintosh EL, et al. MR imaging and PET/CT in diagnosis and management of multiple myeloma. *Radiographics.* 2015;35(2):438–454.

Kyle RA, Elvebrack LR. Management and prognosis of multiple myeloma. *Mayo Clin Proc.* 1976;51:751–760.

Regelink JC, Minnema MC, Terpos E, et al. Comparison of modern and conventional imaging techniques in establishing multiple myeloma–related bone disease: a systematic review. *Br J Haematol.* 2013;162(1):50–61.

■ BONE TUMORS/TUMORLIKE CONDITIONS: LYMPHOMA

KEY FACTS

- ■ Clinical:
  - ● Primary malignant lymphoma accounts for less than 5% of malignant bone lesions. Patients present with pain and swelling in involved region.
- ■ Age: 10 to 80 years of age; most common in those aged in their 60s and 70s
- ■ Sex: Males outnumber females in the ratio 1.8:1.
- ■ Common locations: Distal femur and proximal tibia are most commonly involved followed by the femoral and humeral shafts. Lesions may involve single or multiple sites.
- ■ Imaging features:
  - ● Radiographic features: permeative lytic diaphyseal destruction (70%) and mixed in 28%. May be sclerotic as well, especially in vertebral bodies. Associated soft tissue mass is common (48%). Periosteal reaction in 58% and sequestra in 16%.
  - ● CT: useful to define cortical destruction and soft tissue extension of solitary lesions
  - ● MRI: useful to define cortical destruction and soft tissue extension of solitary lesions. Image features not specific.
- ■ Differential diagnosis:
  - ● Ewing sarcoma
  - ● Osteomyelitis
  - ● Metastasis
  - ● Osteosarcoma
- ■ Treatment: radiation/chemotherapy

(continued)

■ BONE TUMORS/TUMORLIKE CONDITIONS: LYMPHOMA *(Continued)*

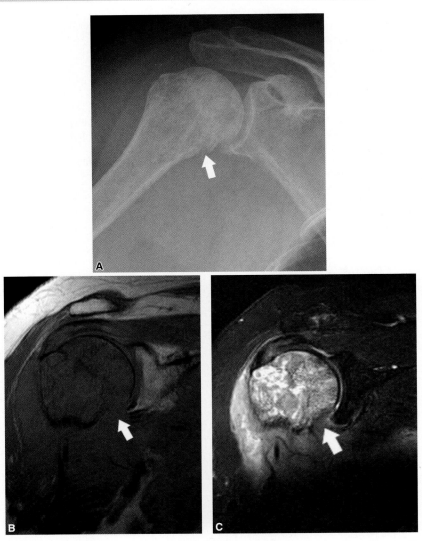

FIGURE 9-37. Lymphoma. Anteroposterior (AP) radiograph **(A)** of the right shoulder shows an ill-defined faintly permeative lesion in the proximal humerus with a focal area of cortical destruction (*arrow*). The diffuse marrow replacement, soft tissue component, and focal area of cortical destruction (*arrows*) are well visualized on the coronal T1-weighted **(B)** and fat-saturated T2-weighted **(C)** magnetic resonance (MR) images. Of note, the small focal area of cortical destruction on the radiograph underestimates the volume of the soft tissue component. Primary osseous lymphomas will often have a large soft tissue component with little or no cortical destruction, sometimes making these lesions difficult to discern on radiographs.

SUGGESTED READING

Daffner RH, Lupetin AR, Dask N, et al. MRI in detection of malignant infiltration of bone marrow. *Am J Roentgenol.* 1986;146:353–358.

Mulligan ME, McRae GA, Murphey MD. Imaging features of primary lymphoma of bone. *Am J Roentgenol.* 1999;173:1691–1697.

Murphey MD, Kransdorf MJ. Primary musculoskeletal lymphoma. *Radiol Clin North Am.* 2016;54(4):785–795.

■ SOFT TISSUE MASSES: LIPOMA

KEY FACTS

- Clinical:
  - Lipomas are the most common soft tissue mass. They are composed of mature adipose tissue. Lesions may grow but usually stabilize. Lipomas may be superficial or deep. Lesions are multiple in 5% to 8% of patients.
- Age: 50 to 70 years
- Sex: Males slightly outnumber females.
- Common locations: deep lipomas—chest wall, retroperitoneum, hands, and feet. Superficial—back, neck, shoulder, abdomen, and gluteal regions.
- Imaging features:
  - Radiographic features: Larger lipomas may be seen as well-defined fat density masses.
  - CT: fat attenuation, well-defined mass. May contain fibrous septations.
  - MRI: fat intensity on all pulse sequences. May have fibrous septa. No enhancement with gadolinium.
- Differential diagnosis:
  - Low-grade liposarcoma
- Treatment: local resection or observe

(continued)

■ SOFT TISSUE MASSES: LIPOMA *(Continued)*

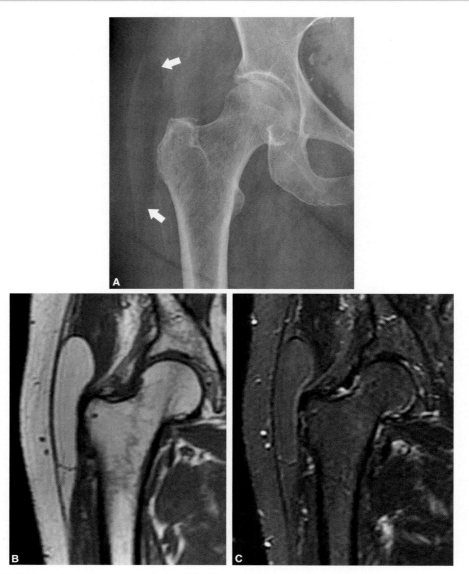

FIGURE 9-38. Lipoma. Anteroposterior (AP) radiograph **(A)** of the right hip demonstrates an elongated tubular soft tissue mass (*arrows*) lateral to the right greater trochanter. The density of the mass is equivalent to the subcutaneous fat. Coronal T1-weighted **(B)** and short-TI inversion recovery (STIR) **(C)** magnetic resonance (MR) images show a well-defined encapsulated mass with homogeneous signal intensity equivalent to normal fat.

SUGGESTED READING

Dooms GC, Hricak H, Sollitta RA, et al. Lipomatous tumors and tumors with fatty components: MR imaging potential and comparison of MR and CT results. *Radiology.* 1985;157:479–483.

Gupta P, Potti TA, Wuertzer SD, et al. Spectrum of fat-containing soft-tissue masses at MR imaging: the common, the uncommon, the characteristic, and the sometimes confusing. *Radiographics.* 2016;36(3):753–766.

Hosono M, Kobayashi H, Fujimoto R, et al. Septum-like structures in lipoma and liposarcoma: MR imaging with pathologic correlation. *Skeletal Radiol.* 1997;26:150–154.

■ SOFT TISSUE MASSES: LIPOSARCOMA

KEY FACTS

- Clinical:
  - Liposarcoma is the second most common soft tissue sarcoma in adults (16% to 18% of malignant lesions) after undifferentiated-unclassified tumors (previously known as undifferentiated pleomorphic sarcoma and malignant fibrous histiocytoma). There are five categories: (i) well differentiated (54%); (ii) myxoid liposarcoma (23%); (iii) dedifferentiated (10%); (iv) pleomorphic (7%); and (v) not otherwise specified (5%). Patients present with an ill-defined mass.
- Age: 40 to 60 years
- Sex: Males slightly outnumber females.
- Common locations: lower extremities (66% to 75%), retroperitoneum (20% to 33%)
- Imaging features:
  - Radiographic features: soft tissue mass. May be partially fat density.
  - CT: fat density mass with areas of increased attenuation with low-grade liposarcoma. High-grade tumors may have little fat density.
  - MRI: Low grade: fat intensity mass with thickened septa and areas of inhomogeneity (decreased signal T1-weighted image and increased signal T2-weighted image). High grade: signal intensity varies. There may be little fat intensity. Irregular enhancement with gadolinium.
- Differential diagnosis:
  - Lipoma variants
  - Malignant fibrous histiocytoma
  - Other soft tissue sarcomas
- Treatment: excision with or without postoperative radiation. The incidence of local recurrence is 25% to 45% in the extremities and 90% to 100% in the retroperitoneum.

(continued)

■ SOFT TISSUE MASSES: LIPOSARCOMA   *(Continued)*

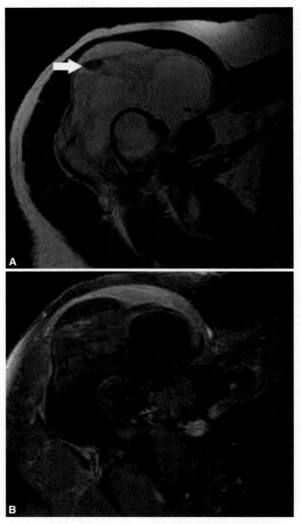

FIGURE 9-39. Well-differentiated liposarcoma/atypical lipomatous tumor. Axial T1-weighted magnetic resonance (MR) image **(A)** of the proximal upper arm demonstrates a large soft tissue mass partially surrounding the humerus. The mass is predominantly composed of fat, but there is a nodular focus of T1 hypointensity *(arrow)* and several thin wispy T1-hypointense septations. These septations demonstrate enhancement on the axial T1-weighted postcontrast MR image **(B)**.

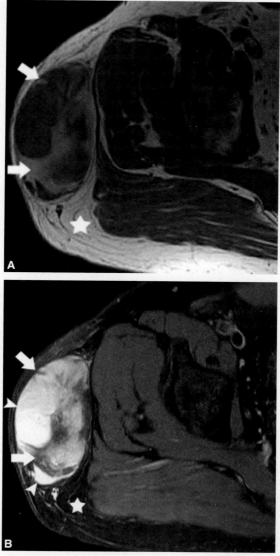

FIGURE 9-40. Myxoid liposarcoma. Axial T1-weighted **(A)** and fat-saturated T2-weighted **(B)** magnetic resonance (MR) images of the right hemipelvis demonstrate a soft tissue mass that contains areas (*arrows*) with T1 and T2 signal intensities that are equivalent to the subcutaneous fat (*star*). The myxoid component of the mass demonstrates prominent T2 hyperintensity (*arrowheads*).

SUGGESTED READING

Gupta P, Potti TA, Wuertzer SD, et al. Spectrum of fat-containing soft-tissue masses at MR imaging: the common, the uncommon, the characteristic, and the sometimes confusing. *Radiographics*. 2016;36(3):753–766.

Kransdorf MJ, Bancroft LW, Peterson JJ, et al. Imaging of fatty tumors: distinction of lipoma and well-differentiated liposarcoma. *Radiology*. 2002;224:99–104.

Peterson JJ, Kransdorf MJ, Bancroft LW, et al. Malignant fatty tumors: classification, clinical course, imaging appearance, and treatment. *Skeletal Radiol*. 2003;32:493–503.

Walker EA, Salesky JS, Fenton ME, et al. Magnetic resonance imaging of malignant soft tissue neoplasms in the adult. *Radiol Clin North Am*. 2011;49(6):1219–1234, vi.

Zoga AC, Weissman BN, Kransdorf MJ, et al. *ACR Appropriateness Criteria—Soft Tissue Masses*. Reston: American College of Radiology; 2012.

■ SOFT TISSUE MASSES: MYXOMA (INTRAMUSCULAR)

KEY FACTS

- Clinical:
  - Patients with this benign mass present with palpable soft tissue mass.
- Age: 40 to 70 years
- Sex: Females outnumber males in the ratio 2:1.
- Common locations: thigh, upper arm and shoulder, gluteal region
- Imaging features:
  - Radiographic features: none. May see soft tissue mass.
  - CT: solid, well-defined intramuscular mass
  - MRI: well-defined mass with low intensity on T1-weighted and homogeneous high intensity on T2-weighted images. There can be thin perilesional fat signal intensity, which is considered a reactive fatty atrophy of the immediately adjacent muscle tissue from exposure to the mucoid material. There can also be perilesional T2 hyperintensity, usually at the poles of the lesion, due to leakage of myxoid material.
- Differential diagnosis:
  - Myxoid liposarcoma
  - Rhabdomyosarcoma
  - Myxoid lipoma
  - Myxoid neurofibroma or schwannoma
- Treatment: local excision

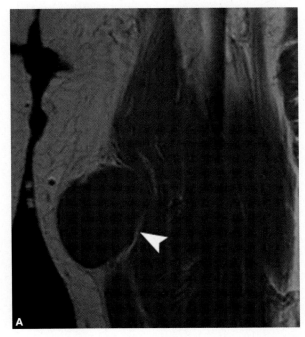

FIGURE 9-41. Myxoma. Coronal T1-weighted **(A)** and fat-saturated T2-weighted **(B)** magnetic resonance (MR) images of the proximal left thigh show a well-defined mass with homogeneous T1 hypointensity and prominent T2 hyperintensity. Note the presence of an incomplete rim of perilesional fat (*arrowhead*) on T1 and perilesional hyperintensity (*arrows*) at the proximal and distal poles of the lesion on T2.

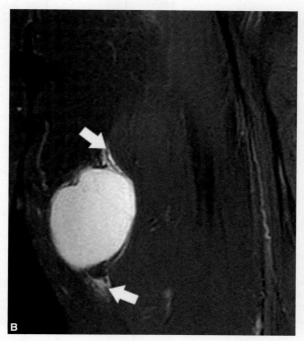

FIGURE 9-41. (*continued*)

SUGGESTED READING

Crombe A, Alberti N, Stoeckle E, et al. Soft tissue masses with myxoid stroma: can conventional magnetic resonance imaging differentiate benign from malignant tumors? *Eur J Radiol.* 2016;85(10):1875–1882.

Peterson KK, Renfrew DL, Fedderson RM, et al. Magnetic resonance imaging of myxoid containing tumors. *Skeletal Radiol.* 1991;20:245–250.

Petscavage-Thomas JM, Walker EA, Logie CI, et al. Soft-tissue myxomatous lesions: review of salient imaging features with pathologic comparison. *Radiographics.* 2014;34(4):964–980.

■ SOFT TISSUE MASSES: SIMPLE VENOUS MALFORMATION (PREVIOUSLY CALLED HEMANGIOMA)

KEY FACTS

■ Clinical:
- Simple venous malformations are common (7% of soft tissue tumors) and represent the most common tumor in children. There are many variants, but most are classified as capillary or cavernous in type. Lesions may change in size and can be painful. There are multiple associated syndromes.
  - ❖ Maffucci: multiple enchondromas and soft tissue venous malformations and spindle cell hemangiomas
  - ❖ Klippel–Trenaunay–Weber: extensive capillary–venous–lymphatic anomaly, bone and soft tissue hypertrophy, varicose veins
  - ❖ Sturge–Weber: facial capillary stain with seizures due to intracranial manifestations of abnormal cerebral venous drainage, glaucoma, buphthalmos, and mental retardation
■ Age: less than 30 years (90% present by 30 years of age)
■ Sex: no sex predilection
■ Common locations: superficial—head and neck; deep—lower extremities
■ Imaging features:
- Radiographic features: normal. Phleboliths may be seen. Bone changes in up to 33% of patients (periosteal reaction, cortical erosion).
- CT: Phleboliths may be seen. Vessels identified with intravenous contrast.
- MRI: serpiginous vessels using conventional spin-echo sequences or magnetic resonance (MR) angiography. There may be large amounts of fat and nonvascular tissue.
■ Differential diagnosis:
- Lipoma
- Angiosarcoma
■ Treatment: observation. Embolization or resection in selected cases.

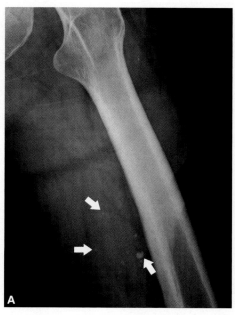

FIGURE 9-42. Simple venous malformation (previously called hemangioma). Frog lateral radiograph of the left hip **(A)** demonstrates several small phleboliths (*arrows*) in the posteromedial soft tissues of the proximal thigh. Axial T1-weighted **(B)** and fat-saturated T2-weighted **(C)** magnetic resonance (MR) images demonstrate a soft tissue mass in the deep adductor compartment with T1 isointensity to muscle and heterogeneous T2 hyperintensity. There is circumferential fat signal intensity (*arrows*) about the malformation. The radiograph was essential for a definitive imaging diagnosis.

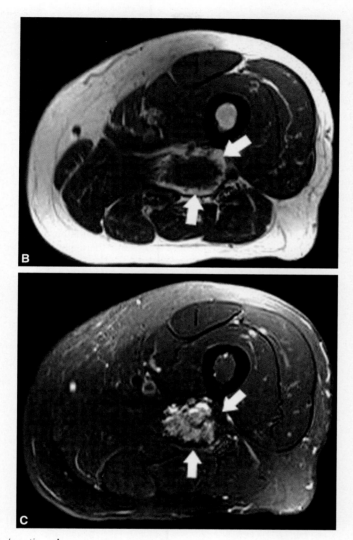

FIGURE 9-42. (*continued*)

SUGGESTED READING

Beutow PC, Kransdorf MJ, Mosen RP, et al. Radiographic appearance of hemangioma with emphasis on MR imaging. *Am J Roentgenol.* 1990;154:563–567.

Flors L, Leiva-Salinas C, Maged IM, et al. MR imaging of soft-tissue vascular malformations: diagnosis, classification, and therapy follow-up. *Radiographics.* 2011;31(5):1321–1340; discussion 1340–1341.

Merrow AC, Gupta A, Patel MN, et al. 2014 revised classification of vascular lesions from the International Society for the Study of Vascular Anomalies: radiologic-pathologic update. *Radiographics.* 2016;36(5):1494–1516.

Sung MS, Kang HS, Lee HG. Regional bone changes in deep soft tissue hemangiomas: Radiographic and MR features. *Skeletal Radiol.* 1998;22:205–210.

Vilanova JC, Barcelo J, Smirniotopoulos JG, et al. Hemangioma from head to toe: MR imaging with pathologic correlation. *Radiographics.* 2004;24:367–385.

Wu JS, Hochman MG. Soft-tissue tumors and tumorlike lesions: a systematic imaging approach. *Radiology.* 2009;253(2):297–316.

■ SOFT TISSUE MASSES: SIMPLE COMMON CYSTIC LYMPHATIC MALFORMATION/LYMPHANGIOMA

KEY FACTS

- Mass composed of multiple endothelial-lined vascular spaces containing proteinaceous fluid. Spaces vary in size (macrocystic, microcystic, and mixed cystic). If spaces measure more than 1 to 2 cm, considered macrocystic.
- Age: birth to 30 years
- Sex: no sex predilection
- Common locations: cystic—head and neck. Other—mediastinum, retroperitoneum, and extremities.
- Imaging features:
  - Radiographic features: soft tissue mass. Calcification rare.
  - CT: macrocystic—soft tissue mass composed of multiple fluid density spaces separated by thin septae
  - MRI: macrocystic—soft tissue mass composed of multiple fluid intensity spaces separated by thin septae. Mild enhancement of septae and outer rims. There may be lobules of enhancing fibroadipose tissue interspersed within the mass.
- Differential diagnosis:
  - Hemangioma
  - Cyst or ganglion
- Treatment: resection, depending on extent and risks

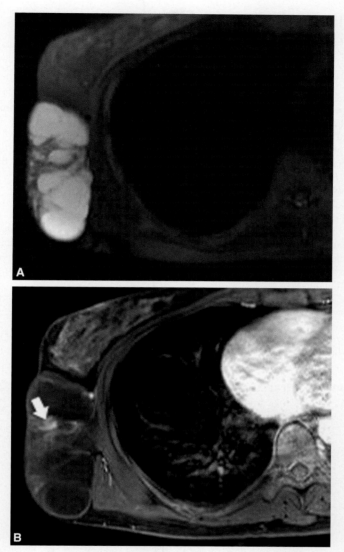

FIGURE 9-43. Simple common cystic (macrocystic) lymphatic malformation (previously called lymph-angioma). Axial HASTE T2 magnetic resonance (MR) image **(A)** of the right axilla demonstrates a mul-tiseptated macrocystic mass with T2 hyperintensity of the cystic spaces. The septae and outer cystic rims are thin and demonstrate mild enhancement on axial fat-saturated T1-weighted MR image **(B)**. The area of nodular enhancement (*arrow*) most likely represents a lobule of interspersed fibrous tissue.

SUGGESTED READING

Elluru RG, Balakrishnan K, Padua HM. Lymphatic malformations: diagnosis and management. *Semin Pediatr Surg.* 2014;23(4):178–185.

Flors L, Leiva-Salinas C, Maged IM, et al. MR imaging of soft-tissue vascular malformations: diagnosis, classification, and therapy follow-up. *Radiographics.* 2011;31(5):1321–1340; discussion 1340–1341.

Merrow AC, Gupta A, Patel MN, et al. 2014 revised classification of vascular lesions from the International Society for the Study of Vascular Anomalies: radiologic-pathologic update. *Radiographics.* 2016;36(5):1494–1516.

Siegel MF, Glazer HS, St. Amour TE, et al. Lymphangiomas in children: MR imaging. *Radiology.* 1989;170:467–470.

■ SOFT TISSUE MASSES: BENIGN PERIPHERAL NERVE SHEATH TUMOR

KEY FACTS

- ■ Clinical:
  - ● Benign peripheral nerve sheath tumors include neurofibromas and schwannomas. Symptoms are similar—slowly growing mass. Pain and paresthesias may be present.
- ■ Age: 20 to 50 years
- ■ Sex: no sex predilection
- ■ Common locations: neurofibroma—cutaneous nerves. Schwannoma—head, neck, flexor surface of extremities, mediastinum, retroperitoneum.
- ■ Imaging features:
  - ● Radiographic features: typically none
  - ● CT: well-defined soft tissue mass
  - ● MRI: neurofibroma—target appearance on T2-weighted images. Low-intensity center with peripheral higher intensity. Central zone enhances on T1-weighted postgadolinium images. Schwannoma—similar to neurofibroma with high intensity on T2-weighted images, target sign and split fat sign.
- ■ Differential diagnosis:
  - ● Cyst
  - ● Myxoma
  - ● Soft tissue sarcoma
- ■ Treatment: resection of schwannoma. Neurofibroma cannot be successfully resected without sacrificing the underlying nerve.

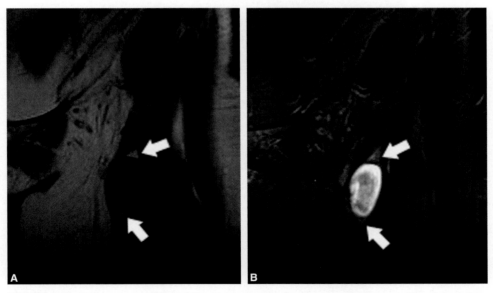

FIGURE 9-44. Schwannoma. Coronal T1-weighted magnetic resonance (MR) image **(A)** of the left inguinal region shows a well-circumscribed ovoid soft tissue mass with T1 isointensity to muscle and an associated split fat sign (*arrows*). The mass demonstrates T2 hyperintensity with central low intensity (target appearance) on the coronal fat-saturated T2-weighted MR image **(B)**.

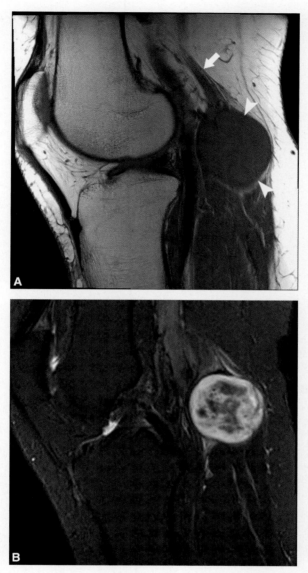

FIGURE 9-45. Neurofibroma. Sagittal T1-weighted magnetic resonance (MR) image **(A)** of the right knee shows a mass (*arrowheads*) eccentrically arising from the posterior tibial nerve (*arrow*) with T1 isointensity to muscle. The mass demonstrates heterogeneous T2 hyperintensity with central low intensity (target appearance) characteristic of neurofibroma on the sagittal short-TI inversion recovery (STIR) MR image **(B)**. There is enhancement of this central zone on the fat-saturated postcontrast T1-weighted MR image **(C)**.

(continued)

■ SOFT TISSUE MASSES: BENIGN PERIPHERAL NERVE SHEATH TUMOR   *(Continued)*

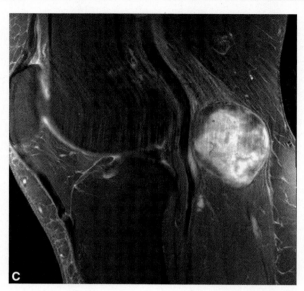

FIGURE 9-45. *(continued)*

SUGGESTED READING

Soldatos T, Fisher S, Karri S, et al. Advanced MR imaging of peripheral nerve sheath tumors including diffusion imaging. *Semin Musculoskelet Radiol.* 2015;19(2):179–190.

Varma DGK, Moulopulos A, Sara AS, et al. MR imaging of extracranial nerve sheath tumors. *J Comput Assist Tomogr.* 1992;16:448–453.

Wasa J, Nishida Y, Tsukushi S, et al. MRI features in the differentiation of malignant peripheral nerve sheath tumors and neurofibromas. *Am J Roentgenol.* 2010;194(6):1568–1574.

Wu JS, Hochman MG. Soft-tissue tumors and tumorlike lesions: a systematic imaging approach. *Radiology.* 2009;253(2):297–316.

■ SOFT TISSUE MASSES: MALIGNANT PERIPHERAL NERVE SHEATH TUMOR

KEY FACTS

- ■ Clinical:
  - ● Malignant peripheral nerve sheath tumors account for 6% to 10% of all soft tissue sarcomas. Half occur in patients with neurofibromatosis. Patients present with enlarging masses with or without pain.
- ■ Age: 20 to 50 years
- ■ Sex: no sex predilection
- ■ Common locations: major nerves or plexus; therefore, upper and lower extremities or trunk
- ■ Imaging features:
  - ● Radiographic features: normal or soft tissue mass
  - ● CT: soft tissue mass in or near major neural structure
  - ● MRI: irregular margins with signal inhomogeneity on T2-weighted images. Irregular bone destruction not uncommon.
- ■ Differential diagnosis:
  - ● Malignant fibrous histiocytoma
  - ● Leiomyosarcoma
  - ● Synovial sarcoma
- ■ Treatment: wide excision. Five-year survival is only 15% to 40%. Prognosis worse if the lesion is larger than 5 cm and in patients with neurofibromatosis.

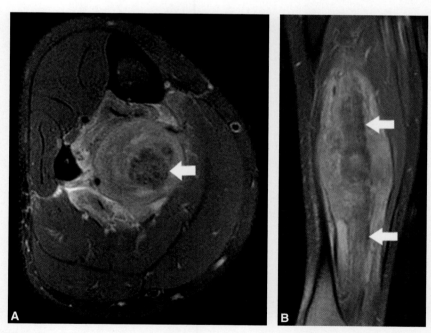

FIGURE 9-46. Malignant peripheral nerve sheath tumor. Axial **(A)** and sagittal **(B)** fat-saturated T2-weighted magnetic resonance (MR) images of the left lower leg show a large ill-defined heterogeneous mass encasing a markedly enlarged tibial nerve (*arrows*).

(continued)

■ SOFT TISSUE MASSES: MALIGNANT PERIPHERAL NERVE SHEATH TUMOR *(Continued)*

SUGGESTED READING

Ducetman BS, Scheithaurer BW, Piepgras DG, et al. Malignant nerve sheath tumors. A clinicopathological study of 120 cases. *Cancer.* 1986;57:2006–2021.

Lin J, Martel W. Cross-sectional imaging of peripheral nerve sheath tumors: characteristic signs on CT, MR imaging, and sonography. *Am J Roentgenol.* 2001;176:75–82.

Soldatos T, Fisher S, Karri S, et al. Advanced MR imaging of peripheral nerve sheath tumors including diffusion imaging. *Semin Musculoskelet Radiol.* 2015;19(2):179–190.

Walker EA, Salesky JS, Fenton ME, et al. Magnetic resonance imaging of malignant soft tissue neoplasms in the adult. *Radiol Clin North Am.* 2011;49(6):1219–1234, vi.

Wasa J, Nishida Y, Tsukushi S, et al. MRI features in the differentiation of malignant peripheral nerve sheath tumors and neurofibromas. *Am J Roentgenol.* 2010;194(6):1568–1574.

■ SOFT TISSUE MASSES: DEEP FIBROMATOSIS (DESMOID TUMOR)

KEY FACTS

■ Clinical:
  ● Fibromatoses may be superficial, which are diagnosed clinically, or deep, which often require imaging for detection and diagnosis. Although benign lesions, they have an aggressive clinical behavior. Multiple lesions are reported in 10% to 15% of cases. Patients present with a soft tissue mass.
■ Age: adolescent to 40 years
■ Sex: no sex predilection
■ Common locations: most in lower extremity, upper extremity, shoulder
■ Imaging features:
  ● Radiographic features: Soft tissue mass may be evident. Pressure erosions of adjacent bone (6% to 16%).
  ● CT: poorly defined soft tissue mass. Good for early bone involvement.
  ● MRI: Variable portions to entire mass may have low signal intensity on all pulse sequences because of fibrous tissue. More often, areas of intermediate signal intensity on T2-weighted images are also present. Prominent enhancement. Irregular margins. Neurovascular and bone involvement easily identified.
■ Differential diagnosis:
  ● Fibrosarcoma
  ● Malignant fibrous histiocytoma
■ Treatment: wide excision when possible. Recurrence rate greater than 75%.

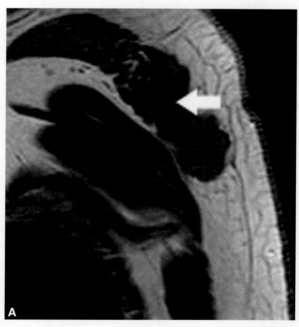

FIGURE 9-47. Desmoid tumor. Sagittal T1-weighted **(A)** conventional T2-weighted **(B)** and fat-saturated postcontrast T1-weighted **(C)** magnetic resonance (MR) images show a poorly defined markedly enhancing mass with areas of low T1 and T2 signal intensity, which is characteristic of fibrous tissue.

(continued)

■ SOFT TISSUE MASSES: DEEP FIBROMATOSIS (DESMOID TUMOR) *(Continued)*

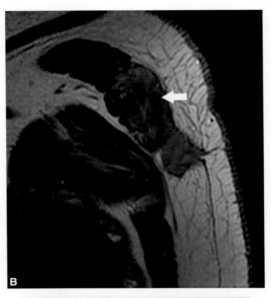

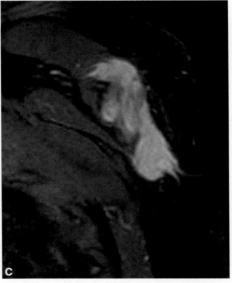

FIGURE 9-47. *(continued)*

SUGGESTED READING

Braschi-Amirfarzan M, Keraliya AR, Krajewski KM, et al. Role of imaging in management of desmoid-type fibromatosis: a primer for radiologists. *Radiographics*. 2016;36(3):767–782.

Lee JC, Thomas JM, Phillips S, et al. Aggressive fibromatosis: MRI features with pathologic correlation. *Am J Roentgenol*. 2006;186:247–254.

Sundaram M, McGuire MH, Schajowicz F. Soft tissue masses: histologic bases for decreased signal (short T2) on T2-weighted MR images. *Am J Roentgenol*. 1987;148:1247–1250.

■ SOFT TISSUE MASSES: ELASTOFIBROMA

KEY FACTS

■ Clinical:
  ● Elastofibroma is a tumorlike mass resulting from friction between the scapula and chest wall. The lesion is not uncommon and is found in 24% of females and 11% of males at autopsy when patients are aged more than 55 years. Half are asymptomatic.
■ Age: more than 55 years; mean 70 years
■ Sex: Females outnumber males in the ratio 2:1.
■ Common locations: between scapula and chest wall in 99%; up to 67% are bilateral
■ Imaging features:
  ● Radiographic features: normal. Rarely, scapula displaced.
  ● CT: soft tissue mass isodense to muscle containing varying amounts of fat. Location more specific for diagnosis than imaging features.
  ● MRI: soft tissue mass with signal intensity similar to muscle on T1- and T2-weighted images containing varying amounts of fat. There is enhancement with gadolinium.
■ Differential diagnosis:
  ● Fibroma
  ● Desmoid
■ Treatment: surgical excision

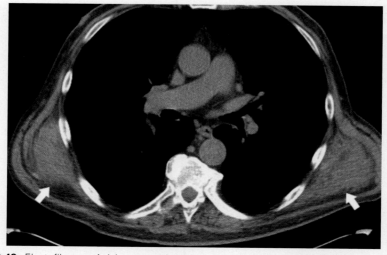

FIGURE 9-48. Elastofibroma. Axial computed tomography (CT) image shows bilateral masses (*arrows*) between the ribcage and serratus anterior muscles that are predominantly isodense to muscle but also contain linear areas of fat density.

(continued)

■ SOFT TISSUE MASSES: ELASTOFIBROMA   *(Continued)*

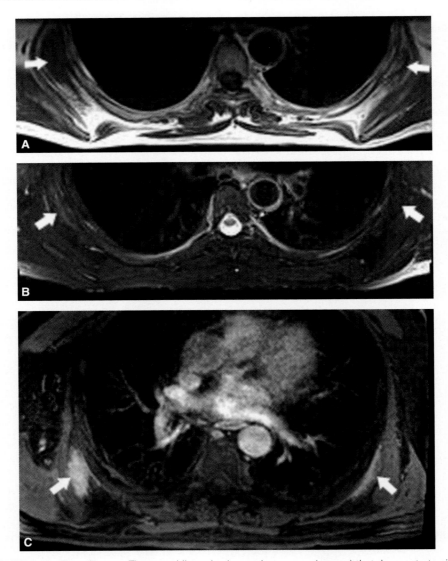

FIGURE 9-49. Elastofibroma. There are bilateral subscapular masses (*arrows*) that demonstrate signal intensities similar to muscle on both axial T1-weighted **(A)** and fat-saturated T2-weighted **(B)** magnetic resonance (MR) images. The characteristic interspersed fat tissue is best seen in the smaller left-sided mass. These masses demonstrate enhancement on axial fat-saturated postcontrast T1-weighted images **(C)**.

SUGGESTED READING

Kransdorf MJ, Meis JM, Montgomery E. Elastofibroma. MR and CT appearance with radiological-pathological correlation. *Am J Roentgenol*. 1992;159:575–579.

Tamimi Mariño I, Sesma Solis P, Pérez Lara A, et al. Sensitivity and positive predictive value of magnetic resonance imaging in the diagnosis of elastofibroma dorsi: review of fourteen cases. *J Shoulder Elbow Surg*. 2013;22(1):57–63.

■ SOFT TISSUE MASSES: GANGLION

KEY FACTS

- ■ Clinical:
  - ● Ganglia are often asymptomatic, well-defined juxta-articular lesions. Some may present with pain. Most are less than 2 cm in size.
- ■ Age: 25 to 45 years
- ■ Sex: much more common in females than in males
- ■ Common locations: wrist and hand most common, but occur around any articular location
- ■ Imaging features:
  - ● Radiographic features: normal or small soft tissue mass
  - ● CT: well-defined soft tissue mass with fluid density
  - ● MRI: well-defined lesion with uniformly high intensity on T2-weighted and low signal intensity on T1-weighted sequences. May vary if complicated by hemorrhage or thick proteinaceous debris. Thin wall enhances with gadolinium.
- ■ Differential diagnosis:
  - ● Synovial sarcoma
  - ● Nerve sheath tumor
- ■ Treatment: aspiration, needle fenestration, or resection

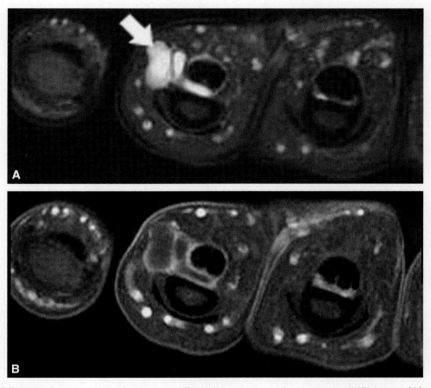

FIGURE 9-50. Ganglion. Axial fat-saturated T2-weighted magnetic resonance (MR) image **(A)** of the fourth finger shows a well-defined septated lesion containing T2-hyperintense fluid (*arrow*). Fat-saturated postcontrast T1-weighted MR image **(B)** shows enhancement of the thin septation and outer wall.

(continued)

■ SOFT TISSUE MASSES: GANGLION   *(Continued)*

SUGGESTED READING

Bermejo A, De Bustamante TD, Martinez A, et al. MR imaging in the evaluation of cystic-appearing soft-tissue masses of the extremities. *Radiographics*. 2013;33(3):833–855.

Feldman F, Surgson SD, Staron RB. Magnetic resonance imaging of para-articular and ectopic ganglia. *Skeletal Radiol*. 1989;18:353–358.

Wu JS, Hochman MG. Soft-tissue tumors and tumorlike lesions: a systematic imaging approach. *Radiology*. 2009;253(2):297–316.

■ SOFT TISSUE MASSES: GIANT CELL TUMOR OF TENDON SHEATH

KEY FACTS

- ■ Clinical:
  - Giant cell tumors of the tendon sheath may be focal or diffuse. The localized lesion is most common in the hand, usually the flexor tendons. Patients present with a slow-growing soft tissue mass.
- ■ Age: 30 to 50 years
- ■ Sex: Females outnumber males.
- ■ Common locations: hand; less commonly, foot, knee, and hip
- ■ Imaging features:
  - Radiographic features: soft tissue mass. Bone erosion in 15%.
  - CT: soft tissue mass associated with tendon. Bone involvement easily appreciated.
  - MRI: mass associated with a tendon and low to isointense to muscle on T1-weighted and low to mildly hyperintense on T2-weighted sequences. Heterogeneous enhancement with gadolinium.
- ■ Differential diagnosis:
  - Granuloma
  - Fibroma
- ■ Treatment: resection. Recurrence occurs in up to 20%.

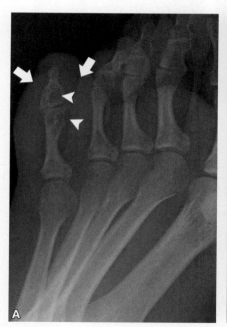 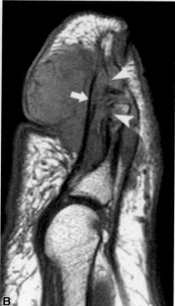

FIGURE 9-51. Giant cell tumor of the tendon sheath. Oblique radiograph **(A)** of the left fifth toe demonstrates a soft tissue mass (*arrows*) with bone erosion (*arrowheads*). Sagittal T1-weighted **(B)** and short-TI inversion recovery (STIR) **(C)** magnetic resonance (MR) images show a mass with T1 isointensity relative to muscle and heterogeneous mild T2 hyperintensity encasing the flexor tendon (*arrow*) with underlying bone erosion (*arrowheads*). The mass demonstrates heterogeneous enhancement on the sagittal fat-saturated postcontrast T1-weighted MR image **(D)**.

(continued)

■ SOFT TISSUE MASSES: GIANT CELL TUMOR OF TENDON SHEATH *(Continued)*

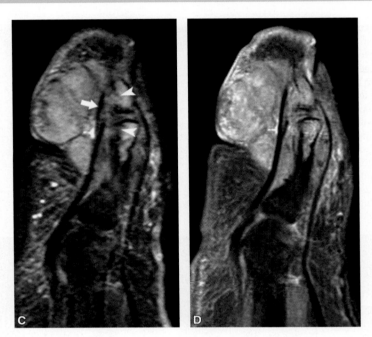

FIGURE 9-51. *(continued)*

SUGGESTED READING

Garner HW, Bestic JM. Benign synovial tumors and proliferative processes. *Semin Musculoskelet Radiol.* 2013;17(2):177–178.

Jelinek JS, Kransdorf MJ, Utz JA, et al. MR imaging of giant cell tumor of the tendon sheath. *Am J Roentgenol.* 1994;162:919–922.

Wu JS, Hochman MG. Soft-tissue tumors and tumorlike lesions: a systematic imaging approach. *Radiology.* 2009;253(2):297–316.

■ SOFT TISSUE MASSES: HEMATOMA

KEY FACTS

- Clinical:
  - Patients present with history of trauma or mass that may be painful. Hematomas may be acute (hours, days), subacute (3 weeks to 3 months), or chronic (more than 3 months).
- Age: occurs at any age
- Sex: no sex predilection
- Common locations: lower extremities
- Imaging features:
  - Radiographic features: normal or soft tissue mass
  - CT: soft tissue mass with areas of increased attenuation caused by blood. Usually well-defined margins.
  - MRI
    - ❖ Acute: muscle density on T1-weighted and variable on T2-weighted sequences
    - ❖ Subacute: increased signal on T1- and T2-weighted sequences. May have low-intensity fibrous rim, internal debris, and fluid–fluid levels
    - ❖ Chronic: similar to subacute
- Differential diagnosis:
  - Sarcoma
  - Abscess
- Treatment: observe or resect, depending on location and symptoms

(continued)

■ SOFT TISSUE MASSES: HEMATOMA   *(Continued)*

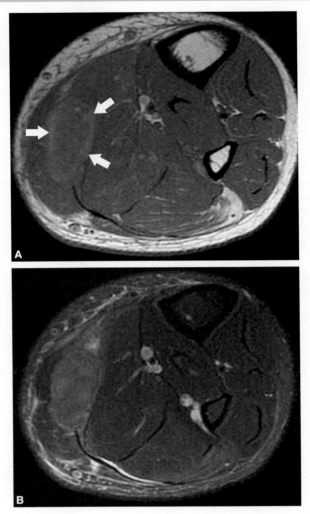

FIGURE 9-52. Acute hematoma. Axial T1-weighted magnetic resonance (MR) image **(A)** of the left lower leg obtained 2 days after injury shows a mass between the medial gastrocnemius and soleus muscles with heterogeneous T1 signal intensity that is isointense to muscle centrally but has an ill-defined rim of T1 hyperintensity (*arrows*). The hematoma demonstrates mild T2 hyperintensity on the fat-saturated T2-weighted MR image **(B)**. Note the associated subcutaneous soft tissue and fascial edema on both sequences.

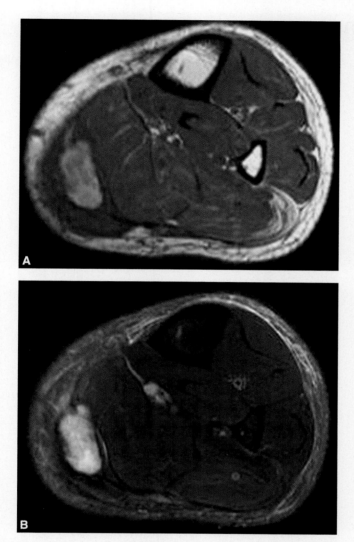

FIGURE 9-53. Subacute hematoma (same patient as Fig 9-52). Axial T1-weighted **(A)** and fat-saturated T2-weighted **(B)** magnetic resonance (MR) images of the left lower leg obtained 18 days after injury now show heterogeneous T1 and T2 hyperintensity within the mass. The mass has a worrisome appearance on the axial fat-saturated postcontrast MR image **(C)**, but axial subtraction MR image **(D)** confirms complete lack of enhancement within the mass and mild reactive enhancement in the surrounding tissues. Note mild interval improvement of the associated subcutaneous soft tissue and fascial edema on T1 and T2 sequences.

(continued)

■ SOFT TISSUE MASSES: HEMATOMA   *(Continued)*

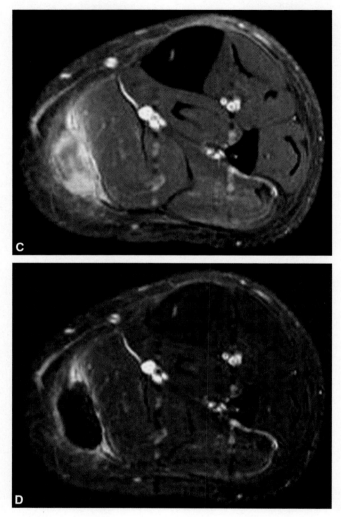

FIGURE 9-53. *(continued)*

SUGGESTED READING

Aoki T, Norkata H, Watanabe H, et al. The radiologic findings of chronic expanding hematoma. *Skeletal Radiol.* 1999;28:396–401.

Wu JS, Hochman MG. Soft-tissue tumors and tumorlike lesions: a systematic imaging approach. *Radiology.* 2009;253(2):297–316.

■ SOFT TISSUE MASSES: MYOSITIS OSSIFICANS

KEY FACTS

- Clinical:
  - Patients may or may not have a history of trauma. Pain, tenderness, and soft tissue mass are common findings.
- Age: children, adults
- Sex: no sex predilection
- Common locations: Eighty percent are in the large muscles of the extremities, especially lower extremities
- Imaging features:
  - Radiographic features: faint soft tissue calcification within 2 to 6 weeks. May have well-defined bony margins by 8 weeks.
  - Separated from periosteum by lucent zone.
  - CT: Characteristic feature is peripheral ossification.
  - MRI: Features vary with age of the lesion. Can have MR features that are confused for malignancy—misdiagnosis is best avoided by correlating MR imaging with radiographs.
  - Early: low intensity on T1-weighted and high intensity on T2-weighted images. Soft tissue edema with similar pattern.
  - Late: peripheral rim of low intensity on all sequences. Irregular areas of increased signal intensity on T2-weighted sequences and fluid–fluid levels centrally. Later, central signal intensity similar to fat on all sequences or areas of low intensity caused by ossification or fibrosis.
- Differential diagnosis:
  - Parosteal sarcoma
  - Juxtacortical osteosarcoma
- Treatment: resection

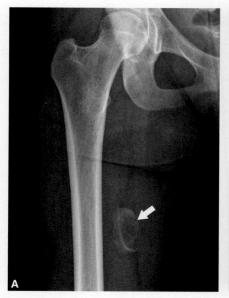 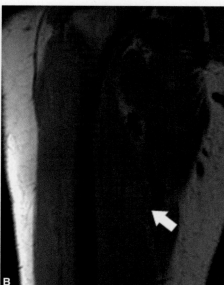

FIGURE 9-54. Myositis ossificans of intermediate age. Anteroposterior (AP) radiograph **(A)** of the right hip shows an area of well-defined ossification (*arrow*) in the medial soft tissues of the proximal thigh. On the coronal T1-weighted magnetic resonance (MR) image **(B)**, the mass (*arrow*) is isointense to muscle and is difficult to discern. Coronal fat-saturated T2-weighted **(C)** and fat-saturated postcontrast T1-weighted **(D)** MR images show an ill-defined mass with prominent surrounding soft tissue edema-like signal and enhancement. There is a subtle rim of decreased T1 and T2 signal (*arrowheads*), which corresponds to the ossification seen on radiographs.

(continued)

■ SOFT TISSUE MASSES: MYOSITIS OSSIFICANS   *(Continued)*

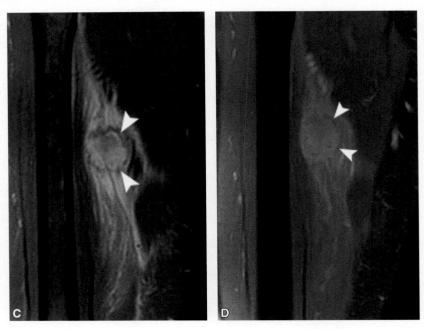

FIGURE 9-54. *(continued)*

SUGGESTED READING

DeSmet AA, Norris MA, Fisher DR. Magnetic resonance imaging of myositis ossificans. *Skeletal Radiol.* 1992;21:503–507.
Tyler P, Saifuddin A. The imaging of myositis ossificans. *Semin Musculoskelet Radiol.* 2010;14(2):201–216.
Wu JS, Hochman MG. Soft-tissue tumors and tumorlike lesions: a systematic imaging approach. *Radiology.* 2009;253(2):297–316.

■ SOFT TISSUE MASSES: UNDIFFERENTIATED-UNCLASSIFIED TUMOR (PREVIOUSLY KNOWN AS UNDIFFERENTIATED PLEOMORPHIC SARCOMA)

KEY FACTS

- Clinical:
  - Undifferentiated-unclassified tumor (previously known as undifferentiated pleomorphic sarcoma) is the most common soft tissue sarcoma in adults more than 45 years of age. Patients usually present with a painless enlarging lower extremity mass.
- Age: 45 to 70 years
- Sex: Males outnumber females in the ratio 2:1.
- Common locations: thigh, lower extremity, upper extremity, and retroperitoneum in decreasing frequency
- Imaging features:
  - Radiographic features: soft tissue mass. Rarely calcifies.
  - CT: soft tissue mass with variable enhancement after intravenous contrast
  - MRI: nonspecific imaging features. Irregular margins with low intensity on T1-weighted and inhomogeneous high signal intensity on T2-weighted sequences. Variable enhancement with gadolinium.
- Differential diagnosis:
  - Pleomorphic liposarcoma
  - Fibrosarcoma
  - Desmoid tumor
- Treatment: wide excision. Radiation and chemotherapy as adjuvant or palliative measures

(continued)

■ SOFT TISSUE MASSES: UNDIFFERENTIATED-UNCLASSIFIED TUMOR (PREVIOUSLY KNOWN AS UNDIFFERENTIATED PLEOMORPHIC SARCOMA) *(Continued)*

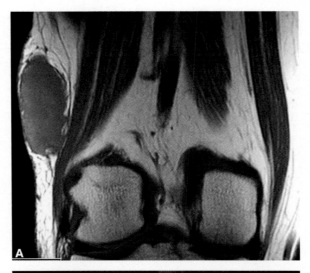

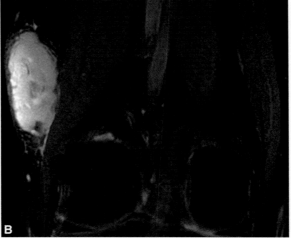

FIGURE 9-55. Undifferentiated-unclassified tumor (previously known as undifferentiated pleomorphic sarcoma). Coronal T1-weighted **(A)** and T2-weighted **(B)** images of the right knee show a heterogeneous mass in the lateral subcutaneous soft tissues that is predominantly hyperintense on T2. There is mild irregularity of the margins of the mass and minimal surrounding soft tissue edema-like signal.

SUGGESTED READING

Baheti AD, O'Malley RB, Kim S, et al. Soft-tissue sarcomas: an update for radiologists based on the revised 2013 World Health Organization classification. *AJR Am J Roentgenol.* 2016; 206(5):924–932.

Walker EA, Salesky JS, Fenton ME, et al. Magnetic resonance imaging of malignant soft tissue neoplasms in the adult. *Radiol Clin North Am.* 2011;49(6):1219–1234, vi.

Weiss SW, Goldblum JR. *Enzinger and Weiss Soft Tissue Tumors.* 4th ed. St. Louis: Mosby; 2001:535–570.

■ SOFT TISSUE MASSES: SYNOVIAL SARCOMA

KEY FACTS

- ■ Clinical:
  - ● Synovial sarcoma is fairly common, accounting for 10% of soft tissue sarcomas. Patients present with a slow-growing, often innocent-appearing mass. The mass typically is near a joint and often associated with a tendon sheath, bursa, or fascial plane. Metastasis is present at time of diagnosis in 25% of patients. Pain is also commonly present.
- ■ Age: 15 to 40 years
- ■ Sex: Males slightly outnumber females.
- ■ Common locations: extremities near larger joints, especially the knee
- ■ Imaging features:
  - ● Radiographic features: normal or well-defined soft tissue mass. Calcification occurs in 33%. Bone involvement occurs in 20%.
  - ● CT: well-defined soft tissue mass near a joint. Subtle calcification is easily appreciated.
  - ● MRI: inhomogeneous signal on T2-weighted sequences. May have cystic appearance and fluid–fluid levels. Calcifications seen as areas of low intensity on all sequences.
- ■ Differential diagnosis:
  - ● Benign cyst
  - ● Hematoma
  - ● Epithelioid sarcoma
  - ● Malignant nerve sheath tumor
- ■ Treatment: wide excision, adjuvant radiation therapy

(continued)

■ SOFT TISSUE MASSES: SYNOVIAL SARCOMA   *(Continued)*

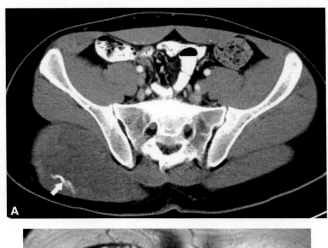

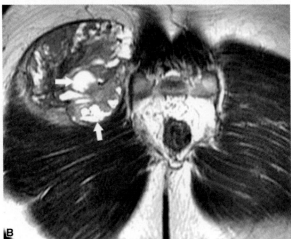

FIGURE 9-56. Synovial sarcoma. Axial computed tomography (CT) image **(A)** of the pelvis shows a large right gluteal soft tissue mass containing a small amount of calcification (*arrow*). The mass is markedly heterogeneous in signal on coronal conventional T2-weighted magnetic resonance (MR) image **(B)** with multiple cystic spaces (*arrows*). Sagittal T1-weighted **(C)** and fat-saturated postcontrast T1-weighted **(D)** MR images show a large heterogeneously enhancing mass containing areas of T1 hyperintense hemorrhage. Note that the T1 hyperintensity does not represent fat because the majority of the T1 hyperintense areas demonstrate enhancement.

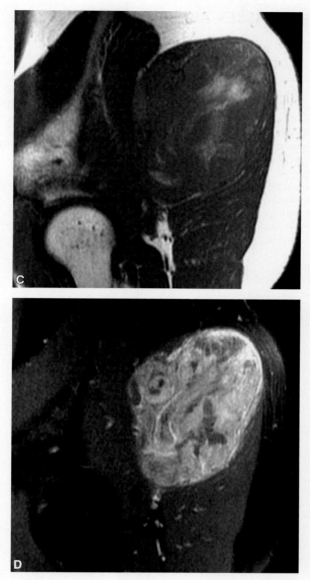

FIGURE 9-56. (*continued*)

SUGGESTED READING

Morton MJ, Berquist TH, McLeod RA, et al. MR imaging of synovial sarcoma. *Am J Roentgenol.* 1990;156:337–340.

Murphey MD, Gibson MS, Jennings BT, et al. From the archives of the AFIP: imaging of synovial sarcoma with radiologic-pathologic correlation. *Radiographics.* 2006;26(5):1543–1565.

Walker EA, Salesky JS, Fenton ME, et al. Magnetic resonance imaging of malignant soft tissue neoplasms in the adult. *Radiol Clin North Am.* 2011;49(6):1219–1234, vi.

■ SOFT TISSUE MASSES: RHABDOMYOSARCOMA

KEY FACTS

- Clinical:
  - Rhabdomyosarcoma is the most common soft tissue sarcoma in children aged less than 15 years, but is also common in adolescents and young adults. Patients present with soft tissue mass when extremities are involved. Metastasis is present at the time of diagnosis in 20%.
- Age: children, young adults
- Sex: Males slightly outnumber females.
- Common locations: head, neck, genitourinary tract, retroperitoneum, and extremities, in decreasing order of frequency
- Imaging features:
  - Radiographic features: vary with location. Most poorly defined masses. Lower genitourinary tract (botryoid sarcoma) may look like multiple cysts in 25% of cases.
  - CT: similar to radiographic
  - MRI: nonspecific imaging features. Typically, high signal intensity on T2-weighted and low on T1-weighted sequences. May be inhomogeneous on T2-weighted sequences, with poorly defined margins.
- Differential diagnosis:
  - Transitional cell (bladder)
  - Leiomyosarcoma
  - Lymphoma
- Treatment: wide excision when possible. Varies with location. Recurrence and metastasis are common.

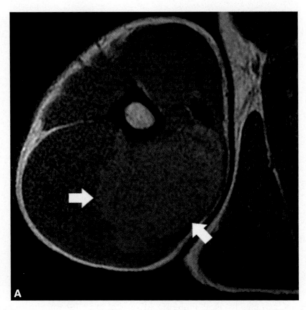

FIGURE 9-57. Rhabdomyosarcoma. Axial T1-weighted **(A)** and fat-saturated T2-weighted **(B)** magnetic resonance (MR) images of the right upper arm show a mass within the triceps muscle with slight T1 hyperintensity and heterogeneous T2 hyperintensity. The mass demonstrates irregular enhancement with areas of necrosis (*star*) on the axial fat-saturated postcontrast T1-weighted MR image **(C)**.

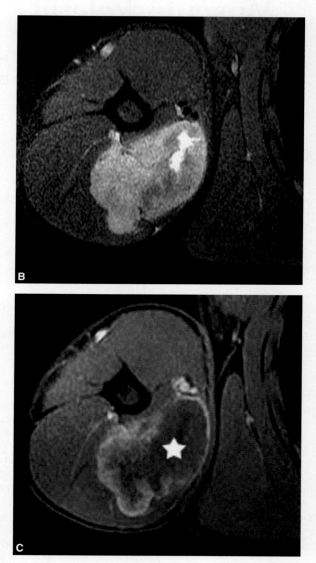

FIGURE 9-57. (*continued*)

SUGGESTED READING

Franco A, Lewis KN, Lee JR. Pediatric rhabdomyosarcoma at presentation: can cross-sectional imaging findings predict pathologic tumor subtype? *Eur J Radiol.* 2011;80(3):e446–e450.

Saboo SS, Krajewski KM, Zukotynski K, et al. Imaging features of primary and secondary adult rhabdomyosarcoma. *Am J Roentgenol.* 2012;199(6):W694–W703.

Weiss SW, Goldblum JR. *Enzinger and Weiss's Soft Tissue Tumors.* 4th ed. St. Louis: Mosby; 2001:785–836.

Musculoskeletal Infection

Stephanie A. Bernard, Jeffrey J. Peterson, and Thomas H. Berquist

■ BASIC CONCEPTS

KEY FACTS

■ Depending on the organism and the patient's immune status, musculoskeletal infections may present with rapidly progressive onset or in a more insidious fashion (Table 10-1). Source of infections may be hematogenous, from contiguous spread (adjacent soft tissues or joint), or from direct implantation (i.e., puncture wound, trauma, or surgery).

■ Insidious onset of infection often follows trauma or surgical intervention or infection with atypical organisms (Tuberculosis, Lyme).

■ Clinical presentation is dependent on patient age, virulence of organisms, patient condition, site of involvement, and circulation (Table 10-2).

■ Early detection and evaluation of the extent of involvement are essential for proper treatment and optimal prognosis.

■ Imaging of musculoskeletal infection usually requires a multimodality approach.

■ Radiography: Soft tissue swelling or joint effusion may be the only findings. Significant bone destruction must be present before radiographs are positive.

Table 10-1 INFECTIONS: TERMINOLOGY AND CATEGORIES

Term/Conditions	Clinical/Image Features
Osteomyelitis	Infections in bone and marrow. Bacterial most common
Infective osteitis	Cortical infection. Often associated with marrow or soft tissue infection
Infective periostitis	Periosteal infection often with marrow and cortex involved
Soft tissue infection	Involves skin, subcutaneous tissues, muscles, tendons, ligaments, fascia, or bursae
Sequestrum	Segment of necrotic bone separated from viable bone by granulation tissue
Involucrum	Living bone around sequestrum
Cloaca	Tract through viable bone
Sinus	Tract from infected region to skin
Fistula	Abnormal communication between two internal organs or internal organs and skin
Brodie abscess	Sharply defined focus of osteomyelitis
Garré sclerosing osteomyelitis	Sclerotic nonpurulent infection with intense periosteal reaction
Chronic recurrent multifocal osteomyelitis	Subacute or chronic infection common in children. May be associated with SAPHO
SAPHO	Palmoplantar pustulosis, articular, and hyperostosis and osteitis (SAPHO) periosteal inflammation
	Chronic course involving chest wall, spine, long bones, large and small joints

SAPHO, synovitis, acne, pustulosis, hyperostosis, osteitis.

Table 10-2 COMMON ORGANISMS IN MUSCULOSKELETAL INFECTIONS

Bacterial Infections	Fungal and Higher Bacterial Infections	Parasitic Infections
Gram-positive	Actinomycosis	Hookworms
Staphylococcal	Nocardiosis	Cysticercosis
Streptococcal	Cryptococcosis	Echinococcosis
Meningococcal	Coccidioidomycosis	
Gonococcal	Histoplasmosis	
Gram-negative bacilli	Sporotrichosis	
Coliform bacterial infections		
Proteus		
Pseudomonas		
Klebsiella		
Salmonella		
Haemophilus		
Brucella		
Mycobacteria		
Tuberculosis		
Atypical mycobacteria		

- Molecular imaging: Bone scanning is sensitive and can detect abnormalities early, but there is less anatomic detail, and findings are not specific. Techniques include three-phase technetium-99m-methylene diphosphate, gallium-67-, and indium- or technetium-labeled white blood cell studies, technetium antigranulocyte antibody scans, and positron emission tomography (PET).
- Computed tomography (CT): Less sensitive than magnetic resonance imaging (MRI) or molecular imaging for most infections. Highest sensitive for soft tissue gas. Contrast aides in identifying abscess. Will detect cortical changes along with sequestra and cloaca in chronic osteomyelitis.
- Ultrasound: Soft tissue infection, abscess formation, foreign body localization, and joint effusions can be identified and can be used for aspiration.
- MRI: MRI is particularly suited for evaluation of early bone or soft tissue infection. Contrast is superior to CT, and anatomic detail is superior to radionuclide scans. When patient is able to receive contrast, contrast-enhanced fat-suppressed T1-weighted images help with identifying extent of infection and tissue viability.
- Aspiration/biopsy: Regardless of the imaging technique used, joint aspiration or synovial or bone biopsy under fluoroscopic or ultrasound guidance may be required to isolate the organism.

SUGGESTED READING

Berquist TH, Broderick DF. Musculoskeletal infections. In: Berquist TH, ed. *MRI of the Musculoskeletal System.* 5th ed. Philadelphia: Lippincott Williams & Wilkins; 2006:916–947.

Palestro CJ, Love C, Miller TT. Infection and musculoskeletal conditions: imaging of musculoskeletal infections. *Best Pract Res Clin Rheumatol.* 2006; 20:1197–1218.

Resnick D. Osteomyelitis, septic arthritis, and soft tissue infection: mechanisms and situations. In: Resnick D. *Diagnosis of Bone and Joint Disorders.* 4th ed. Philadelphia: WB Saunders; 2002:2510–2624.

■ OSTEOMYELITIS

KEY FACTS

■ The imaging appearance is dependent on the virulence of the organism and the stage of disease.
  ● **Acute pyogenic osteomyelitis**: permeative osteolytic destruction with periosteal
  ● **Subacute osteomyelitis** (Brodie abscess): well-defined lytic lesion with sclerotic border
  ● **Chronic osteomyelitis**: sclerosis with central sequestra of osteonecrotic bone, encasing involucrum, and draining cloaca
■ Early diagnosis and management are essential to avoid irreversible bone or articular damage.
■ Hematogenous osteomyelitis is more common in children than in adults and most frequently involves the lower extremities.
■ Metaphyseal regions, near the physis, are most commonly involved.
■ The open physis serves a protective function preventing infection from entering the epiphysis and, depending on joint anatomy, the joint from ages 1 to 16 years.
■ Imaging of osteomyelitis requires a multimodality approach (Table 10-3).
  ● Routine radiographs: may show soft tissue swelling. Bone changes may be inapparent early.
  ● Radionuclide scans: A positive technetium-99m scan is not specific, but a negative scan excludes the diagnosis. Combined indium-111 or technetium-labeled leukocytes and technetium-99m scans are more specific. PET may also be useful, especially for osteomyelitis in the spine.
  ● CT: cortical detail, sequestra, and cloacae
  ● MRI: T1- and T2-weighted magnetic resonance (MR) images are sensitive and can detect changes of infection early. T1-weighted signal abnormalities are most important. Gadolinium-enhanced T1-weighted images are routinely added in our practice. Anatomic detail is superior to radionuclide scans.

Table 10-3   IMAGING APPROACHES FOR OSTEOMYELITIS

Radiographic Features	Next Steps
Positive	Biopsy and treat
Negative; low suspicion	Technetium scan:
	● Negative: stop
	● Positive: MRI or combined radionuclide studies
Negative; high suspicion	MRI or combined radionuclide studies and MRI

MRI, magnetic resonance imaging.

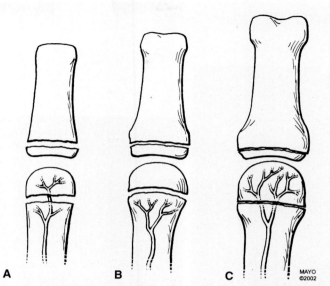

FIGURE 10-1. The vascular supply to the metaphysis and epiphysis in infants **(A)**, children **(B)**, and adults **(C)**. The physis serves a protective function for the epiphysis from ages 1 to 16 years **(B)**.

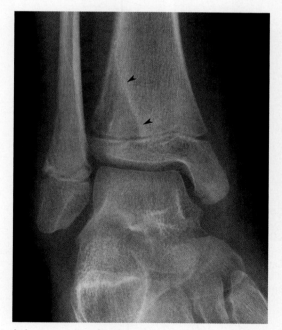

FIGURE 10-2. Characteristic appearance of subacute osteomyelitis as a well-circumscribed metaphyseal lucency in the distal tibia. Radiographic osteolytic lesion with a sclerotic border (*arrowheads*).

(continued)

■ **OSTEOMYELITIS** *(Continued)*

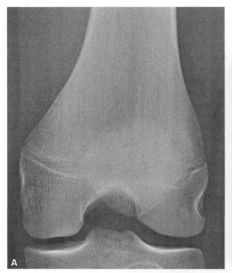
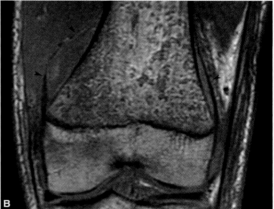
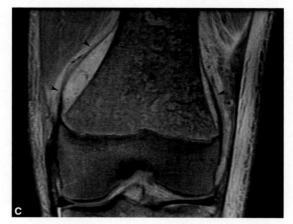

FIGURE 10-3. Acute hematogenous osteomyelitis of the distal femur in a 15-year- old male. **(A)** Radiographically inapparent at time of magnetic resonance imaging (MRI). On MRI, the marrow demonstrates reticulated intermediate **(B)** T1-weighted infiltration of the marrow with increased signal on **(C)** Proton density fat-saturated imaging. Subperiosteal abscess (*arrowheads*) can be seen elevating the periosteum stopping at the level of the physis, where the periosteum is tightly adherent.

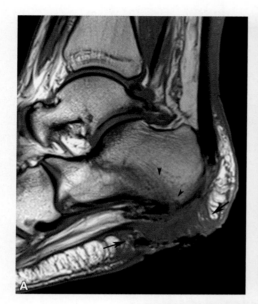
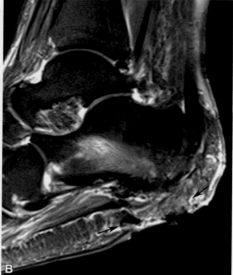
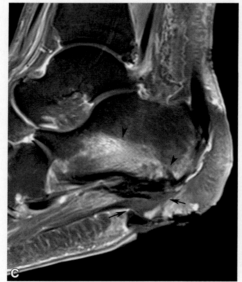

FIGURE 10-4. Osteomyelitis from direct extension from a diabetic foot ulcer in a 51-year-old female. **(A)** T1-weighted, **(B)** short-T1 inversion recovery (STIR), and **(C)** postgadolinium T1-weighted fat-saturated images of the hindfoot demonstrate an ulcer at the plantar aspect of the heel with replacement of the normal subcutaneous fat on T1 image to the bone surface and with contrast outlining sinus tract to skin (*arrows*). Underlying increased T2 signal and enhancement in the marrow with mild T1 marrow infiltration (*arrowheads*).

SUGGESTED READING

Bonakdapour A, Gaines VD. The radiology of osteomyelitis. *Orthop Clin North Am.* 1983;14:21–37.

Collins MS, Schaar MM, Wenger DE, et al. T1-weighted MRI characteristics of pedal osteomyelitis. *Am J Roentgenol.* 2005;185:386–393.

Gold RH, Hawkins RA, Katz BD. Bacterial osteomyelitis: findings on plain film, CT, MRI, and scintigraphy. *Am J Roentgenol.* 1991;157:365–370.

Santiago Restrepo C, Gimenez CR, McCarthy K. Imaging of osteomyelitis and musculoskeletal soft tissue infections: current concepts. *Rheum Dis Clin North Am.* 2003;29:89–109.

■ CHRONIC RECURRENT MULTIFOCAL OSTEOMYELITIS

KEY FACTS

- Characterized by exacerbation and remissions.
- May occur at any age, but most common in children 5 to 10 years of age.
- Patients present with pain, swelling, and tenderness in areas of skeletal involvement.
- The femoral metaphysis, tibia, and medial clavicles are most commonly involved.
- Currently considered an inflammatory, nonpyogenic disorder with possible autoimmune and genetic component.
- Imaging features show sclerosis of the medial clavicles on radiographs and CT. MR features are nonspecific.

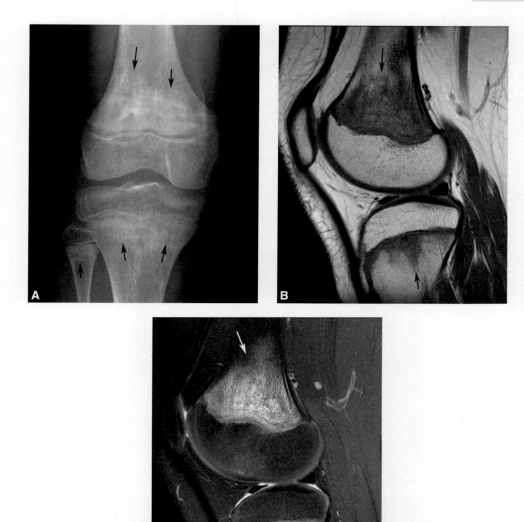

FIGURE 10-5. Chronic recurrent multifocal osteomyelitis (CRMO) in 13-year-old female. **(A)** Anteroposterior (AP) radiograph of the knee demonstrates pyramidal areas of mixed lucency and sclerosis in the metaphyses of the distal femur and proximal tibia and fibula (*arrows*). Similar pyramidal areas (*arrows*) of intermediate to low signal on **(B)** T1-weighted image and bright signal on **(C)** T2-weighted imaging are interspersed with normal marrow fat.

SUGGESTED READING

Demharter J, Bohndorf K, Michl W, et al. Chronic recurrent multifocal osteomyelitis: radiological and clinical investigation in 5 cases. *Skeletal Radiol.* 1997;26:579–588.

Khanna G, Sato TSP, Ferguson P. Imaging of chronic recurrent multifocal osteomyelitis. *Radiographics.* 2009;29:1159–1177.

■ SAPHO (SYNOVITIS, ACNE, PUSTULOSIS, HYPEROSTOSIS, OSTEITIS)

KEY FACTS

■ There is controversy as to whether SAPHO represents a syndrome or group of disorders.

■ Most consider SAPHO a group of disorders that includes chronic recurrent multifocal osteomyelitis. Skin lesions may be present for 2 years before osteoarticular findings appear.

■ Presentations differ depending on patient age.

- Children and young adults: present with features similar to those in chronic recurrent multifocal osteomyelitis. Lytic metaphyseal changes in long bones early. Tibia, fibula, and femur most commonly involved followed by the medial clavicles, sacroiliac joints, and spine.

- Adults: anterior chest wall osteitis in 69% to 90%. Nonspecific discitis in 33%. Unilateral sacroiliac joint involvement in 13% to 52%, long bones in 30%, and flat bones in 10%.

■ CT and MR are most useful for diagnosis.

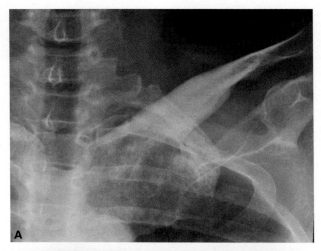

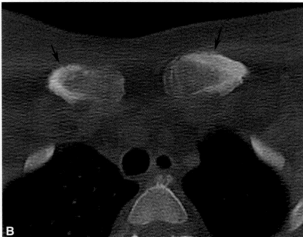

FIGURE 10-6. SAPHO. **(A)** Anteroposterior (AP) radiograph with cortical thickening and enlargement of the medial clavicle. **(B)** Axial computed tomography (CT) image in another patient demonstrates cortical thickening in both clavicular heads (*arrows*).

SUGGESTED READING

Depasquale R, Kumar N, Lalam RK, et al. SAPHO: what radiologists should know. *Clin Radiol.* 2012;67:195–206.

Earwalker JWS, Cotton A. SAPHO: syndrome or concept? Imaging findings. *Skeletal Radiol.* 2003;32:311–327.

Hayem G, Bouchard-Chabot A, Benali K, et al. SAPHO syndrome: long-term follow-up study of 120 cases. *Semin Arthritis Rheum.* 1999;293:159–171.

■ OSTEOMYELITIS—VIOLATED TISSUE

KEY FACTS

- Osteomyelitis may follow trauma, surgery, and puncture wounds with extension from soft tissue foci.
- Clinical presentation is more confusing, and imaging is more difficult, especially when bone and soft tissue anatomy are distorted.
- Orthopedic appliances may cause artifacts on MR and CT images, reducing accuracy.
- Radionuclide scans may remain positive for up to 10 months after trauma or surgery.
- Imaging should begin with radiographs. When there is no metal present, MRI is the technique of choice. Leukocyte or antigranulocyte antibody scans, and more recently PET, provide an alternative with or without metal.

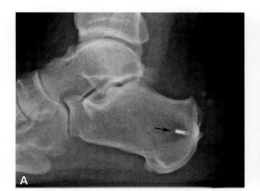
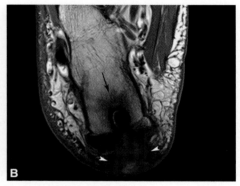
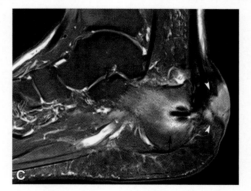

FIGURE 10-7. Infected Achilles tendon anchor with osteomyelitis. **(A)** Lateral radiograph showing metallic anchor (*arrow*) in calcaneus from Achilles tendon repair with posterior soft tissue swelling. T1-weighted axial **(B)** and short-T1 inversion recovery (STIR) sagittal **(C)** magnetic resonance (MR) images demonstrate an abscess extending posteriorly from the metal anchor (*arrowheads*) with intermediate T1 and increased T2 signal marrow changes (*arrows*) surrounding the anchor consistent with osteomyelitis.

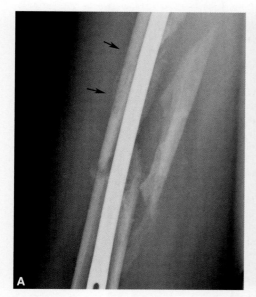 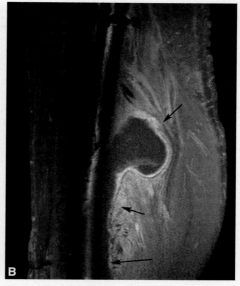

FIGURE 10-8. Posttraumatic acute pyogenic osteomyelitis in 37-year-old male 3 weeks following intramedullary rod fixation of compound femur fracture. Radiograph **(A)** demonstrates permeative osteolysis of the anterior cortex with interrupted periosteal reaction (*arrows*). T1-weighted fat-saturated sagittal image **(B)** following intravenous (IV) gadolinium demonstrates an abscess (*arrows*) along the posterior fracture line with metal susceptibility artifact from intramedullary nail.

SUGGESTED READING

Buhne KH, Bohndorf K. Imaging of posttraumatic osteomyelitis. *Semin Musculoskelet Radiol.* 2004;8:199–204.

Guhlmann A, Recht-Krause D, Suger G, et al. Chronic osteomyelitis detected with FDG PET and correlation with histologic findings. *Radiology.* 1998;206:749–754.

Jacobson AF, Harley JD, Lypsky BA, et al. Diagnosis of osteomyelitis in the presence of soft tissue infection and radiographic evidence of osseous abnormalities: value of leukocyte scintigraphy. *Am J Roentgenol.* 1991;157:807–812.

Kaim A, Ledermann HP, Bongartz G, et al. Chronic posttraumatic osteomyelitis in the lower extremity: comparison of magnetic resonance imaging and combined bone scintigraphy/immune scintigraphy with radiolabeled monoclonal antigranulocyte antibodies. *Skel Radiol.* 2000;29:378–386.

van der Bruggen W, Bleeker-Rovers CP, Boerman OC, et al. PET and SPECT in osteomyelitis and prosthetic bone and joint infections: a systematic review. *Semin Nucl Med.* 2010;40:3–15.

■ JOINT SPACE INFECTION

KEY FACTS

- Infectious arthritis is generally monoarticular and, like osteomyelitis, most commonly involves the lower extremities.
- Children are more likely to present with fever, chills, and inability to bear weight compared with adults in whom presentation may be more subtle.
- Early detection is important to prevent bone loss and joint deformity.
- Joint space and bone changes occur early with pyogenic infection and late with less aggressive infections, such as tuberculosis or atypical mycobacterial infections.
- Imaging features:
  - Radiographs: joint effusion and soft tissue swelling. Joint space widening early, before cartilage destruction.
  - Radionuclide scans: increased uptake early, but nonspecific
  - MRI: joint effusion on T2-weighted images and early bone and cartilage changes. Findings do not provide specific information (Tables 10-4 and 10-5).
  - Joint aspiration: performed under ultrasound or fluoroscopic guidance to isolate organism

Table 10-4 MAGNETIC RESONANCE FEATURES OF JOINT SPACE INFECTION

Image Features	Incidence (%)
Synovial enhancement after contrast	94
Joint effusion	79
Fluid outpouching from capsule	79
Bone erosions	79
Bone marrow edema pattern	74
Synovial thickening	68

Table 10-5 IMAGING APPROACHES TO JOINT SPACE INFECTION

Radiographic Features	Next Steps
Radiographs positive	Aspirate, culture, and treat
Radiographs negative; high index of suspicion	US or fluoroscopic aspiration recommended
Radiograph negative; low index of suspicion	MRI or nuclear medicine imaging (WBC scan/sulfur colloid scan)
	If positive: aspirate and treat
	If negative: clinical follow-up

MRI, magnetic resonance imaging; US, ultrasound; WBC, white blood cell.

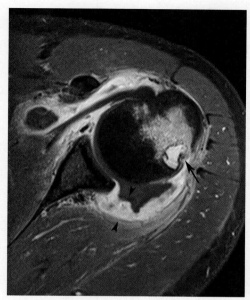

FIGURE 10-9. Pyogenic septic arthritis of the glenohumeral joint following a joint injection with secondary osteomyelitis of the humeral head. T1-weighted fat-saturated axial image following intravenous (IV) gadolinium administration demonstrates synovial thickening and enhancement of the glenohumeral joint with effusion. Infection extending into the marrow at the posterior bare area of the humeral head under the infraspinatus tendon (*arrow*).

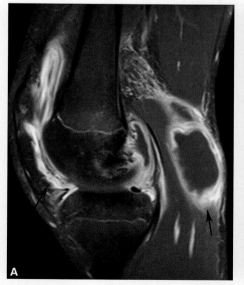
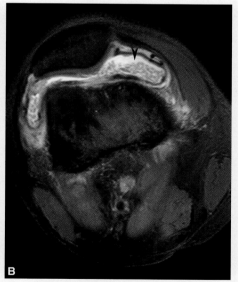

FIGURE 10-10. Joint infection with atypical organism. Fifteen-year-old male with 7 months of recurrent large right knee effusion. T1-weighted fat-suppressed postgadolinium sagittal magnetic resonance (MR) image **(A)** demonstrates joint effusion with synovial thickening and enhancement. Proton density fat-suppressed axial image **(B)** demonstrates layering debris in the form of "rice bodies." While Juvenille idiopathic arthritis and tuberculous were entertained, polymerized chain reaction identified Lyme disease as the cause.

(continued)

▪ JOINT SPACE INFECTION *(Continued)*

SUGGESTED READING

Filippi L, Schillaci O. Usefulness of hybrid SPECT/CT in 99mTc-HMPAO-labeled leukocyte scintigraphy for bone and joint infections. *J Nucl Med*. 2006;47:1908–1913.

Graif M, Schweitzer ME, Deely D, et al. The septic versus nonspecific inflamed joint. MR characteristics. *Skeletal Radiol*. 1999;28:616–620.

Learch TJ. Imaging of infectious arthritis. *Semin Musculoskelet Radiol*. 2003;7:137–142.

■ SOFT TISSUE INFECTION

KEY FACTS

■ Soft tissue infection may be deep or superficial. Most soft tissue infections are related to inoculation by a puncture wound, ulcer, or contamination of a skin abrasion. Cellulitis is an infection of the skin and subcutaneous tissues. The organism is usually *Staphylococcus* or *Streptococcus*. Deep infections may involve muscle (myositis) or fascia (necrotizing fasciitis).

■ Soft tissue abscesses are well-defined fluid collections. Pyogenic abscesses tend to have thick walls compared with thin-walled tuberculous abscesses.

■ Infection may also involve bursae and tendon sheaths.

■ Imaging approaches (Table 10-6):
  ● Routine radiographs: Soft tissue swelling, subcutaneous edema ulceration, or gas in the soft tissues may be identified.
  ● Ultrasound: Fluid collections, foreign bodies, and abscesses can be identified and aspirated or drained.
  ● CT: sensitive to subtle gas in soft tissue planes (necrotizing fasciitis)
  ● MRI: Superior tissue contrast and multiple image planes with T1- and T2-weighted images identify infection and extent of involvement. Gadolinium enhancement occurs in areas of inflammation and walls of abscess cavities.

Table 10-6   IMAGING APPROACHES TO SOFT TISSUE INFECTIONS

Soft Tissue Swelling, Ulceration, or Erythema Clinically	
Radiographic Features	**Next Steps**
Radiograph positive	Biopsy and treat
Radiograph negative; low index of suspicion	Follow
Radiograph negative; high index of suspicion	MRI with contrast
	Negative: stop
	Positive: biopsy and treat

MRI, magnetic resonance imaging.

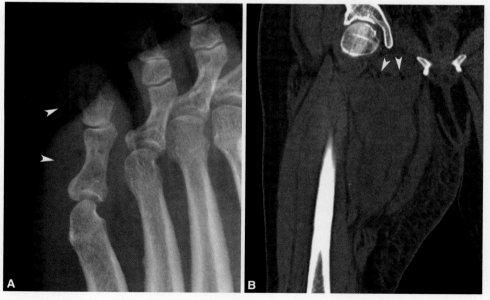

FIGURE 10-11. Soft tissue gas. **(A)** Radiograph shows soft tissue gas (*arrowheads*) and swelling in the 5th toe in a 59-year-old male with diabetes and gangrene. **(B)** Coronal computed tomography (CT) image of the right thigh demonstrates small foci of soft tissue gas (*arrowheads*) that was not radiographically apparent in this 65-year-old female with medial thigh edema from necrotizing fasciitis.

(continued)

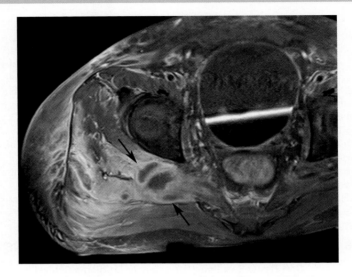

FIGURE 10-12. Right piriformis and gluteal muscle stapholococcal bacterial abscess in a 46-year-old male with untreated dental abscess. Contrast-enhanced fat-suppressed T1-weighted image demonstrates a multilocular thick-walled pyogenic abscess (*arrows*) with surrounding soft tissue inflammation.

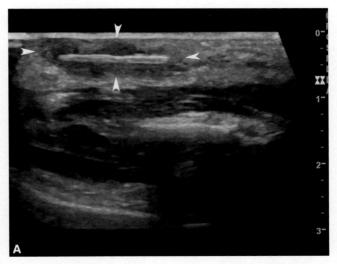

FIGURE 10-13. Foreign body with surrounding inflammation. **(A)** Ultrasound demonstrates an echogenic linear wooden foreign body in thenar eminence with surrounding hypoechoic pus (*arrowheads*). **(B)** Sagittal contrast-enhanced fat-suppressed T1-weighted image demonstrates low signal foreign body with surrounding inflammatory enhancement (*arrowheads*).

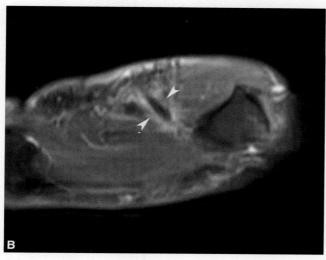

FIGURE 10-13. (*continued*)

SUGGESTED READING

Ma LD, Frassica FJ, Bluenke DA, et al. CT and MRI evaluation of musculoskeletal infection. *Crit Rev Diagn Imaging.* 1997;36:535–568.

Turecki MB, Taljanovic MS, Stubbs AY, et al. Imaging of musculoskeletal soft tissue infections. *Skeletal Radiol.* 2010; 39:957–971.

■ BRODIE ABSCESS

KEY FACTS

- Brodie abscess is a localized osseous infection usually caused by *Staphylococcus aureus*. In up to 50% of patients, no organism is identified.
- Patients often have subtle symptoms and are not systemically ill.
- Most abscesses are metaphyseal (60%) and well marginated with surrounding sclerosis, and range from 4 mm to 4 cm in size. Sequestra are evident in 20%.
- Cortical Brodie abscesses may be confused with osteoid osteoma.
- The distal tibia is the most common site.
- MRI or CT is best for diagnosis.

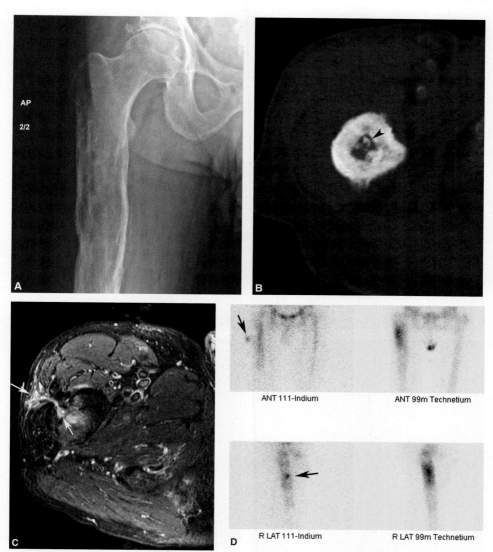

FIGURE 10-14. Chronic osteomyelitis changes in the left proximal femur following prior-healed fracture in a 73-year-old male with a draining skin sinus along the lateral proximal thigh. **(A)** Radiograph demonstrates irregular contoured, cortical formation bone (involucrum) encasing the original proximal femoral diaphysis. **(B)** Axial computed tomography (CT) image shows a sequestrum (*arrowhead*) of necrotic bone in the medullary space. **(C)** Short-T1 inversion recovery (STIR) axial image shows a "cloaca" or sinus tract through cortex (*arrow*). **(D)** Anterior and right lateral planar images from Tc-99m bone scan and Indium-111 24-hour white blood cell (WBC) imaging demonstrates active infection at the site of the draining sinus tract (*arrow*).

(continued)

■ BRODIE ABSCESS *(Continued)*

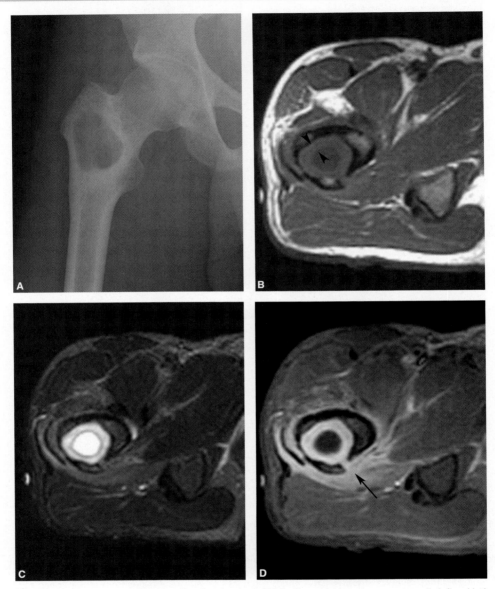

FIGURE 10-15. Subacute infection (Brodie abscess). **(A)** Radiograph demonstrates a well-defined lytic lesion with a sclerotic border. T1-weighted fat-saturated **(B)**, T2-weighted fat-saturated **(C)**, and postg-adolinium T1-weighted fat-saturated **(D)** axial magnetic resonance imaging (MRI) images demonstrate fluid signal centrally. This is surrounded by a mildly hyperintense T1 signal rim of granulation tissue (*arrowheads*) referred to as a "penumbra sign" that enhances following intravenous gadolinium administration. Posterior sinus tract **(D**, *arrow*) with surrounding soft tissue inflammation seen.

SUGGESTED READING

Davies AM, Grimer R. The penumbra sign in subacute osteomyelitis. *Eur Radiol.* 2005;15:1268–1270.
Miller WB, Murphy WA, Gilula LA. Brodie abscess: reappraisal. *Radiology.* 1979;132:15–23.

■ TUBERCULOSIS/ATYPICAL MYCOBACTERIAL INFECTIONS

KEY FACTS

- ■ Musculoskeletal infections from tuberculosis may be from typical (*Mycobacterium tuberculosis*) strains (3% to 5% involve bone and joints) or atypical (*Mycobacterium bovis, Mycobacterium fortuitum, Mycobacterium chelonae, Mycobacterium marinum*) strains (5% to 10% involve the musculoskeletal system).
- ■ *M. tuberculosis:* Musculoskeletal involvement may occur at any age, but it is rare in infants. Infections are more common in patients with debilitating diseases. Fifty percent have pulmonary involvement. The metaphyses and epiphyses are most often involved. In children, multiple lytic lesions may mimic fungal infection or neoplasms.
  - ● Radiographic features: Bone involvement may be difficult to differentiate from pyogenic infection. Joint infections progress more slowly than pyogenic infections. Joint margin erosions are more common, and the joint space is preserved for a longer period compared with pyogenic infections.
  - ● MRI features: low to intermediate signal intensity on T2-weighted and low signal intensity on T1-weighted or higher peripheral signal intensity. Edema pattern and abscesses in 80%.
- ■ Atypical mycobacteria: Atypical mycobacteria are found in soil, water, milk, and animals. Musculoskeletal infections resemble *M. tuberculosis,* but the course is often milder. Diagnosis may be delayed up to 10 months from onset of symptoms (fever, chills, malaise, and weight loss).
  - ● Radiographic features: bone involvement is nonspecific. Spine and joint involvement are similar to that found in *M. tuberculosis.* Unlike tuberculosis, sinus tracts, sequestra, and periostitis occur more frequently. Myositis can be found in patients with acquired immunodeficiency syndrome. Infectious tenosynovitis in the hand and wrist is common.
  - ● MRI features: nonspecific and similar to tuberculosis. May have rice bodies in soft tissue fluid collections.

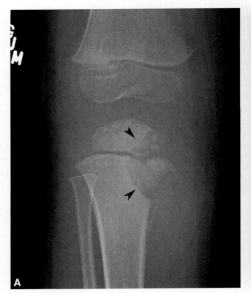
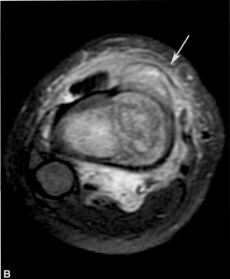

FIGURE 10-16. *Mycobacterium tuberculosis* osteomyelitis in a 7-year-old. **(A)** Radiograph demonstrates a lytic destructive process on either side of the physis in the medial epiphysis and metaphysis (*arrowheads*). **(B)** Axial T2-weighted fat-saturated magnetic resonance imaging (MRI) image shows marrow changes with surrounding soft tissue abscess (*arrow*).

(continued)

■ TUBERCULOSIS/ATYPICAL MYCOBACTERIAL INFECTIONS *(Continued)*

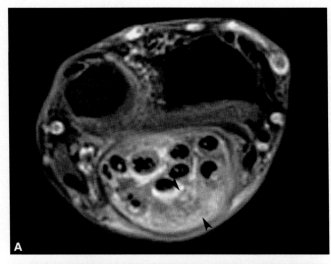

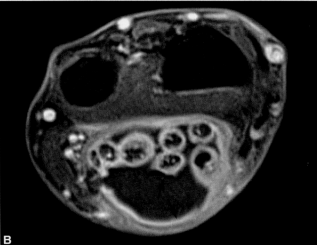

FIGURE 10-17. *Mycobacterium marinum* flexor tenosynovitis in a 62-year-old male from penetrating injury. **(A)** Proton density fat-saturated axial magnetic resonance (MR) image demonstrates intermediate to low signal debris or "rice bodies" (*arrowheads*) distending the flexor tendon sheath. **(B)** Postgadolinium T1-weighted fat-suppressed axial image shows thickened enhancement of the synovium (*arrows*) without enhancement of the debris.

SUGGESTED READING

Amrami KK, Sundarum M, Shin AY, et al. Mycobacterium marinum infections of the distal upper extremity: clinical course and imaging findings in two cases with delayed diagnosis. *Skeletal Radiol.* 2003;32:546–549.

Hong SH, Kim SM, Aku JM, et al. Tuberculosus versus pyogenic arthritis: MR imaging evaluation. *Radiology.* 2001;218:848–853.

Theodorou DJ, Theodorou SJ, Kakitsubata Y, et al. Imaging characteristics and epidemiologic features of atypical mycobacterial infections involving the musculoskeletal system. *Am J Roentgenol.* 2001;176:341–349.

■ FUNGAL INFECTIONS

KEY FACTS

■ Fungal infections are most common in debilitated patients, diabetic patients, patients undergoing steroid therapy, and patients who reside in specific geographic regions.

■ Common fungal infections include

- Actinomycosis (*Actinomyces israelii, Actinomyces bovis*)
  - ❖ Resides in oral cavity.
  - ❖ Bone involvement most common in facial bones.
  - ❖ Distal spread can occur via hematogenous route.
- Cryptococcosis (*Cryptococcus neoformans*)
  - ❖ Organism present in soil.
  - ❖ Infection via direct implantation in open wound (foot common).
  - ❖ Skeletal involvement in 5% to 10%, resulting in destructive bone lesions and draining sinuses.
- Blastomycosis (*Blastomyces dermatitidis*)
  - ❖ Prevalent in Ohio and Mississippi valleys.
  - ❖ Infection via skin or inhalation.
  - ❖ Skeletal involvement in 50% with pulmonary infection.
  - ❖ Radiographic changes include bone destruction and draining sinuses.
- Coccidioidomycosis (*Coccidioides immitis*)
  - ❖ Endemic in southwestern United States.
  - ❖ Infection via inhalation.
  - ❖ Bone involvement in 10% to 20%.
  - ❖ Areas of bony prominence (ligament and tendon attachments) commonly involved.
  - ❖ Destructive lesions with aggressive periostitis are common.
  - ❖ Bilateral extremity involvement is possible.
- Histoplasmosis (*Histoplasma capsulatum, Histoplasma duboisii*)
  - ❖ Present in soil.
  - ❖ Infection via inhalation.
  - ❖ More common in children than adults.
  - ❖ Bone destruction most common in the axial skeleton.
- Echinococcus (*Echinococcus granulosis, Echinococcus multilocularis, Echinococcus vogeli, Echinococcus oligarthus*)
  - ❖ Liver involvement in 65%, lung in 15%, and musculoskeletal in 1% to 4%.
  - ❖ Osseous involvement in the spine in 35%, pelvis in 21%, femora in 10%, tibia in 10%, and ribs in 6%.
  - ❖ Cystic multilocular lesions that may resemble neoplasms.

(continued)

■ FUNGAL INFECTIONS *(Continued)*

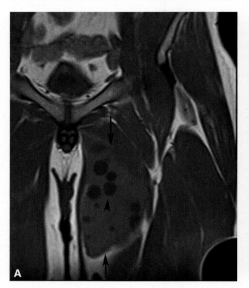 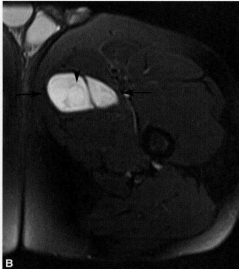

FIGURE 10-18. *Echinococcus multilocularis* infection of the adductor brevis muscle of the left thigh presenting as an intramuscular soft tissue mass in a 36-year-old male. Internal daughter cysts (*arrowheads*) are seen as rounded areas of low signal on **(A)** T1-weighted coronal magnetic resonance (MR) image and high signal thin-walled structures on the **(B)** T2-weighted fat-saturated axial image within a mass that is mildly increased T1 and high T2 signal.

SUGGESTED READING

Corr PD. Musculoskeletal fungal infections. *Semin Musculoskelet Radiol.* 2011;15:506–510.
Holley K, Muldoon M, Tasker S. Coccidioides immitis osteomyelitis: a case review. *Orthopedics.* 2002;25:827–831.
Rhangos WC, Chick EW. Mycotic infections in the bone. *South Med J.* 1964;57:664–674.

11 Marrow Disorders

Jeffrey J. Peterson and Thomas H. Berquist

■ NORMAL MARROW: BASIC CONCEPTS

KEY FACTS

- Bone marrow consists of trabeculae (15%) and cellular constituents (85%) (erythrocytic, leukocytic, fat cells, and reticulum cells).
- Hemopoietic cells (blood cells) comprise red marrow. The remainder, or inactive marrow, is yellow marrow. Red marrow is 40% water, 40% fat, and 20% protein. Yellow marrow is 80% fat, 15% water, and 5% protein.
- At birth, nearly the entire skeleton is composed of red marrow. Red marrow converts to yellow marrow in a predictable pattern from peripheral to central. The adult marrow pattern is usually attained by 25 years of age.
- Adult marrow pattern is primarily red in the axial skeleton (skull, spine, pelvis, ribs, and sternum) and proximal humeri and femora.
  - Magnetic resonance imaging (MRI) features of normal marrow are predictable on T1- and T2-weighted sequences. Yellow marrow has signal intensity similar to subcutaneous fat on T1-weighted sequences and low signal intensity on T2-weighted sequences. Red marrow has lower intensity than fat on T1-weighted and signal intensity near that of fat (high) on T2-weighted sequences. Short-T1 inversion recovery (STIR) sequences show red marrow as even higher intensity compared with T2-weighted sequences.

(continued)

■ NORMAL MARROW: BASIC CONCEPTS *(Continued)*

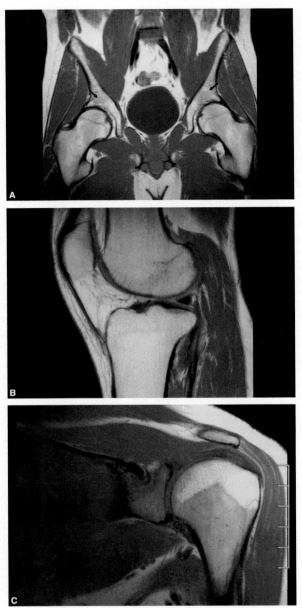

FIGURE 11-1. Marrow patterns. T1-weighted images of the pelvis **(A)**, knee **(B)**, and shoulder **(C)**. The marrow in the pelvis **(A)** is predominantly fatty in this adult except for small areas of red marrow in the acetabular regions (*arrows*). There is also fatty high signal intensity marrow in the knee in an older adult **(B)** and epiphysis of the shoulder in a 20-year-old patient **(C)**. There is red marrow in the humeral shaft and glenoid.

SUGGESTED READING

Chan BY, Gill KG, Rebsamen SL, et al. MR imaging of pediatric bone marrow. *Radiographics.* 2016;36:1911–1930.
Vogler JB, Murphy WA. Bone marrow imaging. *Radiology.* 1988;168:679–693.

■ MARROW RECONVERSION

KEY FACTS

- ■ Hematopoietic demand may result in conversion of yellow to red marrow.
- ■ The sequence of red marrow conversion occurs in reverse of the red to yellow marrow conversion, occurring as one develops adult marrow pattern.
- ■ Reconversion begins in the axial skeleton and moves peripherally.
- ■ Reconversion is symmetric, but not necessarily uniform.
- ■ Patients without bone marrow disorders may develop expanded red marrow termed "hyperplasia."
- ■ Marrow reconversion, or hyperplasia, may be the result of multiple conditions:
  - Chronic anemia
  - Chronic infection
  - Marrow replacement diseases
  - Cyanotic heart disease
  - Marathon running
  - Smoking
- ■ Imaging of red marrow reconversion is best accomplished with MRI. Signal intensity changes may be difficult to differentiate from infiltrative diseases. T1-weighted images show areas of decreased signal intensity. T2-weighted and STIR sequences show signal intensity higher than fat.

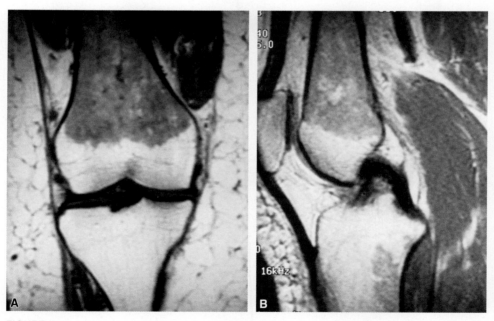

FIGURE 11-2. Marrow hyperplasia in a long-distance runner. Coronal **(A)** and sagittal **(B)** T1-weighted images show low intensity marrow in the femoral diaphysis and metaphysis with a focal area of hyperplasia in the tibia. Cortical bone is normal, and there are no soft tissue abnormalities.

SUGGESTED READING

Shellock FG, Morris E, Deutsch AL, et al. Hematopoietic marrow hyperplasia: high prevalence on MR images of the knee in asymptomatic marathon runners. *Am J Roentgenol.* 1992;158:335–338.

Vande Berg BC, Levouvet FE, Moyson P, et al. MR assessment of red marrow distribution and composition in the proximal femur: correlation with clinical and laboratory parameters. *Skeletal Radiol.* 1997;26:589–596.

■ MYELOID DEPLETION

KEY FACTS

- ■ In patients with myeloid depletion, the hemopoietic (red) marrow is replaced by fatty (yellow) marrow.
- ■ Fat replacement may be diffuse or focal, depending on the extent and duration of the process.
- ■ Conditions leading to myeloid depletion include
  - ● Aplastic anemia
  - ● Chemotherapy
  - ● Radiation
  - ● Marrow toxins
  - ● Viral infections
- ■ Radiation changes are focal, so fat replacement occurs in the treated region. Changes occur as early as 3 to 7 weeks. With low doses, recovery may occur. Patients receiving more than 50 Gy are usually irreversible.
- ■ Fatty marrow has fat signal intensity on T1- and T2-weighted sequences.

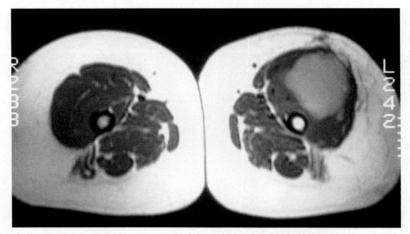

FIGURE 11-3. Radiation therapy. Axial T1-weighted image shows a malignant soft tissue mass with fatty marrow in the femur. Compare with normal lower signal intensity red marrow in the opposite femur.

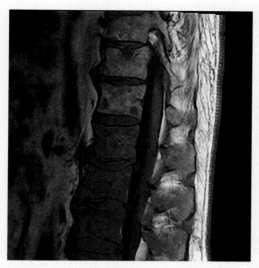

FIGURE 11-4. Sagittal T1-weighted imaging of the lumbar spine depicts fatty marrow in the upper lumbar spine in an area of previous radiation therapy.

SUGGESTED READING

Cavenagh EC, Weinberger E, Shal DW, et al. Hematopoietic marrow reconversion in pediatric patients undergoing spinal irradiation: MR depiction. *Am J Neuroradiol.* 1995;16:461–467.

■ MARROW ISCHEMIA

KEY FACTS

■ Bone marrow ischemic changes are usually focal (see Chapters 3, 4, and 6).

■ Causes of bone marrow ischemia and osteonecrosis are numerous.
- Trauma
- Exogenous steroids
- Systemic diseases
- Gaucher disease
- Sickle cell anemia
- Idiopathic

■ Focal changes are most common in the hip, knee, and shoulder.

■ Avascular necrosis occurs in the subchondral epiphysis, and bone infarction occurs in the metaphysis and diaphysis.

■ Image changes may be evident on radiographs in advanced cases. MRI is the technique of choice for imaging early ischemic changes.

■ Magnetic resonance (MR) imaging often depicts the "double line sign" at the periphery of the osteonecrosis. This consists of an inner high signal intensity line representing granulation tissue and an outer low signal intensity line representing sclerosis. This is reported in up to 80% of cases of osteonecrosis.

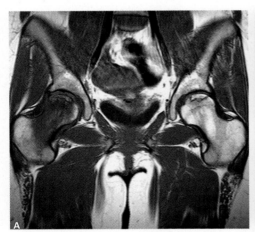 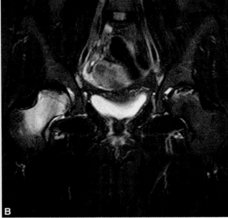

FIGURE 11-5. Avascular necrosis of the hip. Coronal T1-weighted **(A)** and coronal T2-weighted **(B)** magnetic resonance (MR) images show avascular necrosis involving both femoral heads. There is acute collapse of the necrotic femoral articular surface on the right associated with diffuse marrow edema through the right proximal femur. Finding on the left is more chronic with serpiginous sclerosis seen at the margin of the marrow ischemia.

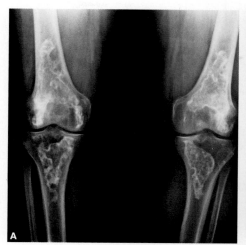
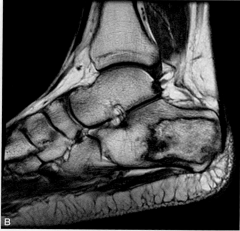

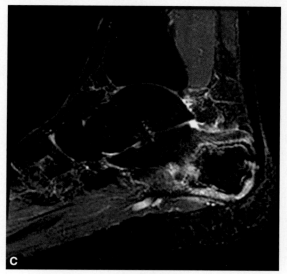

FIGURE 11-6. Bone infarction. **(A)** Standing radiographs of the knees show serpiginous marginal calcifications characteristic of bone infarction in both knees. Sagittal T1-weighted **(B)** and sagittal T2-weighted **(C)** magnetic resonance (MR) images in a different patient depict a large bone infarct in the calcaneus. T2-weighted image nicely depicts the "double line sign" at the periphery of the necrotic focus with an inner high signal intensity line representing granulation tissue and an outer low signal intensity line representing sclerosis. The "double line sign" is seen in up to 80% of cases of osteonecrosis.

SUGGESTED READING

Deely DM, Schweitzer ME. MR imaging of bone marrow disorders. *Radiol Clin North Am.* 1997;35:193–212.
Glickstein MF, Burk DL, Schiebler ML, et al. Avascular necrosis versus other diseases of the hip: sensitivity of MR imaging. *Radiology.* 1988;169(1):213–215.

■ MARROW INFILTRATION: BASIC CONCEPTS

KEY FACTS

- There are numerous marrow infiltrative processes, including inflammatory conditions, neoplastic processes (metastasis, myeloma), lipidosis, histiocytosis, and hyperlipoproteinemias.
- Table 11-1 summarizes infiltrative marrow conditions.
- Routine radiographs may demonstrate marrow expansion, lytic lesions, sclerotic lesions, or mixed lytic and sclerotic changes.
- MR images demonstrate low signal intensity on T1-weighted sequences and increased signal on T2-weighted or STIR sequences in most cases. Contrast enhancement is variable and nonspecific.

Table 11-1   INFILTRATIVE MARROW DISORDERS

Neoplasms
Myeloma
Leukemia
Lymphoma
Myelofibrosis
Lipidosis
   Gaucher disease
   Niemann–Pick disease
   Fabry disease
   Gangliosidosis
Histiocytosis
   Langerhans cell histiocytosis
   Erdheim–Chester disease
Hyperlipoproteinemias

SUGGESTED READING

Resnick D. Lipidosis, histiocytosis, and hyperlipoproteinemias. In: Resnick D, ed. *Diagnosis of Bone and Joint Disorders.* 4th ed. Philadelphia: WB Saunders; 2002:2233–2290.

■ MARROW INFILTRATION: LIPIDOSIS

KEY FACTS

- There are multiple lipidoses. The more common disorders are listed in Table 12-1.
- Gaucher disease is a rare familial disorder of cerebroside metabolism resulting in lipid accumulation in reticuloendothelial cells. The condition affects males and females in childhood or early adulthood. Patients present with hepatosplenomegaly. Infiltration occurs in other regions, including marrow. Radiographs demonstrate marrow expansion, endosteal scalloping, osteonecrosis, and pathologic fractures. Changes are most common in the axial skeleton and proximal long bones. MR images demonstrate decreased signal intensity on T1- and T2-weighted sequences because of fibrosis and glucocerebroside deposition.
- Niemann–Pick disease is a rare genetic disorder with deposition of sphingomyelin in the reticulo-endothelial system. Males and females are equally affected. Many are Jewish.
- There is an acute fatal type and chronic forms with and without central nervous system involvement. Most patients present in infancy with jaundice and hepatosplenomegaly.
- Radiographic features are similar to those for Gaucher disease.
- Fabry disease is a hereditary sex-linked disorder with deposition of ceramide trihexoside.
- Patients present with skin lesions, fever, pain, and paresthesias. Patients may die in later adult life because of renal or cardiac involvement. Radiographic features include periarticular swelling and avascular necrosis.
- Gangliosidosis is an inherited liposomal storage disorder caused by lack of ganglioside β-galactosidase. Ganglioside accumulates in the nervous system and other tissues. Clinical features include mental retardation, a cherry spot in the retina, hepatomegaly, and bony abnormalities. Radiographic features include osteopenia, delayed bone maturation, thickened calvarium, horizontal ribs, flattening of vertebral bodies, flared iliac, and thin long bones.

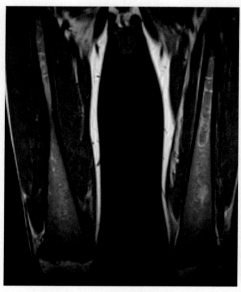

FIGURE 11-7. Gaucher disease. Coronal T1-weighted images of the lower extremities show low signal intensity throughout the marrow containing osseous structures with mild expansion of the medullary canal in the distal femora.

SUGGESTED READING

Resnick D. Lipidosis, histiocytosis, and hyperlipoproteinemias. In: Resnick D, ed. *Diagnosis of Bone and Joint Disorders.* 4th ed. Philadelphia: WB Saunders; 2002:2233–2290.

■ LANGERHANS CELL HISTIOCYTOSIS

KEY FACTS

- Three conditions constitute Langerhans cell histiocytosis (previously known as histiocytosis X): (i) unifocal Langerhans cell histiocytosis (also known as eosinophilic granuloma) (see Chapter 9), (ii) Hand–Schüller–Christian disease, and (iii) Letterer–Siwe disease.
- Common to all is the presence of Langerhans cells containing cytoplasmic inclusion bodies.
- Unifocal Langerhans histiocytosis or eosinophilic granuloma is the mildest form, presenting with single or multiple bone lesions.
  - This condition constitutes 70% of the disorders. Patients present with pain, swelling, and, on occasion, fever and elevated white counts. Radiographic features include lytic lesions with endosteal scalloping and periosteal reaction. Most common sites of involvement are the skull, mandible, ribs, spine, and long bones. Vertebral involvement leads to marked compression.
  - Differential diagnosis includes osteomyelitis, Ewing sarcoma, and lymphoma.
- Hand–Schüller–Christian disease presents with diabetes insipidus, exophthalmus, and single or multiple bone lesions. This condition is most common in children. Multisystem involvement includes otitis media, skin lesions, hepatosplenomegaly, and anemia. Neural, lung, and renal involvement are common. Skeletal lesions are similar to eosinophilic granuloma, but more disseminated. The disease is fatal in up to 30% of cases.
- Letterer–Siwe disease is an acute disorder common in children younger than 3 years. Multisystem involvement (liver, spleen, skin, and anemia) is typical. Most patients survive only 1 to 2 years. Radiographically, there are multiple lytic lesions, most commonly involving the skull.

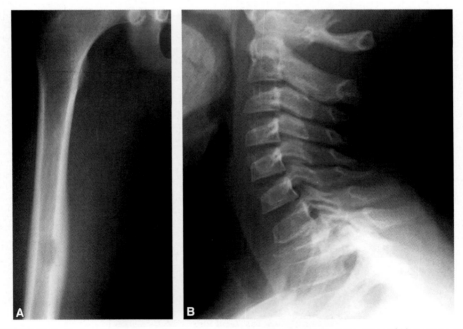

FIGURE 11-8. Eosinophilic granuloma. Anteroposterior (AP) radiograph of the femur **(A)** shows a lytic lesion with endosteal scalloping and periosteal reaction. Lateral radiograph of the cervical spine **(B)** depicts marked compression (vertebra plana) of T1.

SUGGESTED READING

Resnick D. Lipidosis, histiocytosis, and hyperlipoproteinemias. In: Resnick D, ed. *Diagnosis of Bone and Joint Disorders.* 4th ed. Philadelphia: WB Saunders; 2002:2233–2290.

■ ERDHEIM–CHESTER DISEASE

KEY FACTS

■ Non-Langerhans cell histiocytosis most commonly characterized by multifocal osteosclerotic lesions of the long bones.

■ Rare disorder of adults (both male and female) which can also result in histiocytic infiltration of extraskeletal tissues.

- Radiographic features include long bone sclerosis and prominent trabeculae with sparing of the axial skeleton. Bilateral symmetric involvement is common. Histologic changes resemble Hand–Schüller–Christian disease. Biopsy shows sheets of foamy histiocytes.

- Cardiac and pulmonary involvement is common because of release of cholesterol from cells.

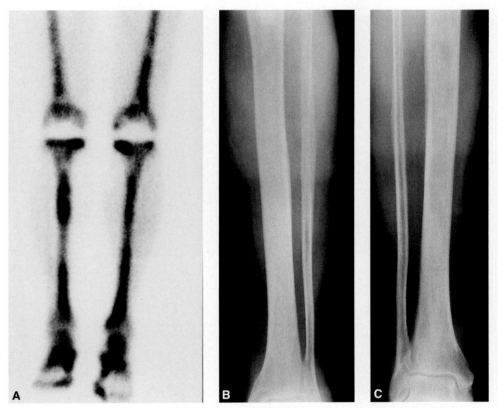

FIGURE 11-9. Erdheim–Chester disease. **(A)** Radionuclide bone scan shows increased tracer in both femora and tibiae. Anteroposterior (AP) **(B, C)** and lateral **(D, E)** radiographs of the tibiae show sclerotic areas with prominent trabeculae.

(continued)

■ ERDHEIM–CHESTER DISEASE *(Continued)*

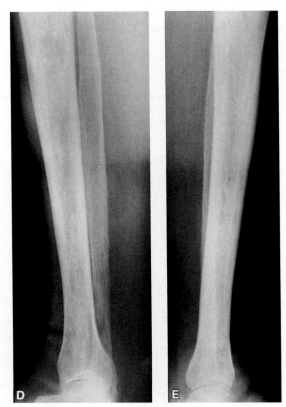

FIGURE 11-9. *(continued)*

SUGGESTED READING

Resnick D. Lipidosis, histiocytosis, and hyperlipoproteinemias. In: Resnick D, ed. *Diagnosis of Bone and Joint Disorders.* 4th ed. Philadelphia: WB Saunders; 2002:2233–2290.

■ HYPERLIPOPROTEINEMIAS

KEY FACTS

■ Hyperlipoproteinemias present with increased plasma cholesterol and triglycerides. Five types are described.
- Type I: deficiency in lipoprotein lipase. Patients are 10 to 30 years old, with lipemia retinalis, hepatosplenomegaly, abdominal pain, and pancreatitis.
- Type II: The most common form, it presents with increased low-density lipoproteins and β-lipoproteins. Patients present in early childhood with xanthomas and premature vascular disease.
- Type III: β-lipoprotein or pre–β-lipoprotein disorders. Patients present with xanthomas and premature vascular disease.
- Type IV: increased low-density lipoproteins and pre–β-lipoproteins. May be secondary to diabetes, pancreatitis, alcoholism, Gaucher disease, and so forth. Patients present after age 20 years with xanthomas, gout, and coronary artery disease.
- Type V: similar to Type IV but with hepatosplenomegaly and paresthesias.

■ Radiographic features include
- Osseous xanthomas
- Soft tissue xanthomas
- Gout
- Soft tissue swelling about joints

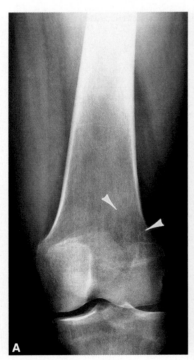 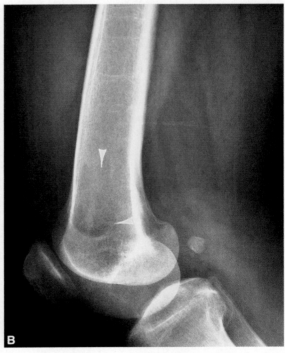

FIGURE 11-10. Osseous xanthomas (Type IV hyperlipoproteinemia). **(A, B)** Routine radiographs show a poorly defined lytic lesion in the distal femur (*arrowheads*). Coronal T1-weighted **(C)** and sagittal T2-weighted **(D)** magnetic resonance (MR) images show a poorly defined lesion that has fatty intensity on T1-weighted image **(C)** and areas of increased intensity on T2-weighted image **(D)**.

(continued)

■ HYPERLIPOPROTEINEMIAS *(Continued)*

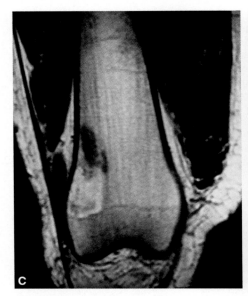 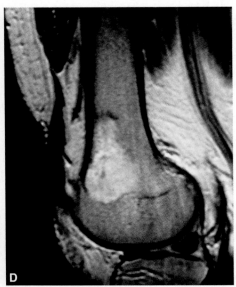

FIGURE 11-10. *(continued)*

SUGGESTED READING

Resnick D. Lipidosis, histiocytosis, and hyperlipoproteinemias. In: Resnick D, ed. *Diagnosis of Bone and Joint Disorders.* 4th ed. Philadelphia: WB Saunders; 2002:2233–2290.

■ MYELOFIBROSIS

KEY FACTS

■ Myelofibrosis is an uncommon disorder resulting in fibrous replacement of marrow and extramedullary hematopoiesis.

■ Patients are typically middle-aged or elderly and present with fatigue, hepatosplenomegaly, and purpura.

■ Secondary gout is evident in 5% to 20%.

■ Radiographic features include bone sclerosis and splenomegaly.

■ MR images demonstrate low signal intensity on T1- and T2-weighted sequences.

■ Differential diagnosis includes Paget disease and metastasis.

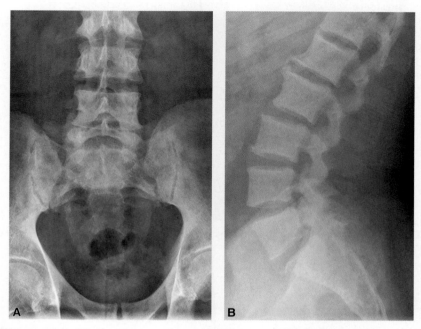

FIGURE 11-11. Myelofibrosis. Anteroposterior (AP) **(A)** and lateral **(B)** radiographs of the lumbar spine show increased bone density and scattered bone sclerosis throughout the axial skeleton.

(continued)

■ **MYELOFIBROSIS**   *(Continued)*

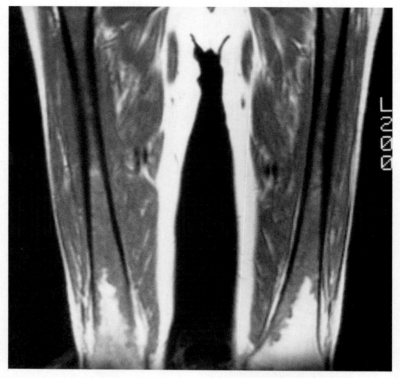

FIGURE 11-12. Myelofibrosis. T1-weighted magnetic resonance (MR) image of the femora shows low signal intensity, except distally.

SUGGESTED READING

Bond JR. Musculoskeletal case of the day. Myelofibrosis. *Am J Roentgenol.* 1993;160(6):1330.

Guermazi A, de Kerviler E, Cazals-Hatem D, et al. Imaging findings in patients with myelofibrosis. *Eur Radiol.* 1999;9(7):1366–1375.

Lanir A, Aghai E, Simon JS, et al. MR imaging in myelofibrosis. *J Comput Assist Tomogr.* 1986;10:634–636.

■ COMPRESSION FRACTURES: BENIGN VERSUS MALIGNANT

KEY FACTS

■ Vertebral compression fractures are common, especially in elderly females.

■ Differentiation of traumatic or osteopenic compression fractures from metastasis or myeloma may be difficult with conventional imaging studies (radiographs, radionuclide scans).

■ MRI is more useful for differentiating compression fractures caused by osteopenia or trauma from malignancy. MR features suggesting malignancy:
  - Focal signal abnormality in multiple vertebrae
  - Diffuse signal abnormality involving the vertebral body and posterior elements
  - Epidural mass
  - Convex posterior vertebral margin on T1-weighted images

■ Benign MR features:
  - Preservation of normal marrow signal
  - Isointense marrow on T2-weighted sequences
  - Isolated vertebral involvement
  - Diffusion-weighted MR images may be most specific. Signal attenuation is evident with osteoporotic compression, and increased signal is evident with malignant lesions or diffusion images (spin-echo or fat-suppressed spin-echo sequences). Dynamic gadolinium-enhanced sequences may also detect pathologic marrow more readily than conventional MR sequences.

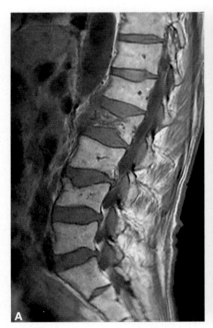 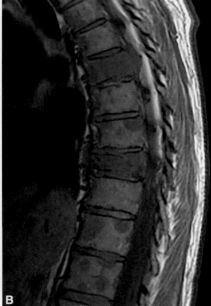

FIGURE 11-13. Sagittal T1-weighted **(A)** shows a subacute vertebral compression fracture at L2 with old compression fractures at L1 and L4 in older patient with steroid-induced osteoporosis. Sagittal T1-weighted **(B)** in another patient with breast cancer shows numerous hypointense lesions at several levels with pathologic compression fracture at T10 related to underlying metastatic disease.

SUGGESTED READING

Rahmouni A, Montazel JL, Divine M, et al. Bone marrow with diffuse tumor infiltration in patients with lymphoproliferative diseases: dynamic gadolinium-enhanced MR imaging. *Radiology.* 2003;229:710–717.

Spuentriep E, Buecher A, Adam G, et al. Diffusion-weighted MR imaging for differentiation of benign fracture edema and tumor infiltration of the vertebral body. *Am J Roentgenol.* 2001;176:351–358.

Arthropathies/ Connective Tissue Diseases

Madhura A. Desai, Jeffrey J. Peterson, and Thomas H. Berquist

■ RHEUMATOID ARTHRITIS

KEY FACTS

- Clinical:
  - Rheumatoid arthritis (RA) affects 1% to 2% of the general population with permanent deformity and disability in 10% to 20%.
- Age: 25 to 55 years
- Sex: Females outnumber males in the ratio 3:1.
- Diagnostic clinical criteria of the American Rheumatism Association are as follows:
  1. Morning stiffness lasting 1 hour before improvement
  2. Soft tissue swelling of three or more joint areas noted on physical examination
  3. Swelling of wrists, metacarpophalangeal joints, and proximal interphalangeal (PIP) joints
  4. Symmetric swelling
  5. Rheumatoid nodules
  6. Positive rheumatoid factor
  7. Radiographic erosions with or without juxta-articular osteopenia in hand, wrist, or both
- Criteria 1 to 4 must be present for 6 weeks. If four or more criteria are present, the criteria are 91% to 94% sensitive and 89% specific for RA.
- Laboratory findings: positive rheumatoid factor, elevated erythrocyte sedimentation rate
- Distribution: hands and wrists, feet, knees, shoulders, hips, elbows, and cervical spine
- Radiographic features: characterized by bilateral symmetric involvement, osteopenia, and an absence of reparative bone or osteophyte formation
  - Early:
    - ❖ Soft tissue swelling around involved joints
    - ❖ Juxta-articular osteopenia
    - ❖ Subtle marginal bone erosions
  - Late:
    - ❖ Osteopenia (diffuse)
    - ❖ Joint space narrowing
    - ❖ Obvious erosions
    - ❖ Joint subluxations
    - ❖ Soft tissue atrophy
    - ❖ Rheumatoid nodules
- Magnetic resonance imaging (MRI) often features marginal bone erosions, osseous and soft tissue edema, and synovitis.
- Cervical spine: Atlantoaxial disease is most common and can include laxity of the transverse ligament and vertical subluxation of the dens.

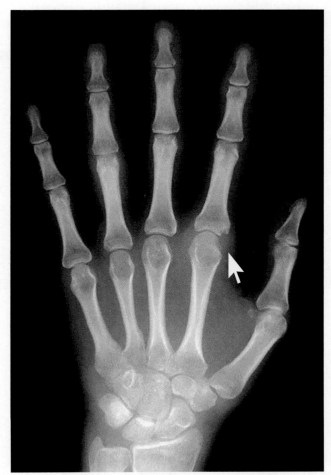

FIGURE 12-1. Early rheumatoid arthritis (RA). Hand radiograph shows early periarticular osteopenia with focal soft tissue swelling about the second metacarpophalangeal (MCP) joint with early erosive marginal erosions (*arrow*).

(continued)

■ RHEUMATOID ARTHRITIS   *(Continued)*

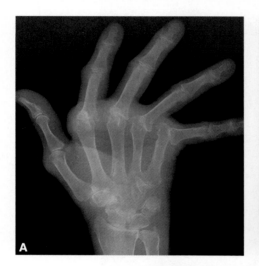
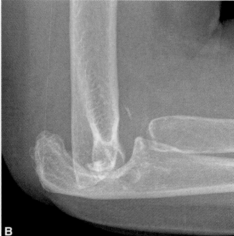

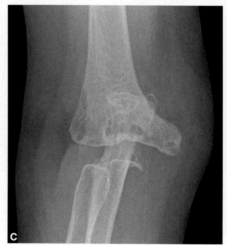

FIGURE 12-2. Advanced rheumatoid arthritis (RA). Hand radiograph **(A)** depicts osteopenia with marked joint space narrowing and erosion with subluxation predominately involving the metacarpophalangeal (MCP) joints. Lateral **(B)** and anteroposterior (AP) **(C)** views of the elbow demonstrate with marked erosive changes at the distal humerus, proximal radius, and proximal ulna which contribute to joint space widening and deformity.

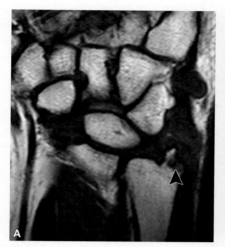
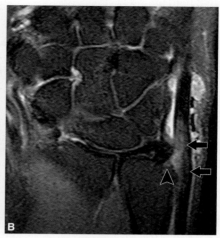

FIGURE 12-3. Early rheumatoid arthritis (RA). Coronal T1-weighted magnetic resonance (MR) **(A)** of the wrist demonstrates low intensity erosion at the ulnar styloid (*arrowhead*), a common location for early erosions. Coronal fat-saturated T2-weighted MR **(B)** shows mild edema at the ulnar styloid (*arrowhead*) with tenosynovitis of the adjacent extensor carpi ulnaris tendon (*arrows*), manifest by tendon thickening, increased internal signal, and complex fluid about the tendon.

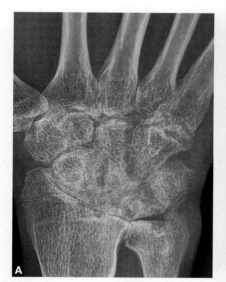
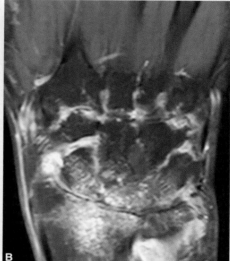

FIGURE 12-4. Carpal rheumatoid arthritis (RA). Extensive erosive changes with loss of joint space at the proximal carpus, distal radius, and ulna **(A)**. Coronal fat-saturated proton density magnetic resonance (MR) **(B)** better demonstrates osseous edema and surrounding soft tissue edema and synovitis.

SUGGESTED READING

Brower AC, Flemming DJ. *Arthritis in Black and White.* 3rd ed. Philadelphia: Elsevier/Saunders; 2012:170–199.

Farrant JM, Grainger AJ, O'Connor PJ. Advanced imaging in rheumatoid arthritis. Part 2: erosions. *Skeletal Radiol.* 2007;36(5):381–389.

Farrant JM, O'Connor PJ, Grainger AJ. Advanced imaging in rheumatoid arthritis. Part 1: synovitis. *Skeletal Radiol.* 2007;36(4):269–279.

Sommer OJ, Kladosek A, Weiler V, et al. Rheumatoid arthritis: a practical guide to state-of-the-art imaging, image interpretation, and clinical implications. *Radiographics.* 2005;25(2):381–398.

■ PSORIATIC ARTHRITIS

KEY FACTS

- ■ Clinical:
  - ● Psoriatic arthritis occurs in 2% to 6% of patients with psoriasis, and may precede or coincide with skin manifestations. Psoriatic arthritis comprises approximately 5% of patients with polyarthropathy.
- ■ Age: 25 to 55 years
- ■ Sex: No sex predilection
- ■ Distribution: hands, feet, sacroiliac joints (50%), and spine, in order of decreasing frequency
- ■ Laboratory findings: negative rheumatoid factor, elevated erythrocyte sedimentation rate, human leukocyte antigen (HLA)-B27 antigen often positive
- ■ Imaging features:
  - ● Bilateral, but asymmetric involvement
  - ● Fusiform (entire digit) soft tissue swelling
  - ● Normal bone density (no osteopenia)
  - ● Marked joint space narrowing
  - ● "Pencil in cup" erosions
  - ● Bone proliferation
  - ● In the hands and feet, distal joint involvement (distal and PIP joints) is more common with psoriatic arthritis than proximal joints involvement (carpal and metacarpal joints), which is more commonly seen with RA.

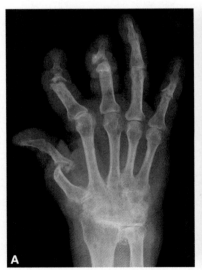 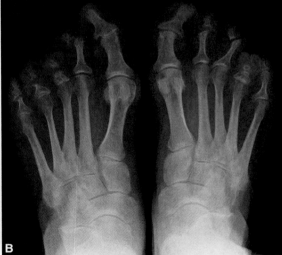

FIGURE 12-5. Psoriatic arthritis. Hand radiograph **(A)** shows proliferative changes and erosions at the second and third interphalangeal (IP) joints with fusiform enlargement of those digits. Classic "pencil in cup" erosion at the first metacarpophalangeal (MCP) joint. There is ankylosis across the fourth distal interphalangeal (DIP) joint. There is also loss of the carpal joint spaces. Radiograph of the feet **(B)** in the same patient demonstrates osteolysis and erosions involving the IP joints diffusely.

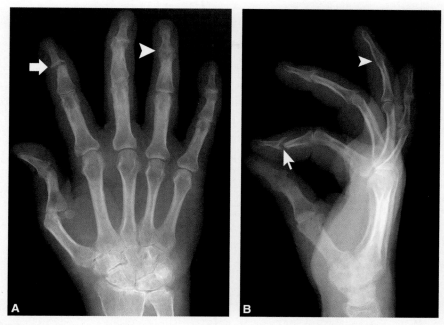

FIGURE 12-6. Psoriatic arthritis. Anteroposterior (AP) **(A)** and lateral **(B)** radiographs of the hand depict ankylosis of the fourth distal interphalangeal (DIP) joint (*arrowhead*) and "pencil in cup" erosions at the second DIP joint (*arrow*).

SUGGESTED READING

Bennett DL, Ohashi K, El-Khoury GY. Spondyloarthropathies: ankylosing spondylitis and psoriatic arthritis. *Radiol Clin North Am.* 2004;42(1):121–134.

Poggenborg RP, Østergaard M, Terslev L. Imaging in psoriatic arthritis. *Rheum Dis Clin North Am.* 2015;41(4):593–613.

Resnick D, Kransdorf MJ. Psoriatic arthritis. In: Resnick D, Kransdorf MJ, eds. *Bone and Joint Imaging.* 3rd ed. Philadelphia: Elsevier-Saunders; 2005:288–297.

■ REACTIVE ARTHRITIS

KEY FACTS

- Formerly known as Reiter syndrome
- Clinical:
  - Reactive arthritis is typically associated with conjunctivitis and urethritis. Patients may also have fever and weight loss. This triad is sexually transmitted. In females, the arthropathy is associated with dysentery.
- Age: 15 to 35 years
- Sex: most common in males
- Distribution: feet, ankles, knees, and sacroiliac joints. Upper extremity involvement is uncommon.
- Laboratory findings: HLA-B27 antigen positive in 75%
- Imaging features:
  - Bilateral asymmetric joint involvement
  - Fusiform (entire digit) soft tissue swelling
  - Joint space narrowing
  - Bone proliferation
  - Ill-defined erosions
  - Normal mineralization

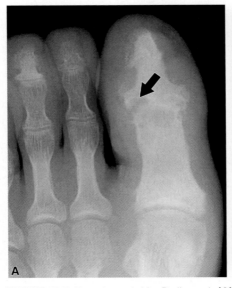 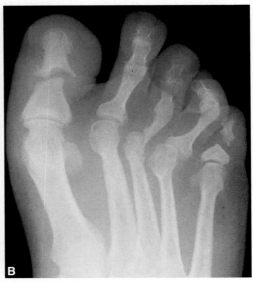

FIGURE 12-7. Reactive arthritis. Radiograph **(A)** in a patient with reactive arthritis shows proliferative changes and erosions (*arrow*) at the first interphalangeal (IP) joint with fusiform swelling of the great toe. Radiograph **(B)** in a different patient, the most notable proliferative and erosive changes are at the first, third, and fifth IP joints. There is ankylosis involving the proximal third phalanx. Mineralization is preserved.

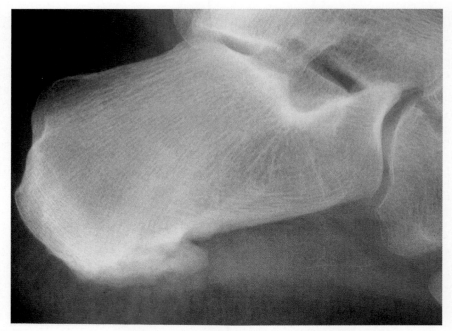

FIGURE 12-8. Reactive arthritis involvement of the calcaneus. Irregular proliferative changes at the plantar aspect of the calcaneus in this patient with reactive arthritis.

SUGGESTED READING

Klecker RJ, Weissman BN. Imaging features of psoriatic arthritis and Reiter's syndrome. *Semin Musculoskelet Radiol.* 2003;7(2):115–126.

■ ANKYLOSING SPONDYLITIS

KEY FACTS

- Clinical:
  - Ankylosing spondylitis is an inflammatory condition that affects primarily the axial skeleton. Patients are typically young males who present with low-back pain. Patients may also have weight loss and low-grade fever.
- Age: 15 to 35 years
- Sex: Males outnumber females in the ratio 4:1 to 10:1.
- Distribution: sacroiliac joints, spine (ascends from lumbar to cervical), hips, knees, shoulders. Peripheral joints of hands and feet are less commonly involved (seen in 10% of those with long-standing disease).
- Laboratory findings: HLA-B27 antigen frequently positive, elevated erythrocyte sedimentation rate
- Imaging features:
  - Bony ankylosis of involved joints
  - Bilateral symmetric involvement of sacroiliac joints
  - Bone mineralization is normal early in the disease process but osteopenic after ankylosis
  - Minimal erosive changes
  - Patients are more susceptible to fractures after ankyloses, notably in the spine.

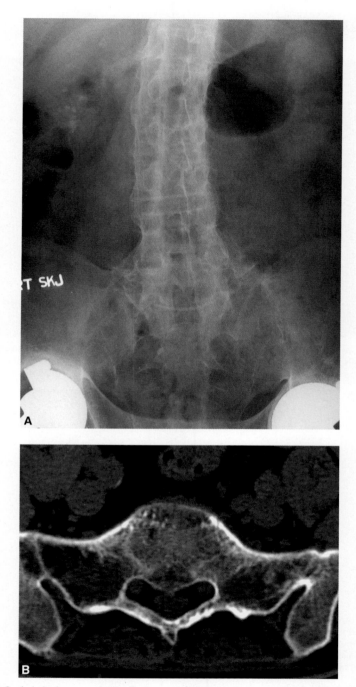

FIGURE 12-9. Ankylosing spondylitis. Radiograph **(A)** shows long-standing ankylosing spondylitis with symmetric sacroiliac (SI) joint ankylosis, syndesmophytes, and spinous ligament ossification. There are bilateral hip replacements. Axial **(B)** computed tomography (CT) shows symmetric ankylosis across bilateral sacroiliac joints.

(continued)

■ ANKYLOSING SPONDYLITIS *(Continued)*

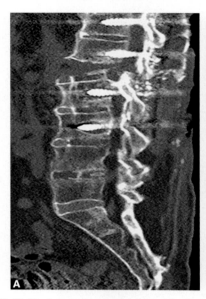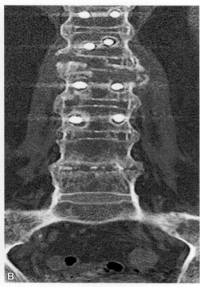

FIGURE 12-10. Ankylosing spondylitis with shear fracture. Coronal **(A)** and lateral **(B)** computed tomography (CT) show ankylosis across the lower thoracic and lumbar spine. Shear fracture at L1–L2 is transfixed with hardware. Lucencies about the screws suggest loosening of the hardware.

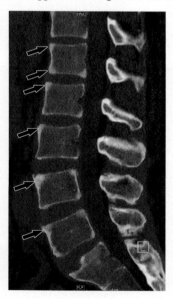

FIGURE 12-11. Ankylosing spondylitis. Early syndesmophytes contribute to squaring of the vertebral bodies on this lateral computed tomography (CT). There are also shiny corners (*arrows*) at the vertebral body margins.

SUGGESTED READING

Brower AC, Flemming DJ. *Arthritis in Black and White*. 3rd ed. Philadelphia: Elsevier/Saunders; 2012:226–242.

Hermann KG, Althoff CE, Schneider U, et al. Spinal changes in patients with spondyloarthritis: comparison of MR imaging and radiographic appearances. *Radiographics*. 2005;25(3):559–569; discussion 569–570.

Lacout A, Rousselin B, Pelage JP. CT and MRI of spine and sacroiliac involvement in spondyloarthropathy. *Am J Roentgenol*. 2008;191(4):1016–1023.

Navallas M, Ares J, Beltrán B, et al. Sacroiliitis associated with axial spondyloarthropathy: new concepts and latest trends. *Radiographics*. 2013;33(4):933–956.

Vinson EN, Major NM. MR imaging of ankylosing spondylitis. *Semin Musculoskelet Radiol*. 2003;7(2):103–113.

■ OSTEOARTHRITIS

KEY FACTS

- Clinical:
  - Osteoarthritis is the most common arthropathy and increases in incidence with age. Osteoarthritis may occur after other arthropathies (secondary osteoarthritis). Degenerative joint disease may be genetic, the result of advancing age or occupational activity, or multifactorial. Patients present with pain and swelling in the involved joints.
- Age: More than 50 years
- Sex: No sex predilection
- Distribution: hands (distal interphalangeal and PIP joints, thumb base), feet, knees, and hips. Elbows and shoulders less commonly involved.
- Laboratory findings: None
- Imaging features:
  - Asymmetric joint space narrowing (uniform joint space narrowing in secondary osteoarthritis)
  - Subchondral sclerosis
  - Subchondral cysts
  - Osteophyte formation
  - Subluxations (less dramatic than RA)
  - Unilateral or bilateral involvement, but asymmetric
  - Absence of erosions
- Erosive osteoarthritis is closely related to primary osteoarthritis but occurs primarily in postmenopausal females with an inflammatory component superimposed on osteoarthritic changes. Distribution in the hand is similar to that of primary osteoarthritis.

(continued)

■ **OSTEOARTHRITIS**   *(Continued)*

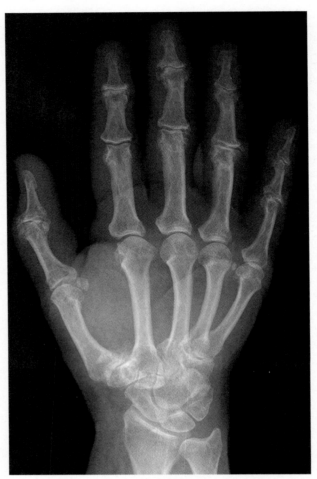

FIGURE 12-12. Osteoarthritis. Posteroanterior (PA) view of the hand and wrist demonstrates the typical distal interphalangeal (DIP) and proximal interphalangeal (PIP) joint involvement with joint space narrowing and osteophyte formation. As in this patient, osteoarthritis commonly also involves the first metacarpophalangeal (MCP) joint and the scaphoid-trapezio-trapezium joints.

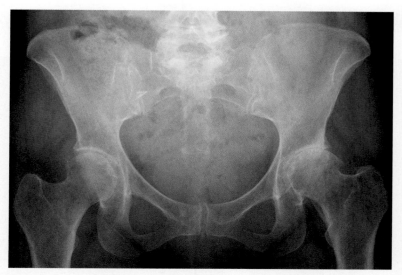

FIGURE 12-13. Osteoarthritis. Anteroposterior (AP) view of the hips with asymmetric osteoarthritic involvement. There is severe joint space narrowing on the left with sclerosis, osteophyte formation, and development of subchondral cysts. Milder joint space narrowing is seen on the right.

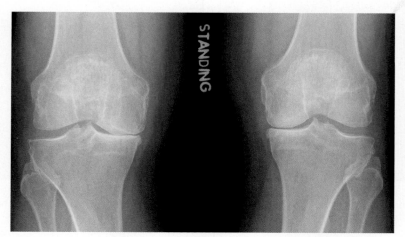

FIGURE 12-14. Osteoarthritis. Standing view of the knees demonstrating typical medial compartment narrowing and osteophyte formation.

(continued)

■ OSTEOARTHRITIS *(Continued)*

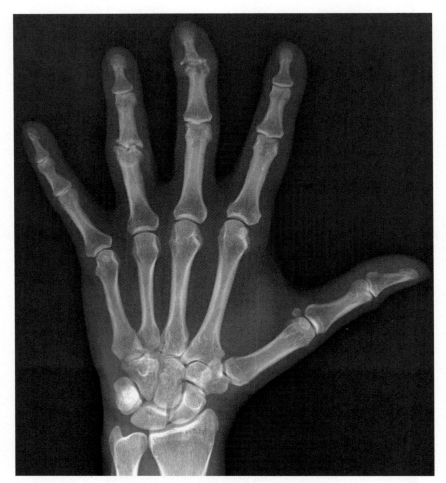

FIGURE 12-15. Erosive osteoarthritis. Asymmetric joint space narrowing, erosions, osteophytes, and soft tissue swelling involving the third distal interphalangeal (DIP) and fourth proximal interphalangeal (PIP) joints in a postmenopausal woman. There is no demineralization.

SUGGESTED READING

Brower AC, Flemming DJ. *Arthritis in Black and White.* 3rd ed. Philadelphia: Elsevier/Saunders; 2012:243–260.

Greenspan A. Erosive osteoarthritis. *Semin Musculoskelet Radiol.* 2003;7(2):155–159.

Gupta KB, Duryea J, Weissman BN. Radiographic evaluation of osteoarthritis. *Radiol Clin North Am.* 2004;42(1):11–41.

Jacobson JA, Girish G, Jiang Y, et al. Radiographic evaluation of arthritis: degenerative joint disease and variations. *Radiology.* 2008;248(3):737–747.

Smith D, Braunstein EM, Brandt KD, et al. A radiographic comparison of erosive osteoarthritis and idiopathic nodular osteoarthritis. *J Rheumatol.* 1992;19:896–904.

■ ENTERIC ARTHROPATHIES

KEY FACTS

- ■ Clinical:
  - ● Arthropathies may accompany enteric conditions, such as Crohn disease, ulcerative colitis, and Whipple disease. Findings may be similar radiographically to ankylosing spondylitis. Incidence of sacroiliitis associated with these conditions varies from 2% to 26%.
- ■ Age: 20 to 40 years
- ■ Sex: No sex predilection
- ■ Distribution: sacroiliac joints, spine, hips, knee; peripheral joints less common
- ■ Laboratory findings: HLA-B27 antigen positive in approximately 90%
- ■ Imaging features:
  - ● Bilateral sacroiliac joint involvement
  - ● Spondylitis similar to ankylosing spondylitis
  - ● Peripheral joint swelling and osteopenia
  - ● Joint space narrowing and erosions rare

(continued)

■ OSTEOARTHRITIS *(Continued)*

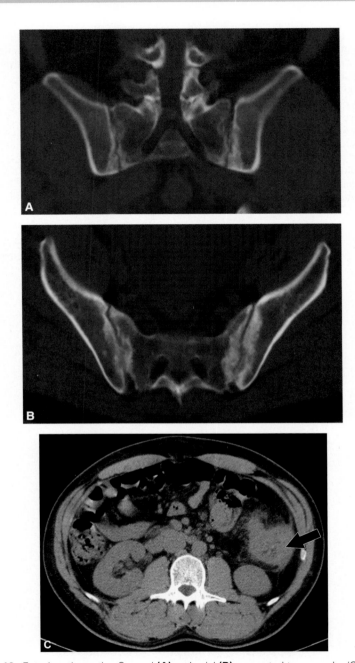

FIGURE 12-16. Enteric arthropathy. Coronal **(A)** and axial **(B)** computed tomography (CT) bone kernel images demonstrate symmetric sacroiliitis with bilateral erosive and sclerotic changes in this patient with inflammatory bowel disease. Axial **(C)** image through the abdomen demonstrates wall thickening involving the descending colon (*arrow*) with stranding in the surrounding fat.

SUGGESTED READING

Resnick D, Kransdorf MJ. Enteric arthropathies. In: Resnick D, Kransdorf MJ, eds. *Bone and Joint Imaging.* 3rd ed. Philadelphia: Elsevier-Saunders; 2005:306–315.

■ SYSTEMIC LUPUS ERYTHEMATOSUS

KEY FACTS

- ■ Clinical:
  - ● Systemic lupus erythematosus is a connective tissue disorder with immunologic abnormalities. Multiple organ systems are involved. Myositis occurs in 30% to 50% of patients, and joint involvement occurs in 75% to 90% of patients.
- ■ Age: 20 to 40 years
- ■ Sex: Females outnumber males by a wide margin. African Americans outnumber Caucasians.
- ■ Distribution: symmetric bilateral involvement of hands, knees, and shoulders
- ■ Laboratory findings: anemia, leukopenia, positive rheumatoid factor, lupus erythematosus cells, and antinuclear antibodies
- ■ Imaging features:
  - ● Soft tissue swelling
  - ● Juxta-articular osteoporosis
  - ● Subluxations and dislocations
  - ● Osteonecrosis
  - ● Bilateral symmetric involvement
  - ● Erosions and joint space loss are absent

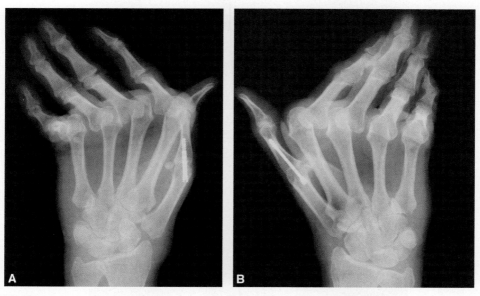

FIGURE 12-17. Systemic lupus erythematosus. Radiographs of the hands **(A, B)** show metacarpophalangeal (MCP) subluxations with no erosions. Note prior fusion of both thumbs.

SUGGESTED READING

Goh YP, Naidoo P, Ngian GS. Imaging of systemic lupus erythematosus. Part II: gastrointestinal, renal, and musculoskeletal manifestations. *Clin Radiol.* 2013;68(2):192–202.

Resnick D, Kransdorf MJ. Systemic lupus erythematosus. In: Resnick D, Kransdorf MJ, eds. *Bone and Joint Imaging.* 3rd ed. Philadelphia: Elsevier-Saunders; 2005:321–327.

Tani C, D'Aniello D, Possemato N, et al. MRI pattern of arthritis in systemic lupus erythematosus: a comparative study with rheumatoid arthritis and healthy subjects. *Skeletal Radiol.* 2015;44(2):261–266.

■ SCLERODERMA

KEY FACTS

- ■ Clinical:
  - ● Scleroderma is a connective tissue disorder that affects multiple organ systems, including the skin, musculoskeletal system, gastrointestinal tract, heart, lungs, and kidneys. Patients often present with pain and pallor of the hands when exposed to cold temperatures. Joint involvement is common initially, and up to 97% eventually have articular disease.
- ■ Age: 30 to 50 years
- ■ Sex: females outnumber males
- ■ Distribution: fingers, wrists, ankles
- ■ Laboratory findings: elevated erythrocyte sedimentation rate, positive rheumatoid factor (30% to 40%), antinuclear antibodies (35% to 96%)
- ■ Imaging features:
  - ● Hand: soft tissue atrophy, calcification, resorption of distal phalangeal tufts
  - ● Osteolysis in other sites, including phalanges, wrist, ribs, clavicle, mandible, and shoulder

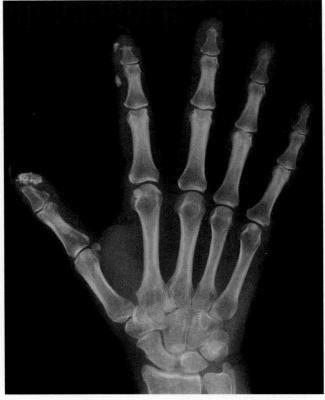

FIGURE 12-18. Scleroderma. Radiograph of the hand shows soft tissue atrophy and tuft resorption at involving the first and second digits with adjacent amorphous soft tissue calcifications. Early tuft resorption is noted in the third digit.

SUGGESTED READING

Bassett LW, Blocka KLN, Furst DE, et al. Skeletal findings in progressive systemic sclerosis (scleroderma). *Am J Roentgenol.* 1981;136:1121–1126.

La Montagna G, Sodano A, Capurro V, et al. The arthropathy of systemic sclerosis: a 12 month prospective clinical and imaging study. *Skeletal Radiol.* 2005;34(1):35–41.

Morrisroe KB, Nikpour M, Proudman SM. Musculoskeletal manifestations of systemic sclerosis. *Rheum Dis Clin North Am.* 2015;41(3):507–518.

■ DERMATOMYOSITIS/POLYMYOSITIS

KEY FACTS

■ Clinical:
- Polymyositis involves skeletal muscle and dermatomyositis muscle and skin. The cause is unknown. Five criteria are established for diagnosis:
  ❖ Progressive proximal muscle weakness
  ❖ Increased serum muscle enzymes
  ❖ Abnormal electromyogram
  ❖ Inflammatory changes on biopsy
  ❖ Skin disease (dermatomyositis)

■ Classifications:
- Typical polymyositis: most common category. More common in females 30 to 50 years old. Proximal muscle weakness in pelvis and thighs. Arthralgias with or without skin involvement.
- Typical dermatomyositis: more common in females. Muscle weakness with erythematosus skin rash. Older age group, typically 50 to 70 years old.
- Dermatomyositis with malignancy: more common in men more than 40 years old. Skin rash, muscle weakness, and malignancy. Tumors found in lung, prostate, breast, and gastrointestinal and genitourinary tracts.
- Childhood dermatomyositis: girls more often affected than boys. Muscle weakness, edema, skin calcification, vasculitis, and joint contractures.
- Acute myolysis: uncommon form with acute myonecrosis. Most common in adolescents and young adults. Outcome often fatal.

■ Imaging features:
- Radiographic features: soft tissue calcification, usually more extensive in children. Swelling about involved joints without bone changes.
- MRI: inflammatory changes in muscles easily detected and useful for biopsy site selection

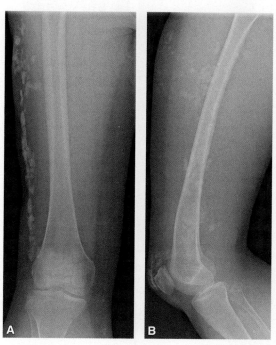

FIGURE 12-19. Dermatomyositis. Anteroposterior (AP) **(A)** and lateral **(B)** radiographs of the thigh with scattered soft tissue calcifications involve the muscle and skin.

(continued)

■ DERMATOMYOSITIS/POLYMYOSITIS *(Continued)*

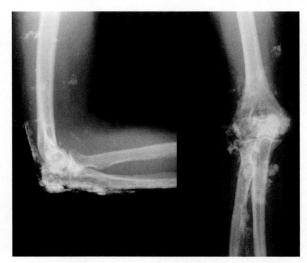

FIGURE 12-20. Dermatomyositis. Radiographs of the elbow show soft tissue calcification that is greater along the extensor surface.

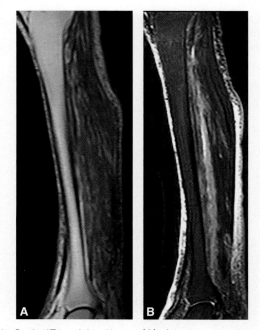

FIGURE 12-21. Myositis. Sagittal T1-weighted image **(A)** of the lower leg demonstrates fatty infiltration and atrophy of the posterior calf musculature from chronic myopathy. Sagittal fat-saturated T2-weighted magnetic resonance (MR) **(B)** shows patchy increased signal compatible with muscular edema suggesting superimposed acute myopathy.

SUGGESTED READING

Frazer DD, Frank JA, Dalakas MC. Inflammatory myopathies: MR imaging and spectroscopy. *Radiology.* 1991;179:341–344.
Garcia J. MRI in inflammatory myopathies. *Skeletal Radiol.* 2000;29(8):425–438.
Schulze M, Kötter I, Ernemann U, et al. MRI findings in inflammatory muscle diseases and their noninflammatory mimics. *Am J Roentgenol.* 2009;192(6):1708–1716.

■ MIXED CONNECTIVE TISSUE DISEASE/OVERLAP SYNDROMES

KEY FACTS

- ■ Clinical:
  - ● Mixed connective tissue disease presents with a combination of features resembling scleroderma, systemic lupus erythematosus, dermatomyositis, and RA. Joints are involved in 90% to 100%.
- ■ Age: children and adults
- ■ Sex: slightly more common in females than males
- ■ Distribution: hands, feet
- ■ Laboratory findings: presence of antibodies to saline extractable nuclear antigen
- ■ Imaging features:
  - ● Juxta-articular osteopenia
  - ● Soft tissue swelling
  - ● Erosions similar to RA
  - ● Scleroderma-like changes in tufts
  - ● Soft tissue calcification
  - ● Joint subluxations

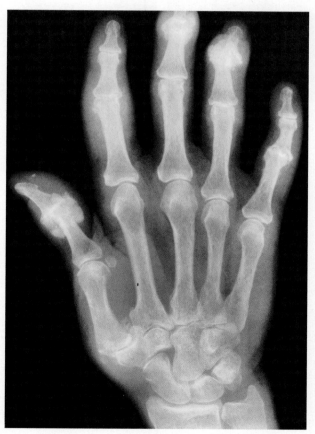

FIGURE 12-22. Mixed connective tissue disease. Anteroposterior (AP) radiograph of the right hand shows periarticular soft tissue calcification, most obvious in the thumb, soft tissue swelling, joint subluxation in the phalangeal joints, and joint space narrowing.

(continued)

■ MIXED CONNECTIVE TISSUE DISEASE/OVERLAP SYNDROMES   *(Continued)*

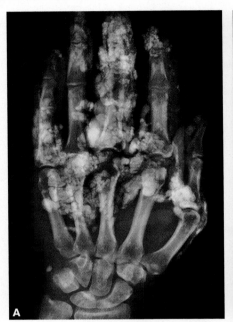 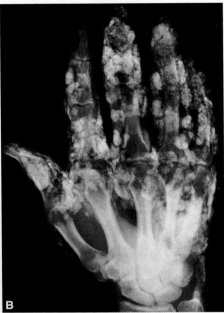

FIGURE 12-23. Mixed connective tissue disease. **(A, B)** Radiographs of both hands show juxta-articular osteopenia and extensive soft tissue calcifications.

SUGGESTED READING

Resnick D, Kransdorf MJ. Mixed connective tissue disease and collagen vascular overlap syndromes. In: Resnick D, Kransdorf MJ, eds. *Bone and Joint Imaging*. 3rd ed. Philadelphia: Elsevier-Saunders; 2005:349–352.

■ JUVENILE CHRONIC ARTHROPATHY

KEY FACTS

- ■ Juvenile chronic arthropathy includes a spectrum of disorders, including juvenile spondyloarthropathies, seropositive RA, and seronegative (Still disease) arthritis.
- ■ Most disorders occur in older children or adolescents and, therefore, have findings similar to the adult disorder.
- ■ Still disease occurs in younger children and accounts for 70% of juvenile chronic arthropathies. Three categories exist with some overlap:
  - ● Systemic disease without joint involvement
  - ● Polyarthropathy with less significant systemic manifestations
  - ● Monoarticular arthropathy without systemic disease
- ■ Distribution: Knee is the most common site for monoarticular disease. Wrists involved more than hands, feet, hips, and cervical spine (similar to RA).
- ■ Imaging features:
  - ● Bilateral symmetric disease for polyarticular form
  - ● Soft tissue swelling
  - ● Osteopenic
  - ● Epiphyseal overgrowth
  - ● Premature physeal closure
  - ● Ankylosis

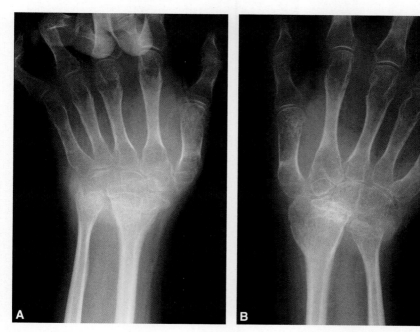

FIGURE 12-24. Juvenile chronic arthropathy. **(A, B)** Anteroposterior (AP) radiographs of the wrists show marked osteopenia with carpal collapse. AP **(C)** and lateral **(D)** radiographs of the knee show epiphyseal hyperemia and soft tissue involvement (synovitis).

(continued)

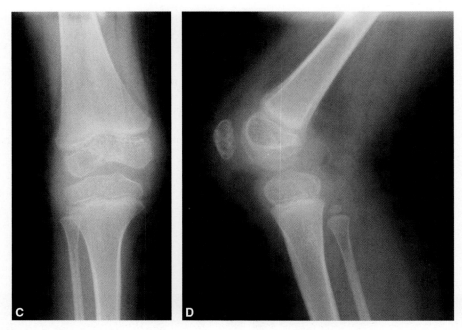

FIGURE 12-24. *(continued)*

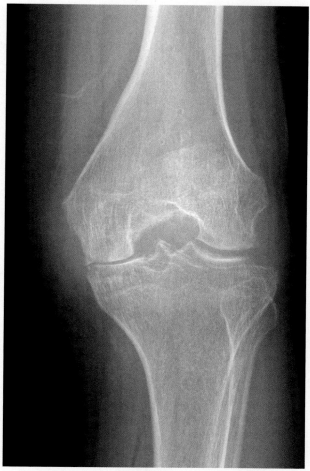

FIGURE 12-25. Juvenile chronic arthropathy. Skeletally mature individual with chronic changes of juvenile chronic arthropathy in the left knee including osteopenia and widening of the intercondylar notch.

SUGGESTED READING

Ansell BM, Kent PA. Radiological changes in juvenile chronic polyarthritis. *Skeletal Radiol.* 1977;1:129–144.
Azouz EM. Arthritis in children: conventional and advanced imaging. *Semin Musculoskelet Radiol.* 2003;7(2):95–102.
Sheybani EF, Khanna G, White AJ, et al. Imaging of juvenile idiopathic arthritis: a multimodality approach. *Radiographics.* 2013;33(5):1253–1273.

■ HEMOPHILIA

KEY FACTS

- ■ Arthropathy of hemophilia is the result of repetitive hemorrhage.
- ■ Hemarthrosis occurs in up to 90% of patients with hemophilia.
- ■ Most hemorrhagic episodes occur in childhood.
- ■ Distribution: knee, elbow, ankle, hip, shoulder
- ■ Imaging features resemble juvenile chronic arthritis:
  - Asymmetric distribution
  - Dense soft tissue swelling (blood)
  - Epiphyseal overgrowth
  - Subchondral cysts
  - Late secondary degenerative changes
  - Osseous pseudotumors

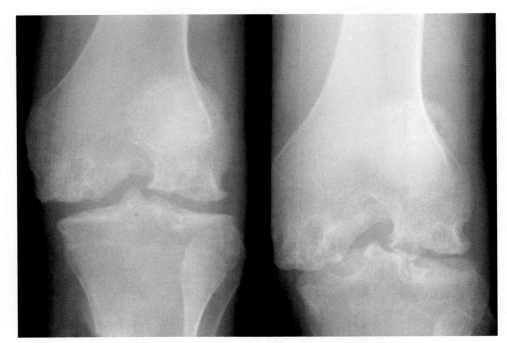

FIGURE 12-26. Hemophilia. Bilateral knees demonstrate epiphyseal overgrowth, widening of the intercondylar notch, and numerous subchondral cysts. Secondary degenerative changes with osteophyte formation are also noted.

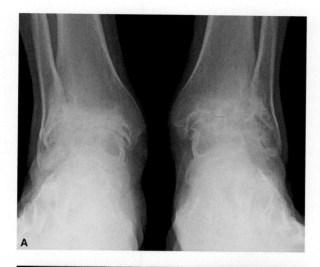

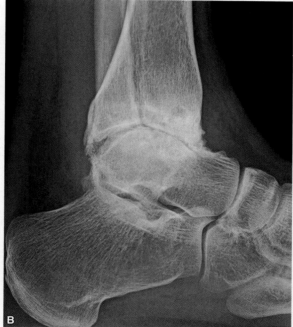

FIGURE 12-27. Hemophilia. **(A, B)** Secondary degenerative changes are predominant with severe tib-iotalar joint space loss, osteophyte formation, subchondral cyst formation, and sclerosis in this patient with chronic hemophilic arthropathy.

SUGGESTED READING

Kerr R. Imaging of musculoskeletal complications of hemophilia. *Semin Musculoskelet Radiol.* 2003;7(2):127–136.

Maclachlan J, Gough-Palmer A, Hargunani R, et al. Haemophilia imaging: a review. *Skeletal Radiol.* 2009;38(10):949–957.

Park JS, Ryu KN. Hemophilic pseudotumor involving the musculoskeletal system: spectrum of radiologic findings. *Am J Roentgenol.* 2004;183(1):55–61.

Pettersson H, Ahlberg A, Nilsson IM. Radiologic classification of hemophilic arthropathy. *Clin Orthop.* 1980;149:153–159.

■ GOUT

KEY FACTS

- Gouty arthropathy is the result of deposition of monosodium urate crystals.
- Males are affected much more frequently than females.
- Laboratory findings: hyperuricemia
- Distribution: feet most common (85%); ankles, hands, wrists, elbows. May present as olecranon bursitis in the elbow.
- Radiographic changes take years to manifest.
- Imaging features:
  - Asymmetric polyarthropathy
  - Tophi
  - Well-defined erosions with sclerotic margins
  - Overhanging edge
  - Normal bone density
- Dual-energy computed tomography (CT) can be useful to diagnose, characterize, and quantify uric acid deposition.

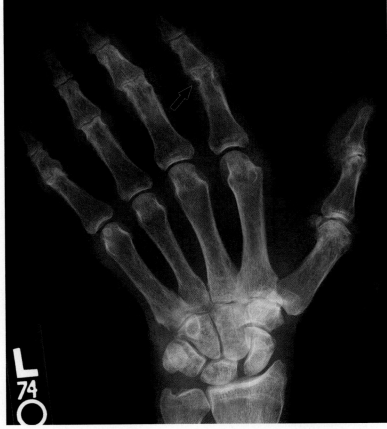

FIGURE 12-28. Gout. Increased density and soft tissue swelling surrounding the second through fourth proximal interphalangeal (PIP) joints and first interphalangeal (IP) joint consistent with gouty tophi. Well-defined periarticular erosion at the head of the second proximal phalanx has a classic "rat bite" appearance.

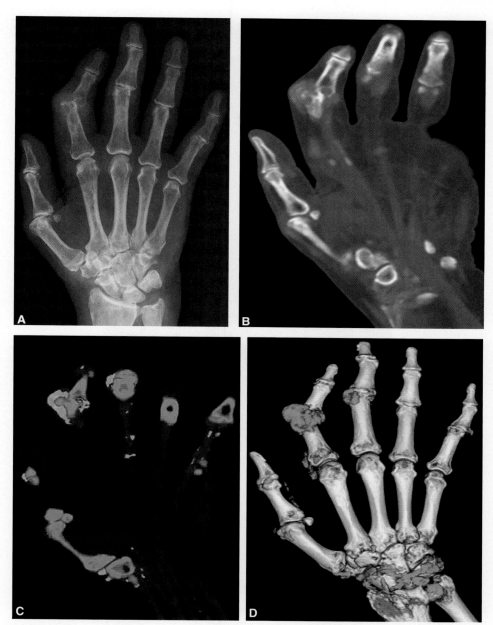

FIGURE 12-29. Gout. Anteroposterior (AP) radiograph **(A)** demonstrates mineralized tophus and periarticular erosions at the second proximal interphalangeal (PIP) joint. Conventional computed tomography (CT) **(B)** better demonstrates the erosions and foci of mineralization. Dual energy CT **(C)** demonstrates the uric acid deposits within tophi as green and distinct from the calcium-containing osseous structures shown in blue. Surface-rendered 3D model **(D)** demonstrates multiple gouty tophi (green) in greater number than suspected on radiographic examination.

(continued)

■ **GOUT**   *(Continued)*

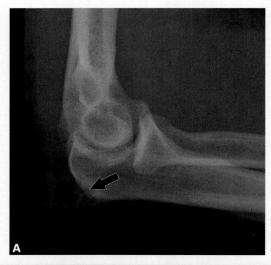

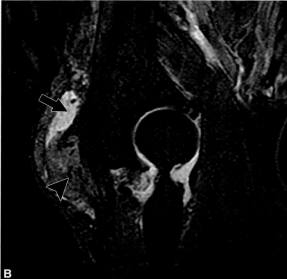

FIGURE 12-30. Gout. Lateral radiograph of the elbow **(A)** demonstrates erosive changes at the olecranon (*arrow*) with overlying soft tissue swelling. Sagittal short-T1 inversion recovery magnetic resonance (STIR MR) **(B)** demonstrates an intermediate density large gouty tophus (*arrowhead*) at the olecranon with adjacent olecranon bursitis (*arrow*).

SUGGESTED READING

Desai MA, Peterson JJ, Garner HW, et al. Clinical utility of dual-energy CT for evaluation of tophaceous gout. *Radiographics*. 2011;31(5):1365–1375.

Gentili A. Advanced imaging of gout. *Semin Musculoskelet Radiol*. 2003;7(3):165–174.

Girish G, Glazebrook KN, Jacobson JA. Advanced imaging in gout. *Am J Roentgenol*. 2013;201(3):515–525.

Monu JU, Pope TL Jr. Gout: a clinical and radiologic review. *Radiol Clin North Am*. 2004;42(1):169–184.

Pascual E. The diagnosis of gout and CPPD crystal arthropathy. *Br J Rheumatol*. 1996;35:306–308.

Soldatos T, Pezeshk P, Ezzati F, et al. Cross-sectional imaging of adult crystal and inflammatory arthropathies. *Skeletal Radiol*. 2016;45(9):1173–1191.

■ HEMOCHROMATOSIS

KEY FACTS

■ Hemochromatosis is an inherited disorder resulting in systemic iron deposition. It may also occur with cirrhosis, multiple transfusions, or excessive iron intake.

■ The disorder is most common in men aged more than 40 years.

■ The arthropathy resembles degenerative joint disease and calcium pyrophosphate deposition disease (CPPD).

■ Distribution: hands and wrists most common, followed by knees and hips.

■ Imaging features:
  - Bilateral asymmetric arthropathy
  - Osteopenia
  - Chondrocalcinosis
  - Subchondral cysts
  - Joint space narrowing
  - Osteophyte formation
  - Subchondral sclerosis

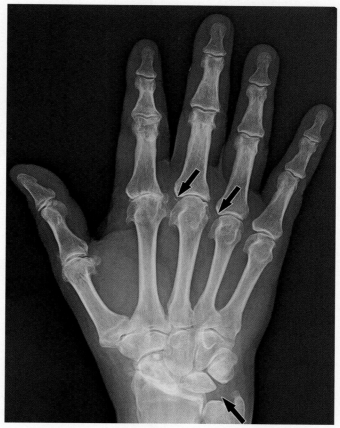

FIGURE 12-31. Hemochromatosis. There is scattered joint space narrowing, most prominent at the radioscaphoid and second metacarpophalangeal (MCP) joints. Note the hooked configuration of the metacarpal head osteophytes. Chondrocalcinosis is seen at the triangular fibrocartilage complex and the third and fourth MCP joints (*arrows*).

(continued)

■ **HEMOCHROMATOSIS** *(Continued)*

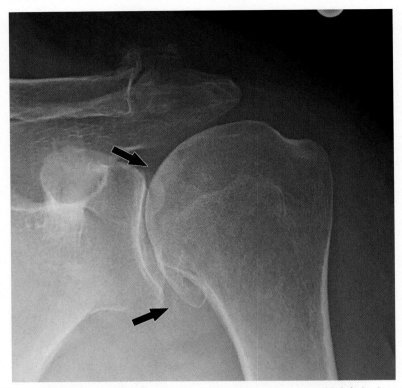

FIGURE 12-32. Hemochromatosis. Glenohumeral joint space narrowing with inferior humeral head osteophyte. There is chondrocalcinosis seen along the glenohumeral joint as well as mineralization in the superior and inferior labrum (*arrows*). Chondrocalcinosis, osteophyte formation, and joint space narrowing are also identified at the acromioclavicular joint.

SUGGESTED READING

Brower AC, Flemming DJ. *Arthritis in Black and White.* 3rd ed. Philadelphia: Elsevier/Saunders; 2012:335–344.

Dallos T, Sahinbegovic E, Stamm T, et al. Idiopathic hand osteoarthritis vs haemochromatosis arthropathy—a clinical, functional and radiographic study. *Rheumatology (Oxford).* 2013;52(5):910–915.

Hirsh JH, Lillen C, Troupin RH. Arthropathy of hemochromatosis. *Radiology.* 1976;118:591–596.

■ CALCIUM PYROPHOSPHATE DEPOSITION DISEASE

KEY FACTS

- CPPD is the most common crystal arthropathy.
- The condition affects 5% of the population, generally the middle-aged or elderly.
- CPPD crystals are deposited in hyaline and fibrocartilage. Patients may have no symptoms or may present with severe pain.
- Distribution: knee, pubic symphysis, and wrist most common, but may involve any joint
- Imaging features:
  - Bilateral asymmetric arthropathy
  - Chondrocalcinosis
  - Joint space loss
  - Normal bone density
  - Multiple subchondral cysts

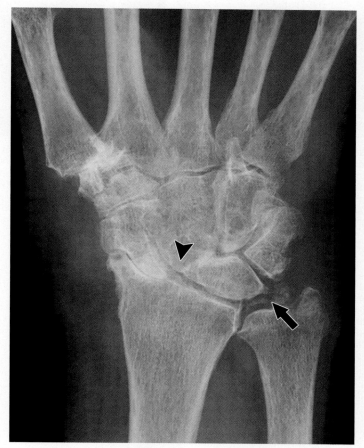

FIGURE 12-33. Calcium pyrophosphate deposition disease (CPPD). There is proximal carpal joint space narrowing, most notable at the radioscaphoid articulation. There is widening of the scapholunate interval and the capitate has migrated proximally (*arrowhead*) consistent with scapholunate advanced collapse (SLAC). Chondrocalcinosis at the triangular fibrocartilage complex (*arrow*). Scattered carpal cysts are evident.

(continued)

■ CALCIUM PYROPHOSPHATE DEPOSITION DISEASE *(Continued)*

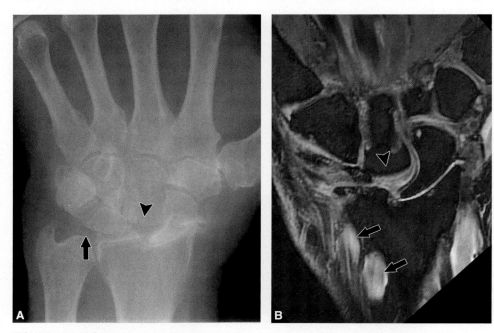

FIGURE 12-34. Calcium pyrophosphate deposition disease (CPPD). Radiograph depicts **(A)** marked radioscaphoid narrowing with osteophyte formation. Scapholunate advanced collapse (SLAC) configuration of the wrist with proximal migration of the capitate (*arrowhead*) through a widened scapholunate interval. Subtle chondrocalcinosis at the triangular fibrocartilage (*arrow*). Coronal short-T1 inversion recovery magnetic resonance (STIR MR) **(B)** of the wrist redemonstrates the proximal migration of the capitate (*arrowhead*). Note the numerous small scattered carpal cysts, better appreciated on MR, as well as the large cysts in the distal radius (*arrows*).

SUGGESTED READING

Adamson TC III, Resnick CS, Gierra J Jr, et al. Hand and wrist arthropathies of hemochromatosis and calcium pyrophosphate deposition disease: distinct radiologic features. *Radiology.* 1983;147:377–381.

Bencardino JT, Hassankhani A. Calcium pyrophosphate dihydrate crystal deposition disease. *Semin Musculoskelet Radiol.* 2003;7(3):175–185.

Steinbach LS. Calcium pyrophosphate dihydrate and calcium hydroxyapatite crystal deposition diseases: imaging perspectives. *Radiol Clin North Am.* 2004;42(1):185–205, vii.

■ WILSON DISEASE

KEY FACTS

- Wilson disease is a rare liver disease resulting in copper deposition in bones, joints, and other tissues.
- Copper interferes with normal osteogenesis, resulting in osteomalacia.
- Up to 50% of patients develop arthropathy.
- Distribution: hands, wrists, feet, shoulders, hips, elbow, knees
- Imaging features:
  - Bone fragmentation
  - Marked irregularity of articular and subchondral bone
  - Osseous loose bodies
  - Resembles osteoarthritis

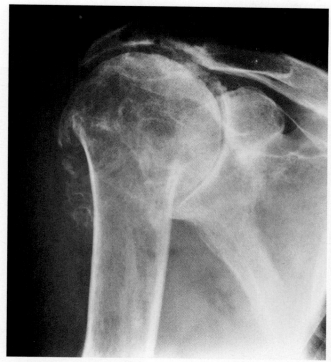

FIGURE 12-35. Wilson disease. Advanced joint destruction with loose bodies, fragmentation, and chronic rotator cuff tear in the right shoulder.

SUGGESTED READING

Brower AC, Flemming DJ. *Arthritis in Black and White*. 3rd ed. Philadelphia: Elsevier/Saunders; 2012:335–344.
Menerey KA, Eides W, Brewer GJ, et al. Arthropathy of Wilson disease: clinical and pathologic features. *J Rheumatol*. 1988;15:331–337.

■ OCHRONOSIS

KEY FACTS

- ■ Ochronosis is a metabolic disease caused by a lack of homogentisic acid oxidase. Homogentisic acid (a dark pigment) is deposited in joints, resulting in cartilage degeneration.
- ■ Patients typically present after age 40 years.
- ■ Distribution: spine—may resemble ankylosing spondylitis. Peripheral joints (knee, hip, shoulder)—similar to CPPD or osteoarthritis.
- ■ Imaging features:
  - ● Bilateral asymmetric arthropathy
  - ● Osteopenia
  - ● Disc degeneration and calcification
  - ● Subchondral sclerosis
  - ● Lack of significant osteophytes
  - ● Loose bodies

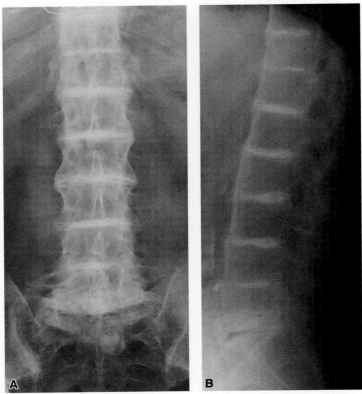

FIGURE 12-36. Onchronosis. Anteroposterior (AP) and lateral radiographs of the lumbar spine **(A, B)** show ankylosis with diffuse degeneration and calcification of the intervertebral discs.

SUGGESTED READING

Brower AC, Flemming DJ. *Arthritis in Black and White*. 3rd ed. Philadelphia: Elsevier/Saunders; 2012:335–344.

■ NEUROTROPHIC ARTHROPATHY

KEY FACTS

- Neurotrophic arthropathy results from repetitive trauma to joint without sensory nerve supply.
- Relaxation of supporting structures results in malalignment of osseous structure fragmentation and, in most cases, subchondral sclerosis.
- Diabetic neuropathy is the most common cause. Multiple sclerosis, syphilis, syringomyelia, meningomyeloceles, and congenital insensitivity to pain may also cause neurotrophic arthropathy.
- Distribution: lower extremity, especially foot and ankle
- Imaging features:
  - Atrophic: bone resorption and demineralization
  - Hypertrophic:
    - ❖ Most common
    - ❖ Articular and osseous fragmentation
    - ❖ Bone sclerosis
    - ❖ Osteophyte formation
    - ❖ Subluxation

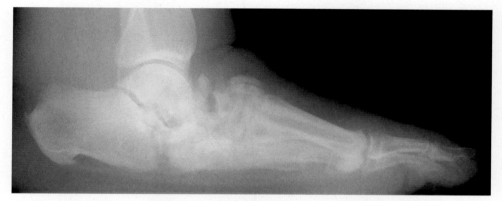

FIGURE 12-37. Diabetic patient with neuropathic arthropathy. Lateral foot radiograph shows destruction of the midfoot with prominent osseous fragmentation and sclerosis. There is loss of the normal longitudinal arch of the foot with multiple subluxations at the level of the tarsometatarsals.

(continued)

■ NEUROTROPHIC ARTHROPATHY *(Continued)*

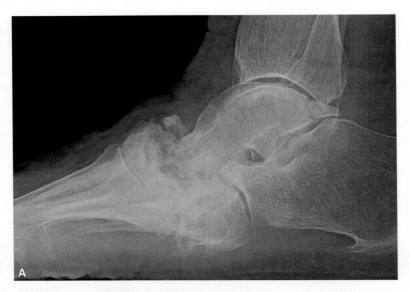

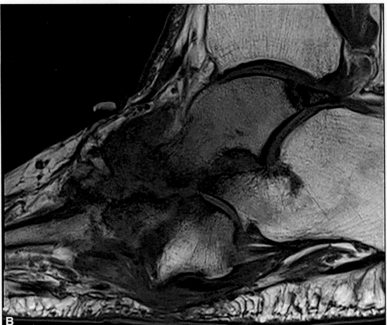

FIGURE 12-38. Diabetic patient with neuropathic arthropathy. Lateral foot radiograph **(A)** shows destruction at the tarsometatarsal joints with osseous fragmentation, sclerosis, and subluxation. T1-weighted magnetic resonance (MR) **(B)** and contrast-enhanced fat-saturated T1-weighted MR image **(C)** demonstrate extensive marrow edema as well as reactive changes including surrounding soft tissue edema and synovitis.

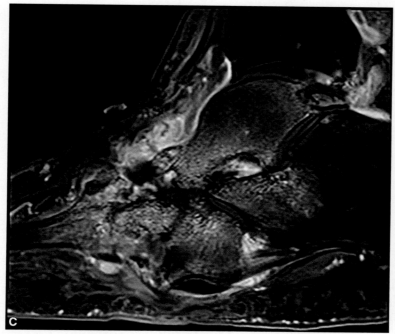

FIGURE 12-38. (*continued*)

SUGGESTED READING

Aliabadi P, Nikpoor N, Alparslan L. Imaging of neuropathic arthropathy. *Semin Musculoskelet Radiol.* 2003;7(3):217–225.

Jones EA, Manaster BJ, May DA, et al. Neuropathic osteoarthropathy: diagnostic dilemmas and differential diagnosis. *Radiographics.* 2000;20(spec no):S279–S293.

Leone A, Cassar-Pullicino VN, Semprini A, et al. Neuropathic osteoarthropathy with and without superimposed osteomyelitis in patients with a diabetic foot. *Skeletal Radiol.* 2016;45(6):735–754.

Sequeira W. The neuropathic joint. *Clin Exp Rheumatol.* 1994;12:325–337.

■ SYNOVIAL CHONDROMATOSIS/OSTEOCHONDROMATOSIS

KEY FACTS

- Primary synovial chondromatosis or osteochondromatosis is a condition of unknown cause. Synovial chondromas or osteochondromas form resulting from synovial metaplasia. There are three phases:
  - Phase 1: active synovial metaplasia with no loose bodies
  - Phase 2: transitional phase with metaplasia and loose bodies
  - Phase 3: no active metaplasia, but loose bodies
- In older patients (>50 years of age), the condition is twice as common in males as females. However, the condition is also common in younger females (aged 20–30 years) and most often involves the hip.
- The condition involves the hip in 50% of cases, but may also involve the knee, elbow, wrist, hand, shoulder, and temporomandibular joint.
- Radiographs may be normal unless the loose bodies are calcified or ossified. Conventional, CT, and magnetic resonance (MR) arthrography are more useful to confirm the diagnosis.
- Secondary degenerative arthritis follows this condition.
- Treatment consists of synovectomy and/or removal of loose bodies.

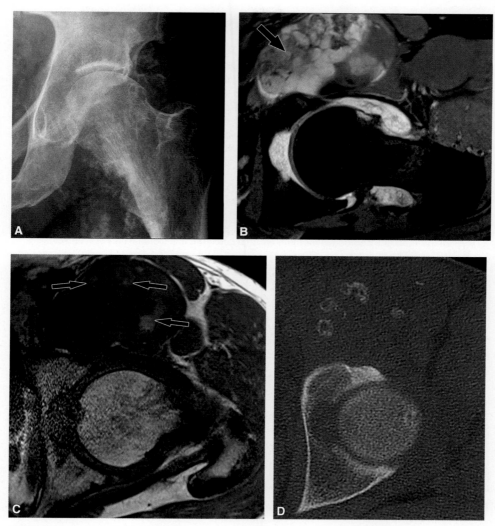

FIGURE 12-39. Primary synovial osteochondromatosis. Anteroposterior (AP) radiograph of the pelvis **(A)** shows numerous calcified bodies projecting over the proximal femur. The hip joint is relatively preserved. Axial fat-saturated T2-weighted magnetic resonance (MR) of the left hip **(B)** shows filling defects extending anteriorly from the joint into a large distended iliopsoas bursa (*arrow*). Axial T1-weighted MR **(C)** shows that several of the loose bodies in the iliopsoas bursa demonstrate fat signal internally (*arrows*) consistent with marrow within the synovial osteochondromas. Axial computed tomography (CT) **(D)** also nicely demonstrates the calcified loose bodies within the iliopsoas bursa.

SUGGESTED READING

Milgram JW. Synovial osteochondromatosis: a histopathologic study of 30 cases. *J Bone Joint Surg.* 1977;59A:792–801.

Murphey MD, Vidal JA, Fanburg-Smith JC, et al. Imaging of synovial chondromatosis with radiologic-pathologic correlation. *Radiographics.* 2007;27(5):1465–1488.

Peh WCG, Shek TWH, Davies AM, et al. Osteochondroma and secondary synovial osteochondromatosis. *Skeletal Radiol.* 1999;28:169–174.

■ PIGMENTED VILLONODULAR SYNOVITIS

KEY FACTS

- Pigmented villonodular synovitis (PVNS) is a relatively uncommon disorder characterized by synovial proliferation with hemosiderin deposition in synovial tissues.
- The condition may involve joints, bursae, or tendon sheaths.
- There are diffuse forms (80% involve the knee) and localized forms such as giant cell tumor of the tendon sheath.
- The condition is diagnosed most commonly in the second through fifth decades.
- PVNS is typically monoarticular involving the knee, followed by the hip, ankle, shoulder, elbow, temporomandibular joint, and spine.
- Radiographic findings are evident in 80% of cases. Findings include swelling, joint effusion (often denser than a simple effusion), and cystic or erosive changes in bone.
- MR features are characteristic with areas of low signal intensity on T1- and T2-weighted sequences resulting from hemosiderin deposition.
- Treatment consists of synovectomy. Recurrence rates are 25% to 50%. Postoperative baseline MR examinations are recommended for more optimal detection of residual PVNS or recurrence.

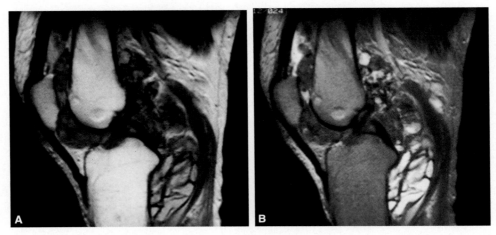

FIGURE 12-40. Pigmented villonodular synovitis (PVNS). Sagittal T1-weighted **(A)** and fat-saturated T2-weighted images **(B)** of the knee demonstrate lobulated soft tissue masses in the knee with areas of low signal intensity on both sequences resulting from hemosiderin deposition.

SUGGESTED READING

Jelinek JS, Kransdorf MJ, Utz JA, et al. Imaging of pigmented villonodular synovitis with emphasis on MR imaging. *Am J Roentgenol.* 1989;152:337–342.

Masih S, Antebi A. Imaging of pigmented villonodular synovitis. *Semin Musculoskelet Radiol.* 2003;7(3):205–216.

Murphey MD, Rhee JH, Lewis RB, et al. Pigmented villonodular synovitis: radiologic-pathologic correlation. *Radiographics.* 2008;28(5):1493–1518.

■ AMYLOID ARTHROPATHY

KEY FACTS

- Amyloid arthropathy is attributed to long-term dialysis using cuprophane dialysis membranes. B2-microglobulin is deposited in the form of amyloidosis.
- Clinically, the condition is unusual in patients on dialysis less than 5 years, but occurs in 80% of patients on dialysis for more than 10 years. Patients present with pain and swelling in the involved joints.
- Radiographs demonstrate large cystic lesions in bone with lobulated soft tissue swelling. Pathologic fractures may occur.
- On MR images, the interosseous lesions demonstrate signal intensity between muscle and fibrous tissue regardless of the pulse sequence. Distention of the joint and bursa is common. Rarely large lytic bone lesions (amyloidoma) may be evident resembling neoplasms.

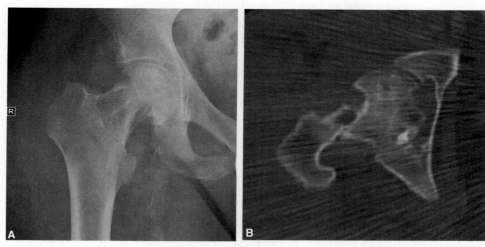

FIGURE 12-41. Amyloidosis in chronic dialysis patient presenting as soft tissue mass. Anteroposterior (AP) radiograph **(A)** shows extensive erosive changes involving the femoral neck. Axial computed tomography (CT) **(B)** shows the erosions are well marginated and also involve the femoral head. Coronal T1-weighted magnetic resonance (MR) **(C)** shows intermediate- to low-density masses within the erosions and extending laterally into the soft tissues (*arrows*) about the iliotibial band where a soft tissue mass could be palpated. The amyloid deposits are heterogeneously intermediate- to low-density on the fat-saturated proton density MR **(D)**. Soft tissue extension of joint disease can resemble neoplasm.

(continued)

■ AMYLOID ARTHROPATHY *(Continued)*

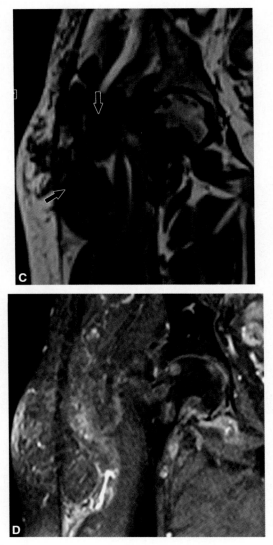

FIGURE 12-41. *(continued)*

SUGGESTED READING

Cobby MJ, Adler RS, Swarz R, et al. Dialysis-related amyloid arthropathy: MR findings in four patients. *Am J Roentgenol*. 1991;157:1023–1027.

Kiss E, Keusch G, Zanetti M, et al. Dialysis-related amyloidosis revisited. *Am J Roentgenol*. 2005;185(6):1460–1467.

Sheldon PJ, Forrester DM. Imaging of amyloid arthropathy. *Semin Musculoskelet Radiol*. 2003;7(3):195–203.

Metabolic Diseases

Jeffrey J. Peterson and Thomas H. Berquist

■ OSTEOPOROSIS: BASIC CONCEPTS

KEY FACTS

- Osteoporosis is a reduction in bone mass. It is the most common clinical bone disease.
- Osteoporosis affects 75 million people in the United States, Europe, and Japan, accounting for 1.5 million fractures per year.
- Osteoporosis is categorized as generalized, regional, or local. Table 13-1 summarizes the causes of osteoporosis.
- Radiographic and imaging features vary with the type of osteoporosis and site.

Table 13-1   CAUSES OF OSTEOPOROSIS

Generalized	Regional/Localized
Senile, postmenopausal	Disuse atrophy
Endocrine disorders	Reflex sympathetic dystrophy
Thyroid dysfunction	Transient regional osteoporosis
Parathyroid dysfunction	Migratory osteoporosis
Cushing disease	
Hypogonadism	
Medications	
Steroids	
Heparin	
Chronic liver disease	
Anemias	
Multiple myeloma	
Environmental factors	
Smoking	
Alcohol abuse	
Nutritional deficiency	
Low calcium intake	
Idiopathic	

SUGGESTED READING

Eastell R. Treatment of postmenopausal osteoporosis. *N Engl J Med*. 1998;338:736–746.
Golob AL, Laya MB. Osteoporosis: screening, prevention, and management. *Med Clin North Am*. 2015;99(3):587–606.
Guglielmi G, Muscarella S, Bazzocchi A. Integrated imaging approach to osteoporosis: state-of-the-art review and update. *Radiographics*. 2011;31(5):1343–1364.

■ OSTEOPOROSIS: GENERALIZED

KEY FACTS

- Generalized osteoporosis may be the result of a long list of disorders (Table 13-1).
- Senile or postmenopausal osteoporosis usually develops in women aged more than 50 years. Fracture risk approaches 60% in females aged more than 50 years.
- Endocrine disorders (Table 13-1) are the most common cause of secondary osteoporosis. The five most common endocrine disorders are hypogonadism, insulinopenia, hyperparathyroidism (HPT), hyperthyroidism, and hypercortisolemia.
- Imaging of osteoporosis is typically accomplished with routine radiographs and bone mineral density measurements (dual-energy X-ray absorptiometry [DXA]). Computed tomography and ultrasound have also been used. However, management decisions and patient monitoring are most often accomplished with DXA.
- Combining DXA data with clinical factors (age, prevalent fractures, family history of fractures, low body mass index, increased risk of falls, and steroids) allows estimation of fracture probabilities over 5- and 10-year periods.
  - Radiographic features: Spine and proximal extremities are primarily involved. Thin cortical bone, vertebral contour abnormalities (endplate compression, compression fractures). Coarsened trabecular pattern in the pelvis and trabecular resorption in the proximal femurs.
  - DXA: Lumbar spine, femoral neck, and wrists are typically studied. Bone density is compared with density in healthy 30-year-old persons (T score) and the patient's age group (Z score).
    - ❖ Normal: > -1
    - ❖ Osteopenia: < -1 to -2.5
    - ❖ Osteoporosis: < -2.5
- Treatment may include ralozifene (mean increase in spine density 2.6% over 4 years), bisphosphonates (mean increase 10% to 15% after 7 to 10 years), teriparatide (13% density increase after 18 months), or strontium ranelate (14.5% density increase after 3 years). Treatments may reduce fracture risk by 30% to 50%. DXA studies are used to monitor therapy at 1- to 2-year intervals.

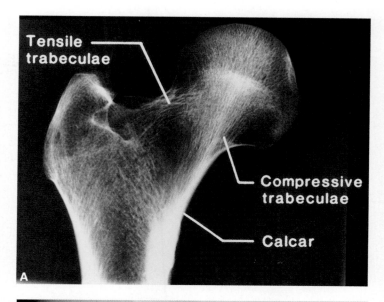

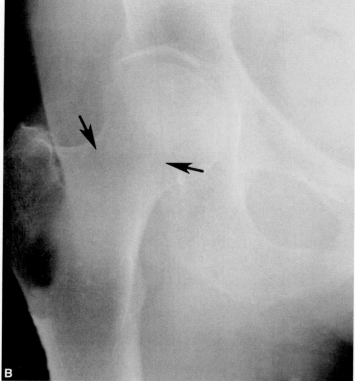

FIGURE 13-1. Osteoporosis. **(A)** Normal right hip with trabecular pattern well demonstrated. **(B)** Osteoporotic right hip with poorly defined trabeculae (*arrows*).

(continued)

■ **OSTEOPOROSIS: GENERALIZED** *(Continued)*

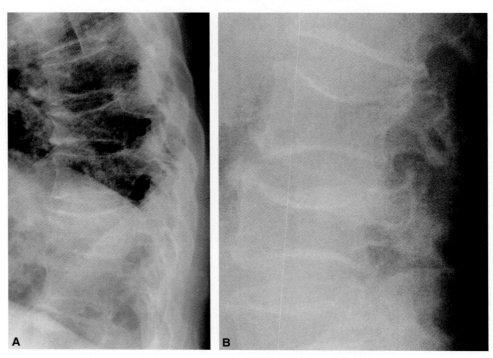

FIGURE 13-2. **(A)** Lateral thoracic spine with osteoporosis and compression fractures. **(B)** Lateral lumbar space shows endplate compression (fish vertebra) with biconcave appearance.

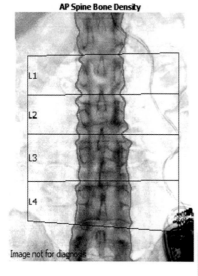

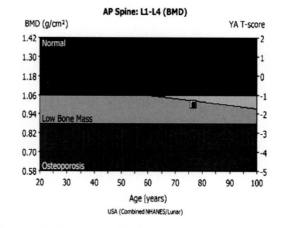

Densitometry: USA (Combined NHANES/Lunar)			
Region	BMD (g/cm²)	YA T-score	AM Z-score
L1	0.768	-3.0	-2.6
L2	1.004	-1.6	-1.3
L3	1.068	-1.1	-0.8
L4	1.091	-0.9	-0.6
L1-L4	0.999	-1.5	-1.2

A

FIGURE 13-3. Dual-energy X-ray absorptiometry (DXA) examination in a 76-year-old man with lumbar **(A)** and hip **(B)** *T* scores of −1.5 and −3.1 for the lumbar spine and right hip, respectively. Findings indicate osteopenia in the spine and osteoporosis for the hip.

Dual Femur Bone Density

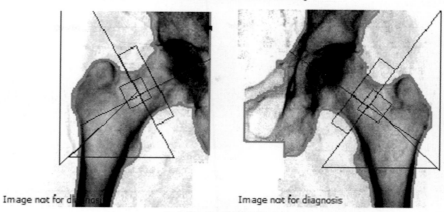

Left Femur: Total (BMD)

BMD (g/cm²)   YA T-score

USA (Combined NHANES/Lunar)

Densitometry: USA (Combined NHANES/Lunar)			
Region	BMD (g/cm²)	YA T-score	AM Z-score
Neck Left	0.611	-3.1	-2.1
Neck Right	0.634	-2.9	-1.9
Neck Mean	0.623	-3.0	-2.0
Neck Diff.	0.023	0.2	0.2
Total Left	0.646	-2.9	-2.2
Total Right	0.696	-2.5	-1.8
Total Mean	0.671	-2.7	-2.0
Total Diff.	0.050	0.4	0.3

HAL chart results unavailable

B

FIGURE 13-3. (continued)

(continued)

■ **OSTEOPOROSIS: GENERALIZED**   *(Continued)*

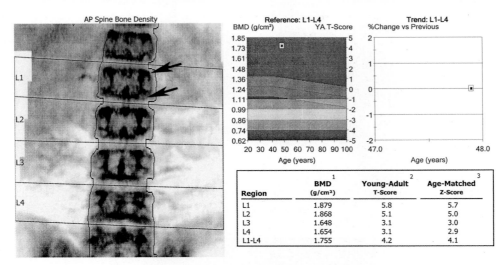

Region	BMD[1] (g/cm²)	Young-Adult[2] T-Score	Age-Matched[3] Z-Score
L1	1.879	5.8	5.7
L2	1.868	5.1	5.0
L3	1.648	3.1	3.0
L4	1.654	3.1	2.9
L1-L4	1.755	4.2	4.1

FIGURE 13-4. Dual-energy X-ray absorptiometry (DXA) study of the spine in a patient with chronic renal failure and renal osteodystrophy. The endplates are dense (*arrows*) and bone density increased with *T* scores of up to 5.8 in L1.

SUGGESTED READING

Alston SH. Bone densitometry and bone biopsy. *Best Pract Res Clin Rheumatol.* 2005;19:487–501.

Briot K, Roux C. What is the role of DXA, QUS, and bone markers in fracture prediction, treatment allocation, and monitoring? *Best Pract Res Clin Rheumatol.* 2005;19:951–964.

Guglielmi G, Muscarella S, Bazzocchi A. Integrated imaging approach to osteoporosis: state-of-the-art review and update. *Radiographics.* 2011;31(5):1343–1364.

■ OSTEOPOROSIS: REGIONAL OSTEOPOROSIS

KEY FACTS

- ■ Osteoporosis may be more localized, affecting single or multiple osseous structures or periarticular regions.
- ■ Changes are most common in the extremities.
- ■ Several disease categories are included in regional osteoporosis.
  - Disuse osteoporosis: Disuse or immobilization osteoporosis is common after trauma with reduced use. Other painful conditions or paralysis may also result in disuse osteoporosis. Radiographic features include generalized osteopenia, subchondral osteopenia, or foci of cortical or medullary lucency.
  - Transient regional osteoporosis: Transient regional osteoporosis has in common focal involvement, rapid onset, and pain, and conditions are self-limited. One of the most common is transient osteoporosis of the hip (see Chapter 3). Radiographic features include rapid-onset osteopenia of the femoral head and neck without acetabular involvement.
  - Complex regional pain syndrome (CRPS) or reflex sympathetic dystrophy: usually follows trauma but may also follow myocardial infarction or hemiplegia. Patients with neoplasms (lung, ovary, breast, and pancreas) may also present with CRPS. Patients present with pain, swelling, and reduced motion.
  - Radiographic features include swelling and prominent juxta-articular osteopenia. Radionuclide scans show increased tracer in the involved osseous structures.

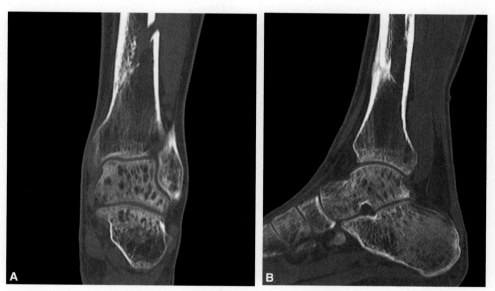

FIGURE 13-5. Disuse osteoporosis. Coronal **(A)** and sagittal **(B)** reformatted computed tomography (CT) images in a patient with a healing distal tibial fracture. The lower extremity shows diffuse loss of bone mineral density related to disuse.

(continued)

■ **OSTEOPOROSIS: REGIONAL OSTEOPOROSIS**   *(Continued)*

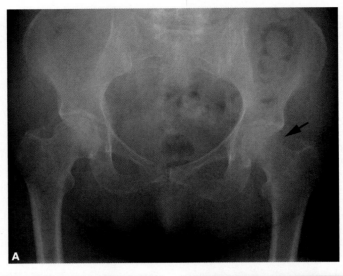

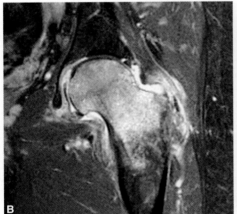
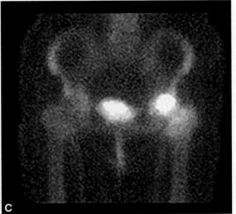

FIGURE 13-6. Transient osteoporosis of the hip: **(A)** Anteroposterior (AP) radiograph of the pelvis shows osteopenia in the left proximal femur (*arrow*). **(B)** Coronal fluid-sensitive magnetic resonance image shows diffuse abnormal signal intensity in the femoral head and neck with a joint effusion. No abnormal signal is seen in the acetabulum, although a small joint effusion is present. **(C)** Radionuclide bone scan shows diffuse increased scintigraphic activity in the femoral head and neck.

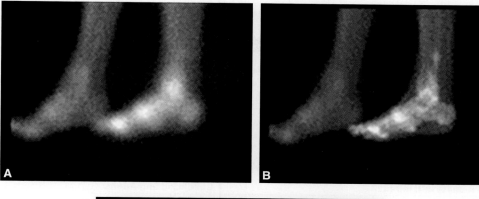

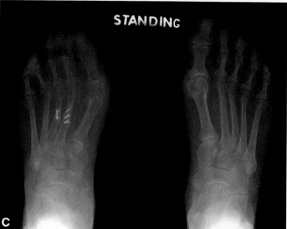

FIGURE 13-7. Chronic regional pain syndrome. Blood pool **(A)** and 3 hours delay **(B)** images from a radionuclide bone scan show hyperemia and increased scintigraphic activity in the left ankle, hind, and midfoot. Anteroposterior (AP) **(C)** radiograph shows advanced osteopenia thoughout the left foot.

SUGGESTED READING

Genant HK, Kozir F, Beherman C, et al. The reflex sympathetic dystrophy syndrome. *Radiology.* 1975;117:21–32.

Hayes CW, Conway WF, Daniel WW. MR imaging of bone marrow edema pattern: transient osteoporosis, transient bone marrow edema, or osteonecrosis. *Radiographics.* 1993;13:1001–1011.

Jones G. Radiographic appearances of disuse osteoporosis. *Clin Radiol.* 1969;20:345–353.

Marinus J, Moseley GL, Birklein F, et al. Clinical features and pathophysiology of complex regional pain syndrome. *Lancet Neurol.* 2011;10(7):637–648.

■ RICKETS AND OSTEOMALACIA: BASIC CONCEPTS

KEY FACTS

- Rickets and osteomalacia are similar histologically. The basic defect is inadequate osteoid mineralization, although osteoid production is also reduced.
- Rickets affects the immature skeleton, with changes most obvious in the growth plate.
- Osteomalacia affects mature bone, although osteomalacia and rickets can coexist in childhood.
- Table 13-2 summarizes the causes of these conditions.
- Figure 13-8 summarizes vitamin D metabolism and associated diseases that lead to rickets and osteomalacia.

Table 13-2   RICKETS AND OSTEOMALACIA

Neonate and Infant	Childhood and Adults
Hypophosphatasia	Dietary calcium and phosphate deficiency
Congenital rubella	Hypophosphatemic (vitamin D resistant)
Vitamin D deficiency	Sprue
Biliary atresia	Pancreatic insufficiency
Celiac disease and malabsorption syndromes	Crohn disease
	Amyloidosis
	Small bowel fistulae
	Small bowel and gastric resections
	Obstructive jaundice
	Chronic liver disease
	Anticonvulsive therapy
	Renal tubular disorders
	Hyperparathyroidism
	Axial osteomalacia

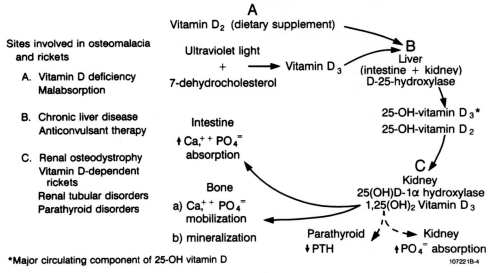

FIGURE 13-8. Vitamin D metabolism and diseases leading to rickets and osteomalacia. (From Berquist TH, ed. *Radiology of the Foot and Ankle.* 2nd ed. Philadelphia: Lippincott Williams & Wilkins; 2000.)

SUGGESTED READING

Kottamasu SR. Metabolic bone diseases. In: Kuhn JP, Slovis TL, Haller JO, eds. *Caffey's Pediatric Diagnostic Imaging*. 10th ed. Philadelphia: Mosby; 2004:2242–2253.

Pitt MJ. Rickets and osteomalacia. In: Resnick D, Bralow L, eds. *Bone and Joint Imaging*. 2nd ed. Philadelphia: WB Saunders; 1996:511–524.

Rasmussen H, Bordier P, Kurokawa K, et al. Normal control of skeletal and mineral homeostasis. *Am J Med*. 1974;56:751–758.

■ RICKETS AND OSTEOMALACIA: RICKETS

KEY FACTS

- ■ Rickets is caused by improper mineralization of the growth plates.
- ■ Radiographic changes of rickets are most obvious in regions of rapid growth. Therefore, changes are most commonly observed in the ribs, proximal humerus, knees, distal tibia, and wrist.
- ■ Radiographic features:
  - ● Osteopenia
  - ● Decreased mineralization in the zone of provisional calcification
  - ● Growth plate widening and irregularity
  - ● Epiphyseal irregularity
  - ● Joint swelling
  - ● "Rachitic rosary" resulting from prominent costochondral junctions of the ribs
  - ● Lower extremity bowing
  - ● Scoliosis

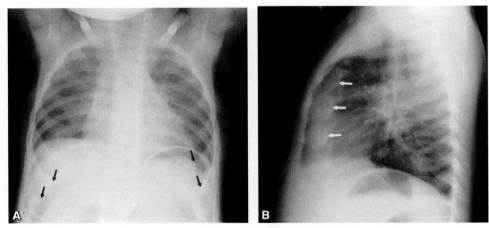

FIGURE 13-9. "Rachitic rosary." Anteroposterior (AP) **(A)** and lateral **(B)** radiographs of the chest show prominence of the costochondral junctions (*arrows*).

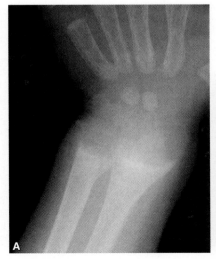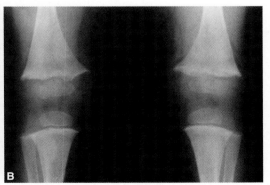

FIGURE 13-10. Rickets in a young child with growth plate widening and irregularity in the wrist **(A)** and knees **(B)**. Note the small epiphyses in the knees.

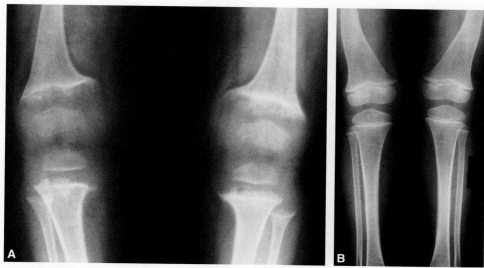

FIGURE 13-11. Vitamin D–resistant rickets in a 1-year-old child. **(A)** Anteroposterior (AP) radiograph of the knees shows irregularity and widening of the growth plates. The epiphyses are small and irregular as well. **(B)** Three years after high-dose vitamin D therapy, the knees appear normal. There is residual femoral bowing. (From Berquist TH, ed. *Radiology of the Foot and Ankle.* 2nd ed. Philadelphia: Lippincott Williams & Wilkins; 2000.)

SUGGESTED READING

Pitt MJ. Rickets and osteomalacia. In: Resnick D, Bralow L, eds. *Bone and Joint Imaging.* 2nd ed. Philadelphia: WB Saunders; 1996:511–524.

Steinbach HL, Noetzli M. Roentgen appearance of the skeleton in osteomalacia and rickets. *Am J Roentgenol.* 1964;91:955–972.

■ RICKETS AND OSTEOMALACIA: OSTEOMALACIA

KEY FACTS

- Osteomalacia and rickets may coexist in the immature skeleton.
- Features of adult osteomalacia include osteopenia, pseudofractures, and bone deformity.
- Pseudofractures (uncalcified osteoid seams) are considered pathognomonic. Pseudofractures are typically bilateral and symmetrical. Common locations include the femoral necks, pubic symphysis, ribs, and scapula.
- Axial osteomalacia is a rare condition involving the axial skeleton with prominent trabeculae, but typically not pseudofractures. The condition typically involves males.
- Osteomalacia and vitamin D-resistant rickets are becoming more frequently recognized with malignancies. Vascular neoplasms predominate.

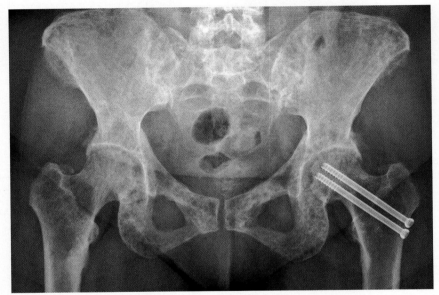

FIGURE 13-12. Osteomalacia. Anteroposterior (AP) radiograph of the pelvis shows osteopenia and disorganized trabeculation with prior left femoral neck pseudofracture.

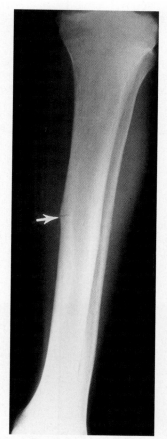

FIGURE 13-13. Osteomalacia. Anteroposterior (AP) radiograph of the tibia shows a midshaft pseudofracture (*arrow*).

SUGGESTED READING

Jawarski ZFG. Pathophysiology, diagnosis, and treatment of osteomalacia. *Orthop Clin North Am.* 1972;3:623–652.
Pitt MJ. Rickets and osteomalacia. In: Resnick D, Bralow L, eds. *Bone and Joint Imaging.* 2nd ed. Philadelphia: WB Saunders; 1996:511–524.

■ RENAL OSTEODYSTROPHY

KEY FACTS

- ■ Osseous changes caused by chronic renal disease are not completely understood, but changes are predominantly the result of secondary HPT and abnormal vitamin D metabolism.
- ■ Vitamin D metabolism is altered because of decreased renal production of the active metabolite (1,25-dihydroxyvitamin D_3).
- ■ Radiographic features vary with age. Brown tumors are less common than with primary HPT. Osteosclerosis is more common. Five basic features may be evident:
  - ● Osteitis fibrosis cystica
  - ● Rickets or osteomalacia
  - ● Osteosclerosis
  - ● Osteoporosis
  - ● Avascular necrosis in patients undergoing steroid therapy
- ■ Features of HPT:
  - ● Periosteal, cortical, subchondral bone resorption; brown tumors; bone sclerosis; chondrocalcinosis
  - ● Rickets and osteomalacia; osteopenia; metaphyseal changes (see section on "Rickets and Osteomalacia"); pseudofractures; slipped capital femoral epiphysis
  - ● Osteoporosis and associated fractures

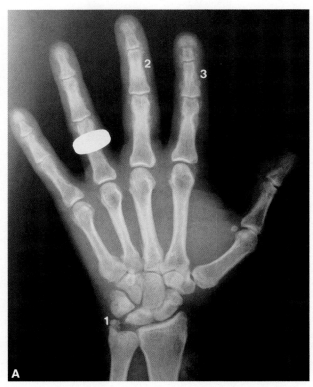

FIGURE 13-14. Renal osteodystrophy in an adult. **(A)** Radiograph of the hand shows chondrocalcinosis (*1*), subperiosteal resorption of the radial aspect of the middle phalanges (*2*), and subtendinous resorption (*3*). **(B)** Lateral radiograph of the lumbar spine shows endplate sclerosis ("rugger jersey spine"). **(C)** Anteroposterior (AP) view of the femur shows bowing with a proximal pseudofracture (*arrow*).

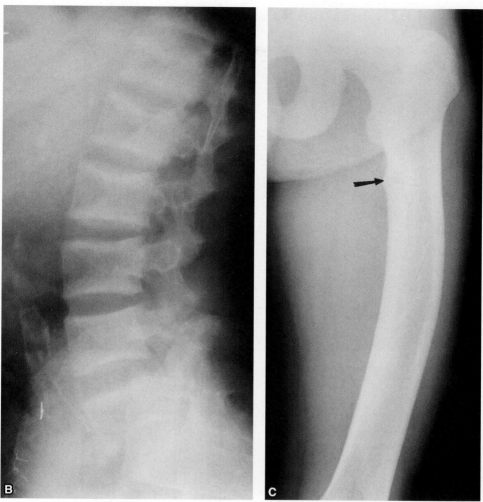

FIGURE 13-14. (*continued*)

(*continued*)

■ RENAL OSTEODYSTROPHY *(Continued)*

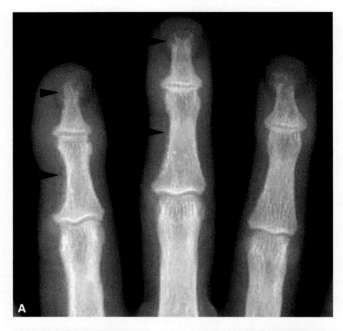

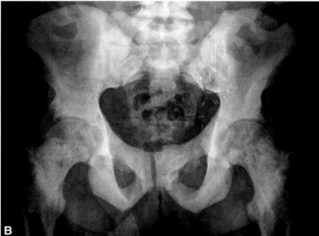

FIGURE 13-15. Renal osteodystrophy. **(A)** anteroposterior (AP) radiograph of the hand shows subperiosteal resorption of the medial aspect of the middle phalanges and terminal tufts of the distal phalanges (*arrowheads*). **(B)** AP radiograph of the pelvis shows osteosclerosis with widening, irregularity, and sclerosis of the sacroiliac joints related to subchondral bone resorption.

SUGGESTED READING

Mankin HJ. Rickets, osteomalacia, and renal osteodystrophy. Part II. *J Bone Joint Surg.* 1974;56A:352–386.

Tigges S, Nance EP, Carpenter WA, et al. Renal osteodystrophy: imaging findings that mimic those of other diseases. *Am J Roentgenol.* 1995;165:143–148.

■ PARATHYROID DISORDERS: HYPERPARATHYROIDISM

KEY FACTS

- ■ Parathyroid hormone is essential for proper transport of Ca^{2+} and related ions in the kidney, bone, and intestinal tract.
- ■ HPT has three categories:
  - Primary parathyroid adenoma, hyperplasia, or carcinoma. Ectopic parathormone may be secreted by lung or renal neoplasms.
  - Secondary decreased Ca^{2+} leads to increased parathormone secretion. The list of causes is long, but the most common include chronic renal disease, decreased intestinal absorption of calcium, and impaired vitamin D metabolism.
  - Tertiary patients on renal dialysis, in chronic renal failure, and with malabsorption. Patients have long-standing secondary HPT, and therefore, the parathyroid glands no longer respond to Ca^{2+} levels.
- ■ Radiographic features of HPT are as follows:
  - Bone resorption (parathormone stimulates osteoclastic resorption)
    - ❖ Subperiosteal (typical in phalanges of the hands)
    - ❖ Cortical endosteal
    - ❖ Subchondral
  - Peritendinous or subligamentous
    - ❖ Paraphyseal
    - ❖ Lamina dura about teeth
  - Osteopenia
  - Pathologic fractures
  - Brown tumors (most common with primary HPT)
  - Osteosclerosis (secondary HPT or renal osteodystrophy)
  - Articular calcification (secondary > primary HPT)
  - Vascular calcification (secondary > primary HPT)
  - Nephrolithiasis
  - Peptic ulcer disease

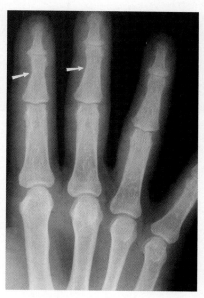

FIGURE 13-16. Primary hyperparathyroidism (HPT). Posteroanterior radiograph of the fingers shows early subperiosteal resorption in the characteristic radial side of the middle phalanges (*arrows*). Cortical bone thickness is also reduced.

(continued)

■ PARATHYROID DISORDERS: HYPERPARATHYROIDISM *(Continued)*

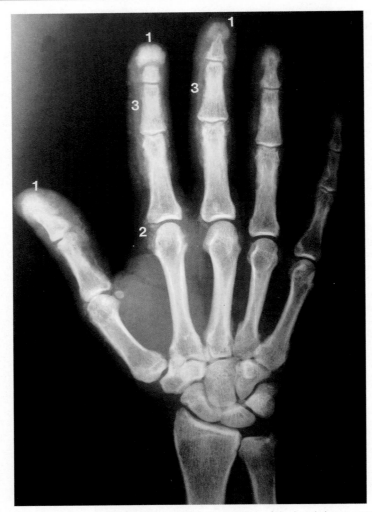

FIGURE 13-17. Secondary hyperparathyroidism (HPT). Radiograph of the hand shows resorption of the first to third tufts with soft tissue calcification (*1*). There is articular calcification (*2*), and subperiosteal and subligamentous resorption (*3*).

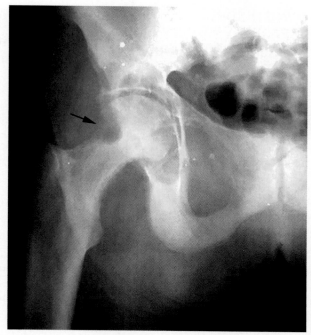

FIGURE 13-18. Primary hyperparathyroidism (HPT). Radiograph of the right femur shows a brown tumor involving the femoral neck (*arrow*).

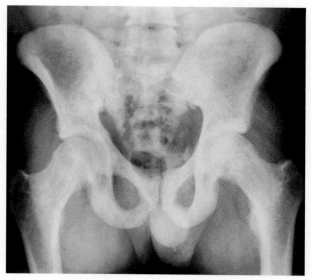

FIGURE 13-19. Secondary hyperparathyroidism (HPT). Radiograph of the pelvis and hips shows diffuse osteosclerosis.

SUGGESTED READING

Resnick D, Kransdorf MJ. Parathyroid disorders and renal osteodystrophy. In: Resnick D, Kransdorf MJ, eds. *Bone and Joint Imaging.* 3rd ed. Philadelphia: Elsevier-Saunders; 2005:603–622.

■ PARATHYROID DISORDERS: HYPOPARATHYROIDISM, PSEUDOHYPOPARATHYROIDISM, AND PSEUDO-PSEUDOHYPOPARATHYROIDISM

KEY FACTS

- Hypoparathyroidism may be the result of resection with thyroidectomy, or it may be idiopathic. The idiopathic form is more common in children (more common in females than males). Patients present with neuromuscular symptoms and decreased serum calcium.
- Pseudohypoparathyroidism differs from hypoparathyroidism in that parathormone levels are normal. Parathyroid glands are normal or hyperplastic, but end-organ resistance is present. Patients present in the second decade with short obese stature, round faces, bradydactyly, and mental retardation. There is sex-linked dominant inheritance. Serum Ca^{2+} is decreased, and PO_4 is increased.
- Pseudo-pseudohypoparathyroidism may be seen in the same families as pseudohypoparathyroidism. Clinical features are similar, but serum Ca^{2+} is normal.
- Radiographic features are summarized as follows:

Radiographic Feature	Hypoparathyroidism	Pseudo and Pseudo-pseudohypoparathyroidism
Osteosclerosis	+	+
Soft tissue calcification	Subcutaneous	Periarticular
Calvarial thickening	+	+
Hypoplastic dentition	+	−
Spinal calcification	+	−
Exostoses	−	+
Bowing deformities	−	+
Premature physeal fusion	+	+
Shortening of metacarpals, metatarsals, phalanges	−	+

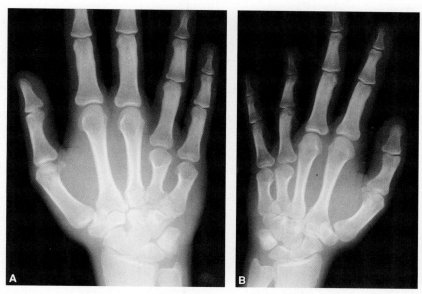

FIGURE 13-20. Pseudohypoparathyroidism. **(A, B)** Anteroposterior (AP) radiographs of the hands show shortening of the fourth and fifth metacarpals.

SUGGESTED READING

Burnstein MI, Kottainaser SR, Pettifar JM, et al. Metabolic bone disease in pseudohypoparathyroidism. *Radiology.* 1985;155:351–356.

■ THYROID DISORDERS

KEY FACTS

- Thyroxine and triiodothyronine are the active forms of thyroid hormone. They affect fat, protein, and carbohydrate metabolism and mineral turnover.
- Hyperthyroidism is most often associated with Graves disease or goiter with active thyroid adenomas. Patients typically present with tachycardia, weakness, and exophthalmus.
- Hypothyroidism is the result of reduced thyroid hormones. Primary hypothyroidism may be related to surgery, thyroiditis, or iodine therapy. Patients present with hoarseness, dry skin and hair, and bradycardia.
- Radiographic features:
  - Hyperthyroidism: osteopenia. Thyroid acropachy (1% of patients): swelling of the hands and feet with diaphyseal periostitis.
  - Hypothyroidism: adults: increased or decreased bone density. Infants and children: delayed skeletal maturation.

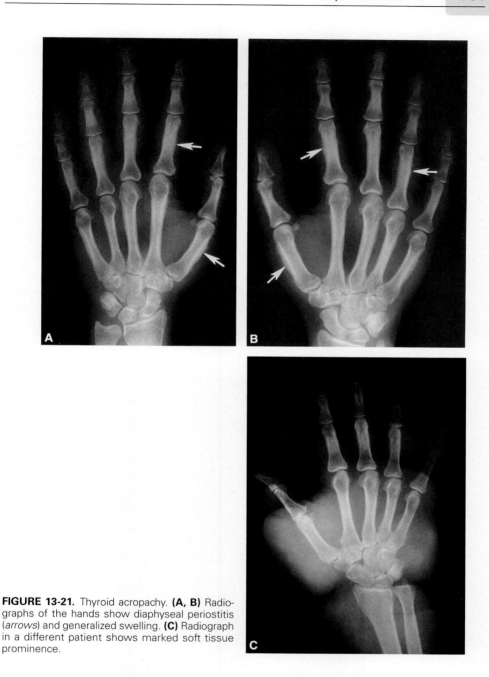

FIGURE 13-21. Thyroid acropachy. **(A, B)** Radiographs of the hands show diaphyseal periostitis (*arrows*) and generalized swelling. **(C)** Radiograph in a different patient shows marked soft tissue prominence.

SUGGESTED READING

Meurier RJ, Bianchi GG, Edouad CM, et al. Bony manifestations of thyrotoxicosis. *Orthop Clin North Am.* 1972;3:745–775.
Scanlon GT, Clemett AR. Thyroid acropachy. *Radiology.* 1964;83(6):1039–1042.

■ PITUITARY DISORDERS

KEY FACTS

■ Growth hormone (somatotropin) is essential for normal skeletal development.

■ Hypopituitarism may be the result of surgery, infection, vascular insufficiency, or neoplasm.

■ Acromegaly and gigantism are the result of hypersecretion of growth hormone. The condition is typically related to acidophilic or chromophobic adenomas. Elevated growth hormone during development leads to gigantism. In the mature skeleton, it results in acromegaly.

■ Patients with acromegaly present with prominent mandibles, frontal bossing, hepatosplenomegaly, and arthropathy with spadelike appearance of the fingers. Up to 25% have diabetes mellitus, and there is an increased incidence of pancreatic adenomas.

■ Radiographic features:

- Hypopituitarism   Delayed skeletal maturation
- Acromegaly: Calvarian   Soft tissue thickening in scalp, fingers, toes, heel pad; calvarial thickening, enlarged sella, prominent frontal sinuses, occipital spurring

Widened disc spaces and osteophytes in the spine

Joint space widening and degenerative changes in the extremities

New bone formation at sites of ligament and tendon attachments

Cortical thickening

Prominent (spadelike) tufts on the distal phalanges

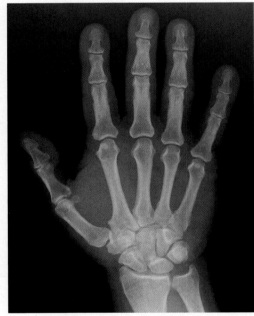

FIGURE 13-22. Acromegaly. Radiograph of the hand shows spadelike tufts and metacarpophalangeal joint space widening.

SUGGESTED READING

Lang EK, Bessler WT. The roentgen features of acromegaly. *Am J Roentgenol.* 1961;86:321–328.

■ PAGET DISEASE

KEY FACTS

- ■ Paget disease is a common condition in older adults causing excessive and disordered bone remodeling. Ninety percent of patients are aged more than 55 years.
- ■ The cause remains unknown.
- ■ The most common sites of involvement are the axial skeleton, femur, and tibia.
- ■ Symptoms are not always present, but are more common in the axial skeleton. Many cases are detected incidentally on radiographs.
- ■ Laboratory data may show elevated alkaline phosphatase and increased serum and urine hydroxyproline.
- ■ Radiographic features are typically divided into four stages:

Initial stage	Predominately lytic with geographic lucent areas
	Skull—osteoporosis circumscripta
	Long bones—"blade-of-grass" appearance
Mixed stage	Mixed lytic and sclerotic changes
Sclerotic stage	Cortical thickening, prominent trabeculae, medullary sclerosis
Malignant degeneration	Occurs in up to 10%: typically osteosarcoma or fibrosarcoma (see Chapter 9)

- ■ Radionuclide scans are intensely positive because of the increased metabolic activity.
- ■ Magnetic resonance imaging (MRI) may present a confusing picture unless radiographs are available for comparison.
- ■ Complications of Paget disease are as follows:
  - ● Pathologic fractures
  - ● Malignant degeneration (MRI superior for imaging when suspected)
  - ● Platybasia
  - ● Cord compression
  - ● Spinal stenosis

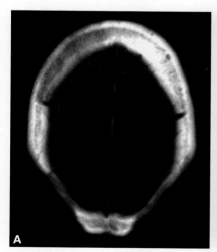 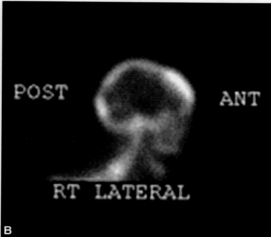

FIGURE 13-23. Osteoporosis circumscripta. **(A)** Computed tomography (CT) of the head shows lucent areas involving the right frontal and bilateral occipital regions. **(B)** Radionuclide bone scan shows increased scintigraphic activity corresponding to these regions.

(continued)

■ PAGET DISEASE   *(Continued)*

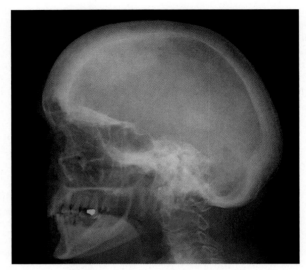

FIGURE 13-24. Paget disease of the calvarium. Lateral radiograph of the skull shows cortical thickening and sclerosis with enlargement of the calvarium.

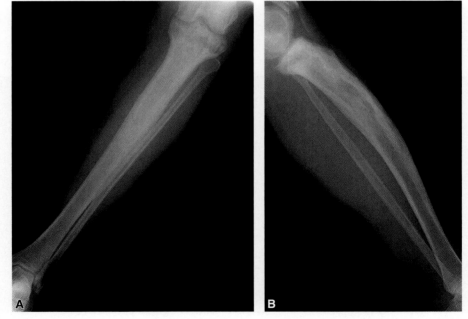

FIGURE 13-25. Paget disease in the tibia. Anteroposterior (AP) **(A)** and lateral **(B)** tibial radiographs show cortical thickening and coarsening of the trabecula extending from the proximal tibia into the mid shaft. There is associated enlargement of the proximal tibia and bowing deformity.

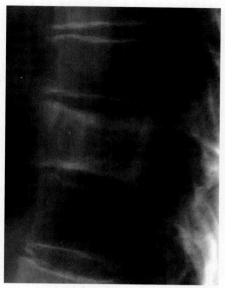

FIGURE 13-26. Paget disease in the spine. Lateral radiograph shows enlargement and cortical thickening of the T10 vertebral body with a "picture frame" appearance.

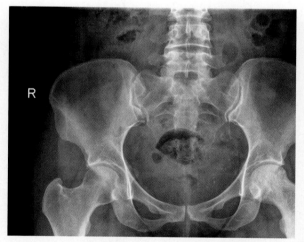

FIGURE 13-27. Paget disease involving the left femur. Anteroposterior (AP) radiograph shows coarsening of the trabecula, cortical thickening, and enlargement of the left proximal femur.

SUGGESTED READING

Roberts MC, Kressel HY, Fallon MD, et al. Paget disease: MR image findings. *Radiology.* 1989;177:341–345.

Sundarum M, Khanna G, El-Khoury GY. T1-weighted MR imaging for distinguishing large osteolysis of Paget disease from sarcomatous degeneration. *Skeletal Radiol.* 2001;30:378–383.

Theodorou DJ, Theodorou SJ, Kakitsubata Y. Imaging of Paget disease of bone and its musculoskeletal complications: review. *Am J Roentgenol.* 2011;196: S64–S75.

CHAPTER 14

Miscellaneous Conditions

Jeffrey J. Peterson and Thomas H. Berquist

■ BONE ISLANDS (ENOSTOSIS)

KEY FACTS

- Bone islands are benign sclerotic areas in bone. They may be single or multiple.
- Bone islands are typically noted incidentally on radiographs.
- Lesions may be seen in patients from 7 to 78 years of age. There is no sex predilection.
- The most common sites are the ribs, pelvis, and femora. Up to 32% may change in size.
- Radiographic features:
  - Round, oval, or spiculated sclerotic areas are typically (66%) 0.5 to 1.5 cm.
  - Appearance is usually characteristic, although the differential diagnosis could include blastic metastasis, osteoma, osteoid osteoma, or infarct.
  - Other imaging studies are usually not required. Radionuclide bone scans are typically normal, but focal increased tracer can occur.
  - Magnetic resonance imaging (MRI) shows low signal intensity on T1- and T2-weighted sequences.

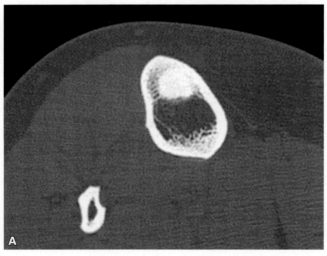

FIGURE 14-1. Bone island in the proximal tibia. Axial **(A)** and coronal **(B)** reformatted computed tomography (CT) images demonstrate a sclerotic focus with speculated margins in the proximal tibia. Coronal T1-weighted **(C)** magnetic resonance (MR) image shows the lesion to be longitudinally oriented. Bone scan **(D)** demonstrates no abnormal scintigraphic activity to correspond to the lesion.

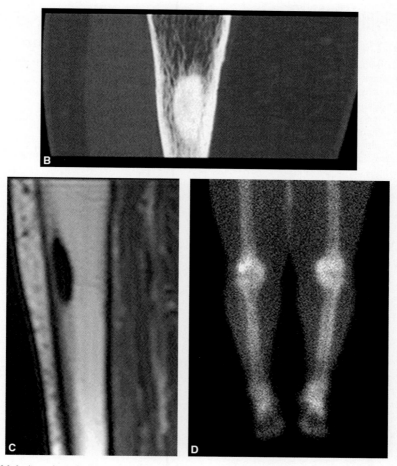

FIGURE 14-1. (*continued*)

SUGGESTED READING

Greenspan A, Steiner G, Knutzon R. Bone island (enostosis): clinical significance and radiologic and pathologic correlations. *Skeletal Radiol.* 1991;20(2):85–90.
Hall FE, Goldberg RP, Davies JAK, et al. Scintigraphic assessment of bone islands. *Radiology.* 1980;135:737–742.

■ OSTEOPOIKILOSIS

KEY FACTS

■ Osteopoikilosis is a sclerotic bone dysplasia presenting in childhood. It has been detected in all bones except the skull.

■ Lesions are smaller than typical bone islands (2 to 10 mm).

■ The condition is considered an autosomal dominant chondrodysplasia.

■ Lesions may grow in children, but stabilize or disappear in adults.

■ Most patients are asymptomatic, although 20% may present with joint pain.

■ Radiographic features:

● Lesions are smaller and more well-defined than bone islands and involve the epiphysis and metaphysis.

● Features are so characteristic that there is usually no difficulty in diagnosis.

● Differential considerations include mastocytosis and tuberous sclerosis.

● Radionuclide scans are typically normal but may be positive in growing lesions.

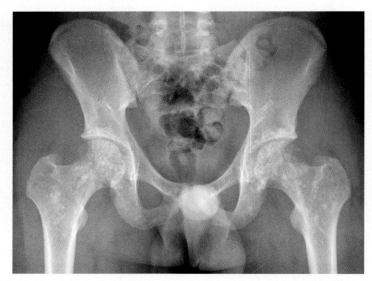

FIGURE 14-2. Osteopoikilosis. Anteroposterior (AP) radiograph of the pelvis and hips shows multiple small sclerotic foci in the proximal femora, ischia, and acetabuli.

SUGGESTED READING

Ellanti P, Clarke B, Gray J. Osteopoikilosis. *Ir J Med Sci.* 2010;179(4):615–616.
Green AE, Ellowood WH, Collins JR. Melorheostosis and osteopoikilosis. *Am J Roentgenol.* 1962;87:1096–1117.

OSTEOPATHIA STRIATA

KEY FACTS

- Osteopathia striata is a rare autosomal dominant inherited condition related to osteopoikilosis.
- Patients are usually asymptomatic.
- Radiographic features:
  - Distinct striations in the metaphysis of long bones parallel to the shaft. Striations may extend into the epiphysis.
  - Changes are usually bilateral.
  - The tibia is the most common site.
  - Radionuclide scans are normal.

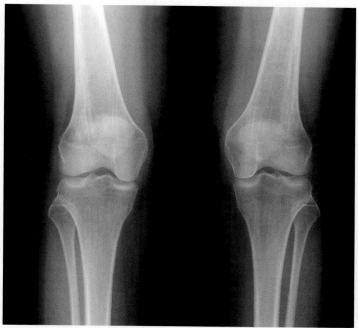

FIGURE 14-3. Osteopathia striata. Anteroposterior (AP) radiograph of the knees shows linear striations in the distal femora and proximal tibia bilaterally.

SUGGESTED READING

Bass HN, Weiner JR, Goldman A, et al. Osteopathia striata syndrome. Clinical, genetic and radiologic considerations. *Clin Pediatr (Phila)*. 1980;19(5):369–373.

Hurt RL. Osteopathia striata—Voorhoeve disease. *J Bone Joint Surg*. 1953;35B:89–96.

■ MELORHEOSTOSIS

KEY FACTS

■ Melorheostosis causes bone sclerosis involving one side of the cortex. The original description looked like dripping candle wax, thus the term "melorheostosis."

■ Cause is unknown. Patients may be asymptomatic or present with pain in the involved region.

■ The condition may be present from birth to late adult life. In 50% of cases, the condition is evident by 20 years of age. There is no sex predilection.

■ The involved extremity may be shorter or, in some cases, longer. Muscle atrophy is also present in some cases.

■ Radiographic features:

● The condition most commonly involves the long bones of the extremities. Most often it is unilateral.

● Sclerosis and cortical thickening involve one side of the involved bone or bones. Typically, the process extends into the metaphysis or epiphysis, but soft tissue and joint involvement can occur. Associated conditions include:

 ❖ Leg length discrepancy
 ❖ Scleroderma
 ❖ Neurofibromatosis
 ❖ Osteopoikilosis
 ❖ Osteopathia striata
 ❖ Hemangiomas

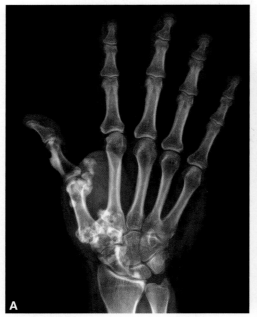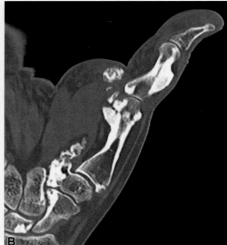

FIGURE 14-4. Melorheostosis. Anteroposterior (AP) radiograph **(A)** and coronal reformatted computed tomography (CT) **(B)** images of the hand show irregular sclerosis and exuberant cortical thickening along the first ray.

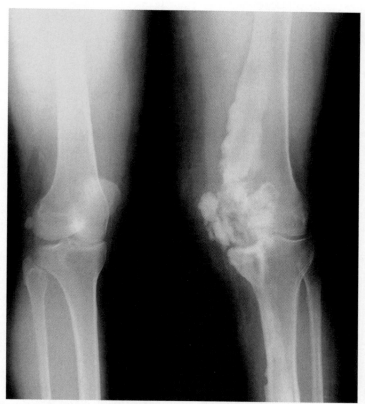

FIGURE 14-5. Melorheostosis. Standing view of the knees shows sclerosis and cortical thickening that crosses the joint into the soft tissues. The tibia is also involved.

SUGGESTED READING

Bansal A. The dripping candle wax sign. *Radiology*. 2008;246(2):638–640.
Morris JM, Samilson RL, Corey CL. Melorheostosis. *J Bone Joint Surg*. 1963;45A:1191–1206.

■ PROGRESSIVE DIAPHYSEAL DYSPLASIA (ENGELMANN DISEASE)

KEY FACTS

- Engelmann disease results in cortical thickening in the diaphysis of long bones progressing proximally and distally in the involved structure.
- Most patients present in infancy or early childhood. It is an autosomal dominant inherited condition.
- Neuromuscular dystrophy and malnutrition are associated with this condition.
- Radiographic features:
  - Symmetric distribution
  - Diaphyseal cortical thickening involving endosteal and periosteal surfaces
  - Normal epiphysis and metaphysis
  - Relative elongation of involved extremities
  - Muscle atrophy
- Differential diagnosis: chronic infection, infantile cortical hyperostosis, fibrous dysplasia

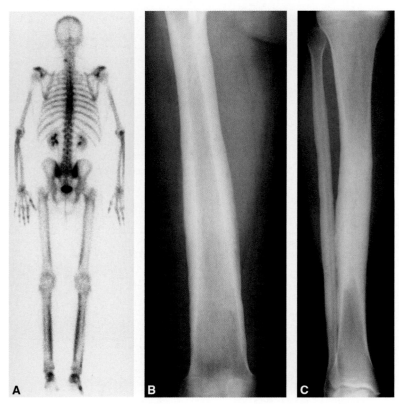

FIGURE 14-6. Engelmann disease. **(A)** Radionuclide bone scan shows symmetric increased cortical uptake in the femora, tibiae, and upper extremities. Anteroposterior (AP) radiographs of the femur **(B)** and tibia **(C)** show marked diaphyseal cortical thickening with sparing of the metaphyses and epiphyses.

SUGGESTED READING

Kumar B, Murphy WA, Whyte MP. Progressive diaphyseal dysplasia (Engelmann disease): scintigraphic-radiographic-clinical correlations. *Radiology.* 1981;140:87–92.

■ CLEIDOCRANIAL DYSPLASIA (CLEIDOCRANIAL DYSOSTOSIS)

KEY FACTS

■ Cleidocranial dysplasia is an uncommon autosomal dominant disorder.

■ Patients present with delayed or incomplete cranial ossification and hypoplastic or aplastic clavicles. Delayed ossification may be evident in the axial skeleton and extremities.

■ The mandible may be large, and delayed tooth development is common.

■ Radiographic features:
  ● Lack of midline ossification and wormian bones in the calvarium
  ● Absent or hypoplastic clavicles
  ● Delayed ossification in the spine, pelvis, and extremities
  ● Femoral necks deformed or aplastic

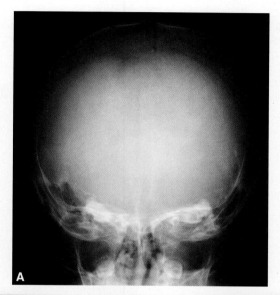

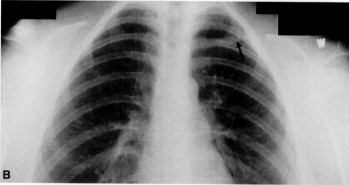

FIGURE 14-7. Cleidocranial dysplasia. **(A)** Anteroposterior (AP) view of the skull shows multiple wormian bones along the suture lines. **(B)** AP view of the upper chest shows an absent right clavicle and small hypoplastic medial segment (*arrow*) on the left.

SUGGESTED READING

Jarvis JL, Keats TE. Cleidocranial dysostosis. A review of 40 new cases. *Am J Roentgenol.* 1974;121:5–16.

■ OSTEOPETROSIS

KEY FACTS

- Osteopetrosis is a disease of uncertain cause that leads to dense brittle bones.
- There are multiple clinical forms of this condition.
  - Osteopetrosis infantile: autosomal recessive with failure to thrive, hepatosplenomegaly, cranial nerve dysfunction, blindness, and deafness. Death frequently occurs in early years of life.
  - Osteopetrosis tarda (delayed): autosomal dominant. Patients are usually asymptomatic. Detection results from mild anemia, cranial nerve palsies, or pathologic fractures.
  - Osteopetrosis intermediate: autosomal recessive with features between infantile and tarda in severity.
- Radiographic features:
  - Infantile: uniformly dense sclerotic bones with changes similar to rickets near the growth plates
  - Tarda: bone-within-a-bone appearance
  - Intermediate: diffuse bone sclerosis, especially of the skull base. Bone-within-a-bone appearance. Avascular necrosis of the femoral heads.

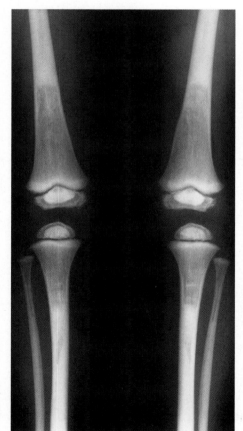

FIGURE 14-8. Osteopetrosis intermediate. Anteroposterior (AP) radiograph of the tibia and femora shows bone sclerosis with bone-within-a-bone appearance in the epiphyses.

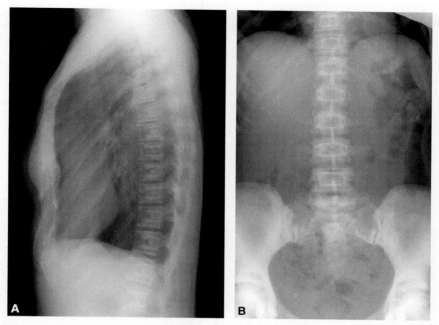

FIGURE 14-9. Osteopetrosis tarda. Lateral **(A)** and anteroposterior (AP) **(B)** radiographs of the lumbar spine show a bone-within-a-bone appearance.

SUGGESTED READING

Shapiro F, Glimcher MJ, Holtrop ME, et al. Human osteopetrosis. *J Bone Joint Surg.* 1980;62A:384–399.
Stark Z, Savarirayan R. Osteopetrosis. *Orphanet J Rare Dis.* 2009;4:5.

■ MASTOCYTOSIS

KEY FACTS

- ■ Mastocytosis is a systemic disease with mast cell accumulation in multiple organs affecting adult males and females.
- ■ Liver, spleen, lymph node, skeletal, and, most commonly, cutaneous organs are involved.
- ■ Patients present with skin lesions resembling urticaria pigmentosa, also diarrhea, vomiting, flushing, or intermittent shocklike episodes.
- ■ Radiographic features occur in 70% of patients:
  - ● Osteopenia and bone destruction most common in the skull, spine, and ribs
  - ● Osteosclerosis, which may resemble metastasis, Paget disease, or myelofibrosis
  - ● Features may be focal or diffuse.

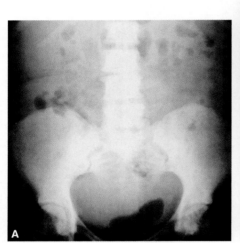

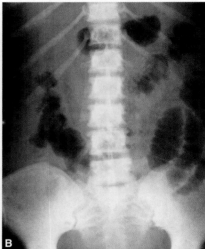

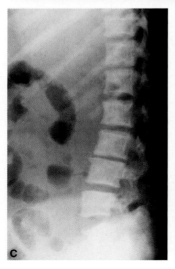

FIGURE 14-10. Mastocytosis. **(A)** Anteroposterior (AP) radiograph of the lumbar spine and pelvis shows generalized bone sclerosis and cortical thickening. There are more focal foci of sclerosis in the femoral heads. AP **(B)** and lateral **(C)** radiographs of the lumbar spine and pelvis in a different patient show diffuse small sclerotic foci.

SUGGESTED READING

McKenna MJ, Frame B. The mast cell and bone. *Clin Orthop.* 1985;200:226–233.
Nguyen BD. CT and scintigraphy of aggressive lymphadenopathic mastocytosis. *Am J Roentgenol.* 2002;178(3):769–770.

■ TUBEROUS SCLEROSIS

KEY FACTS

■ Tuberous sclerosis is an autosomal dominant inherited disorder.

■ Characteristic features include seizure disorders, mental retardation, and cutaneous hamartomas.

■ Radiographic features:

● Skull: foci of sclerosis and trabecular prominence; calvarial thickening; intercerebral calcifications; brain lesions in ventricles, white matter, and cortex 50% to 80%.

● Axial/appendicular skeleton: focal or diffuse cystlike lesions or areas of sclerosis. Subperiosteal and cortical lesions result in irregular cortical appearance.

● Extraskeletal lesions: Fifty percent have renal cysts, angiolipomas, and aneurysms; 30% to 50% have rhabdomyomas of the heart. Pulmonary lesions in 1% commonly lead to pneumothorax.

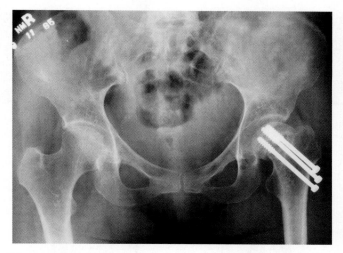

FIGURE 14-11. Tuberous sclerosis. Anteroposterior (AP) radiograph of the pelvis shows oval- or flame-shaped areas of sclerosis in both iliac wings. There is an impacted left femoral neck fracture with pin fixation unrelated to the bone changes of tuberous sclerosis.

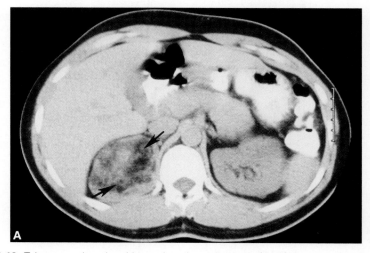

FIGURE 14-12. Tuberous sclerosis with renal angiomyolipomas. **(A, B)** Computed tomography (CT) images show characteristic fat density masses (*arrows*), the largest in the right kidney.

(continued)

■ TUBEROUS SCLEROSIS *(Continued)*

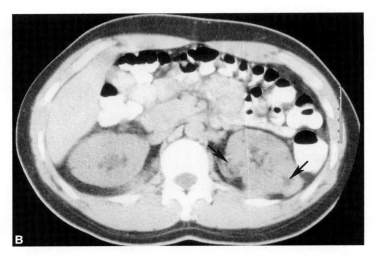

FIGURE 14-12. *(continued)*

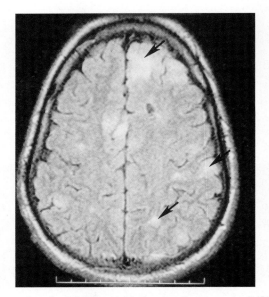

FIGURE 14-13. Tuberous sclerosis. Axial T2-weighted magnetic resonance (MR) image shows multiple areas of signal abnormality *(arrows)* resulting from cortical tubers.

SUGGESTED READING

Medley BE, McLeod RA, Houser OW. Tuberous sclerosis. *Semin Roentgenol.* 1976;11:35–54.
Wood B, Leiberman E, Larding B, et al. Tuberous sclerosis. *Am J Roentgenol.* 1992;158:750.

■ NEUROFIBROMATOSIS

KEY FACTS

- Neurofibromatosis is one of the most common inherited (autosomal dominant) disorders.
- Clinical triad includes skin lesions, mental retardation, and skeletal deformities.
- More than 99% of cases are in the category of neurofibromatosis Type 1 or Type 2.

Type 1 (two or more features)	Six or more café-au-lait skin lesions
	Two or more neurofibromas or one plexiform neurofibroma
	Inguinal or axillary freckling
	Optic glioma
	Two or more iris hematomas
	Osseous lesion
	Parent, sibling, or child with Type 1
Type 2 (one feature)	Bilateral eighth nerve masses

- Type 2 in parent, sibling, or child and an eighth nerve mass, or two of the following: neurofibroma, meningioma, glioma schwannoma, or posterior capsular lenticular capacity
- Radiographic features:
  - Osseous features
  - Orbital and facial bone deformities
  - Spinal deformities (60%)
  - Scoliosis
  - Kyphoscoliosis
  - Vertebral scalloping
  - Pedicle erosion
  - Spindle ribs and transverse processes
  - Extremities
  - Bowing (especially tibia)
  - Pathologic fracture
  - Hypoplastic fibula
  - Pseudoarthrosis with pathologic fracture
- Neural
  - Meningoceles
  - Cranial nerve tumors
  - Peripheral nerve neurofibromas and schwannomas
  - Malignant degeneration of neural lesions 2% to 29%
- Other associated lesions
  - Neuroblastoma
  - Pheochromocytoma
  - Thyroid carcinoma
  - Wilms tumor
  - Rhabdomyosarcoma
  - Leukemia

(continued)

■ **NEUROFIBROMATOSIS** *(Continued)*

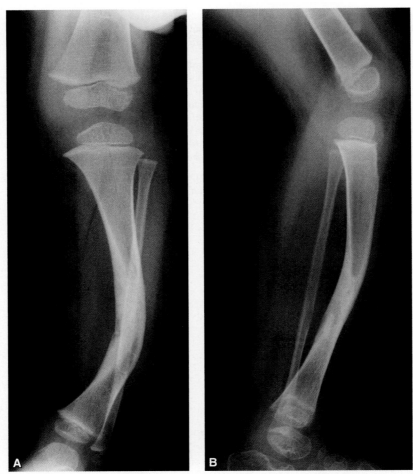

FIGURE 14-14. Neurofibromatosis Type 1. Anteroposterior (AP) **(A)** and lateral **(B)** radiographs show tibial bowing with a healed midtibial fracture.

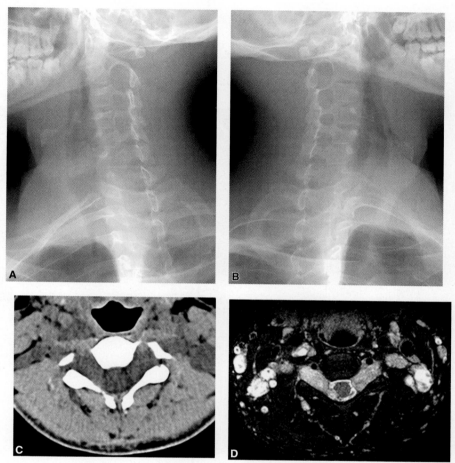

FIGURE 14-15. Neurofibromatosis Type 1. Oblique cervical spine radiographs **(A, B)** depict diffuse widening of the neural foramina at all levels. Axial computed tomography (CT) **(C)** image shows bilateral neurofibromas within the neural foramina and elsewhere through the neck. Axial T2-weighted **(D)** shows the numerous hyperintense neurofibromas to better advantage.

(continued)

■ NEUROFIBROMATOSIS *(Continued)*

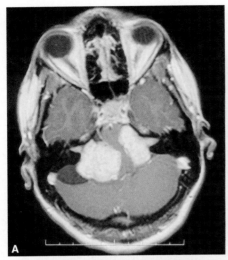

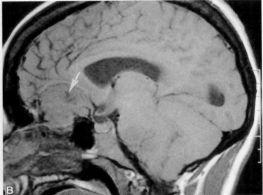

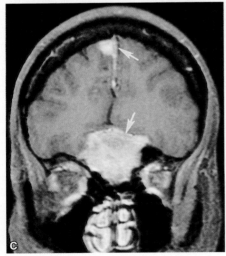

FIGURE 14-16. Neurofibromatosis Type 2. Bilateral vestibular nerve schwannomas and multiple meningiomas. **(A)** Postcontrast axial magnetic resonance (MR) image shows bilateral large vestibular nerve schwannomas extending into the internal auditory canals and compressing the pons. Sagittal **(B)** and coronal enhanced **(C)** T1-weighted images show multiple meningiomas *(arrows)*.

SUGGESTED READING

Aoki S, Barkovich AJ, Nishimura K, et al. Neurofibromatosis types 1 and 2: cranial MR findings. *Radiology.* 1989;172(2):527–534.

Fortman BJ, Kuszyk BS, Urban BA, et al. Neurofibromatosis type 1: a diagnostic mimicker at CT. *Radiographics.* 21(3):601–612.

Sevick RJ, Barkovich AJ, Edwards MS, et al. Evolution of white matter lesions in neurofibromatosis type 1: MR findings. *Am J Roentgenol.* 1992;159:171–175.

■ OLLIER DISEASE (ENCHONDROMATOSIS)

KEY FACTS

- ■ Ollier disease is a noninherited condition resulting in multiple asymmetrically distributed enchondromas.
- ■ Lesions lead to fractures in adults and children.
- ■ In adults, lesions may undergo malignant degeneration to chondrosarcoma (5% to 30%).
- ■ Radiographic features:
  - ● Multiple lytic expanding lesions are located predominantly in the extremities.
  - ● Flat bones of the pelvis may also be involved.
  - ● Lesions may contain calcification.

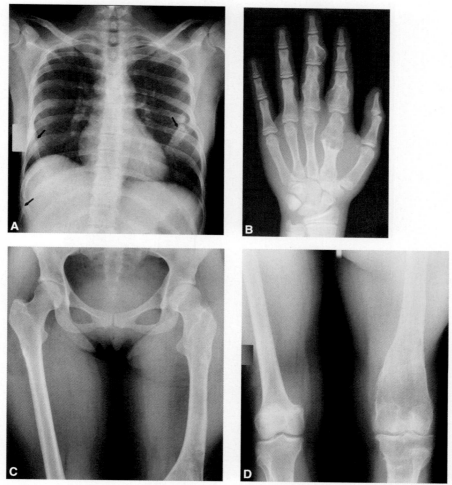

FIGURE 14-17. Ollier disease. **(A)** Posteroanterior (PA) chest radiograph shows multiple expanded calcified rib lesion (*arrows*). **(B)** PA view of the hand shows enchondromas in the second to fourth rays. Anteroposterior (AP) radiographs of the pelvis **(C)** and femora **(D)** show multiple enchondromas in the left femur. The largest expand the distal femur.

SUGGESTED READING

Milgram JW. The origins of osteochondromas and enchondromas. A histopathologic study. *Clin Orthop.* 1983;174:264–284.

■ MAFFUCCI SYNDROME

KEY FACTS

■ Maffucci syndrome is a rare disorder with multiple enchondromas and soft tissue hemangiomas.
■ The syndrome occurs in males and females, beginning in childhood.
■ Half of the cases are unilateral. The hand is most commonly involved.
■ Enchondromas may undergo malignant transformation to chondrosarcoma.
■ Radiographic features:
  ● Multiple expanding lytic lesions that may contain calcifications
  ● Soft tissue masses (hemangiomas) with phleboliths are characteristic.

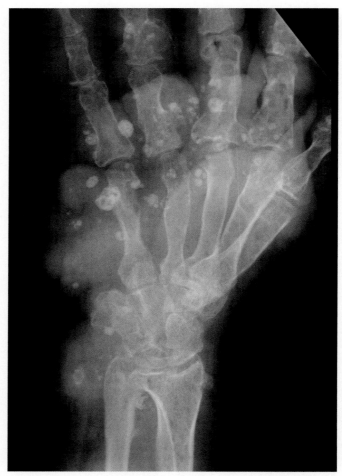

FIGURE 14-18. Maffucci syndrome. Oblique radiograph shows multiple enchondromas and soft tissue masses with vascular calcifications.

SUGGESTED READING

Strang C, Ronnie I. Dyschondroplasia and hemangiomata (Maffucci's syndrome). *J Bone Joint Surg.* 1950;32B:376–383.
Zwenneke Flach H, Ginai AZ, Wolter Oosterhuis J. Best cases from the AFIP. Maffucci syndrome: radiologic and pathologic findings. Armed Forces Institutes of Pathology. *Radiographics.* 2001;21(5):1311–1316.

■ HEREDITARY MULTIPLE EXOSTOSIS

KEY FACTS

■ Hereditary multiple exostosis is an autosomal dominant condition resulting in abnormal bone remodeling and bone deformities.

■ Patients present in childhood with palpable osseous masses, bone shortening, bowing, and joint deformities.

■ Osseous lesions relate to osteochondromas and are bilateral and near the physis.

■ Complications:
  ● Pathologic fracture
  ● Neurovascular injury
  ● Bursa formation
  ● Malignant degeneration (chondrosarcoma in 2% to 27%)

■ Radiographic features:
  ● Osteochondroma-like lesions
  ● Most common in the knee and proximal humerus
  ● Lesions are usually bilateral and symmetric.

(continued)

■ HEREDITARY MULTIPLE EXOSTOSIS   *(Continued)*

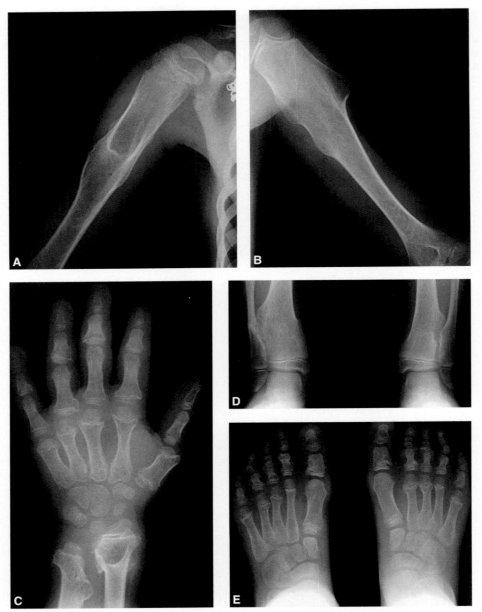

FIGURE 14-19. Hereditary multiple exostosis. Radiographs of the humeri **(A, B)**, left hand and wrist **(C)**, both ankles **(D)**, and feet **(E)** demonstrate multiple exostoses with bone and joint deformities most obvious in the hand and wrist.

SUGGESTED READING

Murphey MD, Choi JJ, Kransdorf MJ, et al. Imaging of osteochondroma: variants and complications with radiologic-pathologic correlation. *Radiographics.* 2000;20(5):1407–1434.

Wilner D. *Radiology of Bone Tumors and Allied Disorders.* Philadelphia: WB Saunders; 1982.

■ EPIPHYSEAL DYSPLASIAS

KEY FACTS

- ■ Epiphyseal dysplasias have two broad categories:
  - ● Spondyloepiphyseal dysplasia: platyspondyly and beaking of the vertebra
  - ● Multiple epiphyseal dysplasia: minimal or no spine abnormalities
- ■ Multiple epiphyseal dysplasia may present in the tarda (childhood) or congenital (first year of life) forms.
- ■ Multiple epiphyseal dysplasia tarda:
  - ● Both sexes equally affected
  - ● Bilateral symmetric involvement of hips, knees, ankles, shoulders, and wrists
  - ● No mental retardation
  - ● Present in early childhood with joint pain and gait disturbances
  - ● Early degenerative joint disease
- ■ Radiographic features:
  - ● Long bone epiphysis appears late
  - ● Irregular and fragmented when ossified
  - ● Slipped epiphysis, coxa vara, and joint deformities common
- ■ Multiple epiphyseal dysplasia congenita has multiple types, including sex-linked and autosomal recessive forms (latter more severe).
  - ● Patients present with calcification of unossified epiphysis in the first year of life.
  - ● Dwarfism, sclerosis, skin lesions, and cataracts are common.
  - ● Mental retardation is present in more severe forms.
- ■ Radiographic features:
  - ● Scattered epiphyseal calcifications
  - ● Shortened long bones

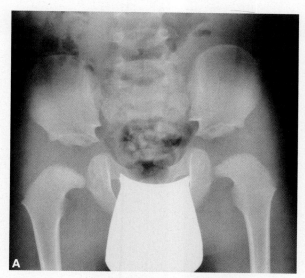

FIGURE 14-20. Multiple epiphyseal dysplasia. Radiographs of the hip **(A)**, left knee **(B, C)**, left foot and ankle **(D, E)**.

(continued)

■ EPIPHYSEAL DYSPLASIAS *(Continued)*

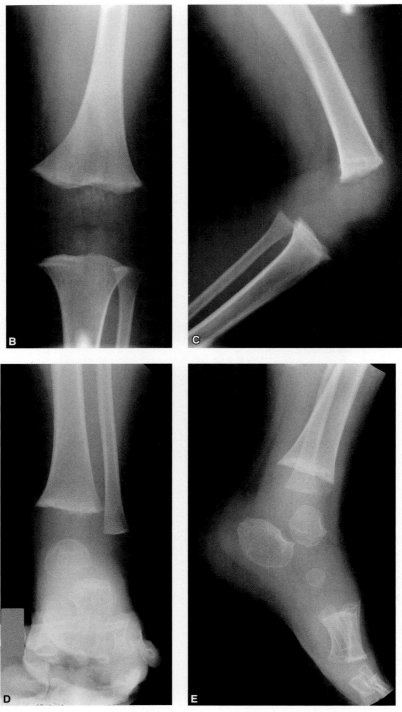

FIGURE 14-20. *(continued)*

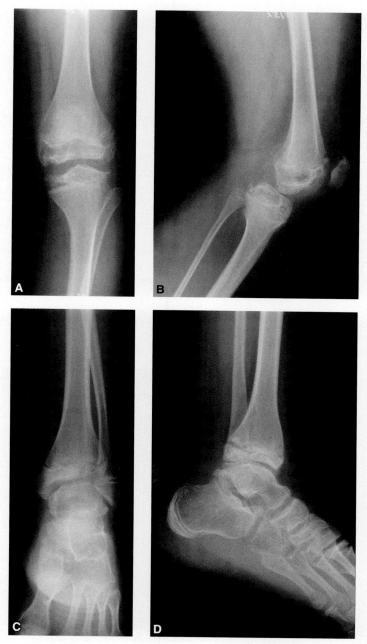

FIGURE 14-21. Multiple epiphyseal dysplasia in an adolescent. Anteroposterior (AP) and lateral radiographs of the knee **(A, B)** and ankle **(C, D)** show irregular epiphysis with joint deformities.

SUGGESTED READING

Berg PK. Dysplasia epiphyseal multiplex. *Am J Roentgenol.* 1966;97:31–38.

■ METAPHYSEAL DYSPLASIAS

KEY FACTS

■ Metaphyseal dysplasias consist of a group of conditions primarily affecting the metaphysis. However, the diaphysis and epiphysis may also be abnormal.

■ Spine involvement is uncommon.

■ Types of metaphyseal dysplasia:

  ● Jansen type: a rare autosomal dominant disorder presenting with dwarfism and bowing of the forearms and legs.

    ❖ Radiographic features: small mandible, prominent frontal sinuses; metaphyseal irregularity and widening extremity bowing with flared metaphysis in childhood

  ● Schmid type: autosomal dominant inheritance. Patients have short stature and bowing of the lower extremities.

    ❖ Radiographic features: metaphyseal irregularity and physeal widening, especially in hips and knees.

  ● McKusick type: autosomal recessive inheritance. Short stature, fine light hair, small hands, joint laxity, and bowing of the lower extremities

    ❖ Radiographic features: metaphyseal cupping and flaring most evident in the lower extremities. Small vertebral bodies.

  ● Shwachman–Diamond type: Patients present with anemia, low white blood cell and platelet counts, and pancreatic insufficiency. Failure to thrive and recurrent pneumonias are part of the syndrome.

    ❖ Radiographic features: coxa vara, osteopenia, metaphyseal irregularity, and irregularity of vertebral bodies.

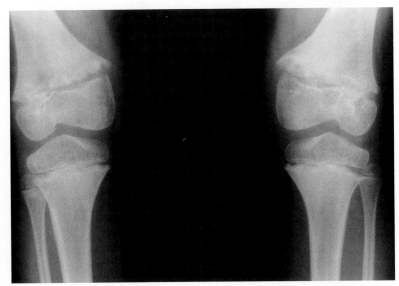

FIGURE 14-22. Metaphyseal dysplasia. Standing radiograph of the knees shows metaphyseal irregularity and flaring with femoral bowing.

SUGGESTED READING

Heselson NG, Raad MS, Hamersma H, et al. The radiological manifestations of metaphyseal dysplasia (Pyle disease). *Br J Radiol.* 1979;52(618):431–440.

McAlister WH, Herman TE. Osteochondrodysplasias, dysostosis, chromosomal aberrations, mucopolysaccharidoses, and mucolipidosis. In: Resnick D, Kransdorf MJ, eds. *Bone and Joint Imaging.* 3rd ed. Philadelphia: Elsevier-Saunders; 2005:1298–1325.

■ MARFAN SYNDROME

KEY FACTS

- ■ Marfan syndrome is a disorder of connective tissue involving the skeleton, cardiovascular system, and eyes. Inheritance is autosomal dominant.
- ■ There is no sex predilection. Patients are typically tall and thin with long limbs. The most evident length disproportion is in the hands and feet.
- ■ Patients may have pectus deformity, scoliosis, and joint laxity.
- ■ Cardiovascular abnormalities (aortic and mitral insufficiency and aortic aneurysms) may shorten life expectancy.
- ■ Ocular abnormalities include myopia and ectopic lentis, with cataract formation in later life.
- ■ Radiographic features:
  - ● Hands and feet—arachnodactyly, pes planus, digital deformities (e.g., hammer toe, claw toe)
  - ● Reduced muscle mass and fat around long bones; slender long bones
  - ● Scoliosis in up to 60% of patients
  - ● Protrusio acetabuli
  - ● Pectus deformity and rib elongation

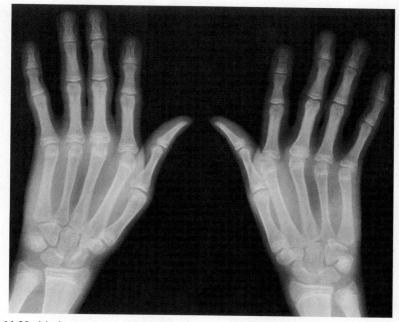

FIGURE 14-23. Marfan syndrome. Posteroanterior (PA) radiograph of the hands shows elongation and thin metacarpals and phalanges.

SUGGESTED READING

Goldman AB. Heritable diseases of connective tissue, epiphyseal dysplasias, and related conditions. In: Resnick D, Kransdorf MJ, eds. *Bone and Joint Imaging*. 3rd ed. Philadelphia: Elsevier-Saunders; 2005:1279–1297.

Ha HI, Seo JB, Lee SH et al. Imaging of Marfan syndrome: multisystemic manifestations. *Radiographics*. 2007;27(4):989–1004.

■ EHLERS–DANLOS SYNDROME

KEY FACTS

- ■ Ehlers–Danlos syndrome is a familial connective tissue disorder.
- ■ Most patients present in childhood.
- ■ Patients present with fragile skin, joint laxity, and bleeding disorders.
- ■ Multisystem involvement may include ocular, pulmonary, gastrointestinal, genitourinary, and cardiovascular disorders.
- ■ Radiographic features:
  - ● Subcutaneous calcifications resembling phleboliths on the extensor surfaces of the forearms and legs
  - ● Joint effusions, hemarthrosis, and subluxations
  - ● Spinal deformity and scoliosis result from ligament laxity
  - ● Posterior vertebral scalloping secondary to dural ectasia

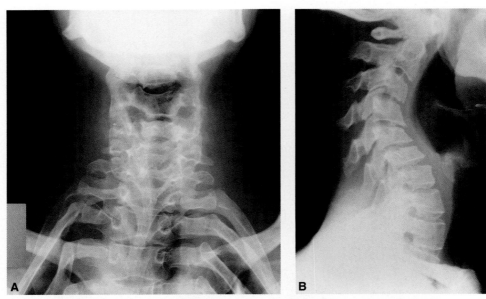

FIGURE 14-24. Ehlers–Danlos syndrome. Anteroposterior (AP) **(A)** and lateral **(B)** radiographs of the cervical spine show exaggeration of the cervical curves.

SUGGESTED READING

Goldman AB. Heritable diseases of connective tissue, epiphyseal dysplasias, and related conditions. In: Resnick D, Kransdorf MJ, eds. *Bone and Joint Imaging.* 3rd ed. Philadelphia: Elsevier-Saunders; 2005:1279–1297.
Zilocchi M, Macedo TA, Oderich GS, et al. Vascular Ehlers–Danlos syndrome: imaging findings. *Am J Roentgenol.* 2007;189(3):712–719.

■ OSTEOGENESIS IMPERFECTA

KEY FACTS

■ Osteogenesis imperfecta is an inherited connective tissue disorder affecting multiple organ systems.

■ There are four clinical features:
  ● Osteoporosis with pathologic fractures
  ● Blue sclera
  ● Dentinogenesis
  ● Premature otosclerosis

■ Classically, the disorder is considered as either congenita or tarda form. More recently, a new classification was developed based on clinical, radiographic, and genetic features (Sillence classification).

Type I	Most common; mildest form
Type II	Lethal; in utero fractures
Type III	Rare; majority have fractures at birth
Type IV	Most variable osseous features

■ Radiographic features:
  ● Diffuse osteoporosis
  ● Thin, gracile bones (Types I and IV)
  ● Short, thick extremities (Types II and III)
  ● Fractures; lower extremity most common
  ● Pseudoarthrosis
  ● Pelvis narrow; triradiate

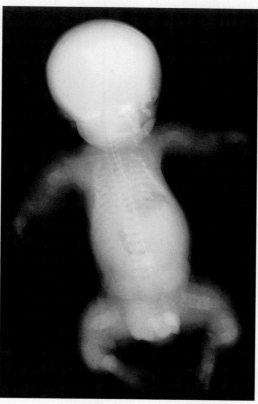

FIGURE 14-25. Osteogenesis imperfecta Type II. Radiograph of a newborn with short, thick osteoporotic extremities and multiple fractures that occurred in utero.

(continued)

■ OSTEOGENESIS IMPERFECTA   *(Continued)*

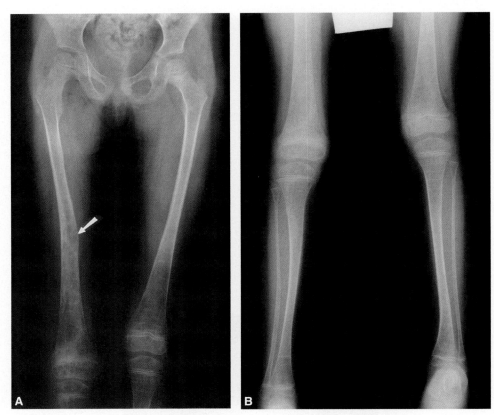

FIGURE 14-26. Osteogenesis imperfecta Type I (tarda). Anteroposterior (AP) radiographs of the femora **(A)** and legs **(B)** show thin, gracile osteoporotic bones with a healed fracture *(arrow)* in the right femur.

SUGGESTED READING

Renaud A, Aucourt J, Weill J, et al. Radiographic features of osteogenesis imperfecta. *Insights Imaging.* 2013;4(4):417–429.
Sillence D. Osteogenesis imperfect: an expanding panorama of variants. *Clin Orthop.* 1981;159:11–25.

■ ACHONDROPLASIA

KEY FACTS

■ Achondroplasia presents in two forms:
  ● Heterozygous (most common): Evident at birth. Dwarfism with normal lifespan.
  ● Homozygous (lethal): Rare. Patients die in early infancy.
■ Patients with typical achondroplasia present with short limbs, more pronounced proximally (rhizomelic micromelia); large head; prominent buttocks; thoracic kyphosis; and exaggerated lumbar lordosis. Hands are short. Spinal changes frequently lead to spinal stenosis.
■ Radiographic features:
  ● Large skull with small foramen magnum
  ● Lumbar interpedicular distance stays the same or decreases from L1 to L5 (normally increases)
  ● Pedicles short and posterior vertebral line concave
  ● Square iliac bones with small sacrosciatic notches and flat acetabular angles
  ● Short proximal long bones with metaphyseal flaring
  ● Shortening of the bones in the hands and feet

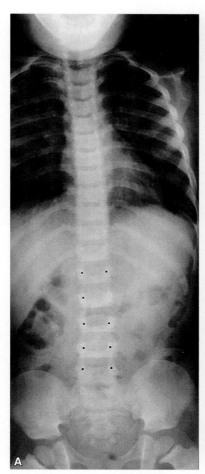
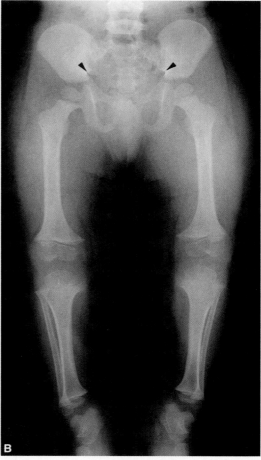

FIGURE 14-27. Achondroplasia. **(A)** Anteroposterior (AP) radiograph of the spine shows no change in lumbar interpedicular distance (*black dots*) progressing from L1 to L5. **(B)** AP radiograph of the pelvis and lower extremities shows small sciatic notches (*arrowheads*), flattening of the acetabular angles, iliac squaring, and short tubular bones with metaphyseal flaring in the knees. **(C)** Lateral radiograph of the spine in an older patient shows short pedicles and concave posterior vertebral margins. The narrowed spinal canal has resulted in laminectomies (*arrows*).

(continued)

■ **ACHONDROPLASIA** *(Continued)*

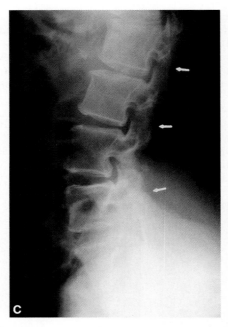

FIGURE 14-27. *(continued)*

SUGGESTED READING

Kao SC, Waziri MH, Smith WL, et al. MR imaging of the craniovertebral junction, cranium, and brain in children with achondroplasia. *Am J Roentgenol.* 1989;153(3):565–569.
Langer LO, Baumann PA, Gorlin RJ. Achondroplasia. *Am J Roentgenol.* 1967;100:12–26.

■ MUCOPOLYSACCHARIDOSES

KEY FACTS

■ Mucopolysaccharidoses (MPS) constitutes a group of disorders that presents with dwarfism and clinical, laboratory, and radiographic features that differentiate the conditions.

■ There are seven separate categories of MPS, with Hurler syndrome (MPS-IH) and Morquio syndrome (MPS-IV) most well known radiographically.

■ Table 14-1 summarizes features and enzyme deficiencies in MPS syndromes.

■ Hurler syndrome (MPS-IH):
  ● Autosomal recessive manifesting in first years of life
  ● Mental retardation, corneal clouding, deafness, cardiac disease
  ● Death in first decade from cardiac disease
  ● Radiographic features:
    ❖ Macrocephaly, J-shaped sella
    ❖ Widening of anterior ribs
    ❖ Hypoplastic vertebra at thoracolumbar junction
    ❖ C11–C12 subluxation
    ❖ Shortening and widening of long bones
    ❖ Pointing of proximal metacarpals

■ Morquio syndrome (MPS-IV):
  ● Severe dwarfism
  ● Spinal kyphoscoliosis
  ● Joint laxity
  ● Prominent mandible and lower face
  ● Short neck
  ● Mentally normal
  ● Corneal clouding and deafness
  ● Radiographic features:
    ❖ Round vertebral bodies with small anterior beak
    ❖ Anterior sternal bowing, increased anteroposterior chest diameter, wide ribs
    ❖ Coxa valga, flared iliac wings, increased acetabular angles
    ❖ Wide metacarpals with proximal pointing, irregular carpal bones
    ❖ Metaphyseal flaring in long bones

(continued)

■ MUCOPOLYSACCHARIDOSES *(Continued)*

Table 14-1   MUCOPOLYSACCHARIDOSES

Type	Enzyme Deficiency	Features
Hurler syndrome (MPS-IH)	α-L-iduronidase	Mental retardation, clouded corneas, coarse facial features, heart disease
Scheie syndrome (MPS-IS)	α-L-iduronidase	Late onset, clouded corneas, aortic valve disease, mentally normal, mild facial changes
Hurler–Scheie syndrome	α-L-iduronidase	Between MPS-IH and MPS-IS
Hunter syndrome (MPS-II)	Iduronidase-Z-sulfatase	Severe: mental retardation, death in second decade Mild: mental retardation, survive until adulthood
Sanfilippo syndrome (MPS-III)	A: Heparin-*N*-sulfatase B: α-*N*-acetyl glucosaminidase C: Glucosaminide-*N*-acetyl transferase D: *N*-acetyl glucosamine-6-sulfate sulfatase	Mental retardation, mild skeletal features
Morquio syndrome (MPS-IV)	Galactosamine-6-sulfate sulfatase	Severe dwarfism, short trunk and neck, mentally normal
Maroteaux–Lamy syndrome (MPS-VI)	*N*-Acetyl galactosamine-4-sulfatase	Dwarfism, coarse facial features, corneal clouding, mentally normal
Sly syndrome (MPS-VII)	β-Glucuronidase	Enlarged liver and spleen, mild to moderate mental retardation

MPS, mucopolysaccharidoses.

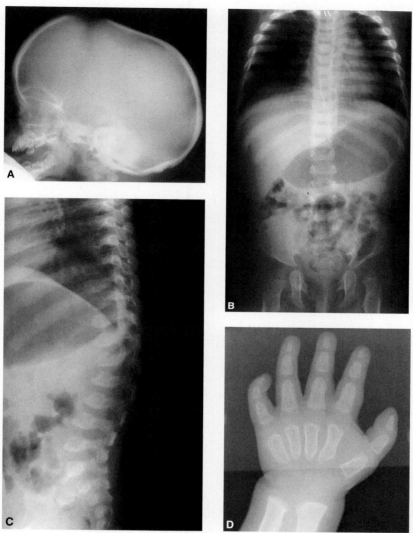

FIGURE 14-28. Hurler syndrome (MPS-IH). **(A)** Lateral radiograph of the skull shows a large "J"-shaped sella and underdeveloped mastoids. Sinuses are hypoplastic. **(B)** Anteroposterior (AP) radiograph of the spine and pelvis demonstrates expanded anterior ribs, hypoplastic ilia, and coxa valga. **(C)** Lateral radiograph of the spine shows hypoplastic vertebrae at the thoracolumbar junction with anterior beaking. **(D)** Hand radiograph demonstrates thick short metacarpals and phalanges with pointing of the proximal metacarpals.

(continued)

■ MUCOPOLYSACCHARIDOSES   *(Continued)*

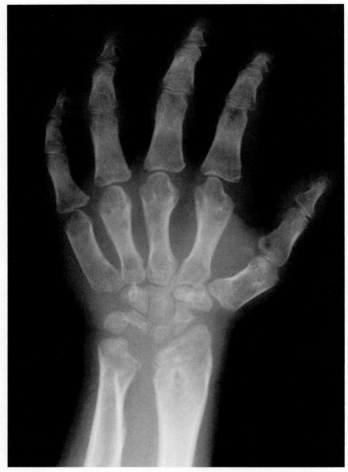

FIGURE 14-29. Morquio syndrome (MPS-IV). Radiograph of the hand shows slanting of the radial and ulnar articular surfaces and small irregular carpal bones. The bones of the hand are short and widened.

SUGGESTED READING

Blighton D. *Heritable Disorders of Connective Tissue.* 5th ed. St. Louis: CV Mosby; 1993.
Reichert R, Campos LG, Vairo F, et al. Neuroimaging findings in patients with mucopolysaccharidosis: what you really need to know. *Radiographics.* 2016;36(5):1448–1462.

■ DYSCHONDROSTEOSIS (LERI–WEILL SYNDROME)

KEY FACTS

- This common syndrome is an autosomal dominant disorder with mesomelic extremity shortening and Madelung deformity.
- The condition is more common in females.
- The condition affects the forearm and legs.
- Radiographic features:
  - Shortened dorsally, bowed radius
  - Distal ulna often subluxed
  - V-shaped radioulnar articular surfaces
  - Shortening of the tibia and fibula
  - Coxa valga
  - Shortening of the bones in the hands and feet

(continued)

■ DYSCHONDROSTEOSIS (LERI–WEILL SYNDROME) *(Continued)*

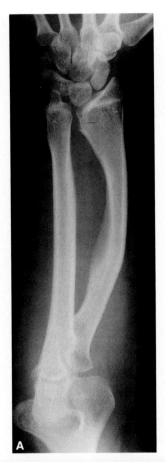

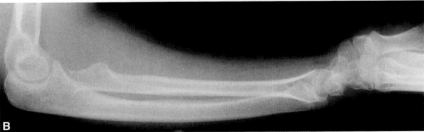

FIGURE 14-30. Dyschondrosteosis (Leri–Weill syndrome). Anteroposterior (AP) **(A)** and lateral **(B)** radiographs of the forearm show Madelung deformity with bowing of the radius and a V-shaped radioulnar articular surface with carpal bones collapsed centrally.

SUGGESTED READING

Langer LO. Dyschondrosteosis of the inherited bone dysplasias with characteristic roentgenographic features. *Am J Roentgenol.* 1965;95:178–185.

Mohan V, Gupta RP, Helmi K, et al. Leri–Weill syndrome (dyschondrosteosis): a family study. *J Hand Surg Br.* 1988;13(1):16–18.

■ PACHYDERMOPERIOSTOSIS

KEY FACTS

- ■ Pachydermoperiostosis, or primary hypertrophic osteoarthropathy, constitutes 3% to 5% of hypertrophic osteoarthropathies.
- ■ Patients present with clubbing on the hands and feet, enlargement of the tabular bones caused by bony proliferation, and pain and swelling in the joints.
- ■ The condition has an autosomal dominant inheritance and is more common in black males.
- ■ Cortical thickening may lead to marrow failure and extramedullary hematopoiesis.
- ■ Radiographic features:
  - ● Clubbing in the hands and feet
  - ● Irregular bony proliferation in the long bones involving the diaphysis, metaphysis, and epiphysis (the last not seen in second-degree hypertrophic osteoarthropathy)

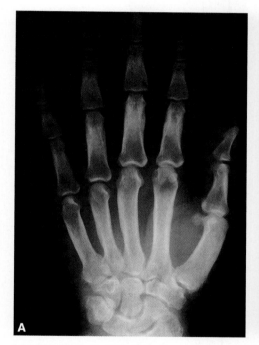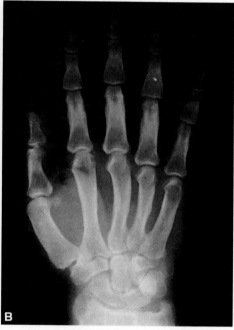

FIGURE 14-31. Pachydermoperiostosis (primary hypertrophic osteoarthropathy). Radiographs of the hands **(A, B)** demonstrate widening and bony proliferation involving the phalanges and metacarpals with involvement of the radial and ulnar epiphyses. Radiographs of the forearms **(C, D)** show cortical thickening and irregularity with widening of the radius and ulna.

(continued)

■ PACHYDERMOPERIOSTOSIS *(Continued)*

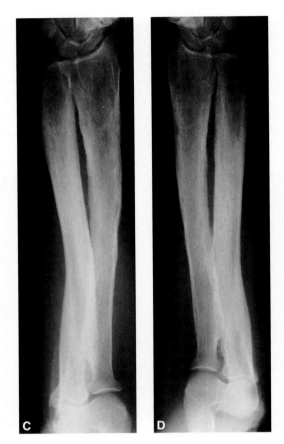

FIGURE 14-31. *(continued)*

SUGGESTED READING

Neiman HL, Gompels BM, Martel W. Pachydermoperiostosis with bone marrow failure and gross extramedullary hematopoiesis. *Radiology.* 1974;110:533–554.

Rastogi R, Suma GN, Prakash R, et al. Pachydermoperiostosis or primary hypertrophic osteoarthropathy: a rare clinicoradiologic case. *Indian J Radiol Imaging.* 2009;19(2):123–126.

■ SECONDARY HYPERTROPHIC OSTEOARTHROPATHY

KEY FACTS

- Secondary hypertrophic osteoarthropathy has replaced the term "pulmonary hypertrophic osteo-arthropathy" because there are numerous nonpulmonary causes.
- Pulmonary disorders are commonly involved (50% of patients with mesothelioma, 12% of patients with bronchogenic carcinoma).
- Gastrointestinal disorders, cystic fibrosis, and congenital heart disease are also associated with hypertrophic osteoarthropathy.
- Patients frequently present with joint pain.
- Radiographic features (Table 14-2):
  - Smooth periostitis
  - Tibiae, fibulae, radii, and ulnae are most commonly involved
  - Proximal extremities may also be involved

Table 14-2   PERIOSTITIS

Condition	Radiographic Features
Primary hypertrophic osteoarthropathy (Pachydermoperiostitis)	Shaggy periostitis, ligament ossification tibia, fibula, tarsal, metatarsal diaphysis, and epiphysis
Secondary hypertrophic osteoarthropathy	Smooth periosteal reaction, tibia, fibula radius, and ulnar diaphysis and metaphysis
Thyroid acropachy (see Chapter 13)	Spiculated periosteal reaction in hands and less commonly the feet
Venous insufficiency	Smooth undulating periosteal reaction most common in the tibia and fibula
Hypervitaminosis A	Undulating periosteal reaction in the tibia, fibula, and metatarsal diaphyses

(continued)

■ SECONDARY HYPERTROPHIC OSTEOARTHROPATHY   *(Continued)*

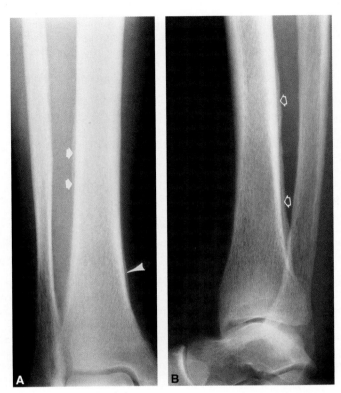

FIGURE 14-32. Secondary hypertrophic osteoarthropathy. Anteroposterior (AP) **(A)** and lateral **(B)** radiographs in a patient with chronic pulmonary disease show periosteal new bone along the lateral tibia (*arrows*), posterior tibia (*open arrows*), and medial tibia (*arrowhead*).

SUGGESTED READING

Morgan B, Coakley F, Finlay DB, et al. Hypertrophic osteoarthropathy in staging skeletal scintigraphy for lung cancer. *Clin Radiol.* 1996;51(10):694–697.

Pineda CJ, Martinez-Lavin M, Goobar JE, et al. Periostitis in hypertrophic osteoarthropathy: relationship to disease duration. *Am J Roentgenol.* 1987;148(4):773–778.

Segal AM, McKenzie AH. Hypertrophic osteoarthropathy: a 10-year retrospective analysis. *Semin Arthritis Rheum.* 1982;12:220–231.

■ VITAMINOSIS: VITAMIN A

KEY FACTS

- Vitamin A is essential for chondrogenesis and longitudinal bone growth.
- Radiographic features are typically not present with low levels of vitamin A.
- Hypervitaminosis A may present as an acute or chronic disorder.
  - Acute: rare today. May be seen with ingested overdoses of polar bear, shark, or chicken liver. Patients present with headache, vertigo, and symptoms of increased intracranial pressure.
  - Chronic: Patients present with anorexia, pruritus, tender subcutaneous nodules over the long bones, fissuring of the legs, and bleeding.
- Radiographic features:
  - Findings confined to the growing skeleton and more often seen with the chronic form
  - Smooth wavy periostitis along the ulna and metatarsals (Table 14-2)
  - Hyperostosis and metaphyseal deformities

SUGGESTED READING

Miller JH, Hayon II. Bone scintigraphy in hypervitaminosis A. *Am J Roentgenol.* 1985;144(4):767–768.
Ruby LK, Mital MA. Skeletal deformities following chronic hypervitaminosis A. *J Bone Joint Surg.* 1974;56:1283–1287.

■ VITAMINOSIS: VITAMIN C

KEY FACTS

■ Vitamin C is required for collagen and matrix formation.

■ Vitamin C is excreted by the kidneys, so excess serum vitamin C is rare.

■ Vitamin C deficiency is uncommon today, but may cause skeletal changes in children and adults.

■ Clinical features are most common in infants and children.

■ Patients present with failure to thrive, petechiae, and hemorrhaging caused by reduced intracellular cement in capillaries.

■ Radiographic features are most dramatic in infants and children.

- Most significant changes occur at the metaphysis, physis, and epiphysis
- Zone of provisional calcification is thick and sclerotic
- Lucent zone (scurvy line) on metaphyseal side of this band
- Corner sign—beaklike metaphyseal extension with lucent metaphyseal changes
- Marked periosteal evolution caused by hemorrhages
- "Ring" epiphyses result from dense provisional zones of calcification at their margins
- Osteoporosis in adults
- Features may return to normal with vitamin C therapy.

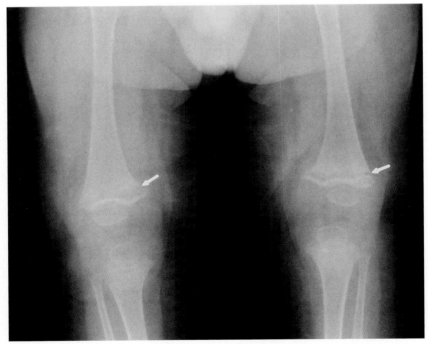

FIGURE 14-33. Hypovitaminosis C in a 10-month-old. Radiographs of the knees show ringed epiphyses and metaphyseal condensation with fractures (*arrows*) proximally.

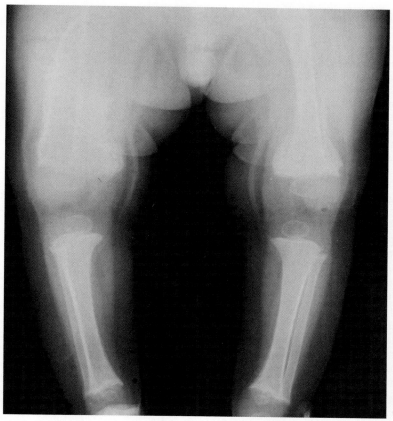

FIGURE 14-34. Hypovitaminosis C in an 8-month-old. Anteroposterior (AP) radiograph of the lower extremities shows healing subperiosteal hemorrhages, more evident along the femora.

SUGGESTED READING

Resnick D, Kransdorf MJ. Hypervitaminosis and hypovitaminosis. In: Resnick D, Kransdorf MJ, eds. *Bone and Joint Imaging.* 3rd ed. Philadelphia: Elsevier-Saunders; 2005:1022–1027.

■ VITAMINOSIS: VITAMIN D

KEY FACTS

- Vitamin D is essential for calcium and phosphorus balance.
- Hypovitaminosis D (osteomalacia and rickets) was discussed in Chapter 13.
- Vitamin D intoxication (hypervitaminosis) can be seen in patients treated for skeletal disorders and adults with Paget disease.
- Patients present with anorexia, vomiting, fever, and abdominal and skeletal pain.
- Radiographic features are primarily related to hypercalcemia and metastatic calcification. Calcifications may occur in vasculature, articular regions, and abdominal viscera.
- Patterns of calcification are not specific (Table 14-3).

Table 14-3   CONDITIONS ASSOCIATED WITH SOFT TISSUE CALCIFICATION

Metastatic Calcification (Calcium/Phosphorus Metabolism)
   Hyperparathyroidism
   Renal osteodystrophy
   Hypervitaminosis D
   Sarcoidosis
   Multiple myeloma
   Metastasis
Calcinosis (Normal Calcium Metabolism)
   Collagen vascular diseases (see Chapter 12)
   Tumoral calcinosis
   Calcinosis universalis
   Dermatomyositis
Dystrophic Calcification (Normal Calcium Metabolism)
   Trauma
   Neoplasms
   Inflammation

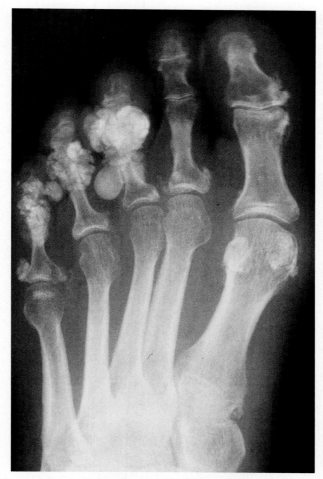

FIGURE 14-35. Vitamin D intoxication. Anteroposterior (AP) radiograph of the foot shows dense amorphous periarticular soft tissue calcification.

SUGGESTED READING

Resnick D, Kransdorf MJ. Hypervitaminosis and hypovitaminosis. In: Resnick D, Kransdor MJ, eds. *Bone and Joint Imaging.* 3rd ed. Philadelphia: Elsevier-Saunders; 2005:1022–1027.

■ TUMORAL CALCINOSIS

KEY FACTS

- Idiopathic tumoral calcinosis typically occurs in males in their 20s and 30s. The condition is more common in black males.
- Trauma is reported in some cases, and 30% to 40% have a family history.
- Radiographs or computed tomography (CT) reveals periarticular calcium masses, often forming multiple lobules. The hips, shoulders, elbows, and ankles are most commonly involved.
- Differential diagnosis includes collagen vascular disorders, chronic renal disease, hyperparathyroidism, and sarcoidosis (Table 14-3).

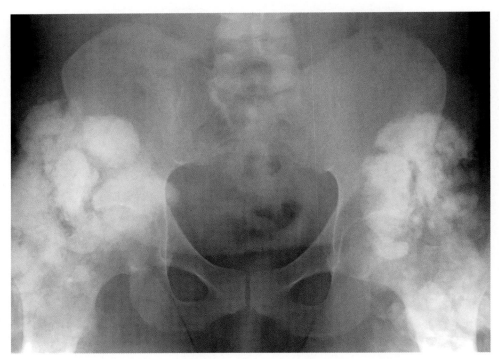

FIGURE 14-36. Tumoral calcinosis. Anteroposterior (AP) pelvis radiograph shows large loculated calcified masses overlying the hip joints.

SUGGESTED READING

Kolawole TM, Bohrer SP. Tumoral calcinosis with fluid–fluid levels in tumoral masses. *Am J Roentgenol.* 1974;120:461–465.
Olsen KM, Chew FS. Tumoral calcinosis: pearls, polemics, and alternative possibilities. *Radiographics.* 2006;26 (3):871–885.

■ HEAVY METAL DISORDERS

KEY FACTS

- ■ Skeletal disorders may be related to lead, aluminum, or copper.
- ■ Lead intoxication occurs in neonates whose mothers have lead intoxication or by ingesting lead-containing paints or inhaling lead-containing fumes. Clinical features may be acute, with neurologic symptoms, seizures, and abdominal pain, or chronic, with fatigue and anemia. Radiographic features occur late. Dense metaphyseal bands are evident radiographically.
- ■ Aluminum intoxication may be seen in patients on dialysis or those taking aluminum hydroxide. Osteomalacia is seen radiographically, but features are not specific.
- ■ Copper deficiency is seen in infants undergoing total parenteral therapy. Radiographic features are similar to those of rickets.

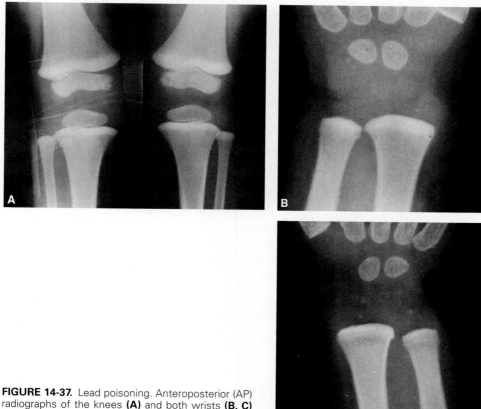

FIGURE 14-37. Lead poisoning. Anteroposterior (AP) radiographs of the knees **(A)** and both wrists **(B, C)** show dense, thick metaphyseal bands.

(continued)

■ HEAVY METAL DISORDERS   *(Continued)*

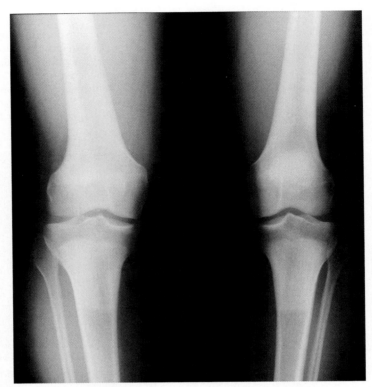

FIGURE 14-38. Heavy metal intoxication. Anteroposterior (AP) radiograph of the knees demonstrates broad bands of sclerosis in the diaphyseal–metaphyseal regions of the tibias and femurs.

SUGGESTED READING

Blickman JG, Wilkinson RH, Graef JW. The radiographic lead band revisited. *Am J Roentgenol.* 1986;146:245–247.

■ HEMOGLOBINOPATHIES/ANEMIAS: BASIC CONCEPTS

KEY FACTS

- Fetal hemoglobin (HbF) comprises 60% to 90% of hemoglobin at birth.
- Adult hemoglobin (HbA) usually replaces HbF at 4 months of age.
- HbA consists of paired polypeptide chains. There are two α chains (141 amino acids) and two β chains (146 amino acids).
- Variations in amino acids on either chain result in a spectrum of clinical diseases, including sickle cell anemia and thalassemia.

SUGGESTED READING

Musely JE. Skeletal changes in the anemias. *Semin Roentgenol.* 1974;9:169–184.

■ HEMOGLOBINOPATHIES/ANEMIAS: SICKLE CELL ANEMIA

KEY FACTS

■ Sickle cell anemia has differing clinical and radiographic features, depending on the hemoglobin structure.

■ Sickle cell anemias:

Homozygous (HbS-S)	α Chain is normal. Valine replaces glutamic acid on the α chain. Present in 1.3% of U.S. African Americans.
Heterozygous (HbC-S)	S gene from one parent and C gene from the other. Present in 1.3% of U.S. African Americans.
Sickle thalassemia	One S gene and one thalassemia gene inherited.

■ Clinical symptoms are most common in the homozygous form.
  ● Symptoms rare during first 6 months
  ● Painful swelling of hands and feet (dactylitis) at 6 months to 2 years
  ● Sickle cell crisis in 20s and 30s, with bone pain, fever, anemia, and abdominal pain
■ Radiographic features are predominately related to bone infarction, marrow hyperplasia, and complications such as osteomyelitis.
  ● Marrow hyperplasia—osteopenia and cortical thinning
  ● Vascular occlusion—bone infarction
  ● Dactylitis (6 months to 2 years)—osteolytic changes and periosteal reaction
  ● Growth deformity—metaphyseal and epiphyseal deformity
  ● Vertebral ischemia—H-shaped vertebral body (also seen in thalassemia, Gaucher disease, and hereditary spherocytosis)
  ● Osteomyelitis—more than 50% of cases are the result of *Salmonella*; *Staphylococcus* is the second most common.

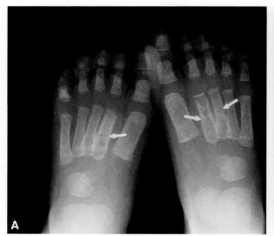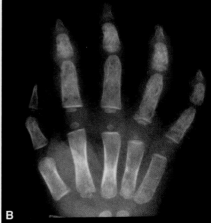

FIGURE 14-39. Sickle cell dactylitis. Anteroposterior (AP) radiographs of the feet **(A)** and right hand **(B)** show necrosis of metatarsals with periosteal reaction (*arrows*) and similar changes in the hand.

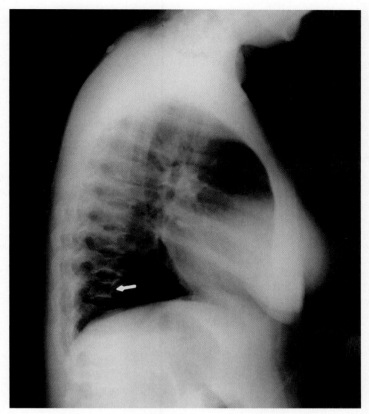

FIGURE 14-40. H-shaped vertebrae. Lateral radiograph of the thoracic spine shows H-shaped vertebral bodies (*arrow*) caused by endplate ischemic changes.

SUGGESTED READING

Diggs LW. Bone and joint lesions in sickle cell anemia. *Clin Orthop.* 1967;52:119–144.

Ejindu VC, Hine AL, Mashayekhi M, et al. Musculoskeletal manifestations of sickle cell disease. *Radiographics.* 2007;27(4):1005–1021.

■ EMOGLOBINOPATHIES/ANEMIAS: THALASSEMIA

KEY FACTS

■ Thalassemia (Cooley anemia) is a term derived from Greek meaning "the sea" because the first patients were of Mediterranean origin.

■ Several forms of thalassemia are recognized.

α Thalassemia	Abnormal α chain. May affect fetus.
β Thalassemia	Abnormal β chain. Manifests after HbF is replaced by HbA.
Homozygous	Thalassemia major
Heterozygous	Thalassemia minor

■ Thalassemia major is diagnosed early, and life expectancy is reduced. α Major (complete absence of α chain) is most severe; infants die in utero. β Thalassemia is diagnosed in infancy or early childhood, and anemia is severe. Patients rarely live beyond their teens.

■ Patients with thalassemia minor have mild anemia and splenomegaly.

■ Radiographic features:
  ● Marrow hyperplasia—osteopenia, "hair-on-end" appearance in the skull
  ● H-shaped vertebrae similar to sickle cell anemia
  ● Cortical thinning, marrow expansion, Erlenmeyer flask deformities in femora
  ● Growth deformities and pathologic fractures
  ● Extramedullary hematopoiesis

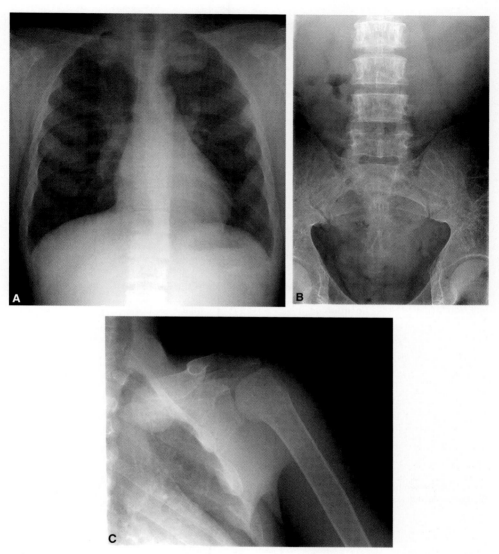

FIGURE 14-41. Thalassemia major. Posteroanterior (PA) radiograph of the chest **(A)** depicts expansion of the medullary canal of the ribs and clavicles with diffuse osteopenia. Anteroposterior (AP) radiograph of the lower lumbar spine and sacrum **(B)** shows marrow expansion, thin corticies with sparse trabeculae, and osteopenia. Radiograph of the shoulder **(C)** demonstrates marrow hyperplasia with expansion of the medullary canal and thinned corticies involving the humerus, clavicle, and ribs.

SUGGESTED READING

Caffey J. Cooley anemia: a review of roentgenographic findings in the skeleton. *Am J Roentgenol.* 1957;78:381–391.
Toumba M, Skordis N. Osteoporosis syndrome in thalassaemia major: an overview. *J Osteoporos.* 2010: 537673.

■ SARCOIDOSIS

KEY FACTS

- Sarcoidosis is a granulomatous disease of unknown origin. The presence of noncaseating granulomas suggests that infection is the likely cause.
- Multiple organ systems are affected (Table 14-4). Symptoms are most common when patients are in their 20s to 40s.
- Pulmonary involvement (bilateral hilar and right paratracheal adenopathy with or without infiltrates) is common (90%), but patients may be asymptomatic.
- Other common symptoms include uveitis, iritis, erythematous rash, and malaise. Fever, weight loss, and hepatosplenomegaly are also common.
- Musculoskeletal involvement (5% to 13%) may be osseous, articular, or muscular in nature.
- Radiographic features:
  - Subcutaneous nodules (5%)
  - Lacelike or cystic changes in the hands and feet (5%)
  - Axial skeleton and long bone lesions may be lytic or sclerotic
  - Muscle granulomas (often asymptomatic, seen on MRI)
  - Joint swelling and narrowing may occur.

Table 14-4 SARCOIDOSIS ORGAN SYSTEM INVOLVEMENT

Location	Incidence (%)
Pulmonary	90
Mediastinum	85
Ocular	80
Liver/spleen	50–80
Muscles	50–80[a]
Cardiac	25
Central nervous system	25
Osseous	5–13
Parotid glands	6
GU tract	5
GI tract	1

[a] Only 1.4% are symptomatic.
GI, gastrointestinal; GU, genitourinary.

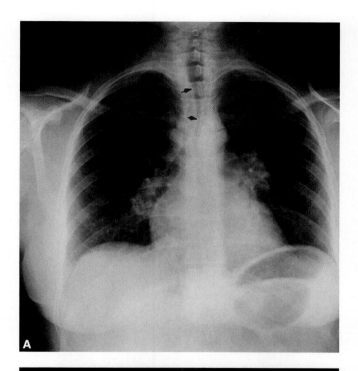

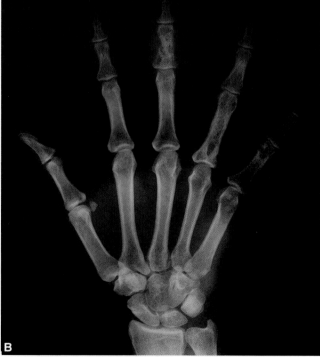

FIGURE 14-42. Sarcoidosis. **(A)** Posteroanterior (PA) radiograph of the chest shows bilateral hilar and right paratracheal adenopathy. Note the tracheal deviation (*arrows*). **(B)** Radiograph of the right hand shows lacelike trabecular pattern and cystic changes in the third middle phalanx and fourth proximal phalanx.

(continued)

■ SARCOIDOSIS *(Continued)*

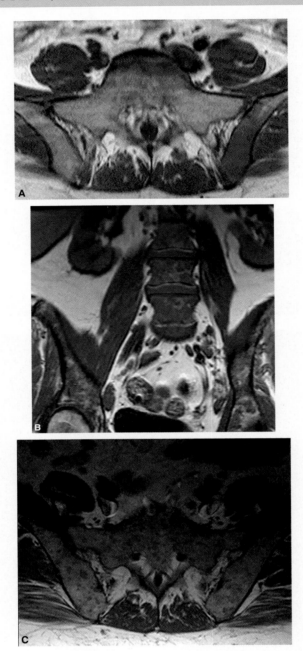

FIGURE 14-43. Various magnetic resonance (MR) imaging patterns of osseous sarcoidosis. Axial T1-weighted **(A)** MR image depicts confluent irregular marrow infiltration involving the left posterior ilium which is a common pattern seen with osseous sarcoid. Coronal T1-weighted **(B)** MR image in another patient shows more patchy, diffuse intramedullary lesions. Axial T1-weighted **(C)** MR image in yet another patient shows innumerable small punctate foci of abnormal signal with a starry sky appearance.

SUGGESTED READING

Gunter B. Sarcoidosis. *Orthopedics.* 1995;18:214–218.

Moore SL, Teirstein AE. Musculoskeletal sarcoidosis: spectrum of appearances at MR imaging. *Radiographics.* 2003;23:1389–1399.

■ DIFFUSE IDIOPATHIC SKELETAL HYPEROSTOSIS

KEY FACTS

- Diffuse idiopathic skeletal hyperostosis (DISH) is an ossifying diathesis of uncertain cause, but distinct in clinical and radiographic features from other disorders such as ankylosing spondylitis.
- Clinical symptoms occur, predominantly in the elderly, but symptoms (tendinitis, restricted range of joint motion, and difficulty swallowing with cervical spine involvement) are often mild compared with radiographic features.
- DISH commonly involves the thoracic spine, but the cervical and lumbar spine may also be involved. Extraspinal changes are most common in the pelvis, knees, elbows, heel, hand, and wrist.
- Heterotopic ossification is common in patients with DISH after hip and knee surgery.
- Radiographic features:
  - Spine (three criteria): (i) flowing ossification anterolaterally involving at least four contiguous vertebrae; (ii) preserved disc height; and (iii) absence of bony ankylosis.
  - Extraspinal features: whiskering at sites of tendon or ligament attachment. Prominent enthesophytes.

(continued)

■ DIFFUSE IDIOPATHIC SKELETAL HYPEROSTOSIS *(Continued)*

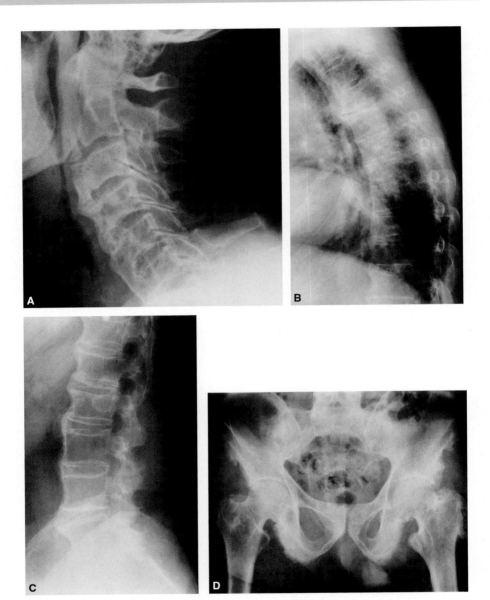

FIGURE 14-44. Diffuse idiopathic skeletal hyperostosis (DISH). **(A)** Lateral view of the cervical spine with prominent anterior ossification causing dysphagia. The disc spaces are preserved and at least four segments are involved. **(B)** Lateral radiograph of the thoracic spine with flowing osteophytic ossification and preserved disc spaces. **(C)** Lateral view of the lumbar spine with anterior ossification and normal disc spaces. **(D)** Anteroposterior (AP) radiograph of the pelvis with ischial whiskering and prominent enthesophytes, especially on the left greater trochanter.

SUGGESTED READING

Haller J, Resnick D, Miller CW, et al. Diffuse idiopathic skeletal hyperostosis: diagnostic significance of radiographic abnormalities of the pelvis. *Radiology.* 1989;172(3):835–839.

Resnick D, Niwayama G. Radiographic and pathologic features of spinal involvement in diffuse idiopathic skeletal hyperostosis (DISH). *Radiology.* 1976;119:559–568.

Taljanovic MS, Hunter TB, Wisneski RJ, et al. Imaging characteristics of diffuse idiopathic skeletal hyperostosis with an emphasis on acute spinal fractures: review. *Am J Roentgenol.* 2009;193(3):S10–S19.

■ GORHAM DISEASE (MASSIVE OSTEOLYSIS)

KEY FACTS

- Gorham disease is of unknown cause. However, pathologic features suggest a vascular derangement.
- The condition can be seen in males and females at any age, but most are diagnosed before age 40 years.
- Patients present with pain and swelling in the involved region.
- Spinal and extra-axial involvement can occur.
- Radiographic features are dramatic with progressive osteopenia and fragmentation of bone that can spread to adjacent osseous or articular structures.
- Serious complications are uncommon unless the spine or chest (respiratory compromise) is involved.

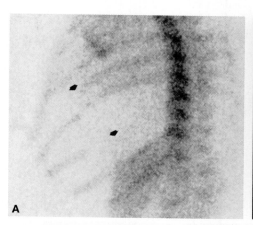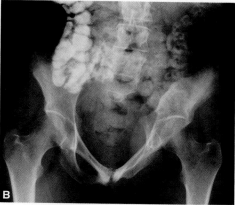

FIGURE 14-45. Gorham disease. **(A)** Radionuclide bone scan shows absent (no uptake) tenth and distal eighth ribs (*arrows*). **(B)** Anteroposterior (AP) radiograph of the pelvis in a different patient with osteolysis of the medial left ilium.

SUGGESTED READING

Collins J. Case 92: Gorham syndrome. *Radiology.* 2006;238(3):1066–1069.

Glass-Royal M, Stull MA. Musculoskeletal case of the day. Gorham syndrome of the right clavicle and scapula. *Am J Roentgenol.* 1990;154(6):1335–1336.

Heyden G, Kindblom LG, Nielsen JM. Disappearing bone disease. A clinical and histologic study. *J Bone Joint Surg.* 1977;59A:57–61.

■ NONACCIDENTAL TRAUMA (BATTERED CHILD SYNDROME)

KEY FACTS

- More than 200,000 incidents of child abuse are reported yearly in the United States.
- Most cases occur in children aged less than 6 years. Up to 70% have radiographic abnormalities.
- Clinical evaluation should include a skeletal survey to search for single or multiple fractures. Radionuclide bone scans are also useful in this regard. CT or MRI is useful when neurologic or central nervous system injury is suspected clinically.
- Extraskeletal findings include cutaneous hemorrhage or bruising, malnutrition, chest and internal abdominal injuries, and subdural hematomas.
- Common fracture sites include the ribs, humerus, femora, tibia, hand, and skull, in order of decreasing frequency.
- Bilateral fractures and abundant calluses are clues to the diagnosis.

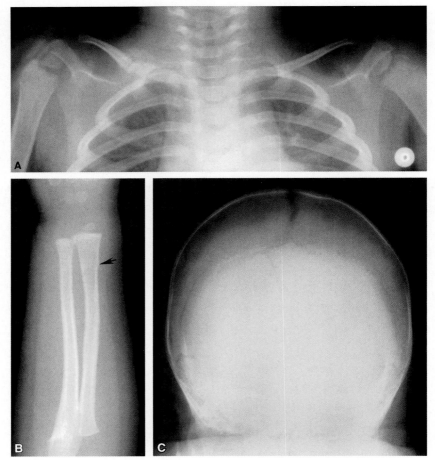

FIGURE 14-46. Nonaccidental trauma. **(A)** Radiograph of the clavicles shows a fracture of the right midclavicle with abundant callus formation. **(B)** Radiograph of the forearm shows a subtle torus fracture (*arrow*). **(C)** Anteroposterior (AP) radiograph of the skull demonstrates a skull fracture. **(D)** Renogram in a 14-month-old shows no perfusion in the left kidney (*arrowhead*). **(E)** Computed tomography (CT) image demonstrates fluid in the abdomen with renal (*arrow*) and splenic (*arrowhead*) injuries.

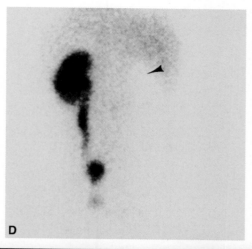

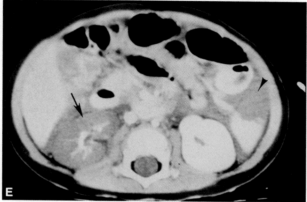

FIGURE 14-46. *(continued)*

SUGGESTED READING

Dias MS, Backstrom J, Falk J, et al. Serial radiography in the infant shaken impact syndrome. *Pediatr Neurosurg.* 1998;29:77–85.

Kogutt MS, Swischuk LE, Fagan CJ. Patterns of injury and significance of uncommon fractures in battered child syndrome. *Am J Roentgenol.* 1974;121:143–149.

Mogbo KI, Slovis TL, Canady AI, et al. Appropriate imaging in children with skull fractures and suspicion of abuse. *Radiology.* 1998;208:521–524.

Index

Page numbers followed by *t* indicate a table; those followed by *f* indicate a figure.

A

Abnormal muscle insertions, 362
Abscess
  Brodie, 620*t*, 638–640, 639*f*–640*f*
  epidural, 75*f*
  paraspinal, 72
Acetabular labral tears, 130, 137–138, 137*f*–138*f*
Achilles tendon
  foot, ankle, and calf, 307–308, 307*f*–308*f*
  infected anchor with osteomyelitis, 630*f*
Achondroplasia, 765–766, 765*f*–766*f*
ACL. *See* Anterior cruciate ligament
Acromegaly, 732, 732*f*
Acromioclavicular dislocation, shoulder and arm,
  378–380, 378*t*, 378*f*–380*f*
Actinomycosis, 621*t*, 643
Acute disseminated encephalomyelitis (ADEM),
  92, 93*f*
Acute inflammatory demyelinating polyneuropathy
  (AIDP), 92, 95*f*
Acute pyogenic osteomyelitis, 622
Adamantinoma, 329, 576, 576*f*
ADEM (acute disseminated encephalomyelitis),
  92, 93*f*
Adhesive capsulitis (frozen shoulder), 419–421,
  419*f*–421*f*
Adult hemoglobin (HbA), 785
AIDP (acute inflammatory demyelinating
  polyneuropathy), 92, 95*f*
AKA supinator syndrome, 472
Albright–McCune, 555
ALL (anterolateral ligament), knee, 189
Aluminum intoxication, 783
Alveolar sarcoma, 151*t*
Amyloid arthropathy, 705–706, 705*f*–706*f*
Amyloidosis, 705*f*–706*f*, 716*t*
Anemias. *See* Hemoglobinopathies/anemias
Aneurysmal bone cyst, 84*f*, 329, 330*f*, 553–554, 554*f*
  hand and wrist, 514*t*
  knee, 249*t*
Ankle fractures. *See also* Foot, ankle, and calf
  adult, 268, 268*f*
    complications, 278, 278*f*
    plafond fractures (pilon), 277, 277*f*
    pronation lateral rotation injuries, 275–276,
      275*f*–276*f*
    pronation–abduction injuries, 273–274, 273*f*–274*f*
    supination lateral rotation injuries, 271–272,
      271*f*–272*f*

    supination–adduction injuries, 269–270,
      269*f*–270*f*
  pediatric, 260–261, 260*f*–261*f*
    complications, 266–267, 267*f*
    juvenile Tillaux, 264–265, 264*f*–265*f*
    Salter–Harris classification, 260, 260*f*–261*f*
    triplane fractures, 262–263, 262*f*–263*f*
Ankylosing spondylitis, 76, 76*f*, 156*t*, 160*t*, 670–672,
  671*f*–672*f*
  foot, ankle, and calf, 339, 339*f*
  knee, 244
Anterior cruciate ligament (ACL)
  chronic tears, 214, 214*f*
  knee, 189, 193*f*
  primary features, 210–211, 210*f*–211*f*
  secondary features, 212–213, 212*f*–213*f*
Anterior disc displacement, temporomandibular
  joint, 4–7, 4*f*–7*f*
Anterior impingement syndrome, 325
Anterior inferior body fracture, 28*t*, 31*f*
Anterior labroligamentous periosteal sleeve
  avulsion, 408
Anterior wedge fracture, 45
Anterolateral impingement syndrome, 325
Anterolateral ligament (ALL), knee, 189
Anteromedial impingement syndrome, 325
Anteroposterior (AP) compression injury, of pelvis,
  110, 112*f*–113*f*
Anticonvulsive therapy, 716*t*
Aplasia, 367–368, 367*f*–368*f*
Arnold–Chiari malformation childhood, 103
Arthropathies, 155, 155*t*
  and connective tissue diseases
    amyloid arthropathy, 705–706, 705*f*–706*f*
    ankylosing spondylitis, 670–672, 671*f*–672*f*
    calcium pyrophosphate deposition disease,
      695–696, 695*f*–696*f*
    dermatomyositis/polymyositis, 681–682,
      681*f*–682*f*
    enteric arthropathies, 677–678, 678*f*
    gout, 690–692, 690*f*–692*f*
    hemochromatosis, 693–694, 693*f*–694*f*
    hemophilia, 688–689, 688*f*–689*f*
    juvenile chronic arthropathy, 685–687, 685*f*–687*f*
    mixed, 683–684, 683*f*–684*f*
    neurotrophic, 699–701, 699*f*–701*f*
    ochronosis, 698, 698*f*
    osteoarthritis, 673–676, 674*f*–676*f*
    pigmented villonodular synovitis, 704, 704*f*

Arthropathies (*continued*)
  psoriatic arthritis, 666–667, 666*f*–667*f*
  reactive arthritis, 668–669, 668*f*–669*f*
  rheumatoid arthritis, 662–665, 663*f*–665*f*
  scleroderma, 680, 680*f*
  synovial chondromatosis/osteochondromatosis, 702–703, 703*f*
  systemic lupus erythematosus, 679, 679*f*
  Wilson disease, 697, 697*f*
  elbow/forearm, 467–469, 467*f*–469*f*
  foot, ankle, and calf
    ankylosing spondylitis, 339, 339*f*
    calcium pyrophosphate deposition disease, 342, 342*f*
    gout, 341, 341*f*
    neurotrophic arthropathy, 340, 340*f*
    osteoarthritis (degenerative joint disease), 334, 334*f*
    psoriatic arthritis, 337, 337*f*
    reactive arthritis, 338, 338*f*
    rheumatoid arthritis, 335–336, 336*f*
  hand and wrist, 518–521, 518*t*, 519*f*–521*f*
    calcium pyrophosphate deposition disease, 518*t*
    gout, 518*t*
    osteoarthritis, 518*t*, 519*f*
    psoriatic arthritis, 518*t*, 521*f*
    rheumatoid arthritis, 518*t*, 519*f*–520*f*
  hip, 156–159, 156*t*, 157*f*–159*f*
    ankylosing spondylitis, 156*t*
    calcium pyrophosphate dihydrate deposition disease, 156*t*
    pigmented villonodular synovitis, 156*t*
    rheumatoid arthritis, 156*t*
    septic arthritis, 156*t*
    synovial chondromatosis, 156*t*
  inflammatory, shoulder and arm, 424–427, 424*f*–427*f*
  knee, 244–248, 245*f*–248*f*
    ankylosing spondylitis, 244
    calcium pyrophosphate deposition disease, 244
    hemophilia, 244
    juvenile chronic arthritis, 244
    osteoarthritis, 244
    pigmented villonodular synovitis, 244
    psoriatic arthritis, 244
    reiter arthritis, 244
    rheumatoid arthritis, 244
    septic arthritis, 244
  pelvis, hips and thighs
    collagen vascular diseases, 155*t*
    connective tissue diseases, 155*t*
    crystalline arthropathies, 155*t*
    infection, 155*t*
    juvenile chronic arthritis, 155*t*
    Paget disease, 155*t*
    pigmented villonodular synovitis, 155*t*
    posttraumatic arthritis, 155*t*
    rheumatoid arthritis, 155*t*
    seronegative spondyloarthropathies, 155*t*
    synovial chondromatosis, 155*t*
  sacroiliac joints, 160–161, 160*t*, 160*f*–161*f*
    ankylosing spondylitis, 160*t*
    infection, 160*t*
    inflammatory bowel, 160*t*
    psoriatic arthritis, 160*t*
    reactive arthritis, 160*t*
    rheumatoid arthritis, 160*t*
  spine, 76–79, 76*f*–79*f*
  temporomandibular joint, 11–12, 12*f*
Arthroscopy, for knee, 203
Aspiration/biopsy, musculoskeletal infections, 621
Astrocytoma, 88
Atlanto-occipital fracture dislocations, of cervical spine, 21, 21*f*
Atlantoaxial dislocations, of cervical spine, 25–27, 25*f*–27*f*
Atypical mycobacterial infections, 621*t*, 641–642, 641*f*–642*f*
Avascular necrosis (AVN), 143–146, 143*t*, 144*f*–146*f*
  hand and wrist, 522–523, 522*f*–523*f*
  pelvis, hips and thighs, 123
  stages, 143*t*
Avulsion fractures
  hip, 126, 126*f*
  pelvis, 107
Axial compression injuries, of cervical spine, 16*t*
Axial osteomalacia, 716*t*

B
Bacterial infections
  gram-negative bacilli
    brucella, 621*t*
    coliform, 621*t*
    haemophilus, 621*t*
    klebsiella, 621*t*
    proteus, 621*t*
    pseudomonas, 621*t*
    salmonella, 621*t*
  gram-positive
    gonococcal, 621*t*
    meningococcal, 621*t*
    staphylococcal, 621*t*
    streptococcal, 621*t*
  higher, fungal and. *See* Fungal infections, higher bacterial infections
  mycobacteria, 621*t*
    atypical mycobacteria, 621*t*
    tuberculosis, 621*t*
Bankart lesions, 408
Barton fracture, 481–482, 481*f*–482*f*
Battered child syndrome (nonaccidental trauma), 796–797, 796*f*–797*f*
Benign nerve sheath tumors, 151*t*
Benign notochordal cell tumor (BNCT), 80, 86*f*
Benign peripheral nerve sheath tumor, 594–596, 594*f*–596*f*
Benign vascular tumors, 514*t*

Bennett fracture, 498*f*
Bertolotti syndrome, 105
Biceps tendon
    elbow/forearm, 455–456, 455*f*–456*f*
    shoulder and arm, 416–418, 416*f*–418*f*
Biliary atresia, 716*t*
Bipartite patella, knee, 179, 179*f*
Blastomycosis, 643
Blount disease, 242, 242*f*
BNCT (benign notochordal cell tumor), 80, 86*f*
Body, head, process fractures, 281–282, 281*f*–282*f*
Bone cyst. *See specific bone cysts*
Bone infarcts, 147, 147*f*
Bone islands (enostosis), 736–737, 736*f*–737*f*
Bone lesions, spine, 80–86, 81*f*–86*f*
Bone marrow
    basic concepts, 645–646, 646*f*
    compression fractures, 661, 661*f*
    edema, 148, 148*f*
    hyperlipoproteinemias, 657–658, 657*f*–658*f*
    infiltration
        basic concepts, 652, 652*t*
        Erdheim–Chester disease, 652*t*, 655–656,
            655*f*–656*f*
        Langerhans cell, 652*t*, 654, 654*f*
        leukemia, 652*t*
        lipidosis, 652*t*, 653, 653*f*
        lymphoma, 652*t*
        myelofibrosis, 652*t*
        myeloma, 652*t*
        neoplasms, 652*t*
    ischemia, 650–651, 650*f*–651*f*
    myelofibrosis, 659–660, 659*f*–660*f*
    myeloid depletion, 648–649, 648*f*–649*f*
    reconversion, 647, 647*f*
Bowstring sign, 509
Brachial plexus, shoulder and arm, 434–435,
    434*f*–435*f*
Bradydactyly, 367, 368*f*
Brodie abscess, 620*t*, 638–640, 639*f*–640*f*
Brucella infection, 621*t*
Buford complex, 415
Bursitis, 130, 133–134, 133*f*–134*f*
    foot, ankle, and calf, 317–318, 317*f*–318*f*
    knee, 255–256, 255*t*, 255*f*–256*f*
Burst fractures
    cervical spine, 35, 35*t*
    thoracolumbar spine, 42
        vertical compression injuries, 48, 48*f*–49*f*
Butterfly vertebra, 105, 105*f*

C
C1 fractures, of cervical spine, 22–24, 23*f*–24*f*
C2 fractures, of cervical spine, 28–31, 28*t*, 29*f*–31*f*
Calcaneal fractures
    extra-articular, 289–290, 289*f*–290*f*
    intra-articular, 287–288, 287*f*–288*f*
Calcinosis universalis, 780*t*

Calcium pyrophosphate deposition disease (CPPD),
    695–696, 695*f*–696*f*
    foot, ankle, and calf, 342, 342*f*
    hand and wrist, 518*t*
Calvarium, Paget disease of, 734*f*
Canadian C-Spine Rule, 14, 15*t*
Capitate fracture, 492*f*
Capitellar fractures, 444, 444*f*
Carpal and carpometacarpal dislocations, 494–496,
    495*f*–496*f*
Carpal fracture, 492–493, 492*f*–493*f*
Carpal instability, hand and wrist, 503–505, 504*f*–505*f*
Carpal tunnel syndrome, 524–525, 524*f*–525*f*
Caudal regression syndrome, 102, 102*f*
Celiac disease, 716*t*
Cerebral palsy, 362
Cervical spine
    atlanto-occipital fracture dislocations, 21, 21*f*
    atlantoaxial dislocations, 25–27, 25*f*–27*f*
    axial compression injuries, 16*t*
    C1 fractures, 22–24, 23*f*–24*f*
    C2 fractures, 28–31, 28*t*, 29*f*–31*f*
    Canadian C-Spine Rule, 14, 15*t*
    compressive hyperextension injuries, 16*t*, 18*f*
    compressive hyperflexion injuries, 16*t*, 17*f*
    disruptive hyperextension injuries, 16*t*, 18*f*
    disruptive hyperflexion injuries, 16*t*, 17*f*
    flexion–rotation injuries, 16*t*, 19*f*
    injuries not clinically significant, 16*t*
    instability, 20*f*
    lateral flexion injuries, 16*t*
    National Emergency X-Radiography Utilization
        Study, 14, 15*t*
    shearing injuries, 16*t*
    subluxation, fracture/dislocation, 38–41, 38*f*–41*f*
    vertebral arch fractures, 32–33, 32*f*–33*f*
    vertebral body fractures, 35–37, 35*t*, 35*f*–37*f*
    vertical compression injuries, 19*f*–20*f*
Chauffeur's fracture, 483, 483*f*
Chiari malformation, 103–104, 103*f*–104*f*
Chip fractures, of cervical spine, 35*t*
Chondroblastoma, 329, 545, 545*f*
    hand and wrist, 514*t*
    knee, 249*t*
    pelvis, hips and thighs, 151*t*
    shoulder and arm, 430
Chondroma
    elbow/forearm, 463*t*
    knee, 249*t*
    pelvis, hips and thighs, 151*t*
    shoulder and arm, 430
Chondromalacia patella, 232, 232*t*, 233*f*
Chondromyxoid fibroma, 329, 547–548, 547*f*–548*f*
    elbow/forearm, 463*t*
    hand and wrist, 514*t*
    knee, 249*t*
Chondrosarcoma, 329
    elbow/forearm, 463*t*
    hand and wrist, 514*t*

Chondrosarcoma (*continued*)
  knee, 249*t*
  pelvis, hips and thighs, 151*t*
  primary, central, 571–572, 572*f*
  secondary, 573–574, 573*f*–574*f*
Chordoma (sacrum), 151*t*
Chronic inflammatory demyelinating polyneuropathy
  (CIDP), 92, 96*f*
Chronic liver disease, 716*t*
  osteoporosis, 707*t*
Chronic osteomyelitis, 622
Chronic overuse/miscellaneous conditions, knee
  bursitis, 255–256, 255*t*, 255*f*–256*f*
  iliotibial band syndrome, 257, 257*f*
  muscle tears, 258–259, 258*f*–259*f*
Chronic recurrent multifocal osteomyelitis (CRMO),
  620*t*, 626–627, 627*f*
CIDP (chronic inflammatory demyelinating
  polyneuropathy), 92, 96*f*
Clavicle fractures, shoulder and arm, 383–384,
  383*f*–384*f*
Cleidocranial dysostosis, 743, 743*f*
Cleidocranial dysplasia, 743, 743*f*
Cloaca, 620*t*
Coccidioidomycosis, 621*t*, 643
Coliform infection, 621*t*
Collagen vascular diseases, 155*t*
  soft tissue calcification and, 780*t*
Colles fracture, 476–479, 477*f*–479*f*
Complex regional pain syndrome (CRPS). *See* Reflex
  sympathetic dystrophy
Compression fractures
  in bone marrow, 661, 661*f*
  of cervical spine, 35*t*
Compressive hyperextension injuries, of cervical
  spine, 16*t*, 18*f*
Compressive hyperflexion injuries, of cervical spine,
  16*t*, 17*f*
Computed tomography (CT)
  arthropathies
    amyloid arthropathy, 705*f*–706*f*
    ankylosing spondylitis, 671*f*–672*f*
    enteric arthropathies, 678*f*
    gout, 690, 691*f*
    synovial chondromatosis, 702, 703*f*
  bone tumors/tumorlike conditions, 530, 533*f*
    adamantinoma, 576
    aneurysmal bone cyst, 553
    chondroblastoma, 545
    chondromyxoid fibroma, 547, 547*f*–548*f*
    chondrosarcoma, 571, 573
    enchondroma, 542, 542*f*–543*f*
    eosinophilic granuloma/langerhans cell
      histiocytosis, 559, 560*f*
    Ewing sarcoma, 570
    fibrosarcoma and malignant fibrous
      histiocytoma, 575, 575*f*
    fibrous dysplasia, 555
    giant cell tumor, 557, 558*f*
    lymphoma, 581

    metastasis, 578
    myeloma, 579, 580*f*
    nonossifying fibroma, 549
    osteoblastoma, 538, 538*f*–539*f*
    osteochondroma, 540, 541*f*
    osteoid osteoma, 536, 536*f*–537*f*
    osteosarcoma, 561
    Paget sarcoma, 577
    parosteal osteosarcoma, 563, 563*f*–564*f*
    periosteal osteosarcoma, 565
    solitary bone cyst, 551
    telangiectatic osteosarcoma, 568
  Brodie abscess, 638, 639*f*
  chronic recurrent multifocal osteomyelitis, 626
  elbow/forearm
    bone tumors, 463
    capitellar fractures, 444
    coronoid fractures, 448
    distal humeral fractures, 436, 439, 442*f*–443*f*
    elbow dislocations, 449
    proximal radius fractures, 445, 446*f*
  foot, ankle, and calf
    body, head, process fractures, 281, 282*f*
    calcium pyrophosphate deposition disease,
      342, 342*f*
    complications, 266
    extra-articular calcaneal fractures, 289, 289*f*
    gout, 341
    impingement syndromes, 325
    intra-articular calcaneal fractures, 287, 288*f*
    midfoot and forefoot syndromes, 328*f*
    midfoot injuries, 292*f*–293*f*
    osteomyelitis, 343, 344*f*
    plafond fractures (pilon), 277
    sinus tarsi syndrome, 323
    skeletal lesions-benign, 329, 331*f*
    soft tissue infection, 345
    talar and subtalar dislocations, 285
    talar dome fractures, 283
    tarsal coalitions, 365, 365*f*–366*f*
    tarsal tunnel syndrome, 321
    triplane fracture, 262, 263*f*
  hand and wrist
    bone tumors, 514
    carpal and carpometacarpal dislocations, 494
    Colles fracture, 476, 478*f*
    distal radioulnar joint subluxation/
      dislocations, 486
    metacarpal fractures, 497
    other carpal fractures, 492
    phalangeal fractures/dislocations, 501
    scaphoid fractures, 487, 490*f*
  knee
    bone tumors, 249
    iliotibial band syndrome, 257
    intra-articular fracture, 194*f*
    osteochondral fractures, 178
    patellar tracking and instability, 230
    proximal tibial fractures, 186
  musculoskeletal infections, 621

neurofibromatosis, 751*f*
nonaccidental trauma, 796*f*–797*f*
osteomyelitis, 622
osteoporosis, 708
pelvis, hips, and thighs
    acetabular fractures, complex, 115, 115*f*–117*f*
    bursitis, 133
    developmental dysplasia of the hip, pediatric,
        167, 170*f*
    femoral anteversion, 176
    fracture/dislocation, 121, 122*f*
    insufficiency fractures, 128
    neoplasms, 151, 152*f*–153*f*
    pelvic fractures, complex, 110
    slipped capital femoral epiphysis, 171
    soft tissue trauma, 131
shoulder and arm
    biceps tendon, 416
    brachial plexus, 434
    impingement, 393
    neoplasms, 430
    posterior instability, 413
    scapular fractures, 388, 388*f*
    sternoclavicular dislocations, 381, 381*f*–382*f*
soft tissue
    infection, 635, 635*f*
    masses. *See* Soft tissue, masses
spine
    bone lesions, spinal, 80
    cervical, trauma, 14, 32*f*–33*f*, 36*f*, 40*f*
    disc herniation, 66, 70*f*
    dorsal arachnoid web, 97, 98*f*
    infection, spinal, 72
    scoliosis, 60
    segmentation anomalies, spinal, 105*f*–106*f*
    spondylolysis/spondylolisthesis, 54, 57*f*
    thoracolumbar, trauma, 42, 45, 47, 47*f*, 48, 49*f*,
        50, 51
synovitis, acne, pustulosis, hyperostosis, osteitis,
    628, 628*f*
temporomandibular joint, 12*f*
    osteoarthritis, 10, 10*f*
tuberous sclerosis, 747*f*–748*f*
tumoral calcinosis, 782
Computed tomography (CT) arthrography
hand and wrist, ligament injuries, 506, 507*f*–508*f*
shoulder and arm
    adhesive capsulitis, 419
    rotator cuff tears, full thickness tears, 395,
        396*f*–397*f*
Congenital anomalies, spinal, 99
caudal regression syndrome, 102, 102*f*
Chiari malformation, 103–104, 103*f*–104*f*
segmentation anomalies, 105–106, 105*f*–106*f*
spinal dysraphism, 99–101, 100*f*–101*f*
Congenital rubella, 716*t*
Congenital scoliosis, 59, 59*t*
Congenital vertical talus, 363, 363*f*
Connective tissue diseases, 155*t*
dermatomyositis/polymyositis, 681–682, 681*f*–682*f*

mixed, 683–684, 683*f*–684*f*
pigmented villonodular synovitis, 704, 704*f*
scleroderma, 680, 680*f*
systemic lupus erythematosus, 679, 679*f*
Cooley anemia. *See* Thalassemia
Copper deficiency, 783
Coronoid fractures, 448, 448*f*
Coxa valga, 174–175, 174*f*–175*f*
Coxa vara, 174–175, 174*f*–175*f*
CPPD. *See* Calcium pyrophosphate deposition disease
CRMO (chronic recurrent multifocal osteomyelitis),
    620*t*, 626–627, 627*f*
Crohn disease, 716*t*
Cruciate ligaments. *See* Anterior cruciate ligament
    (ACL); Posterior cruciate ligament (PCL)
Cryptococcosis, 621*t*, 643
Crystalline arthropathies, 155*t*
CT. *See* Computed tomography
CT arthrography. *See* Computed tomography (CT)
    arthrography
Cysticercosis, 621*t*

D

De Quervain tenosynovitis, 512–513, 512*f*–513*f*
Deep fibromatosis (desmoid tumor), 599–600,
    599*f*–600*f*
Degenerative disc disease, 63–65, 64*f*–65*f*
Degenerative joint disease. *See* Osteoarthritis
Dermatomyositis
    polymyositis, 681–682, 681*f*–682*f*
    soft tissue calcification and, 780*t*
Desmoid tumors
    musculoskeletal neoplasms, 599–600, 599*f*–600*f*
    pelvis, hips and thighs, 151*t*
Developmental dysplasia of the hip, 167–170,
    167*f*–170*f*
Diabetic foot infection, 348–349, 348*t*, 349*f*
Diastematomyelia, 99, 100*f*, 362
Dietary calcium and phosphate deficiency, 716*t*
Diffuse idiopathic skeletal hyperostosis (DISH), 76,
    78*f*, 793–794, 794*f*
Disc herniation, 66–70, 66*f*–70*f*
Discitis, early and late, 72*f*–73*f*
Discoid menisci, 206–207, 207*f*
DISH (diffuse idiopathic skeletal hyperostosis), 76, 78*f*,
    793–794, 794*f*
DISI (dorsal intercalated segment instability),
    503, 504*f*
Dislocations
    cervical spine, 38–41, 38*f*–41*f*
    elbow, 449, 449*f*
    hand and wrist
        carpal and carpometacarpal, 494–496, 495*f*–496*f*
        distal radioulnar joint subluxation/dislocations,
          486, 486*f*
        phalangeal, 501–502, 501*f*–502*f*
    metatarsophalangeal, 296–297, 296*f*–297*f*
    pelvis, hips and thighs, 121–122, 121*f*–122*f*
    shoulder and arm

Dislocations (*continued*)
  acromioclavicular, 378–380, 378*t*, 378*f*–380*f*
  glenohumeral, 374–377, 374*f*–377*f*
  posttraumatic osteolysis, 385–387, 385*f*–387*f*
  sternoclavicular, 381–382, 381*f*–382*f*
  talar and subtalar, 285–286, 286*f*
Disruptive hyperextension injuries, of cervical spine, 16*t*, 18*f*
Disruptive hyperflexion injuries, of cervical spine, 16*t*, 17*f*
Distal humeral fractures
  adult, 439–443, 439*f*–443*f*
  children, 436–437, 436*f*–437*f*
Distal radioulnar joint subluxation/dislocations, 486, 486*f*
Distal radius/ulnar fractures, hand and wrist
  Barton fracture, 481–482, 481*f*–482*f*
  Chauffeur's fracture, 483, 483*f*
  Colles fracture, 476–479, 477*f*–479*f*
  Smith fracture, 480, 480*f*
Distension arthrography, 419, 421*f*
Disuse osteoporosis, 707*t*, 713, 713*f*
Dorsal intercalated segment instability (DISI), 503, 504*f*
Dorsal thoracic arachnoid web, 97, 98*f*
Dual-energy X-ray absorptiometry (DXA), 708, 710*f*–712*f*
Dyschondrosteosis (Leri–Weill syndrome), 771–772, 772*f*

E
Echinococcosis, 621*t*
Echinococcus, 643
Edema, bone marrow, 148, 148*f*
Ehlers–Danlos syndrome, 762, 762*f*
Elastofibroma, 601–602, 601*f*–602*f*
Elbow and forearm
  arthropathies, 467–469, 467*f*–469*f*
  capitellar fractures, 444, 444*f*
  coronoid fractures, 448, 448*f*
  distal humeral fractures
    adult, 439–443, 439*f*–443*f*
    children, 436–437, 436*f*–437*f*
  elbow dislocations, 449, 449*f*
  epicondylar fractures, 438, 438*f*
  forearm fractures, 451–453, 451*f*–453*f*
  infection, 465–466, 465*f*–466*f*
  Monteggia fractures, 450, 450*f*
  neoplasms
    bone tumors, 463, 463*f*, 463*t*
    soft tissue tumors, 464, 464*f*
  nerve entrapment syndromes, 470–475, 470*f*–475*f*
  neurovascular anatomy, 473*f*
  osteochondritis dissecans, 454, 454*f*
  proximal radius fractures, 445–446, 445*f*–446*f*
  soft tissue trauma
    biceps tendon, 455–456, 455*f*–456*f*
    flexor/extensor tendon injuries, 458–459, 458*f*–459*f*
    ligament injuries, 461–462, 461*f*–462*f*
    muscle injuries, 460, 460*f*
    triceps tendon injuries, 457, 457*f*
  ulnar fractures, 447, 447*f*

Enchondroma, 329, 542–544, 542*f*–544*f*
  hand and wrist, 514*t*
Enchondromatosis (Ollier disease), 753, 753*f*
Endocrine disorders, 707*t*
Engelmann disease (progressive diaphyseal dysplasia), 742, 742*f*
Enostosis, 736–737, 736*f*–737*f*
Enteric arthropathies, 677–678, 678*f*
Environmental factors, for osteoporosis, 707*t*
Eosinophilic granuloma. *See* Unifocal Langerhans cell histiocytosis
Ependymoma, 88, 91*f*
Epicondylar fractures, 438, 438*f*
Epidural abscess, 75*f*
Epiphyseal dysplasias, 757–759, 757*f*–759*f*
Epithelioid sarcoma, 151*t*
Erdheim–Chester disease, 652*t*, 655–656, 655*f*–656*f*
Erosive osteoarthritis, 673, 676*f*
Erythema, 348*t*
Ewing sarcoma, 329, 331*f*, 570, 570*f*
  elbow/forearm, 463*t*
  hand and wrist, 514*t*
  knee, 249*t*
  pelvis, hips and thighs, 151*t*
  shoulder and arm, 430
Excessive lateral pressure syndrome, 230
Extra-articular calcaneal fractures, 289–290, 289*f*–290*f*
Extradural tumors, 88, 88*t*

F
Fabry disease, 652*t*, 653
Facet fractures, of cervical spine, 32
Femoral anteversion, 176–177, 176*f*–177*f*
Femoral fractures, 186, 189
Femoral neck fracture, 123–125, 123*f*–125*f*
Femoroacetabular impingement, 139, 139*f*
Femur, Paget disease involving, 735*f*
Fetal hemoglobin (HbF), 785
Fibrosarcoma, 329, 575, 575*f*
  elbow/forearm, 463*t*
  hand and wrist, 514*t*
  knee, 249*t*
  pelvis, hips and thighs, 151*t*
  shoulder and arm, 430
Fibrous defects, hand and wrist, 514*t*
Fibrous dysplasia, 329, 555–556, 555*f*–556*f*
Fifth metatarsal fractures, 294–295, 294*f*–295*f*
Fistula, 620*t*
  spinal dural arteriovenous, 97, 97*f*
  small bowel, 716*t*
Flexion–compression injury, of cervical spine, 35*f*
Flexion–distraction injury
  cervical spine, 38, 38*f*
  thoracolumbar spine, 45, 46*f*
Flexion–rotation injuries
  cervical spine, 16*t*, 19*f*
  thoracolumbar spine, 47, 47*f*
Flexor digitorum longus, 309
Flexor hallucis longus tenosynovitis, 309

Flexor tenosynovitis, 509*f*
Flexor/extensor tendon injuries, 458–459, 458*f*–459*f*
Foot, ankle, and calf
  arthritis
    ankylosing spondylitis, 339, 339*f*
    calcium pyrophosphate deposition disease,
      342, 342*f*
    gout, 341, 341*f*
    neurotrophic arthropathy, 340, 340*f*
    osteoarthritis (degenerative joint disease),
      334, 334*f*
    psoriatic arthritis, 337, 337*f*
    reactive arthritis, 338, 338*f*
    rheumatoid arthritis, 335–336, 336*f*
  fractures
    ankle. *See* Ankle fractures
    calcaneal. *See* Calcaneal fractures
    forefoot injuries. *See* Forefoot, injuries
    midfoot injuries, 291–293, 291*f*–293*f*
    stress fractures, 298–300, 298*t*, 298*f*–300*f*
    talar, 279–284, 279*f*–284*f*
  infection
    diabetic foot, 348–349, 348*t*, 349*f*
    joint space, 346–347, 346*f*–347*f*
    osteomyelitis, 343–344, 344*f*
    soft tissue, 345, 345*f*
  neoplasms
    skeletal lesions, benign, 329–331, 330*f*–331*f*
    soft tissue lesions, benign, 332–333, 332*f*–333*f*
  pediatric disorders
    congenital vertical talus, 363, 363*f*
    forefoot abnormalities, 360–361, 360*f*–361*f*
    Freiberg infraction, 369, 369*f*
    hindfoot abnormalities, 354–357, 355*f*–357*f*
    Köhler disease, 370–371, 371*f*
    normal angles of the foot and ankle, 351–353,
      351*f*–353*f*
    overgrowth/hypoplasia/aplasia, 367–368,
      367*f*–368*f*
    pes planovalgus, 364, 364*f*
    plantar arch abnormalities, 358–359, 358*f*–359*f*
    talipes equinovarus, 362, 362*f*
    tarsal coalitions, 365–366, 365*f*–366*f*
    terminology, 350
  soft tissue trauma
    Achilles tendon, 307–308, 307*f*–308*f*
    anterior tendon injuries, 312–313, 312*f*–313*f*
    bursitis, 317–318, 317*f*–318*f*
    impingement syndromes, 325–326, 325*f*–326*f*
    ligament injuries, 301–303, 301*t*, 301*f*–303*f*
    medial tendon injuries, 309–311, 309*f*–311*f*
    midfoot and forefoot syndromes, 327–328, 327*t*,
      327*f*–328*f*
    os trigonum syndrome, 319–320, 319*f*–320*f*
    peroneal tendon injuries, 304–306, 304*f*–306*f*
    plantar fasciitis, 314–316, 314*f*–316*f*
    sinus tarsi syndrome, 323–324, 323*f*–324*f*
    tarsal tunnel syndrome, 321–322, 321*t*, 322*f*
Forearm. *See* Elbow and forearm

Forefoot
  abnormalities, 360–361, 360*f*–361*f*
  injuries
    fifth metatarsal fractures, 294–295, 294*f*–295*f*
    metatarsophalangeal fracture/dislocations,
      296–297, 296*f*–297*f*
Fracture(s)
  ankle. *See* Ankle fractures
  calcaneal
    extra-articular, 289–290, 289*f*–290*f*
    intra-articular, 287–288, 287*f*–288*f*
    causing tarsal tunnel syndrome, 321*t*
  cervical spine, 38–41, 38*f*–41*f*
    anterior inferior body, 28*t*, 31*f*
    atlanto-occipital, 21, 21*f*
    C1, 22–24, 23*f*–24*f*
    C2 fractures, 28–31, 28*t*, 29*f*–31*f*
    hangman's, 28, 28*t*, 30*f*
    isolated burst, 22
    Jefferson, 23*f*
    lamina, 28*t*
    odontoid, 28, 28*t*, 29*f*
    vertebral arch, 32–33, 32*f*–33*f*
    vertebral body, 35–37, 35*t*, 35*f*–37*f*
  elbow/forearm
    capitellar fractures, 444, 444*f*
    coronoid fractures, 448, 448*f*
    distal humeral fractures, 436–437, 436*f*–437*f*,
      439–443, 439*f*–443*f*
    epicondylar fractures, 438, 438*f*
    forearm fractures, 451–453, 451*f*–453*f*
    Monteggia fractures, 450, 450*f*
    osteochondritis dissecans, 454, 454*f*
    proximal radius fractures, 445–446, 445*f*–446*f*
    ulnar fractures, 447, 447*f*
  forefoot injuries
    fifth metatarsal fractures, 294–295, 294*f*–295*f*
    metatarsophalangeal fracture/dislocations,
      296–297, 296*f*–297*f*
  hand and wrist
    Barton, 481–482, 481*f*–482*f*
    carpal, 492–493, 492*f*–493*f*
    Chauffeur's, 483, 483*f*
    Colles, 476–479, 477*f*–479*f*
    Galeazzi, 484–485, 484*f*–485*f*
    metacarpal, 497–500, 498*f*–500*f*
    phalangeal, 501–502, 501*f*–502*f*
    scaphoid, 487–491, 488*f*–491*f*
    Smith, 480, 480*f*
  midfoot injuries, 291–293, 291*f*–293*f*
  pelvis, hips and thighs
    acetabular, 115–120, 115*f*–120*f*
    complex, 110–114, 111*f*–114*f*
    dislocation, 121–122, 121*f*–122*f*
    femoral neck, 123–125, 123*f*–125*f*
    insufficiency fractures, 128–129, 128*f*–129*f*
    minor, 107–108, 107*f*–108*f*
    single break in pelvic ring, 109, 109*f*
    trochanteric, 126–127

Fracture(s) (*continued*)
  shoulder and arm
    clavicle, 383–384, 383*f*–384*f*
    humeral shaft, 389–390, 389*f*–390*f*
    Neer classification, 372*t*
    proximal humeral, 372–373, 372*f*–373*f*
    scapular, 388, 388*f*
  stress, 298–300, 298*t*, 298*f*–300*f*
    calcaneus, 298*t*
    distal fibula, 298*t*
    distal tibia, 298*t*
    metatarsals, 298*t*
    sesamoids, 298*t*
    tarsals, 298*t*
  talar
    body, head, process fractures, 281–282, 281*f*–282*f*
    talar and subtalar dislocations, 285–286, 286*f*
    talar dome fractures, 283–284, 283*f*–284*f*
    talar neck, 279–280, 279*f*–280*f*
  thoracolumbar spine, 53, 53*f*
Freiberg infraction, 369, 369*f*
Frozen shoulder, 419–421, 419*f*–421*f*
Fungal infections, 643–644, 644*f*
  higher bacterial infections
    actinomycosis, 621*t*
    coccidioidomycosis, 621*t*
    cryptococcosis, 621*t*
    histoplasmosis, 621*t*
    nocardiosis, 621*t*
    sporotrichosis, 621*t*

G
Galeazzi fracture, 484–485, 484*f*–485*f*
"Gamekeeper's thumb," 506
Ganglion, 603, 603*f*
  cysts, 252
    causing tarsal tunnel syndrome, 321*t*, 322*f*
    peroneal tendon, 332*f*
Gangliosidosis, 652*t*, 653
Garré sclerosing osteomyelitis, 620*t*
Gaucher disease, 652*t*, 653, 653*f*
Giant cell tumor, 329
  elbow/forearm, 463*t*
  hand and wrist, 514*t*
  knee, 249*t*
  musculoskeletal neoplasms, 557–558, 557*f*–558*f*
  pelvis, hips and thighs, 151*t*
  shoulder and arm, 430
  tendon sheath, 605–606, 605*f*–606*f*
Gigantism, 732
Glenohumeral dislocation, shoulder and arm, 374–377, 374*f*–377*f*
Gonococcal infection, 621*t*
Gorham disease (massive osteolysis), 795, 795*f*
Gout
  arthropathy, 690–692, 690*f*–692*f*
  elbow/forearm, 469*f*
  foot, ankle, and calf, 341, 341*f*
  hand and wrist, 518*t*

Greater trochanteric pain syndrome, 135–136, 135*f*–136*f*
Guillain–Barré syndrome, 92

H
Haemophilus infection, 621*t*
Hallux rigidus, 327*t*
Hand and wrist
  arthropathies, 518–521, 518*t*, 519*f*–521*f*
  avascular necrosis, 522–523, 522*f*–523*f*
  carpal instability, 503–505, 504*f*–505*f*
  dislocations
    carpal and carpometacarpal, 494–496, 495*f*–496*f*
    distal radioulnar joint subluxation/dislocations, 486, 486*f*
    phalangeal, 501–502, 501*f*–502*f*
  fractures
    Barton, 481–482, 481*f*–482*f*
    carpal, 492–493, 492*f*–493*f*
    Chauffeur's, 483, 483*f*
    Colles, 476–479, 477*f*–479*f*
    Galeazzi, 484–485, 484*f*–485*f*
    metacarpal, 497–500, 498*f*–500*f*
    phalangeal, 501–502, 501*f*–502*f*
    scaphoid, 487–491, 488*f*–491*f*
    Smith, 480, 480*f*
  neoplasms
    bone tumors, 514–515, 514*t*, 515*f*
    soft tissue masses, 516–517, 516*f*–517*f*
  nerve compression syndromes
    carpal tunnel syndrome, 524–525, 524*f*–525*f*
    ulnar nerve compression, 526–527, 526*f*–527*f*
  soft tissue trauma
    de Quervain tenosynovitis and intersection syndrome, 512–513, 512*f*–513*f*
    ligament injuries, 506–508, 506*f*–508*f*
    tendon injuries, 509–510, 509*f*–510*f*
  ulnar lunate abutment syndrome, 528–529, 528*f*–529*f*
Hand–Schüller–Christian disease, 654
Hangman's fracture, of cervical spine, 28, 28*t*, 30*f*
HbA (adult hemoglobin), 785
HbF (fetal hemoglobin), 785
Heavy metal disorders, 783–784, 783*f*–784*f*
Hemangioblastomas, 88
Hemangioendothelial sarcoma, 329
Hemangioendothelioma, 514*t*
Hemangioma, 464*f*. *See also* Simple venous malformation
  pelvis, hips and thighs, 151*t*
  shoulder and arm, 430
  vertebral, 80, 83*f*
Hematoma, 607–610, 608*f*–610*f*
Hemochromatosis, 693–694, 693*f*–694*f*
Hemoglobin
  adult, 785
  fetal, 785

Hemoglobinopathies/anemias
  basic concepts, 785
  osteoporosis, 852*t*
  sickle cell anemia, 786–787, 786*f*–787*f*
  thalassemia, 788–789, 789*f*
Hemophilia, 244, 247*f*, 688–689, 688*f*–689*f*
Hereditary multiple exostosis, 755–756, 756*f*
Hindfoot
  abnormalities, 354–357, 355*f*–357*f*
  calcaneus, 354
  equinus, 354, 357*f*
  valgus, 354, 355*f*
  varus, 354, 356*f*
Hip. *See also* Pelvis, hips and thighs
  avascular necrosis of, 650*f*
  transient osteoporosis of, 714*f*
Histiocytosis, bone marrow
  Erdheim–Chester disease, 652*t*, 655–656, 655*f*–656*f*
  Langerhans cell, 652*t*, 654, 654*f*
Histiocytosis X. *See* Langerhans cell histiocytosis
Histoplasmosis, 621*t*, 643
Hookworms, 621*t*
HPT. *See* Hyperparathyroidism
Humeral osteochondral or ligament avulsions, shoulder and arm, 411–412, 412*f*
Humeral shaft fractures, shoulder and arm, 389–390, 389*f*–390*f*
Hunter syndrome, 768*t*
Hurler syndrome, 767, 768*t*, 769*f*
Hurler–Scheie syndrome, 768*t*
Hyperextension injuries
  cervical spine, 16*t*, 18*f*
  thoracolumbar spine, 50, 50*f*
Hyperflexion injuries
  cervical spine, 16*t*, 17*f*
  thoracolumbar spine, 45–46, 45*f*–46*f*
Hyperlipoproteinemias, 657–658, 657*f*–658*f*
Hyperparathyroidism (HPT), 722, 716*t*, 725–727, 725*f*–727*f*
  soft tissue calcification and, 780*t*
Hyperplasia, 647
Hyperthyroidism, 730
Hypertrophy of abductor hallucis muscle, 321*t*
Hypervitaminosis A, 775*t*, 777
Hypervitaminosis D, 780*t*
Hypoparathyroidism, 728–729, 729*f*
Hypophosphatasia, 716*t*
Hypophosphatemic (vitamin D resistant), 716t
Hypopituitarism, 732
Hypoplasia, 367–368, 367*f*–368*f*
Hypothyroidism, 730
Hypovitaminosis C, 778*f*–779*f*
Hypovitaminosis D, 780

I

Idiopathic osteoporosis, 707*t*
Idiopathic scoliosis, 59, 59*t*
Idiopathic transverse myelitis, 92
Iliopsoas bursa, 133

Iliotibial band syndrome, knee, 257, 257*f*
Impingement syndromes
  foot, ankle, and calf, 325–326, 325*f*–326*f*
  shoulder and arm, 393–394, 393*f*–394*f*
Infections
  arthropathies, 155*t*
  bacterial. *See* Bacterial infections
  elbow/forearm, 465–466, 465*f*–466*f*
  foot, ankle, and calf
    diabetic foot, 348–349, 348*t*, 349*f*
    joint space, 346–347, 346*f*–347*f*
    osteomyelitis, 343–344, 344*f*
    soft tissue, 345, 345*f*
  fungal. *See* Fungal infections
  musculoskeletal. *See* Musculoskeletal infections
  parasitic. *See* Parasitic infections
  pelvis, hips and thighs, 162, 162*f*
  sacroiliac joints, 160*t*
  in spinal, 72–75, 72*f*–75*f*
Infective osteitis, 620*t*
Infective periostitis, 620*t*
Infiltrative marrow disorders
  basic concepts, 652, 652*t*
  histiocytosis
    Erdheim–Chester disease, 652*t*, 655–656, 655*f*–656*f*
    Langerhans cell, 652*t*, 654, 654*f*
  leukemia, 652*t*
  lipidosis, 652*t*, 653, 653*f*
    Fabry disease, 652*t*, 653
    gangliosidosis, 652*t*, 653
    Gaucher disease, 652*t*, 653, 653*f*
    Niemann–Pick disease, 652*t*, 653
  lymphoma, 652*t*
  myelofibrosis, 652*t*
  myeloma, 652*t*
  neoplasms, 652*t*
Inflammatory arthropathies, 424–427, 424*f*–427*f*
Inflammatory bowel, 160*t*
Infrapatellar plica, knee, 226
Instability, shoulder and arm
  basic concepts, 405
  humeral osteochondral or ligament avulsions, 411–412, 412*f*
  labral tears, 408–410, 408*f*–410*f*
  labral variants, 415, 415*f*
  multidirectional, 414, 414*f*
  posterior, 413, 413*f*
  recurrent subluxation/dislocations, capsular abnormalities, 406–407, 406*f*–407*f*
Internal derangement, temporomandibular joint, 2–3, 3*f*
Intersection syndrome, 512–513, 512*f*–513*f*
Intertrochanteric fractures, of hip, 126, 127*f*
Intra-articular calcaneal fractures, 287–288, 287*f*–288*f*
Intradural extramedullary tumors, 88, 88*t*
Intradural intramedullary tumors, 88, 88*t*
Intraosseous nerve syndrome, 474*f*–475*f*
Involucrum, 620*t*

Ipsilateral fractures, 186
Ischemia, bone marrow, 650–651, 650*f*–651*f*
Ischial fractures, of pelvis, 107
Isolated burst fracture, of cervical spine, 22

J
Jefferson fracture, of cervical spine, 23*f*
Joint space infection, 632–633, 632*t*
 foot, ankle, and calf, 346–347, 346*f*–347*f*
 imaging approaches, 632*t*
 magnetic resonance features
  bone erosions, 632*t*
  bone marrow edema pattern, 632*t*
  fluid outpouching from capsule, 632*t*
  joint effusion, 632*t*
  synovial enhancement after contrast, 632*t*
  synovial thickening, 632*t*
Juvenile chronic arthritis, 155*t*
 knee, 244
 temporomandibular joint, 11
Juvenile chronic arthropathy, 685–687, 685*f*–687*f*
Juvenile Tillaux, 264–265, 264*f*–265*f*

K
Kienböck disease, 522
Klebsiella infection, 621*t*
Klippel–Feil anomalies, 103, 106*f*
Knee
 arthropathies, 244–258, 245*f*–248*f*
 bone marrow, 646*f*
 chronic overuse/miscellaneous conditions
  bursitis, 255–256, 255*t*, 255*f*–256*f*
  iliotibial band syndrome, 257, 257*f*
  muscle tears, 258–259, 258*f*–259*f*
 ligament and tendon injuries
  anterior cruciate ligament, acute, 210–214,
   210*f*–214*f*
  basic concepts, 208–209, 208*f*–209*f*
  medial and lateral collateral ligaments, 216–217,
   216*f*–217*f*
  patellar tendon, 220–221, 220*f*–221*f*
  posterior cruciate ligament, 215, 215*f*
  quadriceps tendon, 218–219, 218*f*–219*f*
 ligament and tendon reconstruction, 222–225,
  222*f*–225*f*
 loose bodies, 234–235, 234*f*–235*f*
 meniscal lesions
  discoid menisci, 206–207, 207*f*
  meniscal cysts, 205, 205*f*
  meniscal tears, 197–202, 197*f*–202*f*
  postoperative meniscus, 203–204, 203*f*–204*f*
 neoplasms
  bone tumors/tumorlike conditions, 249–251,
   249*t*, 250*f*–251*f*
  soft tissue tumors and masses, 252–254,
   252*f*–254*f*
 osteochondritis dissecans, 236–238, 236*t*, 236*f*–238*f*
 osteochondroses, 242–243, 242*f*–243*f*

 osteonecrosis, 239–241, 239*f*–241*f*
 patellar disorders
  chondromalacia patella, 232–233, 232*t*, 233*f*
  patellofemoral relationships, 228–229, 228*f*–229*f*
  tracking and instability, 230–231, 230*f*–231*f*
  plicae, 226–227, 226*f*–227*f*
 skeletal trauma
  miscellaneous fractures, 189–196, 189*f*–196*f*
  osteochondral fractures, 178, 178*f*
  patellar fractures, 179–181, 179*f*–181*f*
  proximal tibial fractures, 186–188, 186*f*–188*f*
  supracondylar fractures, 182–185, 182*f*–185*f*
Köhler disease, 370–371, 371*f*

L
Labral tears, shoulder and arm, 408–410, 408*f*–410*f*
Labral variants, shoulder and arm, 415, 415*f*
Lamina fractures, of cervical spine, 28*t*, 32
Langerhans cell histiocytosis, 559–560, 560*f*, 652*t*,
 654, 654*f*
Lateral collateral ligaments (LCL), 216, 216*f*–217*f*
Lateral compression injury, of pelvis, 110, 111*f*
Lateral disc displacement, 8, 8*f*
Lateral flexion injuries, of cervical spine, 16*t*
Lateral patella subluxation, 230
Lateral wedge fracture, of cervical spine, 35*t*, 45, 45*f*
Lateral–medial subluxation, 230
LCL (Lateral collateral ligaments), 216, 216*f*–217*f*
Lead intoxication, 783, 783*f*
Legg–Calvé–Perthes disease, 164–166, 164*f*–166*f*
Leri–Weill syndrome, 771–772, 772*f*
Letterer–Siwe disease, 654
Leukemia, bone marrow, 652*t*
Ligament injuries
 elbow/forearm, 461–462, 461*f*–462*f*
 foot, ankle, and calf, 301–303, 301*t*, 301*f*–303*f*
 hand and wrist, 506–508, 506*f*–508*f*
 knee
  anterior cruciate ligament, acute, 210–214,
   210*f*–214*f*
  basic concepts, 208–209, 208*f*–209*f*
  medial and lateral collateral ligaments, 216–217,
   216*f*–217*f*
  posterior cruciate ligament, 215, 215*f*
 pelvis, hips and thighs, 130
Lipidosis, bone marrow, 652*t*, 653, 653*f*
 Fabry disease, 652*t*, 653
 gangliosidosis, 652*t*, 653
 Gaucher disease, 652*t*, 653, 653*f*
 Niemann–Pick disease, 652*t*, 653
Lipoma, 583–584, 584*f*
 causing tarsal tunnel syndrome, 321*t*
 pelvis, hips and thighs, 151*t*
Liposarcoma, 585–587, 586*f*–587*f*
 pelvis, hips and thighs, 151*t*
Lippman–Cobb measurement, 60, 60*f*
Loose bodies, knee, 234–235, 234*f*–235*f*
Lumbar spine. *See* Thoracolumbar spine
Lymphoma, 329, 581–582, 582*f*

bone marrow, 652*t*
elbow/forearm, 463*t*
hand and wrist, 514*t*
knee, 249*t*
pelvis, hips and thighs, 151*t*
shoulder and arm, 430

M
Macrodactyly, 367, 367*f*
Maffucci syndrome, 754, 754*f*
Magnetic resonance (MR) arthrography
elbow/forearm
ligament injuries, 461
osteochondritis dissecans, 454
hand and wrist, 506, 507*f*–508*f*
pelvis, hips and thighs
acetabular labral tears, 137, 137*f*–138*f*
femoroacetabular impingement, 139, 139*f*
shoulder and arm
adhesive capsulitis, 419, 419*f*–420*f*
humeral osteochondral or ligament avulsions, 411, 412*f*
inflammatory arthropathies, 424, 424*f*–427*f*
labral tears, 408, 408*f*, 410*f*
multidirectional instability, 414*f*
posterior instability, 413, 414*f*
recurrent subluxation/dislocations, capsular abnormalities, 406, 407*f*
rotator cuff tears, 395, 404*f*
Magnetic resonance imaging (MRI)
arthropathies
amyloid arthropathy, 705, 705*f*–706*f*
dermatomyositis/polymyositis, 681, 682*f*
gout, 692*f*
neurotrophic arthropathy, 700*f*–701*f*
pigmented villonodular synovitis, 704
rheumatoid arthritis, 662, 665*f*
synovial chondromatosis, 702, 703*f*
bone islands (enostosis), 736
bone marrow, 645, 647
compression fractures, 661
hyperlipoproteinemias, 657*f*
infiltration, 652
ischemia, 650, 650*f*–651*f*
myelofibrosis, 659, 660*f*
Brodie abscess, 638, 640*f*
elbow/forearm
arthropathies, 467, 468*f*
biceps tendon, 455, 455*f*–456*f*
bone tumors, 463
capitellar fractures, 444
distal humeral fractures, children, 436
epicondylar fractures, 438
flexor/extensor tendon injuries, 458, 458*f*–549*f*
infection, 465, 466*f*
ligament injuries, 461, 461*f*–462*f*
muscle injuries, 460
nerve entrapment syndromes, 474*f*–475*f*
osteochondritis dissecans, 454

proximal radius fractures, 445
soft tissue tumors, 464, 464*f*
triceps tendon injuries, 457, 457*f*
foot, ankle, and calf
Achilles tendon, 307, 308*f*
anterior tendon injuries, 312, 313*f*
bursitis, 317
complications, 266
diabetic foot infections, 348*t*
impingement syndromes, 325
joint space infection, 346
ligament injuries, 301*t*, 303*f*
medial tendon injuries, 309, 311*f*
neurotrophic arthropathy, 340
os trigonum syndrome, 319, 320*f*
osteomyelitis, 343, 344*f*
plafond fractures (pilon), 277
sinus tarsi syndrome, 323
skeletal lesions-benign, 329
soft tissue infection, 345, 345*f*
soft tissue lesions, benign, 332
stress fractures, 298, 298*f*–299*f*
talar dome fractures, 283
talipes equinovarus, 362
tarsal coalitions, 365
tarsal tunnel syndrome, 321
hand and wrist
arthropathies, 518
avascular necrosis, 522, 523*f*
bone tumors, 514
carpal tunnel syndrome, 524, 525*f*
distal radioulnar joint subluxation/dislocations, 486
ligament injuries, 506
other carpal fractures, 492
scaphoid fractures, 487, 490*f*–491*f*
soft tissue masses, 516
tendon injuries, 509
ulnar lunate abutment syndrome, 528, 529*f*
ulnar nerve compression, 526
joint space infection, 632, 633*f*
knee
anterior cruciate ligament, acute, 210
bone tumors, 249
chondromalacia patella, 232
iliotibial band syndrome, 257
ligament and tendon reconstruction, 222
meniscal cysts, 205
meniscal tears, 197, 199*f*
osteochondral fractures, 178
osteochondritis dissecans, 237*f*–238*f*
osteonecrosis, 239
patellar tracking and instability, 230
proximal tibial fractures, 186
soft tissue tumors and masses, 252
musculoskeletal infections, 621
neurofibromatosis, 752*f*
osteomyelitis, 622, 624*f*
violated tissue, 630, 630*f*–631*f*
Paget disease, 733
pelvis, hips, and thighs

Magnetic resonance imaging (MRI) (*continued*)
    bone marrow edema, 148, 148*f*
    bursitis, 133
    developmental dysplasia of the hip, pediatric, 167, 169*f*
    femoral anteversion, 176, 176*f*–177*f*
    greater trochanteric pain syndrome, 135
    infection, 162
    insufficiency fractures, 128, 128*f*–129*f*
    Legg–Calvé–Perthes disease, 164
    neoplasms, 151, 152*f*–153*f*
    osteonecrosis, 141*f*, 143, 144*f*–146*f*, 147, 147*f*
    single break in pelvic ring, 109
    slipped capital femoral epiphysis, 171, 173*f*
    soft tissue trauma, 131
    transient osteoporosis of hip, 149, 149*f*–150*f*
  sarcoidosis, 792*f*
  shoulder and arm
    biceps tendon, 416, 416*f*–418*f*
    brachial plexus, 434, 435*f*
    glenohumeral dislocation, 376*f*
    humeral osteochondral or ligament avulsions, 411
    impingement, 393, 394*f*
    inflammatory arthropathies, 424, 424*f*–427*f*
    labral tears, 408
    labral variants, 415*f*
    neoplasms, 430, 430*f*–433*f*
    nerve entrapment syndromes, 422, 422*f*–423*f*
    osteonecrosis, 428, 428*f*–429*f*
    postoperative changes, 403
    posttraumatic osteolysis, 385, 387*f*
    recurrent subluxation/dislocations, capsular abnormalities, 406, 406*f*
    rotator cuff tears, full thickness tears, 395, 398*f*, 399, 400*f*
    tendinosis, 401, 402*f*
  soft tissue
    infection, 635
    masses. *See* Soft tissue, masses
  spine
    bone lesions, spinal, 80
    caudal regression syndrome, 102, 102*f*
    Chiari malformation, 103, 103*f*–104*f*
    degenerative disc disease, 63, 64*f*–65*f*
    disc herniation, 66, 67*f*–69*f*
    dorsal arachnoid web, 97, 98*f*
    infection, spinal, 72
    neuromyelitis optica spectrum disorder, 92
    scoliosis, 60
    segmentation anomalies, spinal, 105, 105*f*–106*f*
    spinal dural arteriovenous fistula, 97, 97*f*
    spinal dysraphism, 100*f*–101*f*
    spondylolysis/spondylolisthesis, 54, 58*f*
    thoracolumbar, trauma, 42, 48, 51
  synovitis, acne, pustulosis, hyperostosis, osteitis, 628
  temporomandibular joint
    lateral and medial disc displacement, 8, 8*f*
    osteoarthritis, 10, 10*f*
    rheumatoid arthritis, 11, 11*f*

  tuberculosis/atypical mycobacterial infections, 641, 641*f*–642*f*
tuberous sclerosis, 748*f*
tumors/tumorlike conditions
  adamantinoma, 576, 576*f*
  aneurysmal bone cyst, 553, 554*f*
  chondroblastoma, 545, 545*f*
  chondromyxoid fibroma, 547, 547*f*–548*f*
  chondrosarcoma, 571, 572*f*
  enchondroma, 542, 542*f*–544*f*
  eosinophilic granuloma/langerhans cell histiocytosis, 559, 560*f*
  Ewing sarcoma, 570, 570*f*
  fibrosarcoma and malignant fibrous histiocytoma, 575
  fibrous dysplasia, 555, 556*f*
  giant cell tumor, 557, 557*f*–558*f*
  lymphoma, 581, 582*f*
  metastasis, 578, 578*f*
  myeloma, 579
  nonossifying fibroma, 549, 549*f*–550*f*
  osteoblastoma, 538, 538*f*–539*f*
  osteochondroma, 540, 540*f*–541*f*
  osteoid osteoma, 536, 536*f*–537*f*
  osteosarcoma, 561, 561*f*
  Paget sarcoma, 577, 577*f*
  parosteal osteosarcoma, 563, 563*f*–564*f*
  periosteal osteosarcoma, 565, 566*f*
  protocols, 530, 535, 535*f*
  solitary bone cyst, 551, 551*f*–552*f*
  telangiectatic osteosarcoma, 568, 568*f*–569*f*
Malabsorption syndromes, 716*t*
Malignant fibrous histiocytoma, 464*f*
  hand and wrist, 514*t*
  pelvis, hips and thighs, 151*t*
Malignant fibrous histiocytoma of bone, 575, 575*f*
Malignant peripheral nerve sheath tumor, 597, 597*f*
Marfan syndrome, 761, 761*f*
Marginal osteophytes, 76, 77*f*
Maroteaux–Lamy syndrome, 768*t*
Marrow. *See* Bone marrow
Massive osteolysis, 795, 795*f*
Mastocytosis, 746, 746*f*
Mazabraud syndrome, 555, 556*f*
Medial collateral ligaments (MCL), 216, 216*f*–217*f*
Medial disc displacement, 8, 8*f*
Medial patella subluxation, 230
Medial tendon injuries, 309–311, 309*f*–311*f*
Median nerve compression, 471
Mediopatellar plica, knee, 226
Melorheostosis, 740–741, 740*f*–741*f*
Meningiomas, 88
Meningocele, 362
Meningococcal infection, 621*t*
Meniscal cysts, 205, 205*f*
Meniscal lesions
  discoid menisci, 206–207, 207*f*
  meniscal cysts, 205, 205*f*
  meniscal tears, 197–202, 197*f*–202*f*
  postoperative meniscus, 203–204, 203*f*–204*f*

Meniscal tears, 197–202, 197f–202f
Meniscus, postoperative, 203, 203f–204f
Metabolic diseases, 707–735
   osteomalacia, 720–721, 720f–721f
      basic concepts, 716, 716t, 716f
   osteoporosis
      causes, 707t
      generalized, 708–712, 709f–712f
      regional, 713–715, 713f–715f
   Paget disease, 733–735, 733f–735f
   parathyroid disorders
      hyperparathyroidism, 725–727, 725f–727f
      hypoparathyroidism, 728–729, 729f
      pseudo-pseudohypoparathyroidism,
         728–729, 729f
      pseudohypoparathyroidism, 728–729, 729f
   pituitary disorders, 732, 732f
   renal osteodystrophy, 722–724, 722f–724f
   rickets, 718–719, 718f–719f
      basic concepts, 716, 716t, 716f
   thyroid disorders, 730–731, 731f
Metacarpal fracture, 497–500, 498f–500f
Metaphyseal dysplasias, 760, 760f
Metastasis, 88, 578, 578f
   hand and wrist, 514t
   soft tissue calcification and, 780t
   vertebral, 80, 81f
Metatarsalgia, 327t
Metatarsophalangeal fracture, 296–297, 296f–297f
Metatarsus adductus, 360, 360f
Midfoot
   and forefoot syndromes, 327–328, 327t, 327f–328f
   injuries, 291–293, 291f–293f
Migratory osteoporosis, 707t
Mixed connective tissue disease, 683–684, 683f–684f
Monteggia fractures, 450, 450f
Morquio syndrome, 767, 768t, 770f
MPS. See Mucopolysaccharidoses
MR arthrography. See Magnetic resonance (MR)
   arthrography
MRI. See Magnetic resonance imaging
Mucopolysaccharidoses (MPS), 767–770, 768t,
   769f–770f
   Hunter syndrome, 768t
   Hurler syndrome, 767, 768t, 769f
   Hurler–Scheie syndrome, 768t
   Maroteaux–Lamy syndrome, 768t
   Morquio syndrome, 767, 768t, 770f
   Sanfilippo syndrome, 768t
   Scheie syndrome, 768t
   Sly syndrome, 768t
Multidirectional instability, shoulder and arm, 414,
   414f
Multiple epiphyseal dysplasia, 757, 757f–759f
Multiple myeloma, 80, 82f
   osteoporosis, 707t
   soft tissue calcification and, 780t
Multiple sclerosis, 92, 93f
Muscles
   anomalies, 321t

injuries
   elbow/forearm, 460, 460f
   pelvis, hips and thighs, 130, 131–132, 131f–132f
   tears, 258–259, 258f–259f
Musculoskeletal infections
   basic concepts, 620–621, 620t–621t
   brodie abscess, 620t, 638–640, 639f–640f
   chronic recurrent multifocal osteomyelitis, 620t,
      626–627, 627f
   cloaca, 620t
   fistula, 620t
   fungal infections, 643–644, 644f
   Garré sclerosing osteomyelitis, 620t
   infective osteitis, 620t
   infective periostitis, 620t
   involucrum, 620t
   joint space, 632–633, 632t
   organisms in, 621t
   osteomyelitis, 622–625, 622t, 623f–625f
      imaging approaches, 622t
      violated tissue, 630–631, 630f–631f
   sequestrum, 620t
   sinus, 620t
   soft tissue, 620t, 635–637, 635t, 635f–637f
   synovitis, acne, pustulosis, hyperostosis, osteitis,
      620t, 628, 628f
   terminology and categories, 620t
   tuberculosis/atypical mycobacterial infections,
      641–642, 641f–642f
Musculoskeletal neoplasms
   bone tumors/tumorlike conditions
      adamantinoma, 576, 576f
      aneurysmal bone cyst, 553–554, 554f
      chondroblastoma, 545, 545f
      chondromyxoid fibroma, 547–548, 547f–548f
      chondrosarcoma, 571–574, 572f–574f
      enchondroma, 542–544, 542f–544f
      eosinophilic granuloma/langerhans cell
         histiocytosis, 559–560, 560f
      Ewing sarcoma, 570, 570f
      fibrosarcoma and malignant fibrous
         histiocytoma, 575, 575f
      fibrous dysplasia, 555–556, 555f–556f
      giant cell tumor, 557–558, 557f–558f
      imaging approaches, 530
      lymphoma, 581–582, 582f
      magnetic resonance imaging protocols, 535, 535f
      metastasis, 578, 578f
      myeloma, 579–580, 580f
      nonossifying fibroma, 549–550, 549f–550f
      osteoblastoma, 538–539, 538f–539f
      osteochondroma, 540–541, 540f–541f
      osteoid osteoma, 536–537, 536f–537f
      osteosarcoma, 561, 561f
      Paget sarcoma, 577, 577f
      parosteal osteosarcoma, 563–564, 563f–564f
      periosteal osteosarcoma, 565–566, 566f
      radiographic features, 531–533, 531f–533f
      solitary bone cyst, 551–552, 551f–552f
      telangiectatic osteosarcoma, 568–569, 568f–569f

Musculoskeletal neoplasms (*continued*)
  soft tissue masses
    benign peripheral nerve sheath tumor, 594–596,
      594*f*–596*f*
    deep fibromatosis (desmoid tumor), 599–600,
      599*f*–600*f*
    elastofibroma, 601–602, 601*f*–602*f*
    ganglion, 603, 603*f*
    giant cell tumor of tendon sheath, 605–606,
      605*f*–606*f*
    hematoma, 607–610, 608*f*–610*f*
    lipoma, 583–584, 584*f*
    liposarcoma, 585–587, 586*f*–587*f*
    malignant peripheral nerve sheath tumor,
      597, 597*f*
    myositis ossificans, 611–612, 611*f*–612*f*
    myxoma (intramuscular), 588–589, 588*f*–589*f*
    rhabdomyosarcoma, 618–619, 618*f*–619*f*
    simple common cystic lymphatic malformation/
      lymphangioma, 592–593, 593*f*
    simple venous malformation, 590–591, 590*f*–591*f*
    synovial sarcoma, 615–617, 616*f*–617*f*
    undifferentiated-unclassified tumor,
      613–614, 614*f*
Myelofibrosis, 652*t*, 659–660, 659*f*–660*f*
Myeloid depletion, 648–649, 648*f*–649*f*
Myeloma, 579–580, 580*f*
  bone marrow, 652*t*
  elbow/forearm, 463*t*
  hand and wrist, 514*t*
  pelvis, hips and thighs, 151*t*
  shoulder and arm, 430
Myelomeningocele, 362
Myositis ossificans, 611–612, 611*f*–612*f*
Myxoma
  intramuscular, 588–589, 588*f*–589*f*
  pelvis, hips and thighs, 151*t*

N
National Emergency X-Radiography Utilization Study,
  14, 15*t*
Neoplasms. *See also* Musculoskeletal neoplasms;
  Tumors/tumorlike conditions
  bone marrow, 652*t*
  elbow/forearm
    bone tumors, 463, 463*f*, 463*t*
    soft tissue tumors, 464, 464*f*
  foot, ankle, and calf
    skeletal lesions, benign, 329–331, 330*f*–331*f*
    soft tissue lesions, benign, 332–333, 332*f*–333*f*
  hand and wrist
    bone tumors, 514–515, 514*t*, 515*f*
    soft tissue masses, 516–517, 516*f*–517*f*
  knee
    bone tumors/tumorlike conditions, 249–251,
      249*t*, 250*f*–251*f*
    soft tissue tumors and masses, 252–254,
      252*f*–254*f*
  pelvis, hips and thighs, 151–154, 151*t*, 152*f*–154*f*

  shoulder and arm, 430–433, 430*f*–433*f*
  soft tissue calcification and, 780*t*
Nerve compression syndromes, 422
  hand and wrist
    carpal tunnel syndrome, 524–525, 524*f*–525*f*
    ulnar nerve compression, 526–527, 526*f*–527*f*
Nerve entrapment syndromes
  elbow/forearm, 470–475, 470*f*–475*f*
  shoulder and arm, 422–423, 422*f*–423*f*
Nerve roots, inflammatory conditions, 92–96, 93*f*–96*f*
Nerve sheath tumor, 88, 89*f*–90*f*
Neurofibromatosis, 749–752, 750*f*–752*f*
Neuromas, 327*t*
Neuromyelitis optica spectrum disorder (NMOSD),
  92, 94*f*
Neurotrophic arthropathy, 699–701, 699*f*–701*f*
  foot, ankle, and calf, 340, 340*f*
  with/without ulcer, 348*t*
Neurovascular injury, 130
Niemann–Pick disease, 652*t*, 653
NMOSD (neuromyelitis optica spectrum disorder),
  92, 94*f*
Nocardiosis, 621*t*
Nonaccidental trauma, 796–797, 796*f*–797*f*
Nonmarginal osteophyte, 76
Nonossifying fibroma, 329, 549–550, 549*f*–550*f*
Nuclear medicine, bone tumors/tumorlike conditions, 530

O
Obstructive jaundice, 716*t*
Ochronosis, 698, 698*f*
O'Donoghue's triad, 216
Odontoid fracture, of cervical spine, 28, 28*t*, 29*f*
Ollier disease, 753, 753*f*
Os trigonum syndrome, 319–320, 319*f*–320*f*
Osgood–Schlatter disease, 242, 243*f*
Osteoarthritis
  arthropathies/connective tissue diseases, 673–676,
    674*f*–676*f*
  elbow/forearm, 468*f*
  foot, ankle, and calf, 334, 334*f*
  hand and wrist, 518*t*, 519*f*
  hip, 157*f*–158*f*
  knee, 244
  temporomandibular joint, 10, 10*f*
Osteoblastoma, 329, 538–539, 538*f*–539*f*
  hand and wrist, 514*t*
Osteochondral fractures, 178, 178*f*
Osteochondritis, 327*t*
Osteochondritis dissecans
  elbow/forearm, 454, 454*f*
  histologic and magnetic resonance features, 236*t*
  knee, 236–238, 236*t*, 236*f*–238*f*
Osteochondroma, 329, 540–541, 540*f*–541*f*
  elbow/forearm, 463*t*
  hand and wrist, 514*t*
  knee, 249*t*
  pelvis, hips and thighs, 151*t*
  shoulder and arm, 430

Osteochondromatosis, 702–703, 703*f*
Osteochondroses, 242–243, 242*f*–243*f*
Osteogenesis imperfecta, 763–764, 763*f*–764*f*
Osteoid osteoma, 329, 536–537, 536*f*–537*f*
    elbow/forearm, 463*t*
    hand and wrist, 514*t*
    knee, 249*t*, 250*f*
    pelvis, hips and thighs, 151*t*, 152*f*
    shoulder and arm, 430
Osteomalacia, 720–721, 720*f*–721*f*
    basic concepts, 716, 716*t*, 716*f*
Osteomyelitis, 73*f*, 622–625, 622*t*, 623*f*–625*f*
    foot, ankle, and calf, 343–344, 344*f*
    imaging approaches, 622*t*
    infected Achilles tendon anchor with, 630*f*
    violated tissue, 630–631, 630*f*–631*f*
Osteonecrosis, 141, 141*f*
    avascular necrosis, 143–146, 143*t*, 144*f*–146*f*
    bone infarcts, 147, 147*f*
    knee, 239–241, 239*f*–241*f*
    shoulder and arm, 428–429, 428*f*–429*f*
Osteopathia striata, 739, 739*f*
Osteopetrosis, 744–745, 744*f*–745*f*
    infantile, 744
    intermediate, 744, 744*f*
    tarda, 744, 745*f*
Osteopoikilosis, 738, 738*f*
Osteoporosis
    causes, 707*t*
    generalized, 708–712, 709*f*–712*f*
        anemias, 852*t*
        chronic liver disease, 707*t*
        endocrine disorders, 707*t*
        environmental factors, 707*t*
        idiopathic, 707*t*
        medications, 707*t*
        multiple myeloma, 707*t*
        senility, 707*t*
    regional, 713–715, 713*f*–715*f*
        disuse atrophy, 707*t*, 713*f*
        migratory osteoporosis, 707*t*
        reflex sympathetic dystrophy, 707*t*, 715*f*
        transient regional osteoporosis, 707*t*, 714*f*
Osteoporosis circumscripta, 733*f*
Osteosarcoma, 329, 561, 561*f*
    elbow/forearm, 463*t*
    hand and wrist, 514*t*
    knee, 249*t*, 251*f*
    parosteal, 563–564, 563*f*–564*f*
    pelvis, hips and thighs, 151*t*
    periosteal, 565–566, 566*f*
    shoulder and arm, 430
    telangiectatic, 568–569, 568*f*–569*f*
Overgrowth, 367–368, 367*f*–368*f*
Overlap syndromes, 683–684, 683*f*–684*f*

P

Pachydermoperiostosis, 773–774, 773*f*–774*f*, 775*t*
Paget disease, 155*t*, 733–735, 733*f*–735*f*

Paget sarcoma, 577, 577*f*
Pancreatic insufficiency, 716*t*
Parasitic infections
    cysticercosis, 621*t*
    echinococcosis, 621*t*
    hookworms, 621*t*
Paraspinal abscess, 72
Paraspinal osteophyte, 76
Paraspinal tumors, 88, 88*t*
Parathyroid disorders
    hyperparathyroidism, 725–727, 725*f*–727*f*
    hypoparathyroidism, 728–729, 729*f*
    pseudo-pseudohypoparathyroidism, 728–729, 729*f*
    pseudohypoparathyroidism, 728–729, 729*f*
Parosteal osteosarcoma, 563–564, 563*f*–564*f*
Patellar disorders, knee
    chondromalacia patella, 232–233, 232*t*, 233*f*
    fractures, 179–181, 179*f*–181*f*
    patellar tracking and instability, 230–231, 230*f*–231*f*
    patellofemoral relationships, 228–229, 228*f*–229*f*
Patellar tendon injuries, 220–221, 220*f*–221*f*
Patellar tracking and instability, 230, 230*f*–231*f*
Patellofemoral relationships, patellar disorders,
        228–229, 228*f*–229*f*
PCL (posterior cruciate ligament), 215, 215*f*
Pediatric disorders
    foot, ankle, and calf
        congenital vertical talus, 363, 363*f*
        forefoot abnormalities, 360–361, 360*f*–361*f*
        Freiberg infraction, 369, 369*f*
        hindfoot abnormalities, 354–357, 355*f*–357*f*
        Köhler disease, 370–371, 371*f*
        normal angles of the foot and ankle, 351–353,
            351*f*–353*f*
        overgrowth/hypoplasia/aplasia, 367–368,
            367*f*–368*f*
        pes planovalgus, 364, 364*f*
        plantar arch abnormalities, 358–359, 358*f*–359*f*
        talipes equinovarus, 362, 362*f*
        tarsal coalitions, 365–366, 365*f*–366*f*
        terminology, 350
    hip disorders
        coxa vara and coxa valga, 174–175, 174*f*–175*f*
        developmental dysplasia of the hip, 167–170,
            167*f*–170*f*
        femoral anteversion, 176–177, 176*f*–177*f*
        Legg–Calvé–Perthes disease, 164–166, 164*f*–166*f*
        slipped capital femoral epiphysis, 171–173,
            171*f*–173*f*
Pedicle fractures, of cervical spine, 32
Pelvis, hips and thighs
    arthropathies, 155, 155*t*
        collagen vascular diseases, 155*t*
        connective tissue diseases, 155*t*
        crystalline arthropathies, 155*t*
        hip, 156–159, 157*f*–159*f*
        infection, 155*t*
        juvenile chronic arthritis, 155*t*
        Paget disease, 155*t*
        pigmented villonodular synovitis, 155*t*

Pelvis, hips and thighs (*continued*)
   posttraumatic arthritis, 155*t*
   rheumatoid arthritis, 155*t*
   sacroiliac joints, 160–161, 160*f*–161*f*
   seronegative spondyloarthropathies, 155*t*
   synovial chondromatosis, 155*t*
  bone marrow edema, 148, 148*f*
  fractures
   acetabular, 115–120, 115*f*–120*f*
   complex, 110–114, 111*f*–114*f*
   dislocation, 121–122, 121*f*–122*f*
   femoral neck, 123–125, 123*f*–125*f*
   insufficiency fractures, 128–129, 128*f*–129*f*
   minor, 107–108, 107*f*–108*f*
   single break in pelvic ring, 109, 109*f*
   trochanteric, 126–127
  infection, 162, 162*f*
  neoplasms, 151–154, 151*t*, 152*f*–154*f*
  osteonecrosis, 141, 141*f*
   avascular necrosis, 143–146, 143*t*, 144*f*–146*f*
   bone infarcts, 147, 147*f*
  pediatric hip disorders
   developmental dysplasia of the hip, 167–170,
    167*f*–170*f*
   Legg–Calvé–Perthes disease, 164–166, 164*f*–166*f*
   rotational/orientation abnormalities, 174–177,
    174*f*–177*f*
   slipped capital femoral epiphysis, 171–173,
    171*f*–173*f*
  soft tissue trauma, 130
   acetabular labral tears, 137–138, 137*f*–138*f*
   alveolar sarcoma, 151*t*
   benign nerve sheath tumors, 151*t*
   bursitis, 133–134, 133*f*–134*f*
   desmoid tumors, 151*t*
   epithelioid sarcoma, 151*t*
   femoroacetabular impingement, 139, 139*f*
   fibrosarcoma, 151*t*
   greater trochanteric pain syndrome, 135–136,
    135*f*–136*f*
   hemangioma, 151*t*
   lipoma, 151*t*
   liposarcoma, 151*t*
   malignant fibrous histiocytoma, 151*t*
   muscle/tendon tears, 131–132, 131*f*–132*f*
   myxoma, 151*t*
   synovial sarcoma, 151*t*
  transient osteoporosis of hip, 149–150, 149*f*–150*f*
Periosteal osteosarcoma, 565–566, 566*f*
Periostitis, 775*t*
  hypervitaminosis A, 775*t*
  primary hypertrophic osteoarthropathy, 775*t*
  secondary hypertrophic osteoarthropathy, 775*t*
  thyroid acropachy, 775*t*
  venous insufficiency, 775*t*
Peroneal tendon injuries, 304–306, 304*f*–306*f*
  rupture, 304
  subluxation, 304
Perthes lesion, 408
Pes cavus, 358, 359*f*

Pes planovalgus, 364, 364*f*
Pes planus, 358, 358*f*
Phalangeal dislocations, 501–502, 501*f*–502*f*
Phalangeal fracture, 501–502, 501*f*–502*f*
Pigmented villonodular synovitis (PVNS), 155*t*, 156*t*,
   158*f*, 244, 248*f*, 704, 704*f*
Pillar fractures, of cervical spine, 32
Pilon fractures, 277, 277*f*
Pituitary disorders, 732, 732*f*
Plafond fractures (pilon), 277, 277*f*
Plantar arch abnormalities, 358–359, 358*f*–359*f*
Plantar fasciitis, 314–316, 314*f*–316*f*
Plantaris, 258, 258*f*
Platybasia, 106*f*
PLC (posterior ligamentous complex) injury, 42
Plicae, knee, 226–227, 226*f*–227*f*
Polio, 362
Polydactyly, 367, 368*f*
Polymyositis, 681–682, 681*f*–682*f*
Popliteal cysts, 252, 252*f*
Popliteal muscle tears, 258, 259*f*
Popliteus tendon, 208
Positron emission tomography, 340
Posterior cruciate ligament (PCL), 215, 215*f*
Posterior horn, meniscal tears, 198
Posterior impingement syndrome, 325
Posterior instability, shoulder and arm, 413, 413*f*
Posterior interosseous nerve syndrome, 472
Posterior ligamentous complex (PLC) injury, 42
Posteromedial impingement syndrome, 325
Posttraumatic acute pyogenic osteomyelitis, 631*f*
Posttraumatic arthritis, 155*t*
Posttraumatic fibrosis, 321*t*
Posttraumatic osteolysis, 385–387, 385*f*–387*f*
Preiser disease, 522
Primary chondrosarcoma, 430
Primary hypertrophic osteoarthropathy. *See*
   Pachydermoperiostosis
Progressive diaphyseal dysplasia, 742, 742*f*
Pronation lateral rotation injuries, 275–276,
   275*f*–276*f*
Pronation–abduction injuries, 273–274, 273*f*–274*f*
Pronator syndrome, 471
Proteus infection, 621*t*
Proximal humeral fractures, shoulder and arm,
   372–373, 372*f*–373*f*
Proximal radius fractures, 445–446, 445*f*–446*f*
Proximal tibial fractures, knee, 186–188, 186*f*–188*f*
Pseudo-pseudohypoparathyroidism, 728–729, 729*f*
Pseudohypoparathyroidism, 728–729, 729*f*
Pseudomonas infection, 621*t*
Psoriatic arthritis, 76, 77*f*, 518*t*, 521*f*, 666–667,
   666*f*–667*f*
  foot, ankle, and calf, 337, 337*f*
  hand and wrist, 518*t*
  knee, 244
  pelvis, hips and thighs, 160*t*
Psoriatic spondylitis, 76
Pubic rami fractures, of pelvis, 107
Pulmonary hypertrophic osteoarthropathy, 775

PVNS (pigmented villonodular synovitis), 155*t*, 156*t*, 158*f*, 244, 248*f*, 704, 704*f*
Pyogenic septic arthritis, 633*f*

Q
Quadriceps tendon injuries, 218–219, 218*f*–219*f*
Quadrilateral space syndrome, 422

R
RA. *See* Rheumatoid arthritis
Radial nerve
    compression, 471, 472*f*
    motor syndrome, 472
    sensory syndrome, 472
Radial tunnel syndrome, 472
Radiation therapy, 648, 648*f*
Reactive arthritis, 668–669, 668*f*–669*f*
    foot, ankle, and calf, 338, 338*f*
    knee, 244
    pelvis, hips and thighs, 160*t*
    spine, 76
Recurrent subluxation/dislocations, capsular
        abnormalities, 406–407, 406*f*–407*f*
Reflex sympathetic dystrophy, 707*t*, 713, 715*f*
Reiter syndrome. *See* Reactive arthritis
Renal osteodystrophy, 722–724, 722*f*–724*f*
    soft tissue calcification and, 780*t*
Renal tubular disorders, 716*t*
Rhabdomyosarcoma, 618–619, 618*f*–619*f*
Rheumatoid arthritis (RA), 76, 79*f*, 155*t*, 156*t*, 662–665, 663*f*–665*f*
    elbow/forearm, 467*f*
    foot, ankle, and calf, 335–336, 336*f*
    hand and wrist, 518*t*, 519*f*–520*f*
    knee, 244, 246*f*
    pelvis, hips and thighs, 160*t*
    temporomandibular joint, 11–12, 11*f*–12*f*
Rickets, 718–719, 718*f*–719*f*
    basic concepts, 716, 716*t*, 716*f*
"Rocker bottom" deformity, 358, 358*f*
Rotator cuff disease
    basic concepts, 391–392, 391*f*–392*f*
    etiology
        os acromiale, 391*t*
        primary impingement, 391*t*
    impingement, 393–394, 393*f*–394*f*
    postoperative changes, 403–404, 403*f*–404*f*
    rotator cuff tears
        full thickness, 395–398, 395*f*–398*f*
        partial thickness, 399–400, 399*f*–400*f*
    tendinosis, 401–402, 401*f*–402*f*

S
Sacrococcygeal chordoma, 80, 85*f*
Sacroiliac joints, 160–161, 160*t*, 160*f*–161*f*
Salmonella infection, 621*t*
Sanfilippo syndrome, 768*t*

SAPHO (synovitis, acne, pustulosis, hyperostosis, osteitis), 620*t*, 628, 628*f*
Sarcoidosis, 790–792, 790*t*, 791*f*–792*f*
    soft tissue calcification and, 780*t*
Scaphoid fracture, 487–491, 488*f*–491*f*
Scaphoid nonunion advanced collapse (SNAC), 503, 505*f*
Scapholunate advanced collapse (SLAC), 503, 505*f*
Scapular fractures, shoulder and arm, 388, 388*f*
SCFE (slipped capital femoral epiphysis), 171–173, 171*f*–173*f*
Scheie syndrome, 768*t*
Sciatic nerve injury, 362
Scleroderma, 680, 680*f*
Scoliosis
    basic concepts, 59, 59*t*
    imaging, 60–62, 60*f*–62*f*
SDAVF (spinal dural arteriovenous fistula), 97, 97*f*
Seat-belt injuries, 45
Secondary hypertrophic osteoarthropathy, 775–776, 775*t*, 776*f*
Segmentation anomalies, 105–106, 105*f*–106*f*
Senility, 707*t*
Septic arthritis, 156*t*, 244
Sequestrum, 620*t*
Seronegative spondyloarthropathies, 155*t*
Sesamoiditis, 327*t*
Shearing injuries
    cervical spine, 16*t*
    thoracolumbar spine, 51–52, 51*f*–52*f*
Shoulder and arm
    adhesive capsulitis, 419–421, 419*f*–421*f*
    biceps tendon, 416–418, 416*f*–418*f*
    brachial plexus, 434–435, 434*f*–435*f*
    dislocations
        acromioclavicular, 378–380, 378*t*, 378*f*–380*f*
        glenohumeral, 374–377, 374*f*–377*f*
        posttraumatic osteolysis, 385–387, 385*f*–387*f*
        sternoclavicular, 381–382, 381*f*–382*f*
    fractures
        clavicle, 383–384, 383*f*–384*f*
        humeral shaft, 389–390, 389*f*–390*f*
        Neer classification, 372*t*
        proximal humeral, 372–373, 372*f*–373*f*
        scapular, 388, 388*f*
    inflammatory arthropathies, 424–427, 424*f*–427*f*
    instability
        basic concepts, 405
        humeral osteochondral or ligament avulsions, 411–412, 412*f*
        labral tears, 408–410, 408*f*–410*f*
        labral variants, 415, 415*f*
        multidirectional, 414, 414*f*
        posterior, 413, 413*f*
        recurrent subluxation /dislocations, capsular
            abnormalities, 406–407, 406*f*–407*f*
    neoplasms, 430–433, 430*f*–433*f*
    nerve entrapment syndromes, 422–423, 422*f*–423*f*
    osteonecrosis, 428–429, 428*f*–429*f*
    rotator cuff disease

Shoulder and arm (*continued*)
  basic concepts, 391–392, 391*f*–392*f*
  etiology, 391*t*
  full thickness tears, 395–398, 395*f*–398*f*
  impingement, 393–394, 393*f*–394*f*
  partial thickness tears, 399–400, 399*f*–400*f*
  postoperative changes, 403–404, 403*f*–404*f*
  tendinosis, 401–402, 401*f*–402*f*
Sickle cell anemia, 786–787, 786*f*–787*f*
Simple bone cyst. *See* Solitary bone cyst
Simple common cystic lymphatic malformation/
  lymphangioma, 592–593, 593*f*
Simple venous malformation, 590–591,
  590*f*–591*f*
Sinding–Larsen–Johansson disease, 242
Sinus, 620*t*
Sinus tarsi syndrome, 323–324, 323*f*–324*f*
Skeletal lesions, benign, 329–331, 330*f*–331*f*
Skeletal trauma. *See* Trauma, skeletal
Skewfoot, 360, 361*f*
SLAC (scapholunate advanced collapse), 503, 505*f*
SLAP (superior labrum anterior posterior) lesions,
  408, 409*f*
Slipped capital femoral epiphysis (SCFE), 171–173,
  171*f*–173*f*
Sly syndrome, 768*t*
Small bowel
  fistulae, 716*t*
  and gastric resections, 716*t*
Smith fracture, 480, 480*f*
SNAC (scaphoid nonunion advanced collapse),
  503, 505*f*
Snapping tendon syndrome, 130
Soft tissue
  calcification, 780*t*
    calcinosis universalis, 780*t*
    collagen vascular diseases, 780*t*
    dermatomyositis, 780*t*
    hyperparathyroidism, 780*t*
    hypervitaminosis D, 780*t*
    inflammation, 780*t*
    metastasis, 780*t*
    multiple myeloma, 780*t*
    neoplasms, 780*t*
    renal osteodystrophy, 780*t*
    sarcoidosis, 780*t*
    trauma, 780*t*
    tumoral calcinosis, 780*t*
  infection, 620*t*, 635–637, 635*t*, 635*f*–637*f*
    foot, ankle, and calf, 345, 345*f*
    imaging approaches, 635*t*
  lesions-benign, 332–333, 332*f*–333*f*
  masses, 88–91, 89*f*–91*f*
    causing tarsal tunnel syndrome, 321*t*
    hand and wrist, 516–517, 516*f*–517*f*
    knee, 252, 252*f*–254*f*
    musculoskeletal neoplasms. *See* Musculoskeletal
      neoplasms, soft tissue masses
  sarcomas, 88
  swelling, 348*t*

  trauma
    elbow/forearm. *See* Elbow and forearm, soft
      tissue trauma
    foot, ankle, and calf. *See* Foot, ankle, and calf, soft
      tissue trauma
    hand and wrist. *See* Hand and wrist, soft tissue
      trauma
    knee, 252, 252*f*–254*f*
    pelvis, hips and thighs. *See* Pelvis, hips and
      thighs, soft tissue trauma
  ulceration, 348*t*
Solitary bone cyst, 551–552, 551*f*–552*f*
Spina bifida aperta, 99
Spina bifida occulta, 99
Spinal dural arteriovenous fistula (SDAVF), 97, 97*f*
Spinal dysraphism, 99–101, 100*f*–101*f*
Spine
  arthropathies, 76–79, 76*f*–79*f*
  cervical
    atlanto-occipital fracture dislocations, 21, 21*f*
    atlantoaxial dislocations, 25–27, 25*f*–27*f*
    axial compression injuries, 16*t*
    C1 fractures, 22–24, 23*f*–24*f*
    C2 fractures, 28–31, 28*t*, 29*f*–31*f*
    Canadian C-Spine Rule, 14, 15*t*
    compressive hyperextension injuries, 16*t*, 18*f*
    compressive hyperflexion injuries, 16*t*, 17*f*
    disruptive hyperextension injuries, 16*t*, 18*f*
    disruptive hyperflexion injuries, 16*t*, 17*f*
    flexion–rotation injuries, 16*t*, 19*f*
    injuries not clinically significant, 16*t*
    instability, 20*f*
    lateral flexion injuries, 16*t*
    National Emergency X-Radiography Utilization
      Study, 14, 15*t*
    shearing injuries, 16*t*
    subluxation, fracture/dislocation, 38–41, 38*f*–41*f*
    vertebral arch fractures, 32–33, 32*f*–33*f*
    vertebral body fractures, 35–37, 35*t*, 35*f*–37*f*
    vertical compression injuries, 19*f*–20*f*
  congenital anomalies, 99
    caudal regression syndrome, 102, 102*f*
    Chiari malformation, 103–104, 103*f*–104*f*
    segmentation anomalies, 105–106, 105*f*–106*f*
    spinal dysraphism, 99–101, 100*f*–101*f*
  degenerative disc disease, 63–65, 64*f*–65*f*
  disc herniation, 66–70, 66*f*–70*f*
  dorsal thoracic arachnoid web, 97, 98*f*
  infection, 72–75, 72*f*–75*f*
  inflammatory conditions, 92–96, 93*f*–96*f*
  Paget disease in, 735*f*
  scoliosis
    basic concepts, 59, 59*t*
    imaging, 60–62, 60*f*–62*f*
  spinal dural arteriovenous fistula, 97, 97*f*
  spondylolysis/spondylolisthesis, 54–58, 55*f*–58*f*
  synovial cysts, 71, 71*f*
  thoracolumbar
    basic concepts, 42–43, 42*f*–43*f*
    flexion–rotation injuries, 47, 47*f*

hyperextension injuries, 50, 50*f*
hyperflexion injuries, 45–46, 45*f*–46*f*
minor fractures, 53, 53*f*
shearing injuries, 51–52, 51*f*–52*f*
vertical compression injuries, 48–49, 48*f*–49*f*
tumors/tumorlike conditions
bone lesions, 80–86, 81*f*–86*f*
soft tissue masses, 88–91, 89*f*–91*f*
Spinous process fractures, 53
cervical spine, 32
Spondyloepiphyseal dysplasia, 757
Spondylolisthesis, 54–58, 55*f*–58*f*
Spondylolysis, 54–58, 55*f*–58*f*
Sporotrichosis, 621*t*
Sprue, 716*t*
Staphylococcal infection, 621*t*
Stenosing tenosynovitis, 304
Sternoclavicular dislocations, shoulder and arm,
    381–382, 381*f*–382*f*
Streptococcal infection, 621*t*
Stress fractures, 298–300, 298*t*, 298*f*–300*f*, 327*t*
calcaneus, 298*t*
distal fibula, 298*t*
distal tibia, 298*t*
metatarsals, 298*t*
sesamoids, 298*t*
tarsals, 298*t*
Subacute osteomyelitis, 622, 623*f*
Subluxation
cervical spine, 38–41, 38*f*–41*f*
spondylolysis/spondylolisthesis, 54–58, 55*f*–58*f*
Subtrochanteric fractures, of hip, 126, 127*f*
Subungual exostosis, 329
Superior labrum anterior posterior (SLAP) lesions,
    408, 409*f*
Supination lateral rotation injuries, 271–272, 271*f*–272*f*
Supination–adduction injuries, 269–270, 269*f*–270*f*
Supracondylar fractures, knee, 182–185, 182*f*–185*f*
Suprapatellar plica, knee, 226
Suprascapular nerve compression, 422
Syndactyly, 367
Syndesmophyte, 76
Synovial chondromatosis, 155*t*, 156*t*, 159*f*,
    702–703, 703*f*
Synovial cysts, 71, 71*f*
Synovial hypertrophy, 321*t*
Synovial sarcoma, 333*f*, 615–617, 616*f*–617*f*
pelvis, hips and thighs, 151*t*
Synovitis, acne, pustulosis, hyperostosis, osteitis
    (SAPHO), 620*t*, 628, 628*f*
Syringomyelia, 103
Systemic lupus erythematosus, 679, 679*f*

T

Talar and subtalar dislocations, 285–286, 286*f*
Talar body, head, process fractures, 281–282, 281*f*–282*f*
Talar dome fractures, 283–284, 283*f*–284*f*
Talar neck fractures, 279–280, 279*f*–280*f*
Talipes equinovarus, 362, 362*f*

Talocalcaneal coalitions, 321*t*
Tarsal anomalies, 362
Tarsal coalitions, 365–366, 365*f*–366*f*
Tarsal tunnel syndrome
foot, ankle, and calf, 321–322, 321*t*, 322*f*
fractures, 321*t*
ganglion cysts, 321*t*
hypertrophy of abductor hallucis muscle, 321*t*
lipomas, 321*t*
muscle anomalies, 321*t*
posttraumatic fibrosis, 321*t*
soft tissue masses, 321*t*
synovial hypertrophy, 321*t*
talocalcaneal coalitions, 321*t*
trauma, 321*t*
varicosities, 321*t*
Teardop fractures, cervical spine, 35, 35*t*, 36*f*
Telangiectatic osteosarcoma, 568–569, 568*f*–569*f*
Temporomandibular joint (TMJ)
anatomy, 1, 1*f*
anterior disc displacement, 4–7, 4*f*–7*f*
internal derangement, 2–3, 3*f*
juvenile chronic arthritis, 11
lateral and medial disc displacement, 8, 8*f*
miscellaneous arthropathies, 11–12, 12*f*
osteoarthritis, 10, 10*f*
rheumatoid arthritis, 11–12, 11*f*–12*f*
trauma, 9, 9*f*
tumors, 13, 13*f*, 13*t*
Tendinosis, shoulder and arm, 401–402, 401*f*–402*f*
Tendon injuries
elbow/forearm
flexor/extensor, 458–459, 458*f*–459*f*
triceps, 457, 457*f*
foot, ankle, and calf
Achilles tendon, 307–308, 307*f*–308*f*
anterior, 312–313, 312*f*–313*f*
medial, 309–311, 309*f*–311*f*
peroneal, 304–306, 304*f*–306*f*
hand and wrist, 509–510, 509*f*–510*f*
knee
basic concepts, 208–209, 208*f*–209*f*
patellar tendon, 220–221, 220*f*–221*f*
quadriceps tendon, 218–219, 218*f*–219*f*
pelvis, hips and thighs, 130
Tenography, tendon injuries, 509
Tenosynovitis, 304
Tethered cord with lipoma, 101*f*
Thalassemia, 788–789, 789*f*
Thigh. *See* Pelvis, hips and thighs
Thoracolumbar Injury Classification and Severity
    (TLICS) Score, 42
Thoracolumbar spine
basic concepts, 42–43, 42*f*–43*f*
flexion–rotation injuries, 47, 47*f*
hyperextension injuries, 50, 50*f*
hyperflexion injuries, 45–46, 45*f*–46*f*
minor fractures, 53, 53*f*
shearing injuries, 51–52, 51*f*–52*f*
vertical compression injuries, 48–49, 48*f*–49*f*

Thumb fractures, 497

Thyroid acropachy, 731*f*, 775*t*

Thyroid disorders, 730–731, 731*f*

Tibia, Paget disease in, 734*f*

Tibial condylar fractures, 186, 189

Tibial plateau fractures, 182, 186

TLICS (Thoracolumbar Injury Classification and Severity) Score, 42

TMJ. *See* Temporomandibular joint

Transient osteoporosis of hip, 149–150, 149*f*–150*f*

Transient regional osteoporosis, 707*t*, 713, 714*f*

Transverse process fractures, 32, 53

Transverse sacral fractures, of pelvis, 107

Trauma

  causing tarsal tunnel syndrome, 321*t*

  cervical spine

    atlanto-occipital fracture dislocations, 21, 21*f*

    atlantoaxial dislocations, 25–27, 25*f*–27*f*

    axial compression injuries, 16*t*

    C1 fractures, 22–24, 23*f*–24*f*

    C2 fractures, 28–31, 28*t*, 29*f*–31*f*

    Canadian C-Spine Rule, 14, 15*t*

    compressive hyperextension injuries, 16*t*, 18*f*

    compressive hyperflexion injuries, 16*t*, 17*f*

    disruptive hyperextension injuries, 16*t*, 18*f*

    disruptive hyperflexion injuries, 16*t*, 17*f*

    flexion–rotation injuries, 16*t*, 19*f*

    injuries not clinically significant, 16*t*

    instability, 20*f*

    lateral flexion injuries, 16*t*

    National Emergency X-Radiography Utilization Study, 14, 15*t*

    shearing injuries, 16*t*

    subluxation, fracture/dislocation, 38–41, 38*f*–41*f*

    vertebral arch fractures, 32–33, 32*f*–33*f*

    vertebral body fractures, 35–37, 35*t*, 35*f*–37*f*

    vertical compression injuries, 19*f*–20*f*

  nonaccidental, 796–797, 796*f*–797*f*

  pelvis, hips and thighs

    acetabular fractures, 115–120, 115*f*–120*f*

    complex fractures, 110–114, 111*f*–114*f*

    femoral neck fracture, 123–125, 123*f*–125*f*

    fracture/dislocation, 121–122, 121*f*–122*f*

    insufficiency fractures, 128–129, 128*f*–129*f*

    minor fractures, 107–108, 107*f*–108*f*

    single break in pelvic ring, 109, 109*f*

    soft tissue trauma. *See* Pelvis, hips and thighs, soft tissue trauma

    trochanteric fracture, 126–127

  skeletal, knee

    miscellaneous fractures, 189–196, 189*f*–196*f*

    osteochondral fractures, 178, 178*f*

    patellar fractures, 179–181, 179*f*–181*f*

    proximal tibial fractures, 186–188, 186*f*–188*f*

    supracondylar fractures, 182–185, 182*f*–185*f*

  soft tissue calcification and, 780*t*

  temporomandibular joint, 9, 9*f*

  thoracolumbar spine

    basic concepts, 42–43, 42*f*–43*f*

    flexion–rotation injuries, 47, 47*f*

    hyperextension injuries, 50, 50*f*

    hyperflexion injuries, 45–46, 45*f*–46*f*

    minor fractures, 53, 53*f*

    shearing injuries, 51–52, 51*f*–52*f*

    vertical compression injuries, 48–49, 48*f*–49*f*

Triceps tendon injuries, 457, 457*f*

Triplane fractures, 262–263, 262*f*–263*f*

Triquetral fracture, 492*f*

Trochanteric fracture, of hip, 126–127

Tuberculosis, 621*t*, 641–642, 641*f*–642*f*

Tuberculous spondylitis, 72, 74*f*

Tuberous sclerosis, 747–748, 747*f*–748*f*

Tumoral calcinosis, 782, 782*f*

  soft tissue calcification and, 780*t*

Tumors/tumorlike conditions

  bones

    adamantinoma, 576, 576*f*

    aneurysmal bone cyst, 553–554, 554*f*

    chondroblastoma, 545, 545*f*

    chondromyxoid fibroma, 547–548, 547*f*–548*f*

    chondrosarcoma, 571–574, 572*f*–574*f*

    enchondroma, 542–544, 542*f*–544*f*

    eosinophilic granuloma/langerhans cell histiocytosis, 559–560, 560*f*

    Ewing sarcoma, 570, 570*f*

    fibrosarcoma and malignant fibrous histiocytoma, 575, 575*f*

    fibrous dysplasia, 555–556, 555*f*–556*f*

    giant cell tumor, 557–558, 557*f*–558*f*

    imaging approaches, 530

    lymphoma, 581–582, 582*f*

    magnetic resonance imaging protocols, 535, 535*f*

    metastasis, 578, 578*f*

    myeloma, 579–580, 580*f*

    nonossifying fibroma, 549–550, 549*f*–550*f*

    osteoblastoma, 538–539, 538*f*–539*f*

    osteochondroma, 540–541, 540*f*–541*f*

    osteoid osteoma, 536–537, 536*f*–537*f*

    osteosarcoma, 561, 561*f*

    Paget sarcoma, 577, 577*f*

    parosteal osteosarcoma, 563–564, 563*f*–564*f*

    periosteal osteosarcoma, 565–566, 566*f*

    radiographic features, 531–533, 531*f*–533*f*

    solitary bone cyst, 551–552, 551*f*–552*f*

    telangiectatic osteosarcoma, 568–569, 568*f*–569*f*

  elbow/forearm

    chondroma, 463*t*

    chondromyxoid fibroma, 463*t*

    chondrosarcoma, 463*t*

    Ewing sarcoma, 463*t*

    fibrosarcoma, 463*t*

    giant cell tumor, 463*t*

    lymphoma, 463*t*

    myeloma, 463*t*

    osteochondroma, 463*t*

    osteoid osteoma, 463*t*

    osteosarcoma, 463*t*

  foot and ankle

adamantinoma, 329
aneurysmal bone cyst, 329, 330*f*
chondroblastoma, 329
chondromyxoid fibroma, 329
chondrosarcoma, 329
enchondroma, 329
Ewing sarcoma, 329, 331*f*
fibrosarcoma, 329
fibrous dysplasia, 329
giant cell tumor, 329
hemangioendothelial sarcoma, 329
lymphoma, 329
nonossifying fibroma, 329
osteoblastoma, 329
osteochondroma, 329
osteoid osteoma, 329
osteosarcoma, 329
subungual exostosis, 329
hand and wrist
  aneurysmal bone cyst, 514*t*
  benign vascular tumors, 514*t*
  chondroblastoma, 514*t*
  chondromyxoid fibroma, 514*t*
  chondrosarcoma, 514*t*
  enchondroma, 514*t*
  Ewing sarcoma, 514*t*
  fibrosarcoma, 514*t*
  fibrous defects, 514*t*
  giant cell tumor, 514*t*
  hemangioendothelioma, 514*t*
  lymphoma, 514*t*
  malignant fibrous histiocytoma, 514*t*
  metastasis, 514*t*
  myeloma, 514*t*
  osteoblastoma, 514*t*
  osteochondroma, 514*t*
  osteoid osteoma, 514*t*
  osteosarcoma, 514*t*
pelvis, hips and thighs
  chondroblastoma, 151*t*
  chondroma, 151*t*
  chondrosarcoma, 151*t*
  chordoma (sacrum), 151*t*
  Ewing sarcoma, 151*t*
  fibrosarcoma, 151*t*
  giant cell tumor, 151*t*
  lymphoma, 151*t*
  myeloma, 151*t*
  osteochondroma, 151*t*
  osteoid osteoma, 151*t*
  osteosarcoma, 151*t*
shoulder and arm
  chondroblastoma, 430
  chondroma, 430
  Ewing sarcoma, 430
  fibrosarcoma, 430
  giant cell tumor, 430
  hemangioma, 430
  lymphoma, 430

myeloma, 430
  osteochondroma, 430
  osteoid osteoma, 430
  osteosarcoma, 430
  primary chondrosarcoma, 430
soft tissue
  alveolar sarcoma, 151*t*
  benign nerve sheath tumors, 151*t*
  desmoid tumors, 151*t*
  epithelioid sarcoma, 151*t*
  fibrosarcoma, 151*t*
  hemangioma, 151*t*
  lipoma, 151*t*
  liposarcoma, 151*t*
  malignant fibrous histiocytoma, 151*t*
  myxoma, 151*t*
  synovial sarcoma, 151*t*
spine
  bone lesions, 80–86, 81*f*–86*f*
  soft tissue masses, 88–91, 89*f*–91*f*
temporomandibular joint, 13, 13*f*, 13*t*
Turf toe, 327*t*

U
Ulnar fractures, 447, 447*f*
Ulnar lunate abutment syndrome, 528–529, 528*f*–529*f*
Ulnar nerve compression, 470–471, 470*f*–471*f*, 474*f*
  hand and wrist, 526–527, 526*f*–527*f*
Ultrasound
  developmental dysplasia of the hip, pediatric, 167
  elbow/forearm
    biceps tendon, 455
    flexor/extensor tendon injuries, 458
    ligament injuries, 461
    triceps tendon injuries, 457
  foot, ankle, and calf
    Achilles tendon, 307, 307*f*
    anterior tendon injuries, 312
    bursitis, 317
    joint space infection, 346
    osteomyelitis, 343
    sinus tarsi syndrome, 323
    soft tissue infection, 345
    soft tissue lesions, benign, 332
    tarsal tunnel syndrome, 321
  hand and wrist
    carpal tunnel syndrome, 524
    soft tissue masses, 516
    tendon injuries, 509
  musculoskeletal infections, 621
  shoulder and arm
    biceps tendon, 416, 416*f*–417*f*
    impingement, 393
    inflammatory arthropathies, 424
    postoperative changes, 403
    rotator cuff tears, 395, 395*f*–396*f*, 399
    tendinosis, 401
  soft tissue infection, 635, 636*f*–637*f*

Undifferentiated pleomorphic sarcoma. *See* Undifferentiated-unclassified tumor
Undifferentiated-unclassified tumor, 613–614, 614*f*
Undisplaced lunate fracture, 493*f*
Unicameral bone cyst. *See* Solitary bone cyst
Unifocal Langerhans cell histiocytosis, 559–560, 560*f*, 652*t*, 654, 654*f*
Unilateral facet locking, 38, 39*f*

V

Varicosities, 321*t*
Vascular compromise, 362
Venous insufficiency, 775*t*
Vertebral arch fractures, of cervical spine, 32–33, 32*f*–33*f*
Vertebral body
   anomalies, 105
   fractures, of cervical spine, 35–37, 35*t*, 35*f*–37*f*
Vertebral hemangioma, aggressive, 80, 83*f*
Vertebral metastasis, 80, 81*f*

Vertical compression injuries
   cervical spine, 19*f*–20*f*
   thoracolumbar spine, 48–49, 48*f*–49*f*
Vertical shearing injuries, of pelvis, 110, 114*f*
VISI (volar intercalated segment instability), 503, 504*f*
Vitamin A, 777
Vitamin C, 778–779, 778*f*–779*f*
Vitamin D, 780–781, 780*t*, 781*f*
   deficiency, 716*t*
   intoxication (hypervitaminosis), 780, 781*f*
Vitaminosis
   vitamin A, 777
   vitamin C, 778–779, 778*f*–779*f*
   vitamin D, 780–781, 780*t*, 781*f*
Volar intercalated segment instability (VISI), 503, 504*f*

W

Wiberg patellar configurations, 228, 228*f*
Wilson disease, 697, 697*f*